ADVANCED HUMAN NUTRITION

FOURTH EDITION

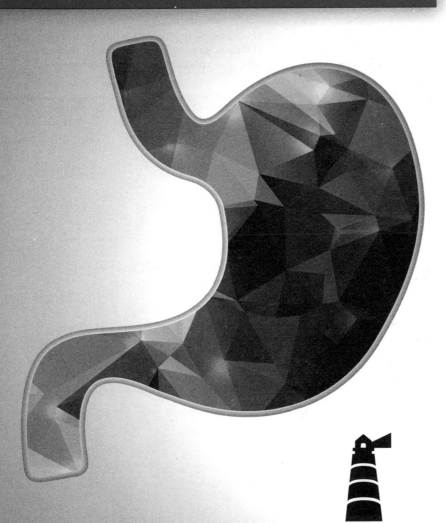

Denis M. Medeiros, PhD, RD, LD

Dean Emeritus of the School of Graduate Studies
Professor Emeritus of Biochemistry and Molecular Biology
University of Missouri at Kansas City
Kansas City, Missouri

And

Professor Emeritus
Department of Food, Nutrition, Dietetics, and Health
Kansas State University
Manhattan, Kansas

Robert E. C. Wildman, PhD, RD, LD, FISSN

Department of Nutrition and Food Sciences
Texas Woman's University
Denton, Texas

JONES & BARTLETT
LEARNING

World Headquarters
Jones & Bartlett Learning
5 Wall Street
Burlington, MA 01803
978-443-5000
info@jblearning.com
www.jblearning.com

Jones & Bartlett Learning books and products are available through most bookstores and online booksellers. To contact Jones & Bartlett Learning directly, call 800-832-0034, fax 978-443-8000, or visit our website, www.jblearning.com.

Substantial discounts on bulk quantities of Jones & Bartlett Learning publications are available to corporations, professional associations, and other qualified organizations. For details and specific discount information, contact the special sales department at Jones & Bartlett Learning via the above contact information or send an email to specialsales@jblearning.com.

Production Credits

VP, Product Management: David D. Cella
Director of Product Management: Cathy L. Esperti
Product Manager: Sean Fabery
Product Assistant: Hannah Dziezanowski
Vendor Manager: Nora Menzi
Director of Marketing: Andrea DeFronzo
VP, Manufacturing and Inventory Control: Therese Connell
Composition and Project Management: SourceHOV LLC

Cover Design: Kristin E. Parker
Rights & Media Specialist: Robert Boder
Media Development Editor: Shannon Sheehan
Cover Image: © winvic/iStock/Getty; © MIKHAIL GRACHIKOV/ Shutterstock.
Printing and Binding: Sheridan Books
Cover Printing: Sheridan Books

Library of Congress Cataloging-in-Publication Data
Names: Medeiros, Denis M., author. | Wildman, Robert E. C., 1964- author.
Title: Advanced human nutrition / Denis M. Medeiros and Robert E.C. Wildman.
Description: Fourth edition. | Burlington, MA : Jones & Barlett Learning,
    [2019] | Includes bibliographical references and index.
Identifiers: LCCN 2017033318 | ISBN 9781284123067 (casebound : alk. paper)
Subjects: LCSH: Nutrition.
Classification: LCC QP141 .W485 2019 | DDC 612.3–dc23 LC record available at https://lccn.loc.gov/2017033318

6048

Printed in the United States of America
23 22 21 20 19   10 9 8 7 6 5 4 3

To my wife, Susan, for her patience and love; and my mother, Rita Wilkie, a proud member of "the greatest generation," for her belief in higher education. Also to my daughter, Kathryn, my stepfather, the late William P. Wilkie, and my father, the late Joseph Medeiros, for their support and love through the years.

—D.M.M.

To my children: Gage and Bryn for your love, patience, and support. Also, to my father, Dave, and nephew, Jack, as well as eternal inspiration from my brother, David, and my mother, Carol.

—R.W.

Brief Contents

Preface   **xiii**

Acknowledgments   **xvi**

About the Authors   **xvii**

Chapter 1   Foundations of the Human Body 1

Chapter 2   Digestion and Absorption 35

Chapter 3   Carbohydrates: Energy, Metabolism, and More 59

Chapter 4   Dietary Fiber: Digestion and Health 95

Chapter 5   Lipids: Fatty Acids, Triglycerides, Phospholipids, and Sterols 111

Chapter 6   Proteins and Amino Acids: Function, Quantity, and Quality 147

Chapter 7   Water 191

Chapter 8   Metabolism, Energy Balance, and Body Weight and Composition 207

Chapter 9   Nutrition, Exercise, and Athletic Performance 245

Chapter 10   Fat-Soluble Vitamins 273

Chapter 11   Water-Soluble Vitamins 305

Chapter 12   Major Minerals 345

Chapter 13   Minor Minerals 373

Chapter 14   Nutraceuticals and Functional Foods 419

Glossary   **439**

Index   **455**

Contents

Preface xiii
Acknowledgments xvi
About the Authors xvii

Chapter 1 Foundations of the Human Body 1

Introduction 2
Elements and Molecules 2
Cell Structure and Organelles 3
   Endoplasmic Reticulum 5
   Golgi Apparatus 6
   Endosomes, Lysosomes, and Peroxisomes 7
   Mitochondria 7
The Nucleus and Genetic Aspects 9
   DNA, RNA, and Genes 9
Protein Synthesis 12
Nutrition and Epigenetics 13
Electron Transport Chain and Oxidative Phosphorylation 13
Cellular Protein Functions 17
   Organelle and Cell Membrane Structure and Cell Receptors 17
   Enzymes 18
   Cell Signaling 18
   Transport 18
   Hormones 19
Tissue 21
Organ Systems 22
   Bone and the Skeleton 22
   Nervous Tissue 23
   Skeletal Muscle 25
   Heart, Blood, and Circulation 26
   Blood Pressure 29
   Renal System 29
Here's What You Have Learned 32
Suggested Reading 32

Chapter 2 Digestion and Absorption 35

Introduction 36
Gastrointestinal Anatomy 37
   Mouth 37
   Stomach 37
   Small Intestine 38
     Rugae, Villi, and Microvilli 39
   Large Intestine (Colon) 39
Gastrointestinal Movement, Motility, and Neural Activity 40
   Smooth Muscle 40
   Smooth Muscle Excitation 40
Enteric Nervous System 40
   Neurotransmitters 41
   Sympathetic and Parasympathetic Innervation 41
Digestive Tract Movements 41
Gastrointestinal Vasculature 42
   Hepatic Portal Vein 42
Gastrointestinal Endocrine and Paracrine Substances 42
   Gastrin 42
   Cholecystokinin 43
   Secretin 43
   Somatostatin 43
   Gastric Inhibitory Polypeptide 43
   Motilin 44
   Peptide YY 45
   Histamine 45
Digestion and Absorption 47
   Phases of Digestion 47
   Oral Cavity 48
     Saliva 48
     Saliva Proteins: Enzymes and Mucus 48
     Saliva Electrolytes 48
   Esophagus 49
     Esophageal Sphincter 49
   Stomach 49
     Gastric Juice and Hydrochloric Acid 50
     Pepsin 50

Intrinsic Factor 50
Gastric Emptying 50
Small Intestine 51
Pancreatic Digestive Juice 51
Pancreatic Juice Delivery 51
The Gallbladder and Bile Storage and Release 52
Bile Composition 52
Gallbladder Contraction 53
Digestive Enzymes of the Small Intestine 53
Small Intestine Absorption 53
Large Intestine 53
Probiotics 54
Prebiotics 54

Lymphatic System 55

Here's What You Have Learned 57

Suggested Reading 58

**Chapter 3   Carbohydrates: Energy,
               Metabolism, and More 59**

Introduction 60

Carbohydrate Types and Characteristics 60
Monosaccharides 60
Monosaccharide Structures 62
Monosaccharide D and L Series 62
Monosaccharide Derivatives 62
Disaccharides 62
Polysaccharides 63
Oligosaccharides 63
Plant Starch 63
Animal Glycogen 65
Glycosaminoglycans 65
Dietary Fiber 66

Carbohydrate Intake, Food Sources,
and Recommendations 67
Carbohydrate Consumption 67
Monosaccharides and Disaccharides 67
Added Sugars and Caloric Sweeteners 68
Cereal Grains 68
Fiber 68
Carbohydrate Recommendations 68
Dietary Fiber 69

Carbohydrate Digestion and Absorption 69
Starch and Disaccharides 69
Absorption of Monosaccharides 70

Carbohydrate Circulation and Cellular Uptake 72
Blood Glucose Regulation 72
Glycemic Index 72
Glycemic Load 74
Glucose Transport into Cells 74
Monosaccharide Activation 75

Major Hormones in Carbohydrate
Metabolism 76
Insulin 76
Insulin Production 76
Insulin Secretion 77
Insulin-Mediated Glucose Uptake 77
Metabolic Roles of Insulin 79
Insulin Receptors 79
Glucagon 79
Insulin-to-Glucagon Molar Ratios 80
Epinephrine 80
Cortisol 81

Major Metabolic Pathways for
Carbohydrate 83
Glycolysis 83
Hexokinase and Glucokinase 83
Phosphofructokinase 83
Pyruvate Kinase 84
Fate of Pyruvate 84
Glycogen Turnover 84
Glycogen Synthesis 85
Glycogen Degradation 86
Pentose Phosphate Pathway 87
Krebs Cycle (Citric Acid Cycle) 87
Gluconeogenesis 88
Lipogenesis 91

Here's What You Have Learned 93

Suggested Reading 94

**Chapter 4   Dietary Fiber: Digestion
               and Health 95**

Introduction 96

Dietary Fiber and Functional Fibers 96
Dietary Fiber 96
Functional Fiber 97

Soluble and Insoluble Fiber 97

Dietary Fiber Types and Characteristics 97
Cellulose 97
Hemicellulose 98
Pectins 100
Lignin 100
Gums 100
β-Glucans 100
Chitin and Chitosan 101
Fructans (Inulin, Oligofructose,
and Fructo-oligosaccharides) 101
Glycosaminoglycans 101
Oligosaccharides 102
Polydextrose 102
Psyllium 102

Resistant Dextrins 102
Resistant Starches 102
Health Benefits of Fiber and Structural
    Carbohydrates 103
Gastrointestinal Fermentation and Health 106
Reduced Glycemic Effect 106
Cholesterol Binding and Reduction of Lipids 107
Fecal Bulking, Constipation,
    and Diverticulosis Support 107
Mineral Binding 108
Daily Intake and Recommendations 108
Here's What You Have Learned 110
Suggested Reading 110

**Chapter 5 Lipids: Fatty Acids,
            Triglycerides, Phospholipids,
            and Sterols 111**

Introduction 112
General Properties and Nomenclature
    of Lipids 112
Fatty Acids 112
Fatty Acid Synthesis, Elongation,
    and Desaturation 114
Pentose Phosphate Pathway 116
cis vs *trans* Fatty Acids 116
Essential Fatty Acids 117
Triglycerides 118
Phospholipids 119
Sterols 120
Molecular Control Mechanisms
    of Fat Metabolism 121
Nuclear Receptors 121
Non-Nuclear Receptors 124
Dietary Lipids: Food Sources, Requirements,
    and Digestion 125
Food Sources 125
Dietary Lipid Requirements 128
Digestion of Lipids 128
Intraluminal Phase 129
Mucosal Phase 130
Secretory Phase 132
Lipid Metabolism 132
Fatty Acid Oxidation 132
Ketone Body Production 133
Eicosanoids 135
Lipoproteins 136
Types of Lipoproteins 136
Metabolism of Lipoproteins 138

The Health Implications and Interpretation
    of Lipoprotein-Cholesterol and Triglyceride
    Levels 141
Alcohol 143
Here's What You Have Learned 144
Suggested Reading 145

**Chapter 6 Proteins and Amino Acids:
            Function, Quantity,
            and Quality 147**

Introduction 148
Amino Acids 148
Protein Structures 150
Dietary Protein and Protein Digestion
    and Absorption 152
Food Protein 152
Meat Protein 152
Fish Protein 152
Milk Protein 152
Egg Protein 153
Wheat Protein 153
Soy Protein 153
Protein Quantity 153
Protein Digestion and Absorption 153
Dietary Protein Quality 158
Roles of Amino Acids and Proteins
    in Metabolism 160
Enzymes 160
Blood Components 161
Blood Clotting 161
Muscle Structure and Function 162
Endocrine Functions 162
Connective Tissue 162
Fluid Balance 162
Acid–Base Balance 162
Immunity, Transport Carriers,
    and Membrane Receptors 162
Energy Supply 163
Precursors to Other Biochemical
    Compounds 163
Role as Carbon and Methyl Donors 163
Other Functions 163
Metabolism of Amino Acids 164
Transamination and Deamination 164
Synthesis of Amino Acids 165
Degradation of Amino Acids 165
Glutamine Metabolism 168
The Alanine–Glucose Cycle 169

Amino Acids and Neurotransmitters.............169
Disposal of Amino Acid Nitrogen.................173
Urea Cycle 173
Protein and Amino Acid Requirements........... 174
Protein....................................174
Amino Acids 176
Amino Acid Inborn Errors of Metabolism........ 178
Issues with Phenylalanine Metabolism:
    Phenylketonuria 178
Issues with Tyrosine Metabolism 178
Issues with Valine, Leucine, and Isoleucine
    Metabolism: Maple Syrup Urine Disease........178
Issues with Methionine Metabolism..............179
Issues with Tryptophan Metabolism..............180
Issues with Lysine, Glycine, and
    Threonine Metabolism.....................181
Leucine and other Branched Chain Amino Acids
    as Related to Body Composition and Obesity.... 182
Protein Quality, Protein Excess, and Protein
    Deficiency................................ 184
Determination of Protein Intakes by Food
    Source Based on Limiting Amino Acids.........184
Excess Dietary Protein.........................185
Protein Undernutrition 185
Here's What You Have Learned 187
Suggested Reading............................ 190

Chapter 7   Water 191

Introduction................................. 192
Properties and Body Distribution of Water........ 192
Properties.................................192
Distribution of Water in the Human Body........192
Sweat Water.................................193
Urinary Water..............................195
Water Balance 199
Edema 202
Mechanisms for Edema Formation 202
Edema in Pathologic States 202
Here's What You Have Learned 205
Suggested Reading............................ 206

**Chapter 8   Metabolism, Energy Balance,
            and Body Weight and
            Composition.................. 207**

Introduction................................. 208
Total Energy Expenditure and Components...... 208
Measurement of Total Energy Expenditure 208
Direct or Human Calorimetry..................209

Indirect Calorimetry..........................209
Doubly Labeled Water 210
Components of Energy Metabolism.............212
Basal Metabolism (Resting Metabolism)............212
Thermic Effect of Activity.....................213
Thermic Effect of Food 214
Adaptive Thermogenesis.......................214
Metabolic States and Integrated
    Energy Metabolism......................... 216
Cellular and Tissue Metabolism....................217
Obligate Glucose Utilization....................218
Transitional Metabolic States 218
Metabolic Crossroads 219
Fed State...................................219
Early Refeeding 219
Intermediate to Longer Fed State 221
Fasting....................................221
Starvation..................................223
Body Weight and Composition 224
Body Weight and Health 224
Body Mass Index............................225
Active People, Body Weight, and Health.............226
Body Composition 226
Elements and Molecules 226
Fat Mass and Fat-Free Mass 226
Body Water 227
Minerals (Ash) 227
Assessment of Body Composition............... 228
Body Densitometry 228
Plethysmography 229
Dual-Energy X-Ray Absorptiometry...............230
Skinfold Assessment 230
Bioelectrical Impedance Analysis.................231
Regulation of Energy Intake, Storage,
    and Expenditure.......................... 232
Futile Cycle Systems..........................232
Chemical Mediators of Energy Homeostasis.......233
Insulin 233
Ghrelin....................................233
Cholecystokinin..............................233
Leptin.....................................233
Neuropeptide Y 234
Galanin 234
Here's What You Have Learned 242
Suggested Reading............................ 243

**Chapter 9   Nutrition, Exercise, and Athletic
            Performance 245**

Introduction................................. 246
Muscle and Exercise Basics.................... 246

Muscle and Neuromuscular Junctions 247
Muscle Action Potentials 248
Sarcomeres and Contraction 248
Muscle Fiber Type 249
Motor Unit Recruitment 249
Exercise and Training Components 251
Muscle Adaptation to Strength Training 251
Muscle Adaptation to Endurance
    Exercise 252
Muscle Fiber Type and Endurance
    Adaptation 252
Hormonal Adaptation to Acute
    and Chronic Exercise 252
    Catecholamines 252
    Insulin and Glucagon 255
    Cortisol, Growth Hormone, and ACTH 255
Energy, Supportive Nutrients, and Exercise 255
    Creatine Phosphate 255
    Carbohydrate Metabolism and Exercise 256
    Muscle Carbohydrate Utilization 258
    Maintaining Blood Glucose Levels
        During Exercise 258
        Cori Cycle 258
        Alanine Cycle 259
    Carbohydrate Oxidation During Exercise 259
    Glycogen Stores and Exercise 260
    Carbohydrate Consumption Before, During,
        and After Exercise 260
    Carbohydrate Supercompensation
        (Glycogen Loading) 261
    Triglyceride and Fatty Acid Metabolism
        and Exercise 261
    Fat Stores and Exercise 261
    Fatty Acid Oxidation in Muscle 263
    Exercise and Fat Utilization 263
    Fat Utilization After Exercise 263
    Protein and Amino Acid Metabolism
        and Exercise 263
        *Effect of Resistance Exercise and Postworkout
        Nutrition on Net Muscle Protein Turnover* 264
        *Effect of Endurance Exercise and Postworkout
        Nutrition on Net Muscle Protein Turnover* 265
    Muscle Amino Acid Metabolism During
        Exercise 266
    General Protein Recommendations 266
    Water and Exercise 267
        Dehydration and Performance 267
        *Water Recommendations for Athletic
        Performance* 267
    Vitamins, Minerals, and Exercise 268
Here's What You Have Learned 270
Suggested Reading 271

Chapter 10 Fat-Soluble Vitamins 273

Introduction 274
    Water and Fat Solubility 274
Vitamin A 274
    Dietary Sources of Vitamin A and Carotenoids 275
    Digestion and Absorption of Vitamin A
        and Carotenoids 275
    Implications of β-Carotene Cleavage
        and Associated Enzymes 277
    Plasma Transport of Vitamin A and Carotenoids 278
    Storage of Vitamin A and Cell Binding Proteins 280
    Functions of Vitamin A and Carotenoids 280
        Vision 280
        Cell Differentiation 281
        Cancer 282
        Glycoproteins 283
        Reproduction 283
        Antioxidant Capacity 283
        Other Functions 283
    Nutrient Relationships for Vitamin A
        and Carotenoids 284
    Excretion of Vitamin A and Carotenoids 284
    Recommended Levels of Vitamin A Intake 284
    Vitamin A Deficiency 284
    Vitamin A Toxicity 284
Vitamin D 285
    Sources of Vitamin D 285
    Absorption and Transport of Dietary Vitamin D 285
    Metabolism of Vitamin D 286
    Vitamin D Receptor and non-Genomic Functions 287
    Recommended Levels of Vitamin D
        Intake 290
    Vitamin D Deficiency 291
Vitamin E 292
    Food Sources of Vitamin E 292
    Vitamin E Absorption and Transport 293
    Vitamin E Storage and Excretion 293
    Function of Vitamin E 294
    Recommended Levels of Vitamin E Intake 294
    Vitamin E Deficiency 296
    Vitamin E and Other Fat Soluble Vitamins in the
        Development of Alzheimer's Disease 296
    Vitamin E Toxicity 297
Vitamin K 297
    Sources of Vitamin K 297
    Absorption and Transport of Vitamin K 298
    Functions of Vitamin K 298
    The Vitamin K Cycle 300
    Recommended Levels of Vitamin K Intake 300
    Vitamin K Deficiency and Toxicity 301

Here's What You Have Learned 302

Suggested Reading 303

Chapter 11   Water-Soluble Vitamins **305**

Introduction 306

Vitamin C (Ascorbic Acid) 306

    Food Sources of Vitamin C 308

    Absorption of Vitamin C 308

    Functions of Vitamin C 309

    Recommended Levels of Vitamin C Intake 309

    Vitamin C Deficiency 311

    Vitamin C Toxicity 311

Thiamin, Riboflavin, Niacin, and Vitamin B$_6$ 312

Thiamin (Vitamin B$_1$) 312

    Dietary Sources of Thiamin 313

    Digestion, Absorption, and Transport
       of Thiamin 313

    Metabolism and Functions of Thiamin 314

    Recommended Levels for Thiamin Intake 316

    Thiamin Deficiency 316

    Thiamin Toxicity 316

Riboflavin (Vitamin B$_2$) 316

    Dietary Sources of Riboflavin 317

    Absorption and Transport of Riboflavin 318

    Metabolism and Roles of Riboflavin 318

    Recommended Levels of Riboflavin Intake 319

    Riboflavin Deficiency and Toxicity 319

Niacin (Vitamin B$_3$) 319

    Sources of Niacin 320

    Digestion and Absorption of Niacin 321

    Metabolism and Functions of Niacin 321

    Recommended Levels for Niacin Intake 322

    Niacin Deficiency 322

    Pharmacologic Use of Niacin and Toxicity 322

Vitamin B$_6$ 323

    Food Sources of Vitamin B$_6$ 323

    Absorption of Vitamin B$_6$ 324

    Metabolism and Function of Vitamin B$_6$ 324

    Recommended Levels of Vitamin B$_6$ Intake 327

    Vitamin B$_6$ Deficiency and Toxicity 327

Folate, Vitamin B$_{12}$, Biotin, and Pantothenic Acid . . 328

Folic Acid (Folate) 328

    Dietary Sources of Folate 328

    Absorption of Folate 328

    Metabolism and Functions of Folate 329

    The Methyl–Folate Trap 331

    Recommended Levels for Folate Intake 331

    Folate Deficiency and Toxicity 331

Vitamin B$_{12}$ 332

    Food Sources, Digestion, and Absorption
       of Vitamin B$_{12}$ 332

    Metabolism and Function of Vitamin B$_{12}$ 333

    Recommended Levels of Vitamin B$_{12}$ Intake 335

    Vitamin B$_{12}$ Deficiency 335

Biotin 337

    Sources of Biotin 337

    Digestion and Absorption of Biotin 337

    Metabolism and Function of Biotin 337

    Recommended Levels for Biotin Intake 338

    Biotin Deficiency and Toxicity 338

Pantothenic Acid 338

    Food Sources of Pantothenic Acid 339

    Digestion and Absorption of
       Pantothenic Acid 339

    Metabolism and Function of
       Pantothenic Acid 339

    Recommended Levels of Pantothenic
       Acid Intake 340

    Deficiency and Toxicity of
       Pantothenic Acid 340

Here's What You Have Learned 341

Suggested Reading 342

Chapter 12   Major Minerals **345**

Introduction 346

Calcium 346

    Dietary Calcium Sources 346

    Calcium Absorption 347

    Blood Calcium Levels and Homeostasis 349

    Physiologic Roles of Calcium 349

    Recommended Levels for Calcium Intake 353

    Calcium Deficiency 353

    Calcium Toxicity 354

Phosphorus 354

    Dietary Phosphorus Sources 354

    Digestion and Absorption of Phosphorus 354

    Serum Phosphorus Levels and Homeostasis 355

    Physiologic Roles of Phosphorus 356

    Recommended Levels of Phosphorus Intake 357

    Phosphorus Deficiency and Toxicity 357

Magnesium 357

    Dietary Magnesium Sources 357

    Magnesium Absorption 357

    Tissue Magnesium Content and Excretion 358

    Physiologic Roles of Magnesium 359

    Recommended Levels for Magnesium Intake 360

    Deficiency and Toxicity of Magnesium 360

Sodium, Chloride, and Potassium 361
    Dietary Sources of Sodium,
        Potassium, and Chloride 361
    Absorption of Sodium, Potassium,
        and Chloride. 362
    Tissue, Urinary, and Sweat Content of Sodium,
        Potassium, and Chloride 364
    Physiologic Functions of Sodium, Potassium,
        and Chloride. 364
    Recommended Levels of Intake for Sodium,
        Potassium, and Chloride 365
    Deficiency, Toxicity, and Health Concerns
        for Sodium, Potassium, and Chloride 365
Sulfur. 368
Here's What You Have Learned 369
Suggested Reading. 370

Chapter 13 Minor Minerals 373

Introduction. 374
Iron. 374
    Dietary Sources of Iron and Iron Absorption 374
        Dietary Iron and Availability. 374
        Dietary Components That Effect Absorption 375
        Iron Absorption Proteins
        and Mechanisms. 376
        Iron Homeostasis. 377
    Metabolism and Function of Iron. 378
        Hemoglobin. 378
        Iron Storage Proteins. 378
        Transferrin. 382
        Cellular Iron Control 382
        Enzyme Activity 382
    Recommended Levels of Intake for Iron 383
    Iron Deficiency. 383
    Iron Toxicity (Overload). 383
        Conditions Under Which Iron Toxicity Occurs. 383
        Mechanism of Iron Toxicity 384
        Iron Toxicity and Diseases 385
Zinc. 386
    Dietary Zinc and Absorption 386
        Food Sources 386
        Dietary Factors That Affect Zinc Absorption 386
        Zinc Absorption Proteins and Mechanism 387
    Metabolism and Function of Zinc 389
        Overall Metabolism 389
        Function of Zinc-Containing Proteins. 389
        Zinc Excretion. 390
    Recommended Levels of Intake of Zinc. 390
    Zinc Deficiency 391
    Zinc Toxicity. 391
Iodine 391

Dietary Sources of Iodide. 391
Absorption of Iodide 392
Metabolism and Function of Iodide 392
Recommended Levels for Iodide Intake 393
Iodide Deficiency 394
Copper. 395
    Dietary Copper and Absorption 395
        Food Sources 395
    Dietary Factors That Affect Copper Absorption 395
    Metabolism and Function of Copper 397
    Copper Transport Proteins and Cell Distribution . . . 399
    Recommended Levels of Intake for Copper. 399
    Copper Deficiency 399
    Genetic Anomalies Influencing Copper Status. 399
Selenium. 401
    Dietary Selenium. 401
    Absorption of Selenium 401
    Metabolism and Function of Selenium 401
    Selenium Incorporation into Proteins. 403
    Relationships Among Selenium and
        Other Nutrients. 404
    Recommended Levels of Intake for Selenium. 404
    Selenium Deficiency 404
    Selenium Toxicity 405
Fluoride 406
    Dietary Sources of Fluoride. 406
    Absorption of Fluoride 406
    Metabolism and Function of Fluoride 407
    Recommended Levels for Fluoride Intake
        and Fluoride Toxicity Concerns. 408
Chromium. 408
    Dietary Chromium 408
    Absorption of Chromium 408
    Metabolism and Function of Chromium. 409
    Recommended Levels of Intake for Chromium
        and Chromium Imbalance 410
Manganese. 410
    Dietary Sources of Manganese 410
    Absorption of Manganese. 410
    Metabolism and Function of Manganese. 410
    Recommended Levels of Intake
        and Manganese Imbalance 411
Ultratrace Minerals. 411
    Cobalt 411
    Boron. 411
        Dietary Sources and Absorption
        of Boron. 411
        Metabolism and Function of Boron. 411
        Recommended Levels of Boron
        Intake and Boron Imbalance 412

Molybdenum 412
   Dietary Sources and Absorption of Molybdenum *412*
   Metabolism and Function of Molybdenum *412*
   *Recommended Levels of Molybdenum Intake
    and Imbalances* *412*
Vanadium 412
   Dietary Sources and Absorption of Vanadium *413*
   Metabolism and Function of Vanadium *413*
   *Recommended Levels of Vanadium
    Intake and Vanadium Imbalances* *413*
Nickel 413
Arsenic 413
Silicon 414
Here's What You Have Learned 415
Suggested Reading 416

**Chapter 14 Nutraceuticals and
              Functional Foods 419**
Introduction 420
Defining Nutraceuticals and Functional Foods . . . 420
Organizational Systems for Nutraceuticals and
   Functional Foods 421

Food Sources 421
   Mechanism of Action *424*
Health Claims 426
Organization of Nutraceuticals by Molecular
   Structure 428
   Isoprenoid Derivatives (Terpenoids) 429
   Phenolic Compounds 430
   Carbohydrates and Carbohydrate Derivatives 433
   Fatty Acids and Structural Lipids 434
   Protein, Amino Acids, and Amino
    Acid Derivatives 434
   Minerals 434
   Microbes (Probiotics) 435
Here's What You Have Learned 436
Suggested Reading 436

Glossary **439**
Index **455**

Preface

In the preface to the last two editions, we posed the question, "Why a book on advanced human nutrition?" We responded that there was, and continues to be, a limited number of intermediate and advanced textbooks that detail why nutrients are important from a biochemical, physiologic, and molecular perspective. Today, the same shortage exists with the exception of *Advanced Human Nutrition*, whose initial success and adoptions exceeded our expectations.

Nutrition is a relatively new science, having evolved from several other scientific disciplines in the 20th century, and it continues to evolve today. The expansion of nutritional knowledge has been astounding. At the beginning of the 20th century, work conducted on food and food components was carried out by only a handful of scientists. As the 20th century progressed into its first few decades, many of the now well-known vitamins were discovered, their structures defined, and synthesis techniques developed. The metabolic mechanisms of macronutrients, particularly carbohydrates, lipids, and proteins, as well as energy metabolism in general, became the subject of intense research. The scientists who carried out such research came from a wide variety of disciplines, including organic and inorganic chemistry, agricultural chemistry, physiological chemistry, medicine, and animal sciences.

Originally, nutritional research was conducted by men and women simply for the love of science. Later, during the 1940s, the federal government took a more active role in scientific research, including nutrition. A high rate of rejection of military conscripts due to nutrition-related conditions prompted the establishment of the first U.S. Recommended Dietary Allowances (RDAs) in 1941. The RDAs have continued to be modified ever since; the Dietary Reference Intakes (DRIs) are the most recent version.

Research had been carried out with the indirect support of the federal government before the establishment of the RDAs. Nutrition research occurred at the land-grant institutions created by Abraham Lincoln in the 1860s through the Morrill Act. Modern nutrition evolved from agricultural, medical, and basic sciences into a discipline of its own. One of the early fathers of nutrition was a Kansas native, E. V. McCollum, who introduced the laboratory rat as a useful model in scientific research when studying vitamin A. Similarly, poultry scientists used chicks as a research model and made contributions to medical sciences. Much of the research on fiber began with animal scientists studying forages and feeds of livestock.

Research pertaining to minerals, their composition in the human diet, and their physiologic roles took form in the 20th century. Most of the earlier mineral research efforts focused on the major minerals, such as calcium, phosphorus, sodium, potassium, chloride, and magnesium. However, some work relating to the role of iron and the development of iron deficiency appeared in the earlier decades of the 20th century.

In the 1960s and 1970s, rapid advances in technology allowed for the ability to detect small quantities of trace minerals, such as selenium, zinc, copper, iron, fluoride, chromium, manganese, and iodine. Although the role of iodine in preventing goiters was already known, as was the potential for deleterious health effects from selenium toxicity, there was limited information on the role of many trace elements in optimizing human health. New technologies, such as neutron activation and atomic absorption spectrophotometry, allowed for detection of trace minerals in the part-per-billion or microgram-per-liter range. An explosion of knowledge regarding trace minerals occurred in the latter part of the 20th century.

As the 20th century came to a close, it was known that many nutrients functioned at the gene level, an idea that was unheard of at the beginning of the 20th century. Today, in the 21st century, new research was and is currently being carried out on the identification of new compounds in the diet, such as plant chemicals (phytochemicals). This area has led to the identification of compounds that promote health and prevent disease.

▶ Approach of this Text

In all of our previous editions, we sought to use a conversational approach in our writing to allow the reader to better grasp nutritional concepts, as opposed to the more encyclopedic writing style common among advanced texts in science disciplines. We have been mindful of pedagogical tools that facilitate student learning. Many students have not mastered the optimal manner in which to read a textbook compared with literary works. A student needs to comprehend what he or she reads. Each chapter contains a series of "Before You Go On…" features in which the reader is asked a series of questions that can be answered from the material covered in the previous section. This tool can be used to help the student comprehend and focus on what is important in the text and to develop better study skills. The student is urged to answer each of the questions before proceeding with the next section of the chapter.

In the third edition of the text, two additional chapters were developed: one on fiber, which was previously part of the carbohydrates chapter; and a second on nutraceuticals and functional foods. Nutraceuticals—nutrients in foods that provide physiologic benefit beyond basic daily needs and/or support disease prevention or treatment—have been studied extensively in the last 15 years, and much has been discovered about their health benefits and mechanism of action. Fiber is one group of phytochemicals (plant-based nutraceuticals) where this information has expanded. Phytochemicals have been used to develop and produce functional foods either as supplements or as food. Thus, separate, in-depth attention to each of these still-evolving topics is needed for the student of nutrition to stay current. We include updated material to these two chapters.

As we did in previous editions, chapters are developed further by combining the scientific basis of why the basic nutrients are required with some applied concepts throughout. We accomplished this by integrating "Special Features" on focused topics to add depth to the chapters and to allow the student to view applications of the basic science. New special features have been added to this edition and existing ones have been updated based on new information in the scientific literature. The first edition was designed both as a textbook and a reference book, but the second, third, and now fourth editions are clearly designed as textbooks for college-level courses in human nutrition. The book assumes that students have completed courses in introductory nutrition, biochemistry, and some anatomy and physiology. Many students who are dietetics and nutrition majors, or who are beginning Master of Science degrees, will find this book appropriate for their level.

We have updated the figures and redesigned the text with the student in mind so that visual and textual, comprehension and study tools are available to reinforce concepts. This new edition has even more figures than the *Third Edition*; these were added after consultation with professors throughout the United States who are actively teaching advanced human nutrition courses, some of whom had been using the previous editions and some of whom had not. The goal here was to broaden the scope of concepts deemed significant for the student to comprehend. However, we took extra care to design the figures to balance simplicity with sufficient detail needed for an advanced treatment of the content.

▶ Organization of this Text

Chapter 1 starts with an overview of the cell and examples of how nutrition can play a role in human health. **Chapter 2** is aimed at a rigorous review of the anatomy and physiology of digestion. Both of these chapters are the foundation on which the rest of the book is built. **Chapter 3** focuses on carbohydrates. However, as in the previous edition, fiber is discussed separately in **Chapter 4**. **Chapters 5 and 6** focus on lipids and proteins, respectively, with the latter becoming one of the highest profile nutrient areas at this time. **Chapter 7** focuses on water as a separate nutrient because it is present in our bodies in the largest quantity of all nutrients. **Chapters 8 and 9** focus on energy, weight control, and exercise. **Chapters 10 and 11** are detailed discussions of the fat-soluble and water-soluble vitamins, respectively. The text proceeds with two chapters on minerals: **Chapter 12** on major minerals and **Chapter 13** on minor minerals. We have added quite a bit of updated information to **Chapters 10 through 13** in response to our peer reviewers. **Chapter 14**, titled, "Nutraceuticals and Functional Foods," proved to be popular by adopters in the *Third Edition*. There have been scores of textbooks written on this topic. For this text, the focus was on understanding what constitutes nutraceuticals and functional foods, how they can be classified, and the nutrient categories of various types.

▶ New to the *Fourth Edition*

Some of the most significant updates to the *Fourth Edition* include the following:

■ Each chapter concludes with a section titled, "Clinical Insights," in which a topic of clinical relevance is presented, linking the basic nutrition science covered in each chapter. Future clinicians will find this useful in connecting the basic and applied elements of human nutrition and dietetics, better preparing each student for future courses in clinical nutrition.

- The use of gene editing (referred to as CRISPR) is discussed in Chapter 1, as this technology has the potential to correct genetic mutations that impact nutrition utilization and metabolism.
- Diseases of the gastrointestinal tract that have nutritional relevance in health and disease are now covered in Chapter 2.
- Bariatric surgery procedures used to treat obesity are discussed in Chapter 2, as their popularity has increased in tandem with some potential nutrition problems.
- The controversy of a possible contributing factor to the obesity epidemic due to increased linoleic acid intake is debated in one of the Special Features in Chapter 5.
- Alcohol, as related to disease, is covered in Chapter 5.
- The new American Heart Association and American College of Cardiology algorithms to determine the risk of a cardiac event are included in Chapter 5.
- Protein requirements have been challenged by some scientists as it relates to the RDA, and Chapter 6 incorporates coverage of this controversy. Newly available methods that determine nitrogen requirements compared with traditional nitrogen balance methods have led some to conclude that the RDA for protein should be increased significantly.
- Protein intake, physical activity, and sarcopenia are discussed in Chapter 6.
- Clinical signs and treatment of dehydration are covered in Chapter 7.
- Energy requirements, as estimated by several different algorithms used in clinical settings, are included in Chapter 8.
- Exercise recommendations for both endurance and weight-bearing exercises are featured in Chapter 9.
- The implications of β-carotene cleavage by different enzymes in the small intestine are covered in Chapter 10.
- Coverage of the role of fat-soluble vitamins, particularly vitamin E, in Alzheimer's disease is included in Chapter 10.
- Transport mechanisms for water-soluble vitamins are discussed in Chapter 11.
- Novel roles of phosphorus in nutrition are featured in Chapter 12.

- The health-promoting effects of a group of phytochemicals—stilbenes—are now discussed in Chapter 14.

▶ Instructor Resources

Comprehensive online teaching resources are available to instructors adopting the *Fourth Edition*, including the following:

- LMS-ready Test Bank, featuring more than 550 questions. This represents an increase of more than 100 questions compared with the previous edition. The level of rigor for each question is now indicated.
- Instructor's Manual, including Learning Objectives, Key Terms, Chapter Outlines, Discussion Questions, Lecture Notes, and In-class Activities. These have been heavily revised from previous editions.
- Slides in PowerPoint format, containing more than 750 slides that can be adapted for in-class lectures. For each topic, sample lectures with PowerPoint slides are included to help save time for the instructor in preparation of class materials. These lectures can be modified easily for each instructor's unique needs.
- Image Bank in PowerPoint format, compiling the figures appearing in this text.

▶ In Conclusion

The order and content of information presented in this book are typical of the curricula at most academic institutions where nutrition and dietetics are taught. Both authors have had experience teaching this information in advanced nutrition courses and the materials included come from years of experience. We expect this course to provide students with the necessary skills and background to pursue higher-level nutrition classes; it can also serve as a capstone class. As we stated in the prefaces of previous editions, we continue to believe that students who use this text will go on to research careers in nutrition, perhaps even making contributions to the field that we will then cover in future editions of this text. There are those who used the *First Edition* of this book and went on to have research careers in nutrition and dietetics, and their findings are reported in this edition. We certainly look forward to and encourage such important works from future students.

Denis M. Medeiros

Robert E. C. Wildman

Acknowledgments

The authors would like to thank the following reviewers for their thoughtful critiques, expert knowledge, and constructive suggestions, which have helped us in improving this edition.

Elizabeth Cuervo, MD
Professor
Florida National University
Miami, FL

Patricia Davidson, DCN, RDN, CDE, LDN, FAND
Assistant Professor
West Chester University
West Chester, PA

Michael A. Dunn, PhD
Associate Professor
University of Hawaii at Manoa
Honolulu, HI

James Gerber, MS, DC
Associate Professor
Western States Chiropractic College
Adjunct Faculty
University of Bridgeport
Bridgeport, CT

Amber Haroldson, PhD, RD
Assistant Professor
Ball State University
Muncie, IN

Jasminka Ilich, PhD, RD
Professor
Florida State University
Tallahassee, FL

Monica Lebre, MS, RDN, LDN
Adjunct Lecturer
Northeastern University
Boston, MA

Dingbo Lin, PhD
Assistant Professor
Oklahoma State University
Stillwater, OK

Pei-Yang Liu, PhD, RD, LD
Assistant Professor
University of Akron
Akron, OH

Mindy Maziarz, PhD, RDN, LD
Assistant Professor
Texas Woman's University
Houston, TX

Susan Muller, PhD
Professor
Stephens College
Columbia, MO

Nina Roofe, PhD, RDN, LD, FAND
Dietetic Internship Director and Assistant Professor
University of Central Arkansas
Conway, AR

Robert B. Rucker, PhD
Distinguished Professor Emeritus
Department of Nutrition and Department of
   Internal Medicine
University of California, Davis
Davis, CA

About the Authors

Denis M. Medeiros, PhD, RD, LD, received his PhD in nutrition from Clemson University in 1981, his MS in physiology from Illinois State University in 1976, and his BS degree from Central Connecticut State University in 1974. He has been on the faculties of Mississippi State University (1981–1984), the University of Wyoming (1984–1989), The Ohio State University (1989–2000), and Kansas State University (2000–2011). He is currently Dean Emeritus of the Graduate School and Professor Emeritus of Molecular Biology and Biochemistry at the University of Missouri at Kansas City. Formerly, Dr. Medeiros was full professor and head of the Department of Human Nutrition, as well as associate dean for scholarship and research, at Kansas State University. He holds the rank of Professor Emeritus of Food, Nutrition, Dietetics, and Health and Associate Dean Emeritus for Scholarship and Research at Kansas State University. He was a former associate dean for research and dean of the College of Human Ecology at The Ohio State University. He has also spent time as a visiting faculty member at the Medical University of South Carolina in Charleston, South Carolina, and at the Washington University School of Medicine in St. Louis, Missouri.

Dr. Medeiros's major research has focused on the role of trace minerals, particularly copper, on the integrity of the cardiovascular system, and on the role of iron in bone integrity. He has received more than $4 million in grants to support his research endeavors from such institutions as the National Institutes of Health, the U.S. Department of Agriculture, and the National Science Foundation. He has authored or coauthored more than 125 scientific peer-refereed articles. Additionally, he has served on numerous editorial boards of prominent journals and has held elective offices in scientific societies. He has taught classes, both at the introductory and advanced levels, for undergraduate students and has taught graduate-level courses throughout his career. In addition, Dr. Medeiros has received outstanding teaching awards for his efforts and is both a registered and licensed dietitian.

Robert E. C. Wildman, PhD, RD, LD, FISSN, received his PhD in human nutrition from The Ohio State University, his MS in foods and nutrition from The Florida State University, and his BS in dietetics and nutrition from the University of Pittsburgh. He is a fellow of the International Society of Sports Nutrition (ISSN) and is an adjunct faculty member in the Department of Food Science and Human Nutrition at Texas Woman's University in Denton, Texas. His major areas of research include nutrition application to metabolism, body composition, weight control and health, and athletic performance. He has authored or coauthored more than 30 papers and several nutrition books, including *The Nutritionist: Food, Nutrition, and Optimal Health* and *Sport and Fitness Nutrition*; he also edited the *Handbook of Nutraceuticals and Functional Foods*. Dr. Wildman is a registered and licensed dietitian with the Academy of Nutrition and Dietetics and is the creator of TheNutritionDr.com.

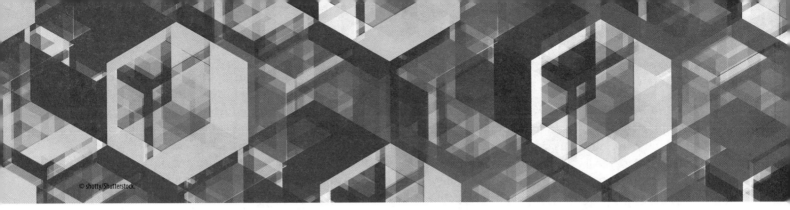

CHAPTER 1
Foundations of the Human Body

1. The human body is composed, in some fashion, of 27 of more than 100 existing elements.
2. The basic unit of life from a nutritional perspective is the cell.
3. Cell components have specialized functions, all of which affect nutritional utilization.
4. Cell proteins have specialized functions, including serving as enzymes, receptors, transporters, and hormones.
5. Not all tissues are created equal. There are more than 200 cell types with the same DNA but with different functions and nutrient requirements.

▶ Introduction

Undeniably, nutrition is of primary importance to the anatomic and physiologic development and maintenance of the human body. This complex multicellular entity consists of organ systems and tissue working together to support growth, maturation, defense, and reproduction. From an evolutionary perspective, humans developed into bipedal primates endowed with enormously expanded cerebral hemispheres, particularly the frontal lobes, which are responsible for intelligent behavior and muscular dexterity. Those characteristics allow humans to move with agility in various directions, investigate their environment, and understand and learn complex behaviors. They also allow humans, unlike other animals, the potential to investigate and comprehend the importance of their own nutrition. In a basic sense, humans are inhalation units, food processors, combustion units for energy molecules as well as storage facilities for excessive energy; and they possess waste removal and defensive systems, internal and external communication systems, locomotive capabilities, and have reproductive capabilities. All of those functions are founded on or influenced by nutritional intake.

Humans comprehend how to nourish the demands of the human body; at the very least, a basic understanding of just what it is that needs to be nourished. But where does one begin to understand this? Perhaps, the most obvious starting point is at the cellular level. Although it is indeed easier for humans to think of themselves as a single unit, the truth of the matter is that a human being is a compilation of some 60 to 100 trillion **cells**. Every one of those cells is a living entity engaging in homeostatic operations to support self-preservation, while in some manner, concurrently engaging in homeostatic mechanisms for the human body as a whole. Each cell is metabolically active, and thus requires nourishment, while, at the same time, produces waste. Therefore, nutrition cannot merely be defined as the study of the nourishment of the human body; rather, it is the nourishment of individual cells and the tissues and organs they make up. An understanding of nutrition also needs to go beyond the living or viable portions of the body to recognize the building blocks of cells themselves—namely, elements and molecules.

▶ Elements and Molecules

Of the more than 100 elements known at this time, the human body uses approximately 27. Oxygen is the most abundant element in the human body, accounting for approximately 63% of its mass. Carbon (18%), hydrogen (9%), and nitrogen (3%) follow oxygen in decreasing order of abundance (**TABLE 1.1**). Carbon, hydrogen, oxygen, and nitrogen atoms are foundations for the most abundant types of molecules in the body, namely, water, proteins, lipids, carbohydrates, and nucleic acids. Water typically accounts for about

TABLE 1.1 Elements of the Human Body					
Major Elements[a]				**Trace Elements**[b]	
Oxygen	63.0%	Potassium	0.4%	Silicon	Boron
Carbon	18.0%	Sulfur	0.3%	Aluminum	Selenium
Hydrogen	9.0%	Sodium	0.2%	Iron	Chromium
Nitrogen	3.0%	Chloride	0.1%	Manganese	Cobalt
Calcium	1.5%	Magnesium	0.1%	Fluorine	Arsenic
Phosphorous	1.0%			Vanadium	Molybdenum
				Iodine	Zinc
				Tin	Copper

[a]Percentages indicate the percentage of body mass composed of a particular element.
[b]Each trace element contributes less than 0.01% to total body mass.

TABLE 1.2	Theoretical Contributors to Body Weight for a Lean Man and Woman	
Component	**Man (%)**	**Woman (%)**
Water	62	59
Fat	16	22
Protein	16	14
Minerals	6	5
Carbohydrate	<1	<1
Total	**100**	**100**

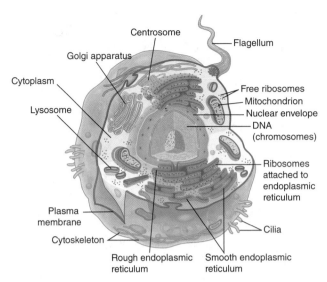

FIGURE 1.1 General Cell Structure. The figure shows the plasma membrane, cytoplasm, mitochondria, ribosomes, lysosomes, endoplasmic reticulum, Golgi apparatus, and the nuclear envelope.

55% to 65% of human mass, whereas proteins and lipids collectively may contribute about 30% to 45%. Finally, nucleic acids, carbohydrates, and other organic molecules contribute about 1% or so to human mass. The remaining portion of the body, approximately 5%, is largely composed of minerals (**TABLE 1.2**).

With the exception of water, the major types of molecules forming the human body are complex and largely constructed of simpler molecules. For example, proteins are composed of **amino acids** linked by peptide bonds. **Deoxyribonucleic acid (DNA)** and **ribonucleic acid (RNA)** are assembled from nucleotides, which themselves are constructed from smaller molecules, namely purine and pyrimidine bases, phosphoric acid, and a carbohydrate (2-deoxy-d-ribose and d-ribose for DNA and RNA, respectively). **Triglycerides** (e.g., triacylglycerol) contain three **fatty acids** esterified to a glycerol molecule, and glucose molecules can be linked together by anhydride bonds to form the carbohydrate storage polymer glycogen.

▶ Cell Structure and Organelles

Although there are over 200 different types of cells in the human body, each performing a unique or somewhat enhanced function, most of the basic structural and operational features are conserved among all cells. This means that although **skeletal muscle** cells and **adipocytes** (fat storage cells) may seem very different in many respects; including primary purpose, color, and shape; the most basic cellular structures and functions of both cell types are similar

but with additional unique functions and roles (**FIGURE 1.1**). This allows us to discuss cells initially as a single entity, and then to expound the unique or highly specialized functions of specific cells in a later discussion.

Human cells have an average size of 5 to 10 micrometers and were first described using light microscopy. Light microscopy allows an imaging magnification of about 1500 times. However, it was not until the advent of electron microscopy that the finer details of cells' **organelles** and ultrastructural aspects were scrutinized. Electron microscopy has the potential to expand imaging magnification up to 250,000 times.

Enveloped in a fluid plasma membrane, the cell can be divided into two major parts: the nucleus and the cytoplasm. The plasma membrane is approximately 7.5 to 10 nanometers thick, and its approximate composition by mass is proteins, 55%; **phospholipids**, 25%; cholesterol, 13%; other lipids, 4%; and carbohydrates, 3%. The plasma membrane is arranged in a lipid bilayer structure, thus making the membrane merely two molecules thick (**FIGURE 1.2**). Phospholipids and cholesterol make up most of the lipid bilayer and are oriented so that their hydrophilic (water-soluble) portion faces the watery medium of the intracellular and extracellular fluids, and their hydrophobic (water-insoluble) portion faces the internal aspect of the bilayer. The major phospholipids in the plasma membrane can vary among cell types; however, they generally include phosphatidylcholine (lecithin), phosphatidylethanolamine,

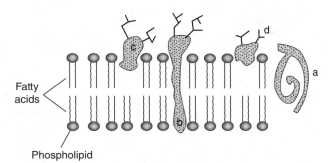

Fatty acids

Phospholipid

FIGURE 1.2 Membrane Structure: The Fluid Mosaic.
A phospholipid bilayer (a) with associated proteins.
Transmembrane proteins (b) can extend all the way
through the membrane, such as the ion channel displayed.
Peripheral proteins (c) are associated with only 1 side of
the bilayer. Carbohydrate extensions (d) from membrane
structures form the glycocalyx.

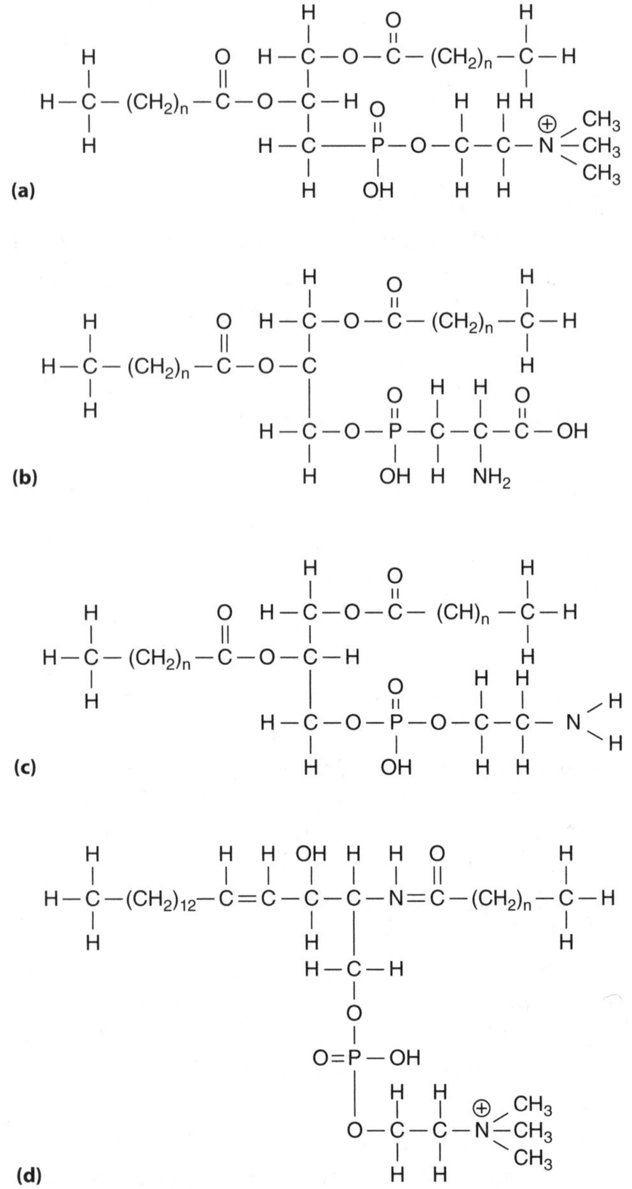

(a)

(b)

(c)

(d)

FIGURE 1.3 Phospholipid Molecular Structures.
Phosphatidylcholine or lecithin (a), phosphatidylserine
(b), phosphatidylethanolamine (c), and sphingomyelin (d).

phosphatidylserine, and sphingomyelin (**FIGURE 1.3**).
Inositol phospholipids are functionally important in
cell signaling operations; however, their quantitative contribution to plasma membrane lipid mass
is relatively small. The hydrophobic inner region of
the bilayer provides a transit barrier impermeable to
hydrophilic substances such as ions, glucose, amino
acids, and urea.

The plasma membrane of a small human cell may
contain 10^9 lipid molecules, approximately half of which
are phospholipids. Cholesterol and glycolipids account
for most of the remaining lipids. The planar cholesterol
molecule is oriented so that its hydrophilic hydroxyl
group is directed toward the polar ends of phospholipids
and their hydrophobic steroid rings and hydrocarbon
tail are directed toward the hydrophobic middle region
of the plasma membrane bilayer (**FIGURE 1.4**). The concentration of cholesterol adds stability to the plasma
membrane by preventing phospholipid fatty acid hydrocarbon chains from crystallizing.

Proteins are a major component of plasma membrane, accounting for about 55% of its mass. However,
with respect to the molecular size differential between
membrane proteins and lipids, the ratio of lipid to
protein molecules is about 50 to 1. Cell membrane
proteins occur either as integral or peripheral proteins
that float within the bilayer. Integral, or transmembrane, proteins extend through the plasma membrane
and function primarily as ion channels, carriers, active
transporters, receptor bases, and enzymes. Typically,
the portion of those proteins that extends through
the hydrophobic core of the plasma membrane is
composed mostly of amino acids with nonpolar side
chains. Transmembrane proteins are mostly glycoproteins, with their carbohydrate moiety extending into
the extracellular fluid. Peripheral proteins are typically
associated with integral membrane proteins on the
intracellular side of the plasma membrane, and their
function is mostly enzymatic.

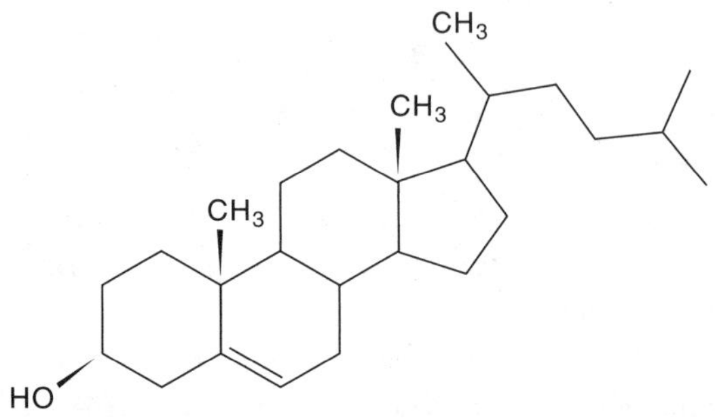

FIGURE 1.4 Cholesterol Molecule. Cholesterol is a
planar molecule that enhances the stability of the plasma
membrane. It is generally a hydrophobic molecule, with
the exception of the hydroxyl group (OH).

Carbohydrates, in the form of polysaccharides attached to plasma membrane proteins (glycoproteins) and lipids (glycolipids), along with proteoglycans make up the glycocalyx (see Figure 1.2). The glycocalyx provides a carbohydrate coat on the extracellular face of the plasma membrane that appears to be involved in receptor activities and cell-to-cell adhesion.

The plasma membrane encloses the cytoplasm, which is composed of the cytosol and organelles. The cytosol is a clear intracellular fluid containing several substances that are either dissolved, suspended, or anchored within the watery medium. These substances include electrolytes, proteins, glucose and **glycogen**, amino acids, and lipids. The concentration of those intracellular substances can differ tremendously from the extracellular fluid (**TABLE 1.3**). For example, the extracellular fluid may be 14 times more concentrated with sodium and 10 times less concentrated with potassium compared with the intracellular fluid. One function of integral membrane proteins is to pump certain substances against their concentration or diffusion gradients to maintain those differences for physiologic purposes.

Many of the highly specialized operations that take place inside cells occur within membrane-contained organelles. Organelles include the endoplasmic reticulum, Golgi apparatus, lysosomes, peroxisomes, endosomes, and mitochondria. Although most types of cells contain all of those organelles or a highly

TABLE 1.4 Overview of Organelle Function

Organelle	Function and Features
Nucleus	Site of most DNA and transcription; site of rRNA production
Mitochondria	Site of most ATP synthesis in cells; some DNA
Lysosomes	Contain acid hydroxylases for digesting most biomolecule types
Endoplasmic reticulum	Synthesizes proteins and lipid substances destined to be exported from cell; site of glucose-6-phosphatase; participates in ethanol metabolism
Golgi apparatus	Further processes molecules synthesized in the endoplasmic reticulum: packaging site for exocytosis-destined molecules; synthesizes some carbohydrates
Peroxisomes	Contain oxidases; participate in ethanol metabolism
Endosomes	Structures produced by the invagination of the cell membrane or Golgi body for degradation or recycling

DNA, deoxyribonucleic acid; rRNA, ribosomal ribonucleic acid; ATP, adenosine triphosphate.

TABLE 1.3 Concentration Differences of General Solutes Across the Plasma Membrane[a]

	Intracellular Fluid (mmol/L)	Extracellular Fluid (mmol/L)
Sodium (Na^+)	12	145
Potassium (K^+)	155	4
Hydrogen (H^+)	13×10^{-5}	3.8×10^{-5}
Chloride (Cl^-)	3.8	120
Biocarbonate (HCO_3^-)	8	27
Organic anions (e.g., lactate)	155	Trace

[a]Electrolyte concentration across the skeletal muscle plasma membrane.

specialized version, the organelles' contribution to the total cell volume can vary. For example, myocytes (**muscle cells**) contain a rich complement of mitochondria, whereas the total surface area of endoplasmic reticulum in a **hepatocyte** (liver cell) is 30 to 40 times greater than the surface area of the plasma membrane. **TABLE 1.4** presents general functions associated with different organelles.

Endoplasmic Reticulum

The **endoplasmic reticulum** is a tubular network that is situated adjacent to the nuclei. In fact, the space inside the tubular network containing the endoplasmic reticulum matrix is connected to the space in between the two membranes of the nuclear envelope.

The membrane of the endoplasmic reticulum is very similar to the plasma membrane, consisting of a lipid bilayer densely embedded with proteins. The endoplasmic reticulum is a major site of molecule formation and metabolic operations within cells.

Visually, the endoplasmic reticulum can be separated into the rough (granular) and smooth (agranular) endoplasmic reticulum due to the presence of ribosomal complexes attached to its outer surface. The electron micrograph in **FIGURE 1.5** displays the ribosomal studding of the endoplasmic reticulum. The ribosomes of the rough endoplasmic reticulum are the site of synthesis for many proteins. As they are being synthesized, growing protein chains thread into the endoplasmic reticulum matrix, where they can undergo rapid glycosylation as well as cross-linking and folding to form more compact molecules. In general, proteins synthesized by the rough endoplasmic reticulum are destined for either exocytosis or to become part of the plasma or organelle membranes. In contrast, the smooth endoplasmic reticulum is a site of synthesis of several lipid molecules, including phospholipids and cholesterol. Once synthesized, those lipids become incorporated into the endoplasmic reticulum membrane, allowing for regeneration of the membrane lost in the form of **transport** vesicles destined for the Golgi apparatus.

Finally, the endoplasmic reticulum engages in other significant cellular operations. The endoplasmic reticulum of specific cells, such as the parenchyma of the liver and kidneys, contains glucose-6-phosphatase, which liberates glucose from glucose-6-phosphate generated by gluconeogenesis as well as glycogen breakdown for release from the cell. The endoplasmic reticulum is also the site of detoxification of potentially harmful substances, such as drugs and alcohol. The cytochrome P450 system is the primary site of detoxification operations in the endoplasmic reticulum.

Golgi Apparatus

The **Golgi apparatus** is composed of several stacked layers of thin, flat, enclosed vesicles and is located in close proximity to both the nucleus and the endoplasmic reticulum. It processes substances produced by the endoplasmic reticulum and also synthesizes some carbohydrates. The carbohydrates include sialic acid and galactose, as well as more complex polysaccharide protein-based molecules such as **hyaluronic acid** and **chondroitin sulfate**. Those are part of the proteoglycan component of mucous and glandular secretions, as well as being primary components of the organic matrix of connective tissue, such as bone, cartilage, and **tendons**. However, it is the molecule-processing and vesicle-formation activities of the Golgi apparatus that are without a doubt its most famous attributes. As molecules, especially proteins, are manufactured in the endoplasmic reticulum, they are transported throughout the tubular system and destined to reach the agranular portion in closest proximity to the Golgi apparatus. At this location, small transport vesicles pinch off and transport those substances to the Golgi apparatus (**FIGURE 1.6**). The vesicles introduce their cargo to the Golgi apparatus by fusing with its membrane.

Once inside the Golgi apparatus, endoplasmic reticulum-derived molecules, which are primarily proteins, can have more carbohydrate moieties added and become incorporated into highly concentrated packets. Eventually, the packets will bud off the Golgi apparatus and diffuse into the cytosol. The packets are then ready to fuse with the plasma membrane to form endosomes (described below) and release their contents into the extracellular space in an exocytotic process. Because of this activity, those packets are

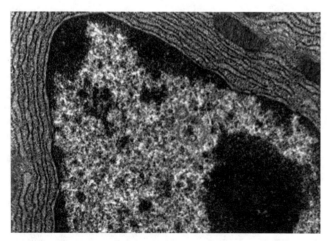

FIGURE 1.5 Rough Endoplasmic Reticulum. Electron micrograph of rough endoplasmic reticulum surrounding a nucleus (28,000×) showing the ribosomal studding.
Courtesy of Louisa Howard, Dartmouth College, Electron Microscope Facility.

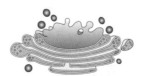 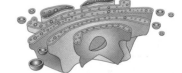

Three-dimensional view   Transverse view

FIGURE 1.6 Golgi Apparatus. Budding of vesicles from the plasma membrane face of the Golgi apparatus. The vesicles generally contain substances that will be secreted from the cell.

often referred to as secretory vesicles or secretory granules. Cells with greater endocrine, exocrine, paracrine, and autocrine activities, such as the pancreas, adrenal glands, and anterior pituitary gland, will show more secretory vesicles when observed with electron microscopy. The contents of those packets may be **hormones**, neurotransmitters, eicosanoids, or ductal secretions. Some of the concentrated packets are not destined for exocytosis; however, because highly specialized buds from the Golgi apparatus become lysosomes.

Endosomes, Lysosomes, and Peroxisomes

Endosomes are produced by an invagination of the cell membrane to transport a variety of compounds (usually lysosomes) for degradation. These structures may also be produced by the Golgi body. Endosomes can transfer materials to the cell membrane for recycling. A good example of this is in the regulation of low-density lipoprotein (LDL). LDL-cholesterol binds to a cell receptor, and the complex is then internalized within the cell in the form of an endosome. The LDL-cholesterol is removed and processed in the lysosome, and the receptor is recycled back to the cell membrane surface for reutilization. Those structures are in many ways responsible for sorting materials within the cell to other cellular organelles or components. The mature endosome is approximately 500 nanometers in diameter.

Lysosomes, which are typically between 250 and 750 nanometers in diameter and loaded with hydrolytic enzyme-containing granules, function as an intracellular digestive system. More than 50 different acid hydroxylases have been found in lysosomes and are involved in digesting various proteins, nucleic acids, mucopolysaccharides, lipids, and glycogen. Lysosomes are very important in cells such as macrophages.

Peroxisomes appear to be produced by specialized buddings of the smooth endoplasmic reticulum and contain oxidases that help detoxify potentially harmful substances. Peroxisomes also participate, to some degree, in ethanol (alcohol) oxidation and the oxidation of long-chain fatty acids.

Mitochondria

Aerobic adenosine triphosphate (ATP) generation takes place in **mitochondria**, self-replicating organelles found in almost every cell type in the human body (see Figure 1.1). Mitochondria can vary in size in different types of cells. In some cells, mitochondria may only be a few hundred nanometers in diameter, whereas in others, they may be as large as 1 micrometer in diameter and as long as 7 micrometers in length. The shape of mitochondria can also vary among cell types. For instance, mitochondria are spherical in brown adipose cells, sausage-shaped in muscle cells, and more oval in hepatocytes. The density of mitochondria within a cell type depends primarily on the oxidative energy demands of that cell. For instance, because of their dedication to the synthesis of chemical compounds, hepatocytes contain approximately 800 mitochondria per cell. Likewise, the high ATP demands of muscle cells also require a rich complement of mitochondria. Mitochondria account for approximately 25 to 35% and 12 to 15% of cardiac and skeletal myocyte volume, respectively.

Mitochondria tend to be located within cells in areas near organelles with high energy demands. Thus, mitochondria may typically appear in close proximity to the nucleus and ribosomes, where protein synthesis occurs, or near contractile myofibril in muscle cells. Also, triglyceride-rich lipid droplets are typically visualized adjacent to or at least in close proximity to mitochondria.

Mitochondria contain two lipid/protein bilayer membranes that are commonly called the outer membrane and the inner membrane (**FIGURE 1.7**). The outer membrane is very porous and is largely unfolded, whereas the inner membrane is relatively impermeable and highly folded, which greatly expands its surface area. Along with the other phospholipids common to cellular membranes, diphosphatidylglycerol or cardiolipin is found in mitochondrial membranes,

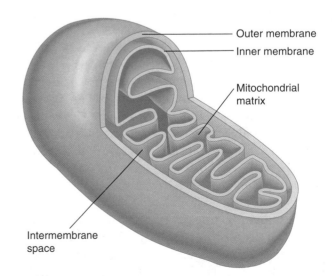

FIGURE 1.7 Mitochondrion. Note the inner and outer mitochondrial membranes.

particularly in the inner membrane. **Enzymes**, such as monoamine oxidase, acyl coenzyme A (acyl CoA) synthetase, glycerophosphate acyltransferase, and phospholipase A_2 are associated with the outer membrane, whereas adenylyl kinase and creatine kinase are found in the intermembrane space.

The inner mitochondrial membrane is the site of oxidative phosphorylation and contains enzymes and cytochrome complexes of the **electron transport chain**. It also provides a barrier enclosing the mitochondrial matrix. The mitochondrial matrix is concentrated with enzymes, largely involved in energy nutrient oxidation, and some DNA. For instance, the enzymes associated with fatty acid oxidation as well as the Krebs cycle are found in the mitochondrial matrix. Oxidative phosphorylation produces mainly ATP, using a series of oxidative enzyme complexes known as the electron transport or respiratory chain.

Mitochondrial biogenesis. The number of mitochondria in any given cell is not static. Some cells, such as those in cardiac tissue, have a high number of mitochondria, whereas cells in the brain have a low number. It could be that the heart relies more on fatty acids for energy, thus requiring more mitochondria. The brain, in contrast, requires more glucose to function, and thus does not need as many mitochondria because it does not prefer to use fatty acids as a source of energy. The creation of more mitochondria under selected conditions is called mitochondrial biogenesis. What are the molecular factors that cause mitochondrial biogenesis?

Mitochondria transcription factor A (mtTFA) is a major transcription factor governing mitochondrial DNA replication and transcription during mitochondrial biogenesis. A transcription factor is normally a protein that binds to the promoter of a gene to begin the process of mRNA synthesis that encodes for a specific protein. Low levels of mtTFA transcript and protein are associated with overall decreased mitochondrial gene transcription in cells. In contrast, expression of human mtTFA in yeast (*Saccharomyces cerevisiae*) devoid of mtTFA restores mitochondrial DNA transcription and function. Functional human mtTFA is a 25-kilodalton protein; its transcriptional activation initiates the synthesis of mitochondrial RNA by mitochondrial RNA polymerase.

The investigation of nuclear control of mitochondrial gene expression has led to the discovery of several other important transcription factors. Nuclear respiratory factor-1 (NRF-1) coordinates nuclear-encoded respiratory chain expression with mitochondrial gene transcription and replication. NRF-1 recognition sites have been found in many genes encoding respiratory functional subunits, such as rat cytochrome c oxidase subunit VIc and the bovine ATP synthase γ subunit. Therefore, NRF-1 activates mitochondrial gene expression by up-regulating mtTFA.

Another nuclear gene product, NRF-2, has also been implicated in the coordination between nuclear and mitochondrial gene expression. Although the majority of genes encoding proteins in respiratory functions have an NRF-1 recognition site, some genes (such as cytochrome c oxidase subunit IV and ATP synthase β subunit) lack an NRF-1 mitochondrial recognition site but contain a NRF-2 recognition site, indicating that these respiratory chain genes may be differentially regulated. In some genes, both NRF-1 and NRF-2 recognition sites have been identified. It is apparent that NRF-1 and NRF-2 may convey nuclear regulatory events to the mitochondria via mtTFA and coordinate the gene expression between the nuclear and mitochondrial genomes.

Peroxisomal proliferating activating receptor-γ coactivator (PGC-1) is thought to be a master regulator of mitochondrial biogenesis, and its interaction with mtTFA, NRF-1, and NRF-2 is the subject of investigation. This transcription factor has the ability to induce the production of mitochondria in brown adipose tissue. The various isoforms of PGC-1 constitute a family: PGC-1α, PGC-1β, and PGC-1-related coactivators. Both PGC-1α and PGC-1β have high expression in tissues rich in mitochondria. Unlike some other transcription factors, PGC-1α does not bind to a DNA promoter directly. Rather, it acts via a protein–protein interaction but does not have enzymatic activity. Transfection of PGC-1α into C_2C_{12} cells (i.e., introduction of PGC-1α into cells) and into myocytes results in turning on mitochondrial biogenesis. PGC-1α may act as a coactivator of NRF-1, which then is thought to bind to the promoter of mtTFA to initiate the concomitant upregulation of both mitochondria- and nuclear-encoded proteins in a coordinated fashion. Another set of transcription factors needed to initiate mitochondrial biogenesis is the transcription specificity factors (TFB1M and TFB2M). Recognition sites are present within the promoters for NRF-1 and NRF-2 for those two transcription factors. It has also been reported that PGC-1α will up-regulate those two transcription factors. Upregulation of mtTFA augments mitochondrial biogenesis with those other transcription factors.

Newer Findings on Mitochondrial Diseases

Genetic, metabolic, and dietary events can result in mitochondrial diseases. Mitochondrial diseases may be due to base-pair substitutions in the mitochondrial genome or may involve defects in the nuclear-encoded mitochondrial proteins. The mechanisms or proteins responsible for ferrying some mitochondrial proteins (chaperone proteins) synthesized in the cytoplasm to the mitochondria can also be defective, and the import of such proteins into the mitochondria can be impaired. All of these factors collectively can lead to mitochondrial dysfunction and pathology.

A number of mitochondrial diseases affect skeletal and cardiac muscle and peripheral and central nervous system tissue, particularly the brain, the liver, bone marrow, the endocrine and exocrine pancreas, the kidneys, and the intestines. Kearns-Sayre syndrome is a mitochondrial disease in which deletion of parts of NADH-coenzyme Q reductase (subunits III and IV), all of ATP synthase subunit VI, and part of ATP synthase subunit VIII occurs. The DNA responsible for encoding cytochrome c oxidase subunit IV is present, but not the DNA of mitochondria-encoded cytochrome c oxidase subunit II. Another disorder, myoclonus epilepsy with ragged red fibers (MERRF), affects both brain and muscle tissue. This disorder causes a notable decrease in cytochrome c oxidase subunit II protein but not in the mRNA. A child afflicted with Leigh syndrome revealed a disorder involving a nuclear mutation in cytochrome c oxidase, but all subunits were present to lesser degrees.

There have been several reports of defects in cytochrome c oxidase in patients suffering from cardiomyopathy, which is a type of heart disease where the muscle fails to contract. More recently, a copper chaperone protein, called SCO2, was found to be mutated in several forms of fatal infantile cardiomyopathy leading to cytochrome c oxidase deficiency. This protein ferries copper from one protein to SCO2, which inserts copper into the cytochrome c oxidase. Apparently, this protein is nonfunctional in some people. In another study, a patient with SCO2 mutations had severe hypertrophic cardiomyopathy that was reversed with copper-histidine supplementation.

⬡ BEFORE YOU GO ON . . .

1. Which cell compound is important for cell signaling?
2. Where within the cell is it likely for carbohydrate and protein to join to become glycoproteins?
3. What are the major phospholipids in cell membranes?
4. In which cell structure would you most likely see cell detoxification occurring via the P450 pathway?
5. Name an organelle that has its own set of DNA.

▸ The Nucleus and Genetic Aspects

The nucleus provides a storage and processing facility for DNA. It is enclosed by the porous nuclear envelope (see Figure 1.1), which is actually two separate membranes, the outer and inner. At certain regions, the outer nuclear membrane connects with the membrane of the endoplasmic reticulum. This allows the space between the two nuclear membranes to be continual with the matrix of the endoplasmic reticulum. Very large protein-associated pores penetrate the nuclear envelope, allowing molecules having a molecular weight of up to 44,000 daltons to move through the envelope with relative ease.

DNA, RNA, and Genes

By and large, the DNA contained within human cells is localized in the nucleus. Small amounts of DNA are also found in mitochondria. All mature human cells, with the exception of erythrocytes (red blood cells), contain 1 or more nuclei. As a rule, cells beget cells; therefore, all nucleated cells will contain the same DNA. Each DNA molecule contains a myriad of regions (**genes**) that code for proteins. Because digestion breaks down ingested food proteins into amino acids prior to absorption into the body, proteins must be constructed within cells from their building blocks—amino acids. Genes contain the instructions for the synthesis of all human proteins, including structural proteins, enzymes, contractile proteins, and protein hormones. Proteins are then involved, either directly or indirectly, in the **metabolism** of all other molecules in the human body.

DNA molecules are extremely long. It has been estimated that the longest human chromosome is over 7.2 centimeters long. Human cells contain 23 pairs of chromosomes (22 autosomal and 1 sex-linked), with the exception of sperm and eggs, which only have 1 of each of the 23 chromosomes. It has been estimated that the DNA in human chromosomes collectively codes for as many as 100,000 proteins.

Despite the fact that human DNA is a polymer consisting of billions of nucleotides linked together, there are only four nucleotide monomers (**FIGURE 1.8**). Adenine and guanine are purine bases, whereas thymine and cytosine are pyrimidine bases. The five-carbon carbohydrate deoxyribose is added to the bases to form adenosine (A), thymidine (T), guanosine (G), and cytosine (C). Those structures, which are called nucleosides, are found in DNA in a phosphorylated form referred to as a nucleotide. DNA links of nucleotides can be written in a shorthand format, for example, ATGGATC.

DNA exists in human cells as double-stranded chains arranged in an antiparallel manner. That is, one DNA polymer runs in a 3′ to 5′ direction whereas the complementary stand runs in a 5′ to 3′ orientation. The strands are held together by complementary base pairing, whereby adenosine on 1 strand hydrogen bonds with thymidine on the other chain, and guanine base-pairs with cytosine (**FIGURE 1.9**). The average length of human genes is about 20,000 base pairs.

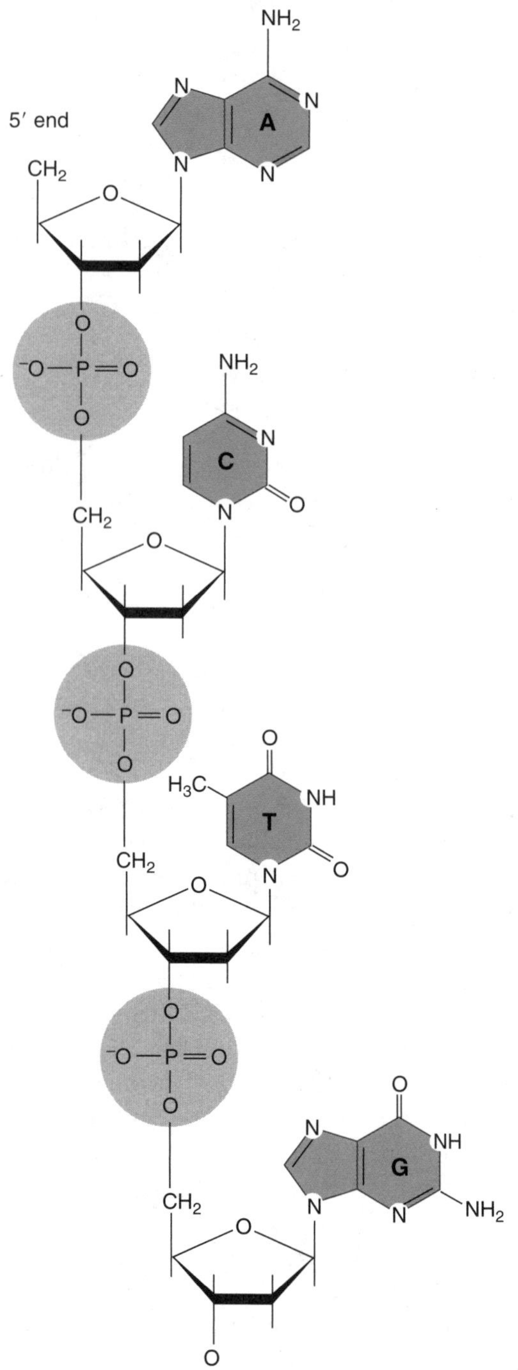

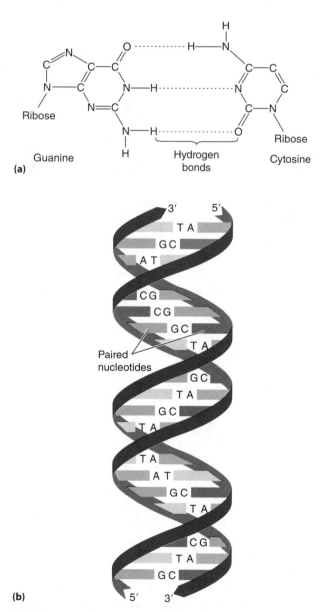

FIGURE 1.8 Single Strand of DNA. DNA bases linked by phosphodiester bonds, indicated by shaded areas.

Data from Doetsch, P. W. *Encyclopedia of Life Sciences.* John Wiley & Sons, Ltd., April 2001. [doi: 10.1038/npg.els.0000557].

FIGURE 1.9 Hydrogen Bonding Between Complementary Nucleotide Bases. The hydrogen-bond link between adenine and thymine (a), and hydrogen bonding between the double helical DNA strands (b).

Whereas DNA in the nucleus is substantial in quantity and strongly associated with histone proteins to form complex chromosomal structures, the DNA in mitochondria contains fewer than 17,000 base pairs and contains a very limited number of coding regions. Mitochondrial DNA contains genes for 13 of the 67 or so protein subunits of the respiratory chain as well as for **ribosomal RNA (rRNA)** and **transfer RNA (tRNA)**.

The processes of protein synthesis have to overcome a few obstacles. First, genes coding for proteins are located primarily within the nucleus. Meanwhile, ribosomal complexes, which are the apparatuses of protein synthesis, exist either within the cytosol or studding the endoplasmic reticulum. Thus, the information inherent to DNA must be delivered from one location to another. This obstacle is overcome by **messenger RNA (mRNA)**. Second, the amino acids necessary to synthesize proteins must be made available at the site of protein synthesis. This obstacle is overcome by tRNA. Amino acids are delivered to ribosomal complexes by tRNA and correctly oriented to allow their incorporation into growing protein chains (**FIGURE 1.10**).

Protein synthesis begins with **transcription**, the process of producing a strand of mRNA that is complementary to the DNA gene being expressed. First, the double-stranded DNA is temporarily opened at the site of the gene, and then ribonucleotides are sequentially base-paired to the DNA template. The process is catalyzed by RNA polymerase II and influenced and regulated by promoter and enhancer sequences of DNA occurring either prior to or after the coding region. The formation of the DNA–RNA complementary base-pairing is the same as for DNA–DNA base-pairing, with one exception: the pyrimidine base uracil (U) substitutes for thymine in base-pairing with adenine. In addition to the substitution of a uracil base for thymine, the nucleotides contain **ribose** instead of deoxyribose (**TABLE 1.5**).

The initial RNA strand created during transcription, called **heterogeneous nuclear RNA (hnRNA)**, is relatively large and generally unusable in this state. Therefore, the newly created hnRNA strand must undergo **posttranscriptional modification**, or change in the original molecule produced following transcription. Segments of the hnRNA strand that do not code for the final protein must be removed, and the remaining segments that do code for the final protein must be joined together. This process is called **splicing**; the removed segments are referred to as **introns**, and the remaining segments are **exons**. Furthermore, the RNA strand is modified at both ends.

The ribosomal complexes providing the site of protein synthesis must be constructed from RNA subunits. DNA contains specific regions that, when transcribed, produce RNA strands that are not used in instructing protein amino acid sequencing but rather are used to construct ribosomal complexes. The enzyme RNA polymerase I transcribes the rRNA 45S precursor, which undergoes a number of cleavages and ultimately produces 18S and 28S rRNA. The latter rRNA is hydrogen-bonded to a 5.8S rRNA molecule. Finally, a 5S rRNA is produced by RNA polymerase III. The 18S rRNA complexes with proteins to form the 40S ribosomal subunit, whereas the 28S, 5.8S, and 5S rRNA complex with proteins to form the 60S ribosomal subunit. The 40S and the 60S ribosomal subunits migrate through the nuclear pores and ultimately condense to

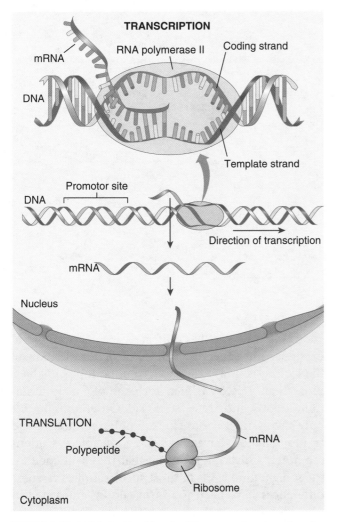

FIGURE 1.10 Protein Synthesis. Diagram of major steps in synthesis of protein as directed by DNA.

TABLE 1.5 Base-Pairing of Nucleic Acid Bases	
DNA–DNA	**DNA–RNA**
A–T	A–U
C–G	C–G

form the 80S ribosome, which, once situated, becomes a site of protein synthesis.

At least three types of RNA are involved in silencing gene expression; they are commonly referred to as **RNA interference (RNAi)**. The first one is called **micro RNA (miRNA)**, and it appears to control translation events in animal cells. miRNA is composed of only a few nucleotide base pairs, approximately 22, and is encoded by the cell's genomic DNA. The human genome encodes more than 1000 types of miRNA. miRNA is mostly involved in suppressing translation by binding to the complementary sequences of mRNA at the 3′ untranslated region (UTR). miRNA sequences are not 100% complementary to the mRNA and may differ by at least one base pair. This difference may block translation of a peptide or protein. Regardless, those processes are sometimes referred to as gene silencing. Approximately 60% of human genes may be targeted by miRNA, and miRNA may be involved in hundreds of biologic processes. Because miRNA is also found in mitochondria, it may also affect the ability of mitochondria to multiply and mature.

The second type of RNAi is referred to as **small interfering RNA (siRNA)**. This type of RNA is very similar to miRNA except that (1) it is synthetic and used for biologic experimentation to silence genes and (2) it is an exact match to the mRNA. Because of the 100% match, when the siRNA pairs with the complementary mRNA, the complex is destroyed, which is different from miRNA, which blocks protein translation.

Finally, there is **small hairpin RNA (shRNA)**, which functions like miRNA but is used more as an experimental agent. shRNA silences genes by introducing them into a cell that is fused to a vector, such as a plasmid or a virus. This shRNA introduction can then lead either to RNA degradation, in the case of a perfect base-pair match, or a block in translation, in the case of an imperfect base-pair match.

▶ Protein Synthesis

For proteins to be constructed, the genetic nucleotide language must be translated into amino acid chains. This fact led to the coining of the term **translation**. Amino acids are specifically linked together as dictated by the sequencing of RNA in the finalized version of mRNA. Messenger RNA contains a series of triplets of bases coding for a given amino acid. Those coding triplets, or codons, are the complementary base triplets originally transcribed in DNA (**TABLE 1.6**). RNA codons in mRNA either indicate a specific amino acid or signal for either the initiation or termination of the synthesis of a protein. Certain amino acids have more than 1 RNA triplet; for example, alanine has four codons, and arginine has six. Other amino acids only have a single codon; for example, methionine and tryptophan both have only one codon apiece. Codons are nearly universal, meaning that they will code for the same amino acids in most species; however, some differences have been found in codons translated in mitochondria.

TABLE 1.6 Genetic Code

First Base (5′)	Second Base				Third Base (3′)
	U	C	A	G	
U	Phe	Ser	Tyr	Cys	U
	Phe	Ser	Tyr	Cys	C
	Leu	Ser	Term[a]	Term	A
	Leu	Ser	Term	Trp	G
C	Leu	Pro	His	Arg	U
	Leu	Pro	His	Arg	C
	Leu	Pro	Gln	Arg	A
	Leu	Pro	Gln	Arg	G
A	Ile	Thr	Asn	Ser	U
	Ile	Thr	Asn	Ser	C
	Ile	Thr	Lys	Arg	A
	Met	Thr	Lys	Arg	G
G	Val	Ala	Asp	Gly	U
	Val	Ala	Asp	Gly	C
	Val	Ala	Glu	Gly	A
	Val	Ala	Glu	Gly	G

[a]Term indicates a stop or termination codon.

Transfer RNA constitutes small cytosolic RNA molecules of about 80 nucleotides in length. Transfer RNA attaches to specific amino acids and delivers them to ribosomal complexes. Transfer RNA is then able to recognize when to include its amino acid into a growing protein chain by codon–anticodon recognition. Each tRNA contains a triplet of bases that will interact with its complementary codon on the mRNA strand being translated. This allows the sequencing of amino acids into growing protein chains to be a very accurate process.

Proteins that are synthesized on ribosomal complexes studding the endoplasmic reticulum thread into the endoplasmic reticulum matrix. As mentioned previously, those proteins are, by and large, modified by the addition of carbohydrate moieties to form glycoproteins. In contrast, proteins formed in association with cytosolic ribosomal complexes mostly remain as free proteins. Again, the free proteins formed in the cytosol remain mostly within the cell, whereas most of the protein formed in association with the endoplasmic reticulum is destined for exocytosis from the cells or to become part of cell membranes.

From an energy standpoint, protein synthesis is a very ATP-expensive operation. To begin with, amino acids must be activated before they can attach to their corresponding tRNA. Thus, if a synthesized protein contains 500 amino acids, 500 ATP molecules must be used simply in forming amino acid–tRNA associations. Furthermore, the initiation of translation, as well as protein elongation, requires even more energy. A portion of the energy demand is provided by the hydrolysis of guanosine triphosphate (GTP). It is estimated that every amino acid–amino acid linkage in a protein requires the energy contribution made by the hydrolysis of four high-energy bonds, provided by ATP and GTP.

▶ Nutrition and Epigenetics

Genetic inheritance of traits has long been accepted by the sequence of base pairs comprising the DNA and their subsequent expression. We now know that factors other than base-pair sequence may affect disease and gene expression. A field of study, epigenetics, adds new information on how factors outside of base-pair sequences can lead to alteration of gene expression. Epigenetics is an evolving field of study whereby factors outside of DNA base-pair sequences can lead to heritable characteristics. Notable epigenetic factors that alter gene expression involve methylation and/or histone modification of DNA.

There are a number of nutrients than may affect methylation of DNA since they may act as methyl donors. Such nutrients include folic acid, vitamin B_{12}, S-adenosylmethionine, choline, and betaine. Over or under methylation may affect gene expression patterns and alter development. Histone acylation is another mechanism by which gene expression may be altered. Methylation of histones may also impact gene expression. Nutrients such as biotin, niacin and pantothenic acid may impact histone methylation. A good example of how such nutrients may impact disease states via epigenetics is with low folic acid intake during pregnancy, which may lead to neural tube defects. Inadequate methylation of DNA due to low dietary intake of folic acid has thought to result in the reprogramming of critical developmental steps in the development. Clearly, the interaction of key nutrients as it relates to methylation and histone acylation opens new doors to understanding the role of nutrients in disease process.

▶ Electron Transport Chain and Oxidative Phosphorylation

Perhaps, the most important function of any cell in the human body is the formation of ATP. ATP is then used by cells to promote three major categories of function: membrane transport, synthesis of molecules, and mechanical work. Substances either directly or indirectly transported by active, or ATP-requiring, processes include sodium, potassium, chloride, urate, and hydrogen ions as well as other ions and organic substances (**FIGURE 1.11**). The cost of active transportation can be extremely heavy in some cells. For example, tubular cells in the kidneys contribute as much as 80% of their ATP expenditure to active transport. The synthesis of chemical compounds in cells, such as proteins, purines, pyrimidines, cholesterol, phospholipids, and a whole host of other compounds, is also extremely energy costly. Some cells may dedicate as much as 75% of their produced ATP to synthetic processes. With regard to mechanical work performed by cells, muscle fiber contraction accounts for most of the ATP used for these specialized processes. The balance comes mostly from the minimal contribution of ameboid and ciliary motion performed by certain cells.

ATP is constantly consumed and regenerated in human cells. The structure of ATP, which is depicted

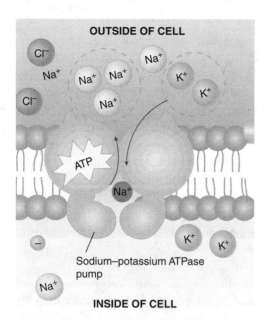

FIGURE 1.11 Sodium–Potassium ATPase Pump.
Adenosine triphosphate (ATP) is hydrolyzed to provide the energy necessary to concomitantly pump sodium and potassium across the plasma membrane against their concentration gradient. For instance, sodium is pumped to the outside of the cell and potassium is pumped to the inside of the cell.

in **FIGURE 1.12**, reveals an adenine base linked to ribose, which itself has a tail of three phosphates linked in series by anhydride bonds. The free energy derived from ATP comes from the hydrolytic splitting of anhydride bonds. Those bonds thus became known as **high-energy bonds**. When ATP is hydrolyzed to produce ADP, the change in standard Gibbs free energy ($\Delta G^{\circ\prime}$) equals –7.3 **kilocalories**/mole. The free energy released when ATP is hydrolyzed is used to drive reactions that require energy. Generally,

adenosine diphosphate (ADP) is formed along with inorganic phosphate (P_i). ADP can be broken down to adenosine monophosphate (AMP) and pyrophosphate (PPi), which releases –3.4 kilocalories/mole. Furthermore, ATP can transfer a phosphate group to compounds such as glucose. ATP, ADP, and AMP are interconvertible by the adenylate kinase reaction:

$$ATP + AMP \leftrightarrow 2\ ADP$$

Carbohydrates, amino acids, triglycerides, ethanol, and their intermediates, derived directly from the diet or mobilized from cellular stores, provide the substrates for ATP formation. As discussed in greater detail later, these fuel molecules must engage in various chemical reaction series or pathways in order for their inherent energy to be used in the formation of ATP. The utilization of carbohydrate begins with a series of chemical reactions occurring in the cytosol known as **glycolysis**. Glycolysis generates a net production of two ATP molecules by substrate-level phosphorylation, an **anaerobic** process. Glycolysis generates pyruvate molecules, which can enter mitochondria and be converted to the activated two-carbon residue acetyl coenzyme A (CoA). Likewise, the breakdown of fatty acids, some amino acids, and ethanol also result in the production of acetyl CoA.

Mitochondrial acetyl CoA condenses with oxaloacetate to form citrate, which then enters the Krebs cycle (**FIGURE 1.13**). The Krebs cycle, also known as the citric acid cycle and the tricarboxylic acid (TCA) cycle, is a series of seven main chemical reactions in which the final reaction regenerates oxaloacetate. Therefore, this pathway is considered cyclic. The net result of these reactions is the production of reduced cofactors that will then transfer the electrons to the electron transport chain. NADH and $FADH_2$ are the reduced forms of NAD^+ (oxidized nicotinamide adenine

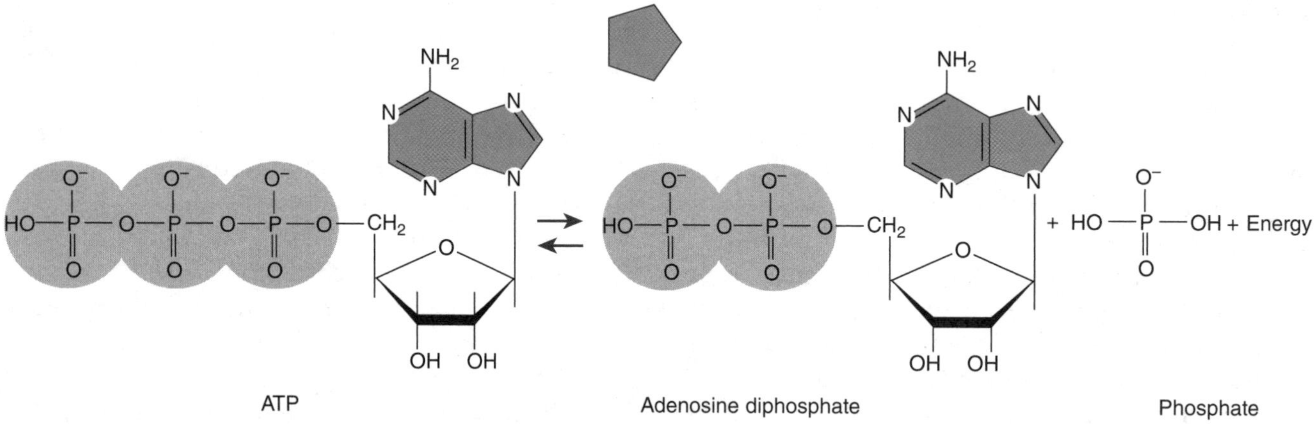

ATP Adenosine diphosphate Phosphate

FIGURE 1.12 Adenosine Triphosphate (ATP). ATP is the primary high-energy molecule produced in human cells. Bonds between the phosphate groups are hydrolyzed to liberate energy, which is applied to cellular processes.

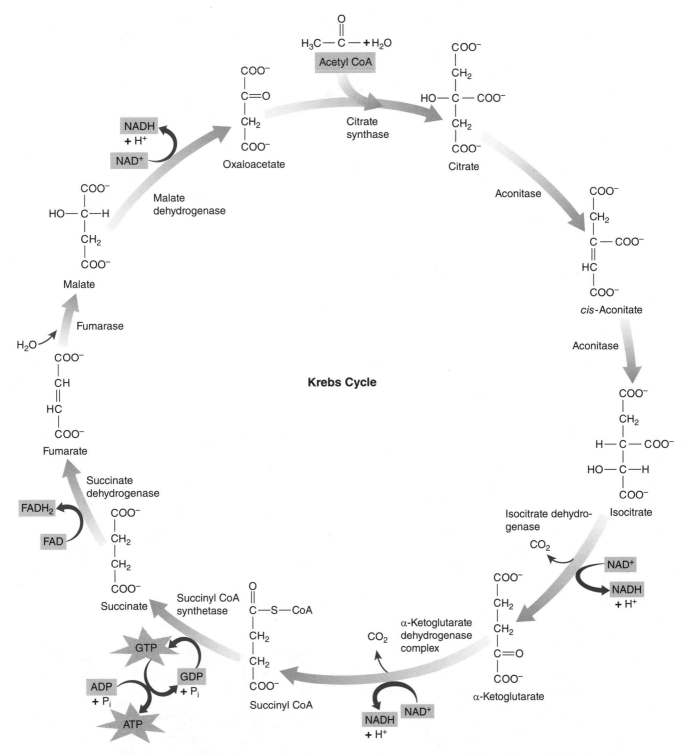

FIGURE 1.13 The Krebs (Citric Acid) Cycle. Basic biochemical reactions to produce NADH + H$^+$ and FADH$_2$ for subsequent ATP synthesis. Acetyl CoA is a major metabolite produced from the oxidation of glucose and fat.

dinucleotide) and FAD (flavin adenine dinucleotide), respectively. Reactions in the Krebs cycle produce three NADH and one FADH$_2$. **Fatty acid oxidation** (β-oxidation) also creates NADH and FADH$_2$; how many of the reduced cofactors are produced depends on the length of a particular fatty acid. Furthermore,

NADH is also produced in the conversion of pyruvate to acetyl CoA in the mitochondria, as well as during glycolysis in the cytosol.

Carbon dioxide is produced in the conversion of pyruvate to acetyl CoA and in two reactions in the Krebs cycle. These reactions are the primary producers

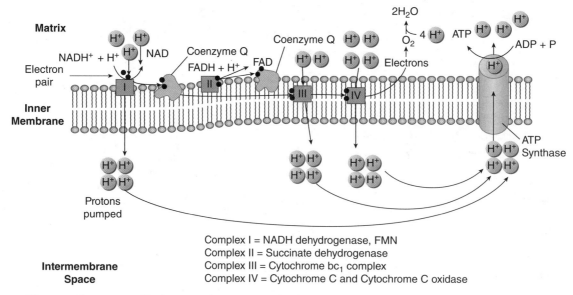

Complex I = NADH dehydrogenase, FMN
Complex II = Succinate dehydrogenase
Complex III = Cytochrome bc$_1$ complex
Complex IV = Cytochrome C and Cytochrome C oxidase

FIGURE 1.14 Electron Transport Chain. Note that O$_2$ is the final electron acceptor.

of this metabolic waste molecule in cells. GTP is also generated by a reaction in the Krebs cycle and functions to drive certain biochemical reactions, such as translation.

As mentioned earlier, ATP is generated **anaerobically** in one chemical reaction of glycolysis. This is an important source of ATP for all cells and is the sole source of ATP for erythrocytes (red blood cells), which lack mitochondria. However, most of the ATP generated within cells occurs via oxidative phosphorylation by the electron transport chain. Oxygen is required for operation of the electron transport chain as the final acceptor of electrons. Without the availability of oxygen, the flow of electrons through the electron transport chain is halted and mitochondrial ATP generation ceases (**FIGURE 1.14**).

The electron transport chain is a series of protein-based complexes stitched into the mitochondrial inner membrane. The inner membrane is highly folded, which increases its surface area and thus the number of electron transport chains per mitochondrion. The folds are known as cristae. Mitochondria of certain cells, such as cardiac muscle cells, are densely packed with cristae (**FIGURE 1.15**).

The reduced cofactors NADH and FADH$_2$ transfer electrons to the electron transport chain. NADH is viewed as free-floating within the mitochondrial matrix as well as the cytosol. Thus, when NAD$^+$ becomes reduced to NADH, it can diffuse to electron transport chains. This certainly seems true of NADH generated within the mitochondria. However, NADH produced in the cytosol probably must rely on an electron-translocation system for its electrons to reach the electron transport chain. Conversely, FAD is

bound tightly to enzymes in the mitochondrial inner membrane. Thus, FAD reduced to FADH$_2$ will not need to endure diffusion and is in theory immediately available to the electron transport chain.

Electrons move forward through the electron transport chain toward O$_2$ because of the large $\Delta G°'$ gradient. The transfer of electrons from NADH to O$_2$ occurs in three stages, each of which is associated with the production of one ATP molecule. Meanwhile, the transfer of electrons from FADH$_2$ to O$_2$ occurs in two principal steps, both of which are associated with the production of one ATP molecule. Therefore, three ATP molecules will be created for each NADH oxidized, and two ATP molecules will be created for each oxidized FADH$_2$.

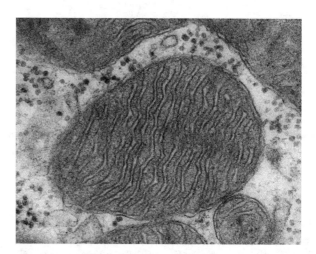

FIGURE 1.15 Electron Micrograph of Cardiac Myocyte Mitochondria (25,000×). Note the densely packed inner membrane, or cristae.

Electrons are passed from NADH to flavin mononucleotide (FMN) as catalyzed by NADH dehydrogenase (Complex I). FMN then passes the electrons through a series of iron-sulfur (Fe-S) complexes to coenzyme Q (CoQ). Coenzyme Q accepts the electrons one at a time, first forming semiquinone and then ubiquinol. The energy liberated by the transfer of electrons at this point is adequate to pump protons to the cytosolic side of the mitochondrial inner membrane. The pumping of electrons at this and other points of the electron transport chain establishes a chemoelectric potential or proton-motive force. Because the mitochondrial inner membrane is generally impermeable to proton diffusion, movement of protons back into the matrix occurs through highly specialized ATP-synthase complexes (F_0-F_1/ATPase). F_0 proteins form a physical channel, allowing proton passage through the membrane, and they are also connected to the F_1 (ATP-synthesizing head) proteins. This is the site of ATP formation. $FADH_2$ also passes its electrons to Complex II and then coenzyme Q; however, because the FMN stage was bypassed, there is no associated pumping of a proton across the mitochondrial inner membrane.

Electrons are transferred from coenzyme Q to cytochrome b and c_1 (Complex III) and then to cytochrome c via the actions of cytochrome reductase. These cytochromes, along with others in the electron transport chain, consist of an iron-containing heme prosthetic group associated with a protein. Enough energy is liberated in the transfer of electrons from coenzyme Q to cytochrome c to pump a proton across the inner membrane.

Cytochrome c transfers electrons to the cytochrome aa_3 complex (Complex IV), which then transfers the electrons to molecular oxygen, creating water. Cytochrome c oxidase is the enzyme involved with the transfer of electrons to oxygen, and again, the energy liberated is significant enough to pump another proton across the mitochondrial inner membrane.

● BEFORE YOU GO ON . . .

1. What are gene-silencing RNAs, and why are they significant?
2. What is meant by posttranscriptional modification?
3. Explain how the breakdown products eventually end up being metabolized in the Krebs cycle?
4. What is the major purpose of NADH and $FADH_2$?
5. What is the chemoelectrical force in regard to electron transport?

▶ Cellular Protein Functions

Thus far, we have learned how a cell makes proteins. As you can imagine, there are thousands of proteins serving a wide variety of functions. Proteins are required for organelle and **cell membrane structure**, are components of **cell receptor**, and play a critical role in **cell signaling** (e.g., protein kinases). Proteins may act as chaperones for other compounds or minerals to other parts of the cell. Proteins are also components of ion channels and, equally as important, make up enzymes to facilitate cellular biochemical reactions. Let's consider each of those protein functions separately.

Organelle and Cell Membrane Structure and Cell Receptors

Organelle and cell membranes are composed of a biphospholipid layer in which proteins are embedded. Many of the proteins embedded in cell membranes may be ion channels or transport proteins. Proteins often exist on cell membranes, where they may crisscross the cell membranes several times. For example, the 5′ (carboxyl) end and 3′ (amino) end of a protein may be at the intracellular or extracellular level (**FIGURE 1.16**). Often, these transport proteins bind to a substrate (e.g., glucose) and the transport protein changes conformation to bring a substrate into the cell (**FIGURE 1.17**) or export material out of a cell. Zinc transporter proteins are a good example of this mechanism. In many cases, such as the sodium–potassium (Na^+–K^+) ATPase pump, energy in the form of ATP is

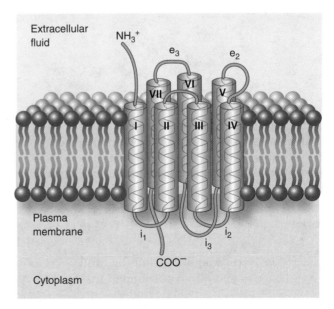

FIGURE 1.16 Structure of a Transmembrane Protein Receptor.

Data from Bockaert, J. *Encyclopedia of Life Sciences*. John Wiley & Sons, Ltd., January 2006. [doi:10.1038/npg.els.0000118].

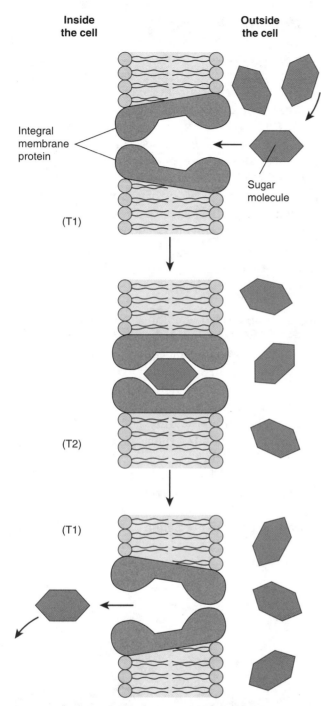

Inside the cell

Outside the cell

Integral membrane protein

Sugar molecule

(T1)

(T2)

(T1)

FIGURE 1.17 Conformation Change of Some Transmembrane Receptors When Importing or Exporting a Substance. In this case, note the change in the transport protein for a sugar molecule as it goes from the outside to the inside of the cell. T1 is the transport protein without a sugar molecule, and T2 is the same protein that has a conformational change when binding to a sugar molecule.

needed to extrude sodium from the inside of the cell to the exterior and pump potassium into the cell.

Enzymes

All enzymes are composed of proteins. Some of those enzymes have carbohydrate components and even

minerals to help them function at an active site. You may remember from biochemistry that an active site is where an enzyme and substrate bind and where the chemical reaction occurs, which normally requires energy. Enzymes facilitate metabolic reactions in a cell and allow the cell to use less energy (normally ATP) to create a reaction. The energy needed to cause a biochemical reaction to occur is often called the energy of activation. An enzyme lowers the energy of activation, which, in essence, means that the cell requires less energy for a reaction to occur. ATP is normally a source of energy involved in enzymatic reactions. For example, consider the following reactions: Glucose is converted to **glucose-6-phosphate** in the presence of ATP; the enzyme glucokinase (sometimes referred to as hexokinase) is essential for this reaction. In contrast, the conversion of malate into oxaloacetate does not require ATP but does require the enzyme malate dehydrogenase.

Cell Signaling

Phosphorylation and dephosphorylation of proteins may activate or deactivate proteins involved with enzymatic reactions and pathways. Certain proteins involved with hormonal regulations have a protein receptor for the hormone. Cyclic AMP, or cAMP ($3'$,$5'$-cyclic adenosine monophosphate), is formed from ATP. cAMP is often called a second messenger because it acts as a messenger for hormones. Inositol–P_3 is another second messenger. The hormone receptor reacts with another intracellular protein, most likely a G protein (**FIGURE 1.18**). G proteins are an integral part of protein signaling to generate a second messenger.

Cell signaling consists of a series of biochemical reactions from the cell surface receptor to convey the message to a DNA promoter to exert the desired effect, for example, transcription of mRNA. Not all signaling has to be genetic; some may simply involve phosphorylation and dephosphorylation, as described earlier. The impact of a G protein is not a simple 1-step reaction of turning a gene off or on, but rather, it is a series of coordinated reactions that act as a cascade leading to a final outcome. A hormone reacting with its receptor may activate a G protein in order to activate adenylate cyclase to produce cAMP, which, in turn, can cause many metabolic reactions.

Transport

As alluded to previously, proteins are vital in the transport of many nutrients within the **enterocyte** and all living cells. Proteins act as conduits to bring compounds into a cell, either by passive diffusion (or **facilitated**

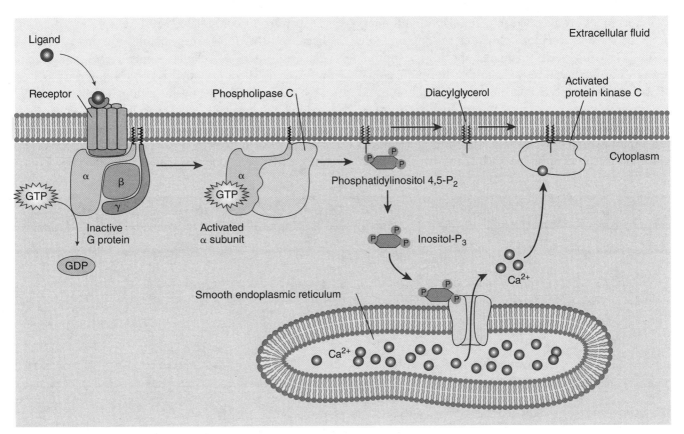

FIGURE 1.18 Cell Signaling Example. A hormone (ligand) interacting with a receptor and a G protein to generate a second messenger, in this case, inositol-P$_3$.

Modified from an illustration by George M. Helmkamp, Jr., School of Medicine, University of Kansas.

diffusion), in which no energy is needed to pass down a concentration gradient, or by **active transport**, for which energy is required. The uptake of amino acids and monosaccharides occurs against a concentration gradient and requires ATP; thus, it is an example of active transport. We mentioned active transport earlier when discussing Na$^+$–Ka$^+$ transport, which is really a cotransport mechanism requiring ATP. (**Cotransport** means one mineral or compound is coming in and one is going out at the same time by the same transport protein.) Carrier-mediated transport is usually saturable, meaning that at some point a concentration of compounds is reached such that further uptake is not possible because all the binding sites of the transporter have been occupied by the solute being transported.

Hormones

There are two ways in which one region of the human body can communicate with another. The first is by way of nerve impulses, and the second is by way of hormones. Hormones are synthesized by endocrine glands of various organs, including the pituitary gland, parathyroid gland, thyroid gland, hypothalamus, pancreas, stomach, small intestine, adrenal glands, placenta, and gonads (ovaries and testicles) (**FIGURE 1.19**). They are large protein and protein-based (i.e., glycoproteins), amino acid-based, or cholesterol-derived steroid molecules. Examples of protein hormones include insulin, growth hormone, glucagon, and antidiuretic hormone. Examples of hormones made from the amino acid tyrosine are epinephrine (adrenalin) and the thyroid hormones (triiodothyronine and thyroxine). Steroid hormones are made from cholesterol and include testosterone, estrogens, cortisol, progesterone, and aldosterone.

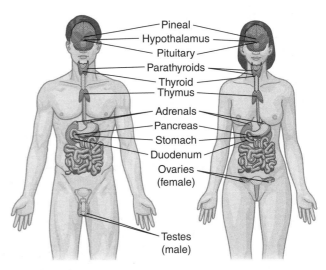

FIGURE 1.19 Endocrine Organs. Major synthesis sites for different hormones.

Hormones are released into circulation and interact with specific receptor complexes on one or more tissues. Only those cells that have a specific receptor for a given hormone will respond to that hormone. Some cell receptors are located on the plasma membrane and are typically part of a larger complex that has an associated intracellular event upon binding. For instance, the binding of the pancreatic hormone glucagon to glucagon receptors on tissue, such as the liver, results in an increase in cytosolic cAMP levels. As noted earlier, because cAMP is responsible for initiating the glucagon-intended cellular events, cAMP is a second messenger. There are other second messengers as well, such as Ca^{2+}, cyclic guanosine monophosphate (cGMP), inositol triphosphate, and diacylglycerol. Other hormones, such as thyroid hormones and steroid-based hormones, have nuclear receptors. Those hormones exert their activity by influencing gene expression (**TABLE 1.7**).

TABLE 1.7 Select Hormones Related to Nutrition and Metabolism and Their General Function		
Source	**Hormone**	**Principal Activity**
Pituitary gland	Growth hormone	Increases growth of most tissue by increasing protein synthesis and increasing fat utilization for energy
	Prolactin	Increases mammary milk formation during lactation
	Antidiuretic hormone	Decreases H_2O loss by kidneys by increasing H_2O reabsorption in nephrons
Thyroid gland	Thyroid hormone	Increases rate of metabolism
	Calcitonin	Decreases blood calcium levels by increasing kidney loss and decreasing digestive absorption of calcium
Parathyroid gland	Parathyroid	Increases blood calcium levels by increasing bone resorption
Adrenal glands	Aldosterone	Increases sodium reabsorption in kidneys
	Cortisol	Increases glucose release into blood from liver by increasing gluconeogenesis
		Increases protein catabolism, which increases amino acid availability for gluconeogenesis
	Epinephrine (adrenalin)	Increases heart rate and stroke volume, increasing glucose release into blood from liver
		Increases glycogen breakdown in liver and muscle
		Increases fat mobilization from fat cells
Pancreas	Insulin	Increases glucose uptake by fat cells and skeletal muscle
		Increases processing of fat and glycogen production and storage
		Increases amino acid uptake and protein production
	Glucagon	Increases fat release from fat cells
		Increases liver glycogen breakdown
		Increases glucose production in liver

SPECIAL FEATURE 1.2

Peroxisomes: The Lost Organelle

Many biology texts only mention peroxisomes in passing and do not focus on their function. However, they play an important role in human health and disease and are metabolically active structures in cells. Peroxisomes contain oxidative enzymes, such as D-amino acid oxidase, urate oxidase, and catalase. In fact, there may be as many as 50 different enzymes in peroxisomes. Under a microscope, peroxisomes have a crystal-line structure inside a sac that contains amorphous gray material. They are self-replicating, much like mitochondria, and may look like granules.

A major function of peroxisomes is to eliminate toxic substances from the body, including hydrogen peroxide. This is notable because peroxisomes can create hydrogen peroxide but also contain the catalase to break it down. Peroxisomes are numerous in liver cells, which is to be expected because toxic by-products tend to accumulate there.

From a nutrition perspective, a major function of peroxisomes is the breakdown of fatty acids. In fact, this breakdown process is what generates hydrogen peroxide. Usually, peroxisomes are the cell organelles in which fatty acids longer than 20 carbons (known as very long chain fatty acids) undergo beta oxidation, followed by transfer to the mitochondria for the remaining oxidation. The number of peroxisomes is under genetic control that is mediated through a nuclear receptor called peroxisome proliferator-activated receptor alpha (PPARα). PPARα is just one type of PPAR. PPARα are very important in controlling lipid anabolism or catabolism by influencing enzymes involved in lipid metabolism, as discussed in Chapter 5. Clinically, peroxisomes have been known to possess inborn errors of metabolism whereby enzymes needed for the breakdown of fatty acids are deficient or lacking. Such diseases can lead to lipid buildup in the liver and have serious medical outcomes.

Some hormones may have receptors on cells of only one kind of tissue, whereas others may have receptors on cells of several different types of tissues. For example, the hormone prolactin stimulates milk production in female breasts. Therefore, the cells associated with the milk-producing mammary glands have receptors for prolactin, whereas cells of most other kinds of tissue do not have prolactin receptors. In contrast, growth hormone receptors are found on cells of many kinds of tissue in the body.

Steroid hormones have a much different way of exerting an influence. A steroid receptor binds in the cytoplasm or nucleus to a receptor that then binds to the promoters of a gene or DNA. The influence of most of those complexes is to turn a gene on, or initiate the transcription process.

● BEFORE YOU GO ON . . .

1. What does an enzyme essentially do to facilitate a biochemical reaction in a cell?
2. What are some of the functions proteins play within a cell membrane?
3. How do protein hormones differ from steroid hormones in exerting their effect?
4. Name a key protein involved with cell signaling.
5. What is facilitative diffusion compared with active transport?

▶ Tissue

Similar cells performing similar or supportive tasks constitute tissue. All of the 200 or so cell types in the human body are generally classified as belonging to four basic kinds of tissue. Many biochemistry students study biochemical pathways without an appreciation that not all of those pathways occur to the same degree in each cell or all tissues.

Epithelial cells line surfaces, such as blood vessels; reproductive, digestive, and urinary tracts; ducts; and skin. They are subclassified into four types of epithelial cells: simple squamous, stratified squamous, columnar (**FIGURE 1.20**), and cuboidal. **Muscle** tissue is primarily composed of contractile muscle cells (myocytes) and includes skeletal, cardiac, and smooth muscle cell types (**FIGURE 1.21**). Although the general purpose of muscle tissue is to contract, the different types of muscle have structural and physiologic differences. **Nervous tissue**, such as in the central and autonomic nervous systems and other nerves, allows for communication and sensory perception. Finally, **connective tissue** is the most abundant, widely distributed, and varied tissue type. It exists as a thin mesh or webbing that helps hold tissue and organs together as well as providing strong fibers for bones, cartilage, and tendons. Blood is considered a form of connective tissue.

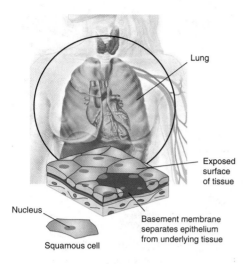

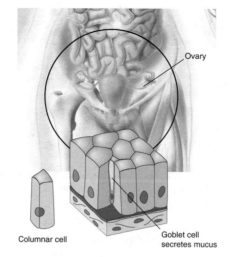

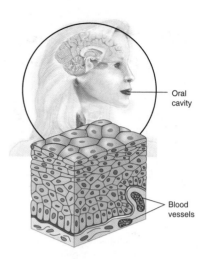

Simple squamous epithelium
Lining of blood vessels, air sacs of lungs, kidney tubules, and lining of body cavities
A

Columnar epithelium
Lining of the digestive tract and upper part of the respiratory tracts, auditory and uterine tubes
B

Stratified squamous epithelium
Skin, mouth, and throat lining; vaginal lining; anal lining; and cornea
C

FIGURE 1.20 Epithelia. Different types of epithelia include simple squamous (a), columnar (b), and stratified squamous (c).

Smooth muscle
Walls of hollow organs, pupil of eye, skin (attached to hair), and glands

DESCRIPTION Tissue is not striated; spindle-shaped cells have a single, centrally located nucleus
FUNCTION Regulation of size of organs, forcing of fluid through tubes, control of amount of light entering eye, production of "gooseflesh" in skin; under involuntary control

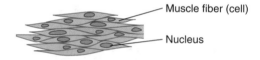

Skeletal muscle
Attachment to bone

DESCRIPTION Tissue is striated; cells are large, long, and cylindrical with several nuclei
FUNCTION Movement of the body, under voluntary control

Cardiac muscle
Heart

DESCRIPTION Tissue is striated; cells are cylindrical and branching with a single centrally located nucleus
FUNCTION Pumping of blood, under involuntary control

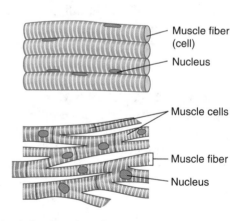

FIGURE 1.21 Muscle Cell Types. Muscle cell types in the human body: smooth, skeletal, and cardiac.

▶ Organ Systems

Organs are structures that are made up of two or more kinds of tissue. The contributing tissues are organized in such a way that they can perform more functions than the single tissue alone. Organ systems are groups of organs arranged in a manner such that they can perform a function more complex than any of the organs independently. **TABLE 1.8** lists the 10 organ systems in the human body and their component organs.

Bone and the Skeleton

The human **skeleton** is a combination of 206 separate bones as well as supporting ligaments and cartilage. The bones of the skeleton are attached to muscles, which allows for locomotion. Bones are also used for protection. The skull and the vertebrae enclose the brain and spinal cord, respectively, thereby protecting the central nervous system. Twelve pairs of ribs extend from the vertebrae and protect the organs of the chest.

TABLE 1.8 Organ Systems

Organ Systems	Tissue or Organs Involved
Integumentary	Skin, hair, nails, sense receptors, oil glands
Skeletal	Bones and joints
Muscular	Muscles
Nervous	Brain, spinal cord, nerves
Circulatory	Heart, blood vessels
Lymphatic	Lymph nodes, lymph vessels, thymus, spleen, tonsils
Respiratory	Nose, pharynx, larynx, trachea, bronchi, lungs
Digestive	Mouth, teeth, salivary glands, tongue, pharynx, esophagus, stomach, small intestine, large intestine, rectum, anal canal, gallbladder, pancreas
Urinary	Kidneys, ureters, urinary bladder, urethra
Reproductive (male)	Testes, ductus deferens, urethra, prostate, penis, scrotum
Reproductive (female)	Ovaries, uterus, uterine (fallopian) tubes, vagina, vulva, breasts

Bone also serves as a storage site for several minerals, such as calcium and phosphorus and is the site of formation for red blood cells (**erythropoiesis**).

By approximately 6 weeks of gestation, the skeleton is rapidly developing and visually noticeable with imaging instrumentation. Bone continues to grow until early adulthood, complementing the growth of other body tissue. Up until this point, bones grow in both length and diameter. However, around this time, the growth of longer bones; such as the femur, humerus, tibia, and fibula; ceases, and the adult height is realized. Some of the bones of the lower jaw and nose continue to grow throughout an individual's life, although the rate of growth slows dramatically.

The longest, heaviest, and strongest bone in the human body is the femur, which in an adult is about one-fourth of an individual's height. It is designed to handle physical stresses, such as vigorous jumping, greater than 280 kilograms per square centimeter (approximately 2 tons per square inch). Meanwhile, the three small bones in the inner ear are among the smallest bones. The pisiform bone of the wrist is very small as well, having a size approximate to that of a pea.

Bone contains several different types of cells, which are supported by a thick fluid called the **organic matrix**. The organic matrix is about 90 to 95% collagen protein, with the remainder being a homogeneous medium called ground substance. The collagen fibers are typically oriented along lines of tensile force, which provides bone with its tensile strength. The ground substance contains extracellular fluid with proteoglycans, especially chondroitin sulfate and hyaluronic acid. Also deposited within the organic matrix are mineral deposits called **hydroxyapatite**. Hydroxyapatite is composed of calcium and phosphate salt crystals: $Ca_{10}(PO_4)_6(OH)_2$. A typical crystal is about 400 angstroms long, 100 angstroms wide, and 10 to 30 angstroms thick. These crystals have the geometric shape of a long, thin plate. Magnesium, sodium, potassium, and carbonate ions are associated with hydroxyapatite crystals; however, they appear to be peripheral rather than an integral part of the structure. Small blood vessels also run throughout bone and deliver substances to and away from bone.

Bone is constantly experiencing **turnover**. That is, specific cells are constantly remodeling bone by absorbing and depositing bone components. **Osteoclasts**, which are large phagocytic cells, secrete proteolytic enzymes that digest proteins in the organic matrix, as well as acids (i.e., lactic and citric acids) that solubilize the minerals. In contrast, **osteoblasts**, found on the surface of bone, secrete bone components. Turnover allows bone to adapt or be remodeled according to the demands placed on it. For example, one of the benefits of weight training is an increased stress placed on bone, which then adapts by increasing its density. In contrast, prolonged exposure to zero gravity in space travel decreases the stress on bone and results in a loss of bone density.

Nervous Tissue

Nervous tissue is composed mostly of nerve cells (**neurons**), which serve as a very rapid communication system in the human body (**FIGURE 1.22**). The central nervous system includes the brain and spinal cord and represents the thinking and responsive portion of human nervous tissue. Links of neurons extend from the central nervous system to various organs and other tissue, thereby allowing for regulation of their

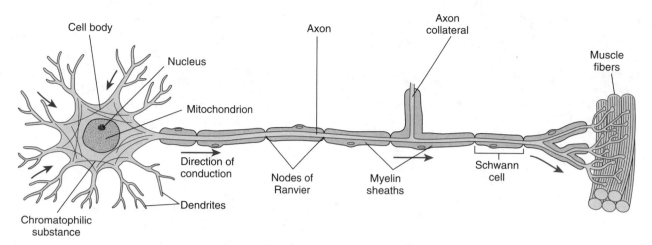

FIGURE 1.22 General Neuron Structure. Structure of nerve cell and overview of signal transmission from the cell body via the axon to the target structure.

function. Also, links of neurons extend to all skeletal muscle, allowing the central nervous system to initiate and control movement. Special neurons function as sensory receptors and are located in the skin and in sensory organs (e.g., tongue, nose, ears, eyes) and inside the body. Those receptors send afferent impulses to the brain to provide information (e.g., pain, smell, taste, temperature) regarding the external and internal environment. Neurons are **excitable cells** that are able to respond to a stimulus by changing the electrical properties of their plasma membrane. Only muscle and nerve cells possess this ability and thus are deemed excitable.

Electrolytes are dissolved in extracellular and intracellular fluids. However, their concentrations are unequal across the plasma membrane (see Table 1.3). The concentrations of sodium (Na^+), chloride (Cl^-), and calcium (Ca^{2+}) are greater in the extracellular fluid, whereas the concentration of potassium (K^+) is greater in the intracellular fluid. For instance, the concentration of sodium in the extracellular fluid is about 14 times greater than in intracellular fluid, whereas potassium is about 10 times more concentrated in the intracellular fluid relative to the extracellular fluid. The concentration differences provide the potential for electrolytes to diffuse across the plasma membrane through their respective ion channels when those are opened (**FIGURE 1.23**).

At rest, a leaking of potassium ions through channels allows for the development of a net negative charge in the intracellular fluid close to the plasma membrane and a positive charge in the extracellular fluid near the plasma membrane. This polarizes the membrane. The charge difference is referred to as the **resting potential**, which is –90 millivolts, as measured in the intracellular fluid. When neurons, as well

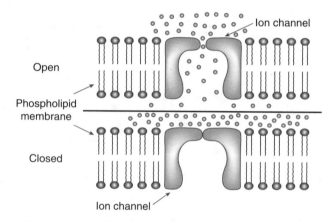

FIGURE 1.23 Ion Channel. The regulated opening of ion channels allows for rapid diffusion across the membrane.

as muscle (i.e., excitable cells), are stimulated, the resting membrane electrical potential is rapidly and transiently reversed and then returns to the resting state. This event, called an **action potential**, is propagated along the plasma membrane like a ripple on a pond.

Although some neurons are very long and may extend several meters or so, the trek of a neural impulse traveling either from a sensory neuron to the brain or from the brain to skeletal muscle or organs, or simply within the brain itself, requires the transmission of the impulse along several neurons linked together. An impulse reaching the end of one neuron is transferred to the next neuron by way of **neurotransmitters**. Numerous neurotransmitters are employed by nervous tissue, including serotonin, norepinephrine, dopamine, histamine, and acetylcholine. Terminal branches of neurons come in close contact with other neurons or tissue such as skeletal tissue or various organs (**FIGURE 1.24**). This near connection is the **synapse**.

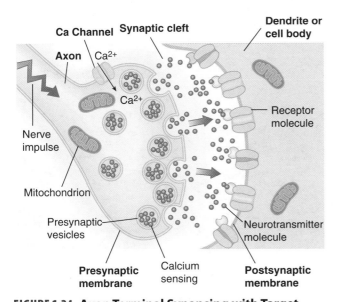

FIGURE 1.24 Axon Terminal Synapsing with Target Cell. The axon is shown. Neurotransmitter release and action on adjacent cells occur via receptor molecules on the postsynaptic membrane. Here the neurotransmitter is acetylcholine, which will react with a receptor molecule on skeletal muscle cells and elicit an action potential.

Neurotransmitters are released from the signaling neuron and interact with receptors on the receiving cell, as depicted in Figure 1.24. This can initiate or inhibit the firing of an action potential on that cell.

The brain is an organ that is very densely packed with neurons. It weighs about 1,600 grams in an adult man and 1,450 grams in an adult woman and is protected by the skull. It is designed to interpret sensory input and decipher other incoming information, to develop both short- and long-term memory, to originate and coordinate most muscular movement, and to regulate the function of many organs. The brain can be subdivided into the cerebral hemispheres; the diencephalon (thalamus, hypothalamus, and epithalamus); the brain stem (midbrain, pons, and medulla); and the cerebellum. Although nutrition is directly involved in the proper development and function of all these regions, certain locations are especially important. For example, the hypothalamus is discussed to a greater extent than other regions with respect to its involvement in appetite regulation.

The spinal cord is approximately 42 centimeters (17 inches) long and extends from the foramen magnum of the skull, is continuous with the medulla of the brain stem, and reaches the level of the first lumbar vertebrae. The spinal cord in essence is a two-way neural impulse conduction pathway to and from the brain. It is encased by protective vertebrae.

Skeletal Muscle

Skeletal muscle is composed mostly of very specialized cells that have the ability to shorten or contract upon command by the motor cortex of the brain. Because these cells are very long, they are often referred to as **muscle fibers**. Each muscle fiber is encased in a fine sheath of connective tissue called the endomysium. Several fibers that are bundled up in parallel and encased in a connective tissue sheathing are called fascicles. The several fascicles are themselves bundled within dense, coarse connective tissue called the epimysium. Skeletal muscle is so named because it is anchored at both ends to different bones of the skeleton. One anchoring site is called the origin, where the bone is generally immobile; the other attachment is called the insertion, in which the pulled bone is moved.

Like neurons, skeletal muscle fibers are excitable. In fact, the excitability of skeletal muscle fibers is very similar to that of neurons. However, the end result of excitability in a muscle fiber is the contraction or shortening of that cell. There are two principal types of muscle fibers: type I (slow-twitch) fibers and type II (fast-twitch) fibers.

Light and electron microscopy provide insight regarding the structural differences between muscle fibers and other cells. Each muscle fiber contains hundreds to thousands of small fiber-like units called **myofibrils**. Myofibrils can account for as much as 80% of a muscle cell's volume. Each myofibril is a stalk-like collection of protein (**FIGURE 1.25**). The predominant proteins are **actin** and **myosin**, which are referred to as thin and thick filaments, respectively. They are organized into a tiny contraction region called a **sarcomere**, which sits next to adjacent and connected sarcomeres (**FIGURE 1.26**). Other proteins associated with the sarcomeres are **troponin** and **tropomyosin**. Those proteins are involved in regulating the contraction of sarcomeres.

When skeletal muscle cells are stimulated, calcium (Ca^{2+}) ion channels open and calcium floods into the region of myofibrils and bathes the sarcomeres. Calcium enters the intracellular fluid from either the extracellular fluid or from storage within an organelle called the **sarcoplasmic reticulum**. Most of the calcium enters from the sarcoplasmic reticulum, which is a modified version of the smooth endoplasmic reticulum. Calcium then interacts with troponin proteins and initiates contraction by removing tropomyosin from the actin-myosin binding site (**FIGURE 1.27**). Myosin then slides actin fibers toward the center of the sarcomere, thereby shortening the sarcomere. The concomitant shortening of adjacent

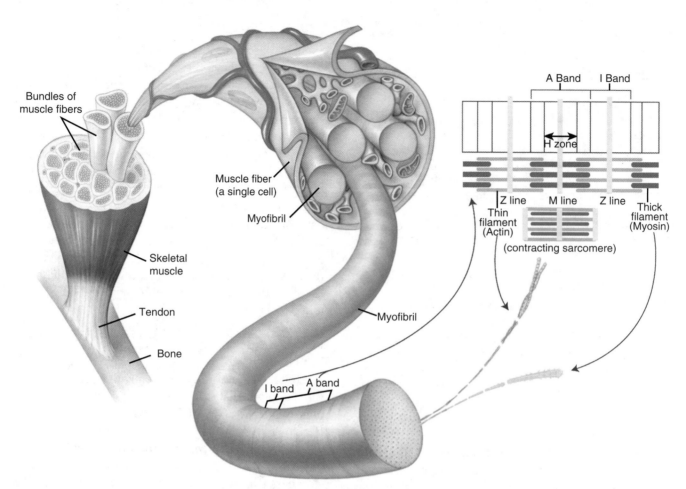

FIGURE 1.25 **Skeletal Muscle Components.** Diagram represents the ultrastructure aspects of the muscle (actin and myosin) and how it relates to a myofibril The diagram then demonstrates how the myofibril composes muscle fiber bundles, and how the bundles compose the skeletal muscle.

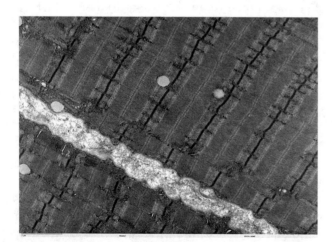

FIGURE 1.26 **Electron Micrograph of Adjacent Sarcomeres (27,000×).** Note the banding arrangement.
Courtesy of Louisa Howard, Dartmouth College, Electron Microscope Facility.

sarcomeres within a myofibril shortens the myofibril. Myofibrils in parallel shorten, thereby shortening a myofiber. The shortening of bundled myofibers allows for the shortening of a muscle as a whole.

For muscle fibers to contract, a lot of ATP must be used; some of the released energy is harnessed to power the contraction. ATP is also necessary for a contracted muscle cell to relax. When the stimulus is removed, ATP is needed to pump calcium out of the intracellular fluid of the muscle fiber into the sarcoplasmic reticulum or across the plasma membrane.

Heart, Blood, and Circulation

The adult heart is about the size of a fist and weighs about 250 to 350 grams. It serves to pump blood through miles and miles of blood vessels to all regions of the human body. Blood leaves the heart through the great arteries, namely, the aorta and pulmonary trunk, which feed into smaller arteries, which, in turn, feed into smaller arterioles and subsequently into tiny capillaries that thoroughly infiltrate tissue. Blood drains from capillaries into larger venules, which themselves drain into larger veins, which ultimately return blood

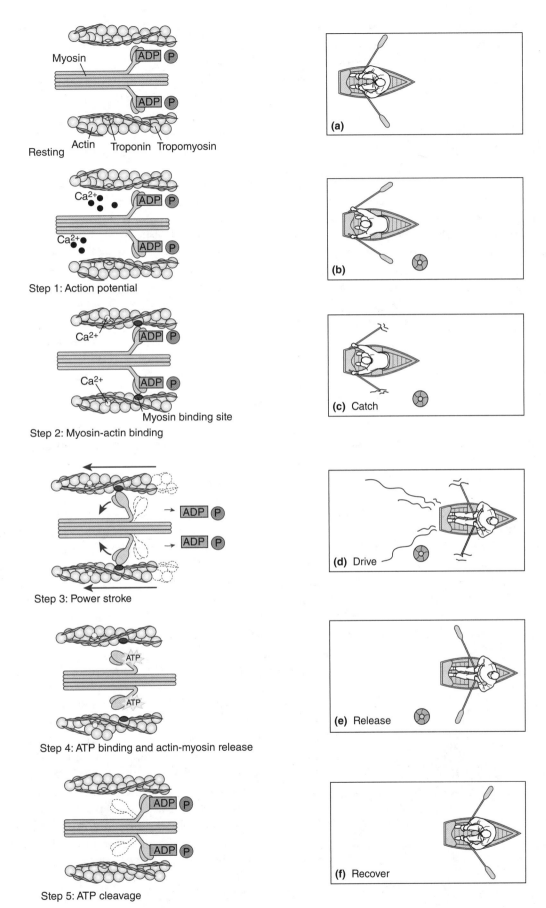

FIGURE 1.27 Calcium Binding to Troponin. Calcium binding to troponin results in the movement of tropomyosin and the revealing of myosin binding sites on actin. This allows myosin to bind and myofibrils to contract.

to the heart. The blood is a delivery system. It delivers oxygen, nutrients, and other substances to cells throughout the human body. At the same time, blood serves to remove the waste products of cell metabolism (such as CO_2 and heat) from tissue. Capillaries are the actual site of the exchange of substances and heat between cells and the blood.

The heart consists of four chambers (two atria and two ventricles) and can be divided into a left and right half (**FIGURE 1.28**). The left half, consisting of the left atrium and ventricle, serves to receive oxygen-rich blood returning from the lungs and pump it to all tissue throughout the body. The right half of the heart, consisting of the right atrium and ventricle, serves to receive oxygen-poor blood returning from tissue throughout the body and pump it to the lungs. Therefore, the heart functions as a relay station for moving blood throughout the body in one large loop.

The heart is composed primarily of muscle cells that are mostly similar to skeletal muscle cells yet retain certain fundamental differences. Although most of the events involved in contraction of the cardiac muscle are the same as the skeletal muscle, the heart is not attached to bone. Furthermore, the heart does not require stimulus from the motor cortex to initiate contraction. The stimulus invoking excitability in the heart comes from a specialized pacemaker region called the atrioventricular (AV) node. The heart may beat in excess of two billion times throughout a human being's life.

The blood is composed of two main parts: solid cells and liquid plasma. **Erythrocytes** (red blood cells) function primarily as a shuttle transport for oxygen. **Hematocrit** is the percentage of the blood volume that is red blood cells. A typical adult hematocrit may be 40 to 45%. **Plasma** constitutes approximately 55% of the blood. About 92% of the plasma is water, while the remaining 8% includes over 100 different dissolved or suspended substances, such as nutrients, gases, electrolytes, hormones, and proteins, such as albumin and clotting factors.

The remaining components of blood are the **leukocytes** (white blood cells) and **platelets**, which collectively make up approximately 1% of blood. White blood cells are the principal component of the immune system and provide a line of defense against bacteria, viruses, and other intruders, whereas platelets participate in blood clotting.

Red blood cells transport oxygen throughout the human body. About 33% of the weight of a red blood cell is attributed to a specialized protein called **hemoglobin**. Hemoglobin is a large molecule that contains four atoms of iron. Hemoglobin's job is to bind to oxygen so that it can be transported in the blood. There are about 42 to 52 million red blood cells per cubic millimeter of blood, and each healthy cell contains about 250 million hemoglobin molecules. Because each hemoglobin molecule can carry four O_2 molecules, each red blood cell has the potential to transport 1 billion molecules of O_2.

When the heart pumps, blood is propelled from the right ventricle into the **pulmonary arteries** for transport to the lungs. Upon reaching the lungs and the pulmonary capillaries, CO_2 exits the blood and enters into the lungs. It is then removed during exhalation. At the same time, O_2 enters the blood from the lungs and binds with hemoglobin in red blood cells. The oxygen-containing blood leaves the lungs and travels back to the left side of the heart.

As the heart contracts, blood is pumped from the left ventricle into the **aorta**. Blood moves from the aorta into the arteries, then into the arterioles, and finally, into tiny capillaries in tissue. Blood that has perfused tissue is drained into small venules, which drain into larger veins and, subsequently, into the vena cava. The blood leaving the heart is rich with oxygen, whereas the blood returning to the heart from tissue is relatively poor in oxygen. Carbon dioxide from tissue dissolves into the blood, with some being converted to carbonic acid via erythrocyte **carbonic anhydrase**. The venous blood is then pumped by the heart to the lungs to reload with O_2 and release CO_2. The measurement of the blood pumped out of the heart, directed toward either the lungs or body tissue, during one heart beat is the **stroke volume**. By multiplying stroke volume by heart rate, **cardiac output** can be determined.

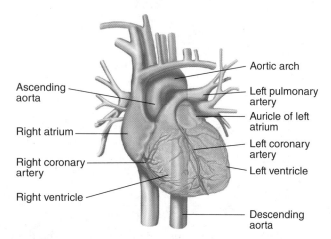

FIGURE 1.28 Human Heart. The major blood vessels are also shown.

Labels: Aortic arch; Ascending aorta; Left pulmonary artery; Auricle of left atrium; Right atrium; Left coronary artery; Right coronary artery; Left ventricle; Right ventricle; Descending aorta

Cardiac output   = Stroke volume × Heart rate
(milliliters/minute)   (milliliters/beat) (beats/minute)

Cardiac output is the volume of blood pumped out of the heart, either to the lungs or toward body tissue, in 1 minute. It should not matter which of the two destinations one considers because they occur simultaneously and will have a similar stoke volume of about 5 liters per minute. During exercise, both heart rate and stroke volume increase, which consequently increases cardiac output. In some people, cardiac output may increase as much as five to six times during heavy exercise. This allows for more oxygen-rich blood to be delivered to working skeletal muscle.

Under resting and comfortable environmental conditions, approximately 13% of the left ventricular cardiac output goes to the brain, 4% to the heart, 20 to 25% to the kidneys, 10% to the skin, and the rest to the remaining tissue in the body, such as the digestive tract, liver, and pancreas. During heavy exercise, a greater proportion of this cardiac output is routed to working skeletal muscle. This requires some redistribution of blood routed to other, less-active, areas at that time, such as the digestive tract. In contrast, during a big meal and for a few hours afterward, a greater proportion of cardiac output is routed to the digestive tract, which steals a portion of the blood directed to areas having no immediate need, such as skeletal muscle.

Blood Pressure

Whether blood is in the heart or in blood vessels, it has a certain pressure associated with it. In fact, blood moves through the circulation from an area of greater **blood pressure** to an area of lower blood pressure. When the heart contracts, the pressure of the blood in the heart increases enough to drive the movement of blood throughout the circulatory system. Pressure is the force that is exerted upon a surface and is measured in millimeters of mercury (mm Hg). Blood pressure is typically measured in a large artery, such as the brachial artery in the arm, and is expressed as systolic pressure over diastolic pressure. For instance, when blood pressure is measured at 120/80 mm Hg ("120 over 80"), the pressure exerted by systemic arterial blood is 120 mm Hg during left ventricular contraction (systolic) and 80 mm Hg when the left ventricle is relaxing (diastolic) between beats.

Renal System

Typically understated in function, the kidneys regulate the composition and volume of the extracellular fluid, which includes the blood. The two kidneys, along with their corresponding ureters, the bladder, and urethra, make up the renal (or urinary) system (**FIGURE 1.29**). Although the kidneys make up less than 1% of total body weight, they receive about 20 to 25% of the left ventricular cardiac output. Together, the kidneys filter and process approximately 180 liters of blood-derived fluid daily.

Each kidney contains about 1 million **nephrons**, which are the blood-processing sites (**FIGURE 1.30**). Each nephron engages in two basic operations: (1) it filters plasma into a series of tubes, and (2) it processes

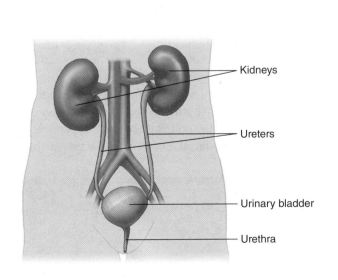

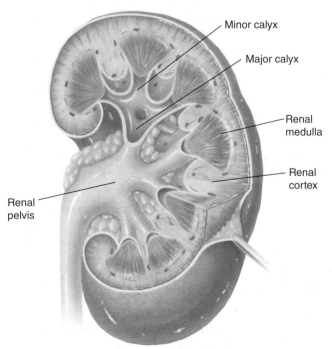

FIGURE 1.29 The Urinary System. Structures or components responsible for the production and elimination of urine produced by cells.

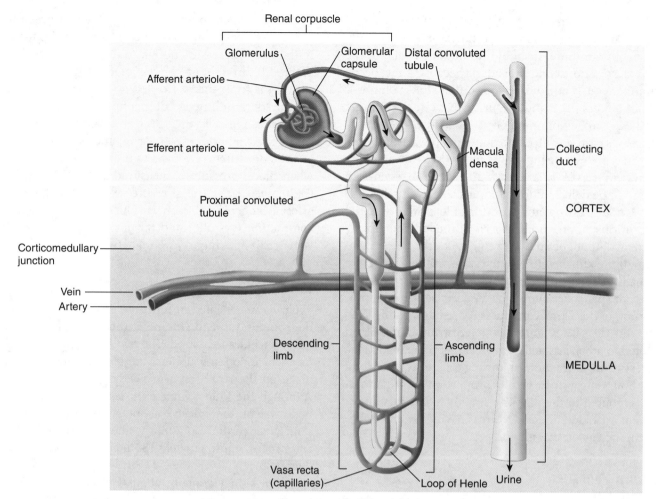

FIGURE 1.30 The Nephron. The basic structure of the nephron and its relationship to the renal cortex and medulla, along with the blood supply, are shown. The Bowman (or glomerular) capsule, the proximal and distal tubules, the loop of Henle, and collecting ducts compose the nephron.

the filtered fluid, reabsorbing needed substances while excreting unwanted or extra substances as urine. A relatively high capillary pressure (60 mm Hg) in the glomerulus drives the formation of plasma-derived fluid (**ultrafiltrate**) into the first aspect of the nephron tubule system, the Bowman, or glomerular, capsule. Ultrafiltrate is a water-based solution containing electrolytes, sulfites, bicarbonate, phosphates, amino acids, glucose, urea, creatinine, and other substances. Blood cells and most plasma proteins are too large and are not filtered.

The components of the ultrafiltrate have two possible fates: they are either reabsorbed into the blood or become part of urine. Normally, the reabsorption of substances such as glucose and amino acids is extremely efficient. In contrast, the reabsorption of water and electrolytes involves hormonal regulation (e.g., aldosterone and atrial natriuretic polypeptide). The active processes in the renal tubule system engaged in reabsorbing glucose, amino acids, and some electrolytes require a significant amount of energy.

Of the 180 liters of fluid filtered and processed by the nephrons daily, less than 1% actually becomes urine.

Thus, the reabsorptive processes of the kidneys are extremely powerful. Beyond regulating the composition of the extracellular fluid, the kidneys engage in other homeostatic operations. The kidneys are very sensitive to hypoxia of low oxygen level and secrete the endocrine factor erythropoietin, which stimulates erythropoiesis in bone marrow. Furthermore, renal parenchyma contains a vitamin D-metabolizing enzyme that converts a less-active form of vitamin D to its most active form.

◆ **BEFORE YOU GO ON . . .**

1. Within which tissue is red blood cell production most likely to occur?

2. What is cardiac output, and how is it calculated?

3. What is meant by the term *AV node*?

4. How do you distinguish between bone osteoclasts and osteoblasts?

5. List the proteins associated with the sarcomeres of muscle.

✏ *CLINICAL INSIGHT*

Gene Therapy

The foundation of the human body is best understood at the biochemical and gene levels in most cases. These understandings are the result of years of basic research from a wide variety of disciplines. The ultimate goal is to provide insight into what contributes to both health and disease. Not all nutrition deficiencies have a dietary origin. Many human and animal diseases/disorders have a genetic component. In nutrition there are genetic diseases that affect nutrient absorption, such as Menkes disease, where copper is unable to be absorbed. From a disease such as muscular dystrophy to nutrient malabsorption, much research has been directed toward correcting genetic mutations by deleting the aberrant genes and replacing them with functional genes that produce the correct protein needed for optimal health. Replacing a defective gene with a healthy gene is gene therapy. This can be done by replacing the defective gene, knocking the expression of the gene out (knock-out), or adding a new gene to combat the product of the defective gene. Diseases such as Parkinson's, Alzheimer's disease, cardiovascular diseases of various types and, of course, various cancer types, as cancer in essence is often referred to as a disease of genes.

Early approaches to gene therapy produced mixed results, and, in fact, some human trials ended with deaths or other undesirable effects. Due to risks, clinical trials on gene therapy are only currently allowed where there are no other cures available. Techniques that have been employed include modifying the mRNA produced and correcting the few codons of the strand where the mutation occurs. Another approach is to use viruses (or vectors) to repair the DNA itself. Gene silencing that targeting either the DNA from producing a mutated protein or silencing the mRNA produced is another approach. The latter involves using a ribozyme that are simply RNA sequences that function enzymatically and destroy the mRNA so the protein is not made. However, this does not always solve the ultimate problem of inserting a normal protein to replace the abnormal one.

The use of viruses to insert genes may produce problems of its own such as immune response to the virus, the possibility that the virus could insert the new gene in an incorrect area on the gene leading to tumor formation.

Clustered regularly interspaced short palindromic repeats (CRISPR) is a technology that is gaining attention. This is a strand of DNA with short repeats of DNA sequences that are sometimes called "spacers." This has gained attention as a gene editing tool. CRISPR is found naturally in bacteria where it functions as a defense mechanism against viruses. Another piece of how CRISPR works is that it is associated with an enzyme referred to as a CRISPR associated protein or Cas. Sequences to produce a Cas is found near the CRISPR areas. Together, these two entities are referred to as CRISPR–Cas. There are two important features that have been developed with respect to gene therapy that arose from this system (**FIGURE 1.31**). First, the Cas enzymes are directed to chop the DNA where mutations or unwarranted sequences are located. The most common enzyme to chop the DNA is called Cas9. A second feature is that a piece of RNA that is complementary to the DNA sequence you want to remove is required. This is referred to as a guide RNA and, essentially, is the tool to tell the complex where to find the defective gene and cut it. The structure of this guided RNA has something referred to as the stem loop structure and the Cas enzyme associates with this part of the RNA. The RNA–Cas complex, when aligned with the complementary DNA, will allow the Cas enzyme to destroy the defective gene. At this point, the two ends of the DNA can rejoin without the defective sequences or sequences with a normal copy of the gene can be inserted. This tool is much more precise than other tools, such as ones using embryonic stem cells.

It is not entirely clear how safe this new technology is. The enzymes could cut DNA in unwarranted areas, for instance. An advantage appears to be the much lower costs this technology offers experimentally over other traditional approaches. Regardless, it is clear that gene therapy using this new technology will be at the forefront of technology to correct diseases caused by mutations, including those where nutrient function is altered.

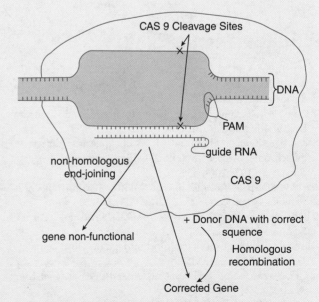

FIGURE 1.31 CRISPR–Cas 9 System. Illustration denoting how a defective gene can be removed from a cell and replaced with the corrected gene.

▶ Here's What You Have Learned

1. Fifty-five percent to 60% of the adult human body is composed of water; the remainder is protein and lipid

2. The human body has more than 200 cell types, each of which has specialized functions but identical DNA

3. Cell membrane and organelle membranes are composed of a bilipid layer. Cell membranes are 50% protein

4. Carbohydrates may be part of a cell membrane linked to a protein to form a glycocalyx

5. Ribosomes are the site of protein synthesis and are found in the endoplasmic reticulum

6. Connective tissue, bone, cartilage, and tendons are composed of proteoglycan and chondroitin sulfate, which are synthesized in the Golgi apparatus of the cell

7. Tissues with a high dependence on aerobic metabolism or fatty acid oxidation have more mitochondria

8. Protein synthesis is dependent on DNA and RNA. Replication, transcription, translation, and posttranslational modification are coordinated events within cells to produce unique proteins for each gene

9. Mitochondrial DNA encodes for 13 of the 67 protein subunits that compose the electron transport chain for ATP production

10. Production of protein is a very energy-expensive process. For example, 500 ATP molecules are needed to form 500 amino acid–tRNA associations

11. Proteins are important in the structure of the cell, as cell receptors and hormones, in cell signaling, and in transport of nutrients across cell membranes

12. Bone is mostly acellular; collagen is its major component

13. Neurons are excitable tissue in which neurotransmitters such as serotonin, norepinephrine, dopamine, histamine, and acetylcholine are synthesized

14. Skeletal muscle and cardiac muscle have specialized structures referred to as sarcomeres that possess a specialized protein involved with muscle contraction

15. Oxygenation and disposal of waste from cells depends not only on cardiac function but also on an adequate cardiac output

16. Discovery and application of the CRISPR to gene therapy offers the promise of elimination of inherited diseases, including those interfering with normal nutrient function

▶ Suggested Reading

Alberts B, Johnson A, Lewis J, Raff M, Roberts K, Walter P. *The Molecular Biology of the Cell.* 5th ed. London: Garland Press, Taylor and Francis; 2007.

Choi SW, Friso S. Epigenetics: a new bridge between nutrition and health. *Adv Nutr.* 2010:1(1):8–16.

DiMauro S, Zeviani M, Rizzuto R, et al. Molecular defects in cytochrome oxidase in mitochondrial diseases. *J Bioenerg Biomembr.* 1988;20(3):353–364.

Ebert MS, Sharp PA. Roles for microRNAs in conferring robustness to biological processes. *Cell.* 2012;149(3):515–524.

Hall JE, Guyton AC. *Textbook of Medical Physiology.* 11th ed. St. Louis, MO: Elsevier; 2005.

Jackson CL. Mechanisms of transport through the Golgi complex. *J Cell Sci.* 2009;15:443–452.

Jang H, Serra C. Nutrition, epigenetics, and diseases. *Clin Nutr Res.* 2014;3(1):1–8.

Lieberman MA, Marks DB. *Marks' Basic Medical Biochemistry: A Clinical Approach.* 3rd ed. Philadelphia: Lippincott Williams & Wilkins; 2009.

Medeiros DM. Assessing mitochondria biogenesis. *Methods.* 2008;46(4):288–294.

Müller-Höcker J, Johannes A, Droste M, Kadenbach B, Hübner G. Fatal mitochondrial cardiomyopathy in Kearns-Sayre syndrome with deficiency of cytochrome–c-oxidase in cardiac and skeletal muscle. An enzymehistochemical–ultra–immunocytochemical–fine structural study in longterm frozen autopsy tissue. *Virchows Arch B Cell Pathol Mol Pathol Incl Mol Pathol.* 1986;52(4):353–367.

Murray RK, Rodwell VW, Granner DK. *Harper's Illustrated Biochemistry.* 27th ed. New York: McGraw-Hill; 2006.

Puigserver P, Wu Z, Park CW, Graves R, Wright M, Spiegelman BM. A cold-inducible coactivator of nuclear receptors linked to adaptive thermogenesis. *Cell.* 1998;92(6):829–839.

Rossi AE, Boncompagni S, Dirksen RT. Sarcoplasmic reticulum-mitochondrial symbiosis: bidirectional signaling in skeletal muscle. *Exerc Sport Sci Rev.* 2009;37(1):29–35.

Scheffler IE. *Mitochondria.* Berlin: Wiley; 2009.

Schwartzkopff B, Zierz S, Frenzel H, et al. Ultrastructural abnormalities of mitochondria and deficiency of myocardial cytochrome c oxidase in a patient with ventricular tachycardia. *Virchows Arch A Pathol Anat Histopathol.* 1991;419(1):63–68.

Silverstein A, Silverstein V, Nunn LS. *Cells.* Minneapolis, MN: Twenty-First Century Books; 2009.

Virbasius JV, Scarpulla RC. Activation of the human mitochondrial transcription factor A gene by nuclear respiratory factors: a potential regulatory link between nuclear and mitochondrial gene expression in organelle biogenesis. *Proc Natl Acad Sci USA.* 1994;91(4):1309–1313.

Zhu J, Luo BH, Barth P, Schonbrun J, Baker D, Springer TA. The structure of a receptor with two associating transmembrane domains on the cell surface: integrin alpha IIbbeta3. *Mol Cell.* 2009;34(2):234–249.

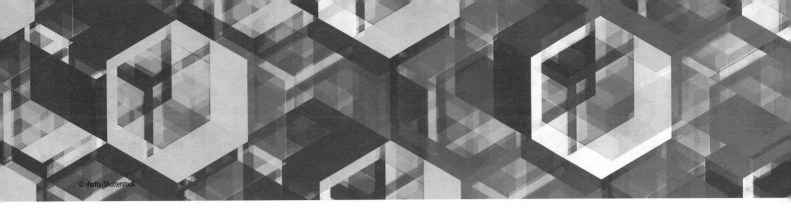

CHAPTER 2

Digestion and Absorption

◄ HERE'S WHERE YOU HAVE BEEN

1. The basic unit of human life is the cell, which operates independently and in concert with other cells to sustain human life.
2. There are approximately 200 different types of cells in the human body, each one with different roles and nutrient requirements.
3. Cell structural and operational components have specialized functions that affect nutrient processing, storage, and requirements.
4. Many nutrients play a role in protein synthesis by influencing gene expression or various steps in protein manufacturing.
5. Proteins have many specialized functions, including serving as enzymes, transporters, receptors, and hormones.

HERE'S WHERE YOU ARE GOING ➤

1. Digestion is a complex synergy of the physical actions of chewing, mixing, and movement and the chemical actions of acids, enzymes, and detergent-like emulsifiers.
2. Absorption refers to the movement of nutrients from the digestive tract into the blood or lymphatic circulation, whereas the concept of bioavailability also includes the uptake and use of a nutrient by cells or tissue.
3. Perceptions of hunger and satiety involve multiple hormonal and neurologic signals, including cholecystokinin, neuropeptide Y, ghrelin, obestatin, insulin, and leptin.
4. Different types of bacteria are found throughout the entire digestive tract; the specific conditions of the different segments (e.g., mouth, stomach, colon) determine which species will thrive.

▶ Introduction

With the exception of intravenous infusion, nutrient entry into the body takes place by way of the gastrointestinal, or alimentary, tract. This tract is basically a tube that extends from the mouth to the anus, and the lumen is considered to be outside of the body

(**FIGURE 2.1**). The gastrointestinal tract, or simply "the gut," and several organs (the salivary glands, pancreas, liver, and gallbladder) that empty supportive substances into the gut make up the gastrointestinal system. The primary objectives of the gastrointestinal system are to break down complex food components into substances appropriate for absorption into the body as well as

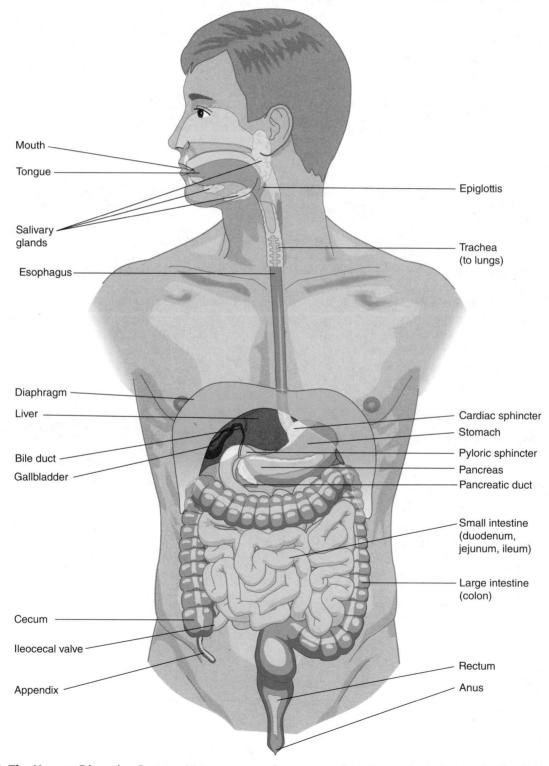

FIGURE 2.1 The Human Digestive System. Major organs and structures of the human body involved in food digestion and nutrient absorption.

to provide a means of waste removal from digestive and metabolic operations. To meet those objectives, the gastrointestinal system must engage in digestive, motility, secretory, and absorptive operations.

▶ Gastrointestinal Anatomy

From a histologic perspective, the wall of the gastrointestinal tract is fairly consistent throughout its length (**FIGURE 2.2**). Although some variation does exist, allowing the specialized operations inherent to different segments of the gastrointestinal tract, the structure of the wall can be discussed in general terms. The gastrointestinal tract wall is characterized by several distinct layers. The layer closest to the lumen is the mucosa. The outermost region of the mucosa, the muscularis mucosae, is mostly composed of smooth muscle. Adjacent to the muscularis mucosae is the submucosa. Situated outside of the submucosa is a layer of circular smooth muscle that is covered by a layer of longitudinal smooth muscle. The outermost layer of the gastrointestinal wall is the serosa. Buried within the different layers of the gastrointestinal tract wall are blood vessels, which transport nutrients, oxygen, and hormones to and from the wall, as well as nerve plexuses, which control wall activity.

Mouth

The mouth and the pharynx provide entry to the gastrointestinal tract. Several secretory glands located in the mouth release saliva, which begins the chemical

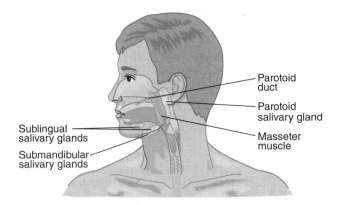

FIGURE 2.3 Location of Primary Salivary Glands. Glands responsible for saliva production and some enzymes to initiate food digestion. Masseter muscle aids in mastication, or chewing of food.

digestion of food while also supporting chewing (mastication) and swallowing (deglutination) mechanisms (**FIGURE 2.3**). Swallowed content enters the stomach by traversing the 25-centimeter (10-inch) muscular esophagus. The esophagus ends with a thickened muscular ring called the lower esophageal sphincter (LES) or cardiac sphincter, with respect to its close anatomic proximity to the heart.

Stomach

The stomach is approximately 25 centimeters long and is J-shaped, with its curvature toward the right (**FIGURE 2.4**). It is situated just beneath the diaphragm and is separated from the esophagus by the

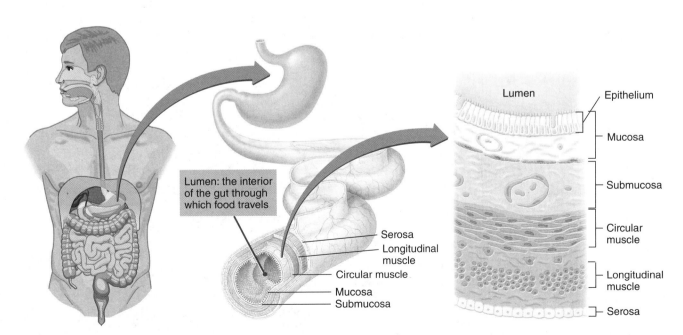

FIGURE 2.2 General Anatomic Structure of the Digestive Tract Wall. Illustration on the epithelium, mucosa, submucosa, circular muscle, longitudinal muscle, and serosa that comprise the digestive tract.

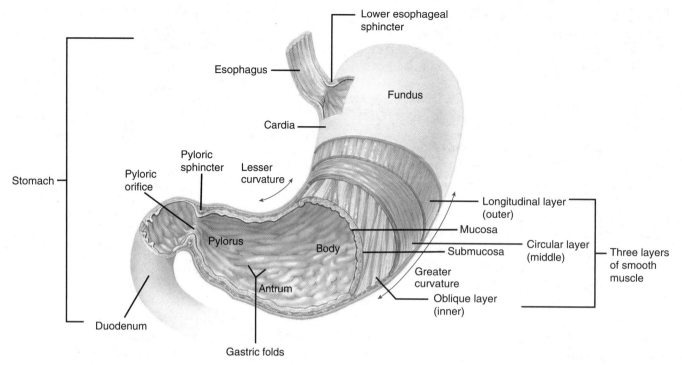

FIGURE 2.4 The Stomach. Areas of the stomach: fundus, cardia, and antrum. Note that the stomach structures, including sphincter muscles and cross-sectional views of the mucosa, submucosa, and muscles.

LES; distally, the stomach is separated from the small intestine by another smooth muscular ring called the **pyloric sphincter**. The volume of an empty adult stomach is only about 50 milliliters (about 1.67 ounces); however, it can accommodate as much as 1.5 liters (52 ounces) or more during a meal.

The stomach is subdivided into three segments: the fundus, cardia (or body), and antrum. Those segments and their walls are characterized by the presence of several exocrine and endocrine glands. The oxyntic glands are the primary type of **gastric** gland;

those structures contain exocrine cells that secrete a hydrochloric acid (HCl) solution, pepsinogen, intrinsic factor, mucus, and other substances (**FIGURE 2.5**). The density of the glands, along with the histology, can vary regionally in the stomach.

Small Intestine

The contents of the stomach are slowly released into the small intestine, which is approximately 3 meters (10 feet) in length and can be divided into three

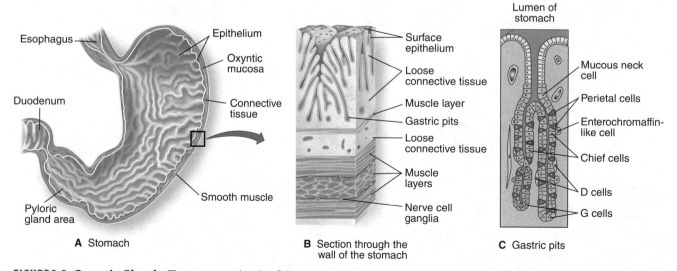

FIGURE 2.5 Oxyntic Glands. The oxyntic glands of the stomach secrete hydrochloric acid (HCl), pepsinogen, intrinsic factor, mucus, and other substances into the lumen of the stomach.

segments. The **duodenum** is the most proximal segment to the stomach and is typically approximately 30 centimeters (1 foot) in length. Secretions from the liver and gallbladder, via the hepatic bile ducts and cystic duct, respectively, combine in the common bile duct, which empties into the duodenum through the sphincter of Oddi. Secretions from the pancreas, via the pancreatic duct, flow into the terminal aspect of the common bile duct and subsequently flow into the duodenum via the sphincter of Oddi. The **jejunum** and the ileum, in that order, are the distal segments of the small intestine and combine for approximately 2.75 meters (9 feet) in length.

Rugae, Villi, and Microvilli

The small intestine is the primary site of digestion and absorption in the gastrointestinal tract. To optimize digestive and absorptive operations, the surface area of the small intestine wall is greatly enhanced by three mucosal modifications. First, the small intestine wall is thrown into folds (rugae) called valvulae conniventes (folds of Kerckring). Those semicircular folds, which extend as much as 8 millimeters into the lumen, increase the surface area of the small intestine wall 3-fold (**FIGURE 2.6**). Next, millions of fingerlike projections called **villi** protrude from the small intestine wall and enhance the surface area another 10-fold. The villi themselves are lined primarily with small intestine epithelial cells called enterocytes, which are highly specialized for digestive and absorptive operations.

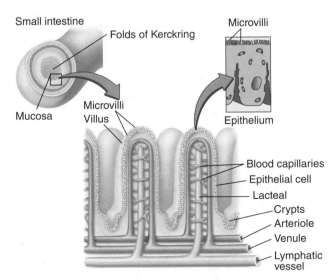

FIGURE 2.6 Three Levels of Folding of the Small Intestine. The folds of Kerckring are merely a folding of the mucosa. Extending from the folds of Kerckring are fingerlike projections (villi) that are lined with enterocytes. The luminal face of the plasma membrane of enterocytes has thousands of bristle-like extensions called microvilli.

Finally, the plasma membranes of the enterocytes contain fine evaginations called **microvilli** on their luminal surface. A single enterocyte may contain approximately 1700 microvilli, each typically being about 1 micrometer in length and 0.1 micrometer in diameter. Microscopically, this gives the lining of the small intestine a brush border appearance. Microvilli expand the surface area another 20-fold. Cumulatively, the folds of Kerckring, villi, and microvilli enhance the surface area of the small intestine about 600 times, to approximately 300 square meters, or roughly the size of a tennis court.

In the gastrointestinal tract, villi are unique to the small intestine and are specifically designed to provide nutrients entrance to the body. Internally, each villus contains a capillary and a central lacteal, which together provide the means for nutrient absorption (see Figure 2.6). In general, small absorbed water-soluble substances will enter the systemic circulation by crossing the capillary wall. In contrast, most absorbed lipid-soluble substances are destined to enter the blood indirectly by first draining into the central lacteal as part of a **lipoprotein** (chylomicron) and flowing through the lymphatic circulation.

In the depths between villi are the crypts of Lieberkühn. The cells found in these crypts undergo rapid mitosis, and the new cells then migrate up the villi to allow continual replacement of enterocytes that are being sloughed off the tip of the villi. Enterocyte turnover is approximately 3 to 5 days. Other cells in the crypts include protein-secreting Paneth cells, mucus-secreting goblet cells, and enterochromaffin cells, which perform endocrine activities. Finally, lymphoid tissue, called Peyer patches, is also found in the wall of the small intestine and contains both T lymphocytes and B lymphocytes. Peyer patches provide a line of defense against bacteria and other ingested foreign substances.

Large Intestine (Colon)

The small intestine is separated from the large intestine, or **colon**, by the ileocecal valve. The large intestine is approximately 1.5 to 1.8 meters (5 to 6 feet) long, with an average diameter of 6 centimeters (~2.5 inches); the diameter decreases moving distally. The large intestine can be segmented, in order, into the cecum, colon, rectum, and anal canal. With respect to the directional movement of content through the colon in an upright human, regions of the colon are often referred to as ascending, transverse, and descending. The large intestine is the site of a rich bacterial population and is involved in absorbing water and some electrolytes as well as in the activities involved in defecation.

● **BEFORE YOU GO ON . . .**

1. What is the entry point for the digestive tract, and what is the role of saliva in digestion?

2. What portion of the small intestine do secretions of the liver and gallbladder enter?

3. What is the shape and design of the stomach, and what are the stomach's key segments?

4. What are the three segments of the small intestine, and what are the three ways that the surface area is enhanced?

5. What are the crypts of Lieberkühn?

▶ Gastrointestinal Movement, Motility, and Neural Activity

Contents are moved throughout the length of the digestive tract in a strategic and coordinated manner. Smooth muscle contractions both mix and propel digesting contents throughout the digestive tract. Digestive tract motility is largely controlled by the **enteric nervous system (ENS)**.

Smooth Muscle

The motility of substances throughout the length of the gastrointestinal tract is provided by the smooth muscle found in the wall. Longitudinal smooth muscle fibers extend along the length of the gastrointestinal tract, and the circular smooth muscle fibers wrap around the tract. Individual muscle fibers approximately 200 to 500 micrometers in length and 2 to 10 micrometers in diameter are arranged in bundles containing up to 1,000 fibers each. Adjacent bundles of smooth muscle fibers are separated by a thin region of connective tissue, but they are fused together at several points, which allows for muscle bundle contraction to occur as a syncytium. Therefore, when an action potential is fired anywhere within the muscle mass, it has the potential to be conducted throughout the muscle, thereby allowing the muscle to contract as a unit.

Contraction of the smooth muscle in the gastrointestinal tract wall appears to occur rhythmically and is associated with the presence of waves in the smooth muscle membrane potentials. Two types of electric waves occur in smooth muscle cells: slow waves and spikes. Slow waves, which it is assumed are caused by the undulating activity of Na^+-K^+ pumps, alter the membrane potential by 5 to 15 millivolts. Their frequency can vary, depending largely on the location in the gastrointestinal tract. For instance, slow waves occur at a frequency of about 3 per minute in the stomach while occurring at a rate of 12 per minute in the duodenum.

Smooth Muscle Excitation

Slow waves are not actually action potentials and, therefore, do not directly evoke contraction of smooth muscle. However, when slow waves exceed −40 millivolts, they give rise to spikes, which are indeed true action potentials and thus stimulate muscle contraction. Spikes, or spike potentials, differ from the action potentials characteristic of neurons in at least two ways. First, spike potentials, which last 10 to 20 milliseconds, are about 10 to 40 times longer than neuron action potentials. Second, the ion channels involved in the spike potential are unique as well. Spike potentials appear to be caused by slow-opening and slow-closing Ca^{2+}-Na^+ channels, which are different from the rapidly opening and closing Na^+ channels involved in the action potentials of neurons. Spike potentials can also be distinguished from slow waves based on ion channel activity. Slow waves are not associated with an increase in intracellular calcium and, therefore, do not evoke fiber contraction. Like other muscle fibers, smooth muscle cells of the gastrointestinal tract wall contract in response to an increase in intracellular calcium concentration acting through a calmodulin-controlled mechanism.

In addition to rhythmic contraction, gut smooth muscle exhibits tonic contraction. Although demonstrating fluctuations in intensity, tonic contractions are continual and protracted, lasting as long as several minutes to hours. The origin of a tonic contraction may be the result of a repetitive series of spike potentials or the influence of certain hormones or other factors that allow for continual depolarization of the membrane potential.

▶ Enteric Nervous System

The gastrointestinal tract is endowed with the enteric nervous system (ENS), which is functionally distinct yet inter-connected with the central nervous system (CNS). That means that although the ENS can function on its own, its activity is still influenced by the autonomic extensions of the CNS. Furthermore, sensory neurons originating in the intestinal wall epithelium communicate with both the enteric and CNS.

The ENS extends from the esophagus to the anus, contains approximately 100,000,000 neurons, and is characterized by two main plexuses. The myenteric plexus, or Auerbach plexus, is the outer plexus and is located between the longitudinal and circular smooth muscle layers and runs the entire length of the enteric nervous system. The proximity of this complex relative to smooth muscle layers makes the myenteric plexus ideal to control motor activity along the length of the gastrointestinal tract. Stimulation of the myenteric plexus generally results in increased wall tone, rate and intensity of rhythmic contractions, and velocity of excitatory wave conduction along the wall of the gastrointestinal tract.

In contrast to those operations, stimulation of the myenteric plexus can also result in some inhibitory activity as well. For instance, some of its neurons release inhibitory neurotransmitters, such as vasoactive inhibitory polypeptide (VIP), when stimulated. The significance of this activity includes relaxation of intestinal sphincter muscles, such as the pyloric sphincter and the ileocecal valve, thus allowing passage of intestinal content from one gut segment into another. The second plexus, which is known as the submucosa plexus, or Meissner plexus, is situated within the submucosa and is mainly involved in gastrointestinal secretions and local blood flow regulation.

Neurotransmitters

Neurons of the ENS produce a variety of potential neurotransmitter substances, including acetylcholine, epinephrine, ATP, dopamine, serotonin, VIP, γ-aminobutyric acid (GABA), glycine, cholecystokinin (CCK), leu-enkephalin and met-enkephalin, substance P, secretin, neurotensin, motilin, and gastric-releasing peptide (GRP), which is the mammalian analogue of the amphibian peptide bombesin. Although the role of a few of these substances in ENS activity has been well established, the presence of other substances has not necessarily been linked to physiologic function.

Acetylcholine mediates contraction of the smooth muscle in the gut as well as secretions from the salivary glands, stomach, pancreas, and small intestine. Norepinephrine, in contrast, generally inhibits smooth contraction, secretion, and blood flow. GRP is a 27-amino acid peptide that is released from neurons in the gastric antrum and fundus, as well as the pancreas; and stimulates the release of gastrin, CCK, pancreatic polypeptide, insulin, glucagon, and somatostatin. VIP is a 28-amino acid peptide that is produced by neurons throughout the gastrointestinal tract, salivary glands, and pancreas. VIP release causes relaxation of the LES, the proximal stomach, and the internal anal sphincter.

Sympathetic and Parasympathetic Innervation

The gastrointestinal tract is extrinsically innervated by both the sympathetic and parasympathetic systems. Both systems elicit a response in the gastrointestinal system by synapsing with neurons of the ENS first. Furthermore, chemoreceptors and mechanoreceptors in the mucosa of the gastrointestinal tract can relay afferent impulses to the CNS or elicit a reflex by way of ENS plexuses. Because the activities of the ENS and the sympathetic and parasympathetic nervous systems are not under conscious control, those systems are collectively referred to as the autonomic nervous system.

The vagus nerve supplies almost all of the parasympathetic activity down to the level of the transverse colon, whereas fibers supplied by the pelvic nerve innervate the descending colon, sigmoid colon, rectum, and the anal canal. Cholinergic fibers innervating the striated muscle in the upper third of the esophagus and external anal canal are also delivered by the vagal and pelvic nerves, respectively. Parasympathetic fibers are especially dense in the oral cavity and the most analward segments of the gastrointestinal tract, while not being particularly as dense in the small intestine. Parasympathetic stimulation generally increases gastrointestinal activity, although some inhibitory processes do result.

Contrary to parasympathetic innervation, the density of sympathetic innervation is more consistent throughout the length of the gut. Sympathetic fibers originate in the T5 through L2 regions of the spinal cord, and preganglionic fibers synapse in either the celiac, superior or inferior mesenteric, or hypogastric ganglia. From there, postganglionic fibers innervate regions of the myenteric and submucosal plexuses. Neurons of the ENS then relay signals to smooth muscle, secretory cells, and endocrine cells of the gastrointestinal tract and generally elicit a response that decreases gastrointestinal activity.

▶ Digestive Tract Movements

The gastrointestinal tract exhibits two basic types of movement. Propulsive movements move contents forward, whereas mixing movements allow for a thorough blending of gastrointestinal contents. Peristalsis is the basic propulsive movement. A ring of muscular constriction encircling the gut is initiated and then begins to move forward (analward) by pushing the intestinal matter in front of the ring forward. Distention is a strong stimulus for the origin of a peristaltic wave. For instance, if intestinal matter stretches the gut wall, a contractile ring is initiated about 2 to 3 centimeters behind the point of distention, and peristalsis is propagated in the direction of the anus. In addition, the gut can relax several centimeters on the anus side of the distention to ease transit of matter into that area. Parasympathetic signals can also initiate peristalsis along with irritation of the mucosal lining of the gut. An intact myenteric plexus is necessary for effective peristaltic waves in an associated area.

Mixing movements differ from one segment of the gastrointestinal tract to another. In areas just prior to a sphincter closure, forward movement of intestinal matter is blocked and thus peristaltic waves take on a more distinctive mixing role. In other regions, local constrictive contractions occur approximately every several centimeters in a regimented fashion to help chop and blend intestinal contents.

▶ Gastrointestinal Vasculature

The gastrointestinal tract receives blood from several arterial branches of the abdominal aorta. For instance, the celiac artery delivers blood to the stomach, the superior mesenteric artery delivers blood to the small intestine and proximal portion of the large intestine, and the inferior mesenteric artery supplies blood to the more distal aspects of the large intestine. Small arterial branches of superior mesenteric artery ultimately serve individual villi because a capillary network is centralized inside each of those mucosal projections (see Figure 2.6).

Hepatic Portal Vein

Once blood has perfused those regions, it drains into its respective veins, which then drain into the **hepatic portal vein**. By design, blood that has perfused the gut, as well as the pancreas and spleen, is destined to flow to the liver before returning to the heart. This allows the liver to have the first shot at substances absorbed into intestinal wall capillaries. Furthermore, as the blood courses through hepatic sinusoids, gut-derived bacteria and other debris can be removed by reticuloendothelial cells before entering the circulation at large.

● BEFORE YOU GO ON...

1. What type of muscle is found in the wall of the digestive tract and how is it arranged?
2. How do substances move through the digestive tract, and how are they mixed with digestive juices?
3. What is the nervous system of the digestive tract, and how does it interact with the CNS?
4. What is the special function of the vagus nerve?
5. What are the special features of circulation serving the gastrointestinal system?

▶ Gastrointestinal Endocrine and Paracrine Substances

Distributed throughout the gastrointestinal tract are cells possessing endocrine or paracrine functions or both. Those cells manufacture and secrete substances such as serotonin, cholecystokinin, gastrin, secretin, gastric inhibitory polypeptide (GIP), motilin, neurotensin, and somatostatin. Interestingly, many of those substances are also found in the neural end of the enteric nervous system.

Gastrin

Gastrin is secreted by gastrin cells (G cells), which are located primarily in the glands of the gastric antrum and also in the mucosa of the duodenum. Several polypeptides of varying lengths possess gastrin activity. All of those polypeptides possess an identical carboxyl (COOH) terminal amino acid sequence (Try-Met-Asp-Phe-NH_2), with the terminal phenylalanine (Phe) residue being aminated (NH_2). The most abundant forms are G-17 (I and II) and G-34 (big gastrin), with the number denoting the quantity of amino acids in the polypeptide. **FIGURE 2.7** presents the amino acid sequence of G-17. G-14 (minigastrin) is also physiologically active, whereas pentagastrin (G-5) is a synthetic form of gastrin. During interdigestive periods or fasting, gastrin levels in the plasma are on the order of 50 to 100 picograms per milliliter and are mostly attributable to G-34. However, when G cells are stimulated during a meal, more G-17 is released. G-17 and G-34 are equipotent; however, the half-life of G-34 is approximately 38 minutes, whereas the half-life of G-17 is only 7 minutes.

Gastrin (G-17)

Glu-Gly-Pro-Trp-Leu-Glu-Glu-Glu-Glu-Ala-Tyr-Gly-Trp-Met-Asp-Phe-NH$_2$

HSO_3

Cholecystokinin

Lys-(Ala,Gly,Pro,Ser)-Arg-Val-(Ile,Met,Ser)-Lys-Asn-(Asn,Gln,His, Leu$_2$,Pro,Ser$_2$)-Arg-Ile-(Asp,Ser)-Arg-Asp-Tyr-Gly-Trp-Met-Asp-Phe-NH$_2$

HSO_3

Secretin

His-Ser-Asp-Gly-Thr-Phe-Thr-Ser-Glu-Leu-Ser-Arg-Leu-Arg-Asp-Ser-Ala-Arg-Leu-Gln-Arg-Leu-Leu-Gln-Gly-Leu-Val-NH$_2$

FIGURE 2.7 Amino Acid Composition of Gastrin, Cholecystokinin, and Secretin. Major amino acid composition of polypeptides that initiate digestion. Gastrin and cholecystokinin have polypeptides that vary in length, with this figure illustrating the "parent" compounds. Secretin is present with only one form of the polypeptide.

The stimulus for gastrin release from G cells includes the presence of small peptides, certain amino acids (especially phenylalanine and tryptophan), and calcium in the lumen of the stomach. Neural stimulation, either mediated directly by the vagus or indirectly by gastric distention-initiated ENS reflexes, also evokes gastrin release. Gastrin-releasing peptide (GRP) appears to be the neurotransmitter released as a result of vagal stimulation. The primary role of gastrin is to regulate gastric acid secretion while also mediating pepsinogen and intrinsic factor secretion. Gastrin is approximately 1500 times more potent than histamine in stimulating acid release from oxyntic glands. Gastrin also stimulates the growth of the oxyntic glands. Gastrin release is reduced relative to increasing acidity in the lumen of the stomach.

Cholecystokinin

Similar to gastrin, the polypeptide cholecystokinin (see Figure 2.7) is also present in multiple forms and is secreted from cells located in the mucosa of the duodenum and jejunum. Molecules exhibiting CCK activity have the same active COOH-terminal tetrapeptide sequence as gastrin. Isolated forms of CCK include CCK-58, CCK-39, CCK-33, CCK-22, and CCK-8. CCK release is stimulated by the presence of intraluminal fatty acids having a chain length of nine or more carbons and their corresponding monoglycerides. Partially digested proteins and individual amino acids such as phenylalanine and tryptophan, as well as intraluminal glucose, promote CCK release. GRP

also seems to stimulate the release of CCK. Among the well-established roles of CCK are to stimulate the release of pancreatic enzyme secretion, gallbladder contraction, and relaxation of the sphincter of Oddi. CCK also has an effect on gastric and intestinal motility and a trophic effect on the pancreas.

Secretin

In contrast to gastrin and CCK, secretin only has one circulating form, a 27-amino acid polypeptide (see Figure 2.7). It is released from secretin-containing cells located in the mucosa of the duodenum and jejunum when the hydrogen ion content of the proximal small intestine increases. Circulating levels of secretin increase when intraluminal pH falls below 4.5. Intraluminal fatty acids may also evoke the release of secretin. The major function of secretin is to stimulate the pancreas to release a bicarbonate-rich alkaline solution into the pancreatic duct. Secretin also promotes water and bicarbonate secretion from the biliary system. Secretin exhibits other functions as well, such as inhibition of gastric emptying, inhibition of gastric acid secretion, and the release of pepsinogen in the stomach. However, whether those functions are physiologically significant remains uncertain.

Somatostatin

Beyond mucosa cells throughout the intestinal tract, somatostatin is also manufactured and released from D cells in the pancreatic islets of Langerhans as well as nerve fibers in both the central and enteric nervous systems. Somatostatin occurs as either SS-14 or SS-28, and circulatory levels are increased due to the presence of fat and protein in the intestines and to some degree by an acidic pH in the antrum region of the stomach, as well as in the duodenum. Although it has many functions outside of digestive physiology, somatostatin is involved in the inhibition of gastrin release from G cells, in pancreatic enzyme release, and in the secretion of stomach acid. Beyond those roles, somatostatin is involved in inhibiting the release of secretin, motilin, and CCK, as well as inhibiting the absorption of amino acids, water, and electrolytes and gut motility.

Gastric Inhibitory Polypeptide

Gastric inhibitory peptide (GIP) is produced and released from cells located primarily in the duodenum and jejunum. GIP is a 42-amino acid polypeptide released in response to an intraluminal presence of several substances, including glucose, amino acids, and hydrolyzed triglycerides, as well as being released in response to an increase in duodenal hydrogen ion concentration. Although its name suggests a regulatory role in gastric acid secretion, this function has not been proven to be physiologic. However, GIP does have a physiologic role in intensifying the glucose-stimulated release of insulin. Because of this role, GIP is also called glucose-dependent insulinotropic peptide, thus retaining the GIP abbreviation.

Motilin

Motilin, a 22-amino acid linear polypeptide, is released from mucosal cells of the upper small intestine. The

---

SPECIAL FEATURE 2.1

Gastroesophageal Reflux Disease (GERD)

A growing medical problem is gastroesophageal reflux disease, commonly referred to as GERD. GERD occurs when there is reflux of acidic stomach contents back into the esophagus. This will cause heartburn and can also result in contents refluxing to the back of the throat, which leaves it sore. Without treatment, ulceration of the esophageal lining can occur. Difficulty in swallowing will result if the esophagus narrows as a result of chronic irritation. GERD may also lead to a precancerous condition known as Barrett syndrome. Regurgitation of food is not uncommon with GERD. Symptoms of GERD are more likely to occur during the night, but they may occur at other times.

GERD occurs when the lower esophageal sphincter muscle does not close properly due to a decreased tone. Under normal situations, the sphincter muscle opens upon swallowing and then closes after the food contents enter the stomach. Risk factors associated with GERD include:

- Obesity
- Alcohol intake
- Hiatal hernia
- Pregnancy
- Smoking

Medications can also lead to the development of GERD or worsen the condition and symptoms. Medications that can cause or worsen GERD include tricyclic antidepressants, asthmatic bronchodilators, dopamine-related drugs used to treat Parkinson's disease, and β-blockers used to treat heart disease.

Although certain food types can modulate the symptoms, lifestyle modifications may alleviate them. In addition to decreasing alcohol intake, people with GERD should stop smoking and lose weight. It may also be helpul to not lay down for 2 to 3 hours after consuming a meal. Eating dinner and then laying down to watch television will only exacerbate the symptoms. Sitting up following a meal will allow the food contents to be digested more effectively in the stomach first followed by further digestion when the partially digested food enters the duodenum. Snacks before bedtime, especially those that are high in fat, also increase the likelihood of GERD.

Certain foods tend to be more problematic than others. The best way for a person to determine which foods are causing a problem is to keep a food diary and then determine if GERD episodes occur after eating certain foods. In general, spicy foods tend to be more problematic. Acidic foods, such as tomatoes and citrus beverages, may need to be avoided prior to bedtime. Onion and garlic may also cause GERD episodes. Chocolate and certain oils, such as spearmint oil, are contraindicated because those tend to lessen the lower esophageal sphincter pressure. Coffee and fatty foods may also lessen the sphincter pressure. Generally speaking, foods that are good sources of protein will increase the lower esophageal pressure and are recommended. Also, small, more frequent meals are another dietary recommendation to decrease the incidence of reflux.

Many health professionals recommend use of antacids to help alleviate the symptoms of GERD. Both over-the-counter and prescription antacid medications are available. Many antacids are salts of calcium, magnesium, or aluminum with hydroxyl or bicarbonate groups to help neutralize the acids. Another class of medications used to treat GERD is the proton pump inhibitors, which include Prilosec, Prevacid, Protonix, Aciphex, and Nexium, which are available by prescription. Prilosec is also available over the counter in lower dosage forms. H_2 blockers are another class of medications. H_2 blockers include Tagamet, which has a long track record in treating GERD; Pepcid AC proton pump inhibitors appear more effective than H_2 blockers, and almost all individuals with GERD will have favorable responses.

If lifestyle modifications and medications are unable to relieve GERD, surgical intervention is required. Surgical techniques can be used to strengthen the sphincter muscle. In one technique, burning the lower esophageal sphincter results in the production of scar tissue that can strengthen the muscle.

level of motilin increases during interdigestive periods. Motilin is believed to initiate migrating myoelectric complexes (MMCs) in the duodenum, which occur every 90 minutes or so during interdigestive periods and function as a sweeping mechanism moving digestive residue analward. Motilin also stimulates the production of pepsin. Often, motilin is referred to as the "housekeeper of the gut" because it supports peristalsis in the small intestine, thereby clearing this space for the next meal.

Peptide YY

Peptide YY (or PYY) is a 36-amino acid protein produced and released by cells in the ileum and colon in response to a meal and appears to reduce appetite. In addition, a structurally similar version is produced and released by the pancreas in response to feeding. PYY works by binding to neuropeptide Y (NPY) receptors located in the autonomic nervous system (ANS) and the brain. PYY inhibits gastric motility and, therefore, functions to slow the transit of contents through the small intestine to increase the efficiency of digestion and nutrient absorption. In addition, PYY increases water and electrolyte absorption in the colon and may also suppress pancreatic secretion.

Histamine

Histamine is derived from the amino acid histidine by the actions of histidine decarboxylase. In addition to its established activities as a neurotransmitter, histamine is secreted from gastric mast cells. Although the mechanisms leading to the release of histamine from those cells are relatively unclear, the paracrine function of histamine in evoking gastric acid secretion is well known. Therapeutically, histamine H_2-receptor antagonists, such as cimetidine, inhibit parietal cell hydrochloric acid secretion as stimulated by gastrin, acetylcholine, and histamine analogues.

⬣ BEFORE YOU GO ON . . .

1. What is gastrin? How is it released and is there more than one form?
2. Where is secretin released, and what is its role in digestion?
3. What are the principal stimulants of CCK, and what is the function of this hormone?
4. What role do GIP, motilin, and PYY play in digestion?
5. What role does histamine play, and where and how is it released?

SPECIAL FEATURE 2.2

Mediators of Appetite

Hormonal Influences

Insulin

Barring anomaly, the level of circulating insulin appears to be proportionate to the volume of adipose tissue. In addition to insulin's effect on energy substrate metabolism, it also influences appetite and food intake. Insulin is able to cross the blood–brain barrier by way of a saturable transport system and may reduce feeding by inhibiting the expression of neuropeptide Y (NPY), enhancing the effects of cholecystokinin (CCK), and inhibiting neuronal norepinephrine reuptake. Thus, teleologically, the correlation between adiposity and plasma insulin levels may be an adaptive mechanism to support decreased caloric consumption. Interestingly, the influence of insulin on NPY expression is not seen in the genetically obese Zucker (*fa/fa*) rats. Because the *fa* gene codes for the leptin receptor, it is likely that some of the effects of insulin on reducing appetite are leptin mediated.

Cholecystokinin

As discussed previously, cholecystokinin is secreted by mucosal cells of the proximal small intestine in response to the presence of food components. Postprandial circulating CCK levels are related to satiety and feeding in humans. There appear to be two types of CCK receptors (A and B), and both may be involved in regulating food intake. CCK-A receptors are present within the gastrointestinal system, whereas CCK-B receptors are present in the brain.

By way of interaction with CCK-A receptors in the pylorus, CCK promotes contraction of the pyloric sphincter, which increases gastric distention. This initiates vagal afferents from the stomach that terminate in the nucleus of the solitary

(continues)

SPECIAL FEATURE 2.2 *(continued)*

tract within the brain stem. Impulses are then transmitted to the parabrachial nucleus, which is then connected to the ventromedial hypothalamus, resulting in decreased food intake. This mechanism is diminished by experimental vagotomy.

Although CCK-B receptors are found in the brain, CCK circulating in the systemic circulation does not cross the blood–brain barrier. Therefore, it has been suggested that because the brain also produces some CCK, afferent neural signals may result in the release of CCK in the cerebral spinal fluid, which binds with CCK-B receptors and decreases feeding.

Neuroendocrine Influences

Leptin

In 1995, leptin, a protein chain of 167 amino acids, was discovered as a product of the obese (*ob*) gene. Its receptor was cloned shortly thereafter. The name *leptin* is derived from the Greek word *leptos*, meaning "thin." In obese hyperphagic, homozygote *ob/ob* mice; two prominent mutations have been identified that lead either to a lack of mRNA expression or to production of an ineffective product. Leptin has been shown to reduce food intake and increase energy expenditure in both obese and lean animals. In humans, adipose cells also synthesize and secrete this protein relative to the amount of stored body fat. Leptin receptors have been found in various body tissues, such as the kidneys, liver, heart, skeletal muscle, hypothalamus, pancreas, and anterior pituitary. Leptin receptors found in the arcuate nucleus of the hypothalamus have led researchers to hypothesize that leptin may somehow regulate satiety. Leptin appears to also decrease NPY synthesis and release from that same region. In addition, leptin has been shown to increase corticotropin-releasing factor (CRF) expression and release from the hypothalamus.

It is possible that serum leptin levels are elevated in some obese subjects due to the receptor's resistance to leptin's action. This is supported by another model of genetic **obesity** in mice. The so-called obese diabetic mouse has a mutation in the diabetes (*db*) gene. It is typical for those mice to have a 10-fold greater level of leptin in comparison with lean control mice. Because it has not been determined that there is an anomaly in the *ob* gene in these animals, a defect in the receptor is suspected at present. Some human cross-sectional studies have revealed that obese individuals may also have elevated levels of leptin; however, it is not clear whether there is a defect in the hypothalamic leptin receptor in these individuals. Thus, it has been speculated that there may be leptin resistance.

The presence of receptors in the pancreas has also led researchers to hypothesize that serum leptin may somehow regulate insulin metabolism. Whether this is indeed the case is unresolved. In vitro studies have demonstrated that leptin does not alter the uptake of glucose in the absence of insulin, nor does it influence glucose's sensitivity to insulin. Other studies appear to strongly correlate a counter-regulatory effect of leptin with insulin resistance.

Leptin may also play a role in energy substrate metabolism, because there may very well be an inverse correlation between leptin and energy intake, fat intake, resting energy expenditure, carbohydrate oxidation, and **respiratory exchange ratio (RER)**. Therefore, those resistant to leptin may encounter two metabolic obstacles: (1) the link between the central nervous system and appetite regulation is disturbed, and (2) resting energy expenditure is decreased, facilitating weight gain. Also, there is evidence to suggest that leptin levels decrease in response to weight loss and remain decreased as long as the weight loss is maintained. Furthermore, increased levels of leptin have been found in normal-weight and obese women compared with their male counterparts, as well as in female-patterned obesity (or peripheral fat stores). This is an expected finding because females have a greater percentage of body fat mass than males.

Ghrelin

Ghrelin is a hunger-stimulating hormone; its level increases before meals and decreases after meals. Ghrelin is produced by P/D1 cells lining the fundus of the stomach and epsilon cells of the pancreas and is considered the counterpart of leptin. In addition, ghrelin is produced in the hypothalamus and acts to stimulate the secretion of growth hormone from the anterior pituitary gland. In fact, much of ghrelin's ability to increase hunger is based on its interaction with the hypothalamus by activating NPY neurons in the arcuate nucleus. Both leptin and insulin influence the sensitivity of those neurons to ghrelin. Furthermore, ghrelin also plays a role in the mesolimbic cholinergic-dopaminergic system, which communicates "reward" in the presence of food as well as alcohol.

Neuropeptide Y

Neuropeptide Y is a peptide synthesized and secreted by the neurons of the arcuate nucleus of the hypothalamus, partially in response to leptin binding to its receptors. Increased activity of those neurons has been demonstrated in animal studies during periods of energy deficit, and; therefore, obesity may develop in response to abnormally increased production. NPY appears to stimulate food intake, especially carbohydrate sources. The paraventricular nucleus appears to be particularly sensitive to NPY. Interestingly, NPY is also synthesized and released by the adrenal gland and sympathetic nerves into circulation; however, it does not cross the blood–brain barrier.

When NPY is injected directly into the medial hypothalamus of satiated animals, feeding is stimulated. Furthermore, there is a preference for carbohydrates. NPY seems to increase the percentage of carbohydrate used for energy while simultaneously being associated with a reduction in energy expenditure. It is believed that the NPY-induced, increased use of carbohydrate allows for the production of more acetyl CoA for lipogenesis. NPY also seems to support fat storage in white adipose tissue, while decreasing brown adipose tissue activity. Interestingly, NPY may have a stimulatory effect on the secretion of insulin, vasopressin, and leuteinizing hormone.

Peptide YY

Peptide YY is related to NPY. Peptide YY is a 36 amino acid peptide produced by cells of the ileum and colon. Upon feeding, the level of this peptide increases 15 minutes after a meal. When the peptide is administered from an exogenous source, its major effect is to inhibit energy intake as well as body weight in both rodent models and humans. Apparently, a possible mechanism by which this functions is to block the effect of NPY neurons while binding to other neurons to signal satiety.

Galanin

Galanin is another peptide factor that, along with its receptors, is found in greater concentrations in the hypothalamus. Animal studies suggest that galanin increases feeding as well as the preference for carbohydrate and fat. In addition, galanin is associated with a reduction in energy expenditure because it inhibits sympathetic nervous system activity; however, it does not seem to influence the proportion of fuel used (e.g., carbohydrate vs fat). Two subclasses of receptors have been identified in rats but only one in humans. Unlike leptin and NPY, plasma galanin concentrations and activity do not appear to be regulated by weight. Galanin also has an inhibitory effect on insulin secretion, and synthesis of galanin is inhibited in response to increased serum insulin.

▶ Digestion and Absorption

The foundation of human nourishment is the consumption of other living entities or their products to obtain elements and molecules common to both. Essential nutrients are substances that humans are unable to produce, either at all or in adequate quantities, and thus must be provided by the diet. Because of the complex integration of nutrients into their sources, digestive activities are necessary to liberate nutrients, such as freeing minerals from proteins; to reduce the size of nutrients, such as breaking down complex proteins to amino acids or complex **starch** to monosaccharides; and to modify nutrients so that they can be recognized by transport systems involved in their absorption.

Phases of Digestion

Digestive operations are influenced by several factors. For instance, the mere thought or smell of food can initiate activities in the digestive tract. In addition, many physical and chemical interactions modify digestive activities. Based on this, digestion can be separated into three phases:

1. *Cephalic phase.* The cephalic phase occurs when food stimulates pressure-sensitive mechanoreceptors in the mouth and chemo-receptors in the mouth and nasal cavity. The mere thought of food can also trigger central pathways that relay impulses to vagal efferent nerves that reach the stomach. Thus, the cephalic phase can be blocked by vagotomy.

2. *Gastric phase.* The gastric phase begins when distention of the stomach wall stimulates mechanoreceptors. This action elicits vagovagal and intramural reflexes that stimulate the release of gastrin and other hormones, thereby increasing stomach secretions as well as intestinal secretions.

3. *Intestinal phase.* The intestinal phase occurs as a result of both mechanical and chemical events. Duodenal luminal distention leads to the release of a hormone called entero-oxyntin. Meanwhile, interaction between nutrients and receptors elicits the release of other hormones, such as CCK and secretin.

Oral Cavity

Once food enters the mouth, it is chewed (masticated) and bathed in salivary juice. Incisors are anterior in the mouth and provide a strong cutting action, whereas the more posterior molars provide a grinding mechanism. **FIGURE 2.8** shows the structure of a tooth. Chewing is controlled by nuclei in the brain stem, which innervates the muscles of the jaw via the fifth cranial nerve. A coordinated effort by all muscles in the jaw can generate a force of 55 pounds on the incisors and 200 pounds on the molars. Chewing physically tears food apart while actions of the tongue help position food between the teeth; the combination of actions mixes food with saliva.

Saliva

Saliva lubricates food for easier swallowing, solubilizes food components for taste perception, cleans the mouth and teeth to prevent caries, and initiates chemical digestion. Approximately 1 to 1.5 liters of saliva are produced daily by the glands of the oral cavity. The parotid, submandibular, and sublingual glands, along with well-distributed buccal glands, are the principal glands involved in producing a complex compilation of enzymes, mucus, R proteins, growth factors, antibacterial and antiviral factors, ions, and water (see Figure 2.3). Finally, saliva contains the blood group substances A, B, AB, and O.

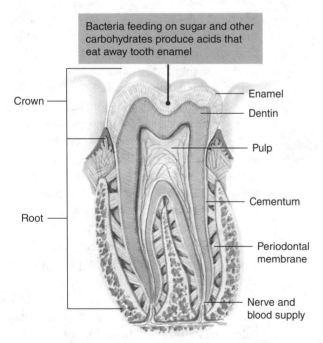

FIGURE 2.8 General Anatomy of a Tooth. Poor nutrition may compromise the integrity of teeth. The enamel portion is susceptible to erosion by bacteria feeding on sticky carbohydrates. Enamel erosion allows other structures to be compromised, leading to dental caries.

Saliva Proteins: Enzymes and Mucus

Two types of protein secretions are found in saliva: serous and mucous. The serous type of protein secretion, which is secreted by the parotid, submandibular, and sublingual glands; contains ptyalin (**α-amylase**) and lingual lipase and is also secreted by the sublingual glands. α-Amylase begins the chemical digestion of starches by cleaving α1-4 links between glucose monomers. Lingual lipase hydrolyzes certain ester bonds of triglycerides and is of particular significance in infants. Another salivary enzyme, kallikrein, does not have catabolic properties but supports the digestive process by converting a plasma protein into bradykinin, which increases blood flow to salivary glands. The mucous type of protein secretion contains the lubricating glycoprotein mucin. Along with the submandibular and sublingual glands, the buccal glands also secrete mucus.

Saliva Electrolytes

The inorganic component of saliva includes sodium, potassium, chloride, bicarbonate, calcium, magnesium, and phosphate. At rest, saliva is hypotonic; however, the potassium concentration (30 milliequivalents per liter [mEq/L]) is greater than plasma levels. In contrast, the concentrations of sodium, chloride, and bicarbonate, all about 15 mEq/L, are below plasma levels. The concentrations of sodium and chloride in saliva at rest may be only about 10 to 15% of their levels in plasma. When saliva flow is stimulated, the concentration of potassium decreases, although not below plasma levels. In contrast, the concentrations of sodium, chloride, and bicarbonate increase, with the latter rising above plasma concentration. This increases salivary pH to approximately 7.8 from a resting pH of between 6.0 and 7.0.

Saliva is very important for oral hygiene. With the exception of periods of sleep, saliva is secreted at a basal rate of about 0.5 milliliter per minute, with the protein being predominantly of the mucous type. The secretion of saliva helps wash away pathogenic bacteria and residual food particles from teeth. Saliva also contains antibacterial factors such as thiocyanate ions, several proteolytic enzymes (including lysozyme), and antibodies, which collectively destroy a significant quantity of bacteria in the oral cavity.

Although the concentration of sodium and potassium can be influenced by aldosterone and antidiuretic hormone, the rate of salivary flow is controlled autonomically. That is to say that hormones that influence the release of other digestive secretions have little effect on salivary flow. Furthermore, the autonomic control of salivary secretion is different from many other organs in that both parasympathetic and sympathetic activity will elicit flow. However, parasympathetic activity has a far greater influence on flow.

Esophagus

The act of swallowing involves both voluntary and involuntary activity. Three overlapping layers of striated muscle—the superior, middle, and inferior pharyngeal constrictors—make up the muscular wall of the pharynx. The inferior constrictor also thickens at a point to form a muscular ring that constitutes the upper esophageal sphincter. The striated muscle continues down about one-third of the length of the esophagus and gives way to circular and longitudinal smooth muscle. Circular smooth muscle thickens at the distal aspect of the esophagus, forming the lower esophageal sphincter.

The act of swallowing is complex and involves coordinated and unvarying efforts of both voluntary and involuntary actions. At rest, the upper esophageal sphincter is contracted to close the esophageal inlet. In contrast, the pharyngeal muscle exhibits only a low level of tone. The act of swallowing involves a series of voluntary and even some involuntary motions occurring in sequence, beginning with the clenching down of the jaws. Subsequently, the tongue is elevated against the hard palate, and elevation of the soft palate allows the nasopharynx to separate from the oropharynx. Next, there is a voluntary and then an involuntary contraction of the pharyngeal muscles that moves in the direction of the esophageal inlet. Concomitantly, strap muscles in the neck move the pharyngoesophageal junction, thereby properly aligning the esophageal inlet with the pharynx. The 1- to 2-second relaxation of the upper esophageal sphincter allows the bolus of food to pass into the esophagus after being forced through the mouth by the tongue and through the pharynx by its peristaltic contraction.

Esophageal Sphincter

A powerful contraction of the upper esophageal sphincter is associated with the initiation of a peristaltic wave that propels food along the length of the esophagus. There is no delay in the transition from striated muscle to smooth muscle contraction, and a bolus of food can smoothly traverse the length of the esophagus in about 6 to 9 seconds. Relaxation of the lower esophageal sphincter occurs as the peristaltic wave is initiated and propagates to the length of the esophagus. It remains relaxed until the peristaltic wave meets the sphincter; then, after a brief interlude to allow the bolus to move into the stomach, it contracts forcefully.

Stomach

The primary operations of the stomach are to provide a depot for ingested food and to regulate its release into the small intestine; provide an acidic environment supportive of protein digestion and bacteriocidal activities; secrete a proteolytic enzyme; and secrete substances that assist in vitamin B_{12} absorption.

The outer longitudinal, middle circular, and inner oblique layers of smooth muscle in the wall of the stomach can relax and allow for the accommodation of approximately 1.5 liters of content without significantly increasing intragastric pressure. Furthermore, the musculature of the stomach wall provides both mixing movements as well as the propulsive movements that allow for a regulated release of gastric contents into the small intestine. Those layers (see Figure 2.4) can differ from one another with regard to distribution throughout the stomach as well as in their thickness in different regions of the stomach. For instance, whereas the circular layer is for the most part found completely throughout the stomach wall, the longitudinal layer is absent from the anterior and posterior surfaces. Also, the thickness of both the circular and longitudinal layers increases in a proximal to distal manner in the stomach.

Glands located largely in the body and fundus contain a variety of exocrine cell types. Those include parietal (oxyntic) cells, which secrete HCl and intrinsic factor; peptic cells, which secrete mainly pepsinogen; and mucous neck and surface cells, which produce large amounts of mucus (see Figure 2.5). Some endocrine cells can also be found lining the oxyntic gland. Quantitatively, parietal cells make up approximately one-third of the cells lining the gland; gastric chief cells make up about 20 to 25%; and mucous neck and surface cells make up about 20 and 10%, respectively.

The general release of gastric secretions is primarily under the control of acetylcholine, gastrin, and histamine, all of which perform their function by first binding with their respective receptors on secretory cells. Acetylcholine stimulates the release of secretions from all gastric secretory cell types. This includes pepsinogen from peptic cells, HCl from parietal cells, mucus from mucous neck cells, and gastrin from G cells. In contrast, gastrin and histamine strongly stimulate the release of HCl from parietal cells but have little stimulatory impact on other secretory cell types.

Gastric Juice and Hydrochloric Acid

Hydrochloric acid, which has a pH of 0.8, is released by parietal cells and creates an acidic environment in the stomach. The pH of stomach juice is approximately 1.5 to 2.5, which is important for (1) denaturing complex three-dimensional proteins, (2) activating pepsin, (3) liberating various nutrients from organic complexes, and (4) destroying ingested microbes. The mixture of ingested material and gastric secretions is known as chyme.

During interdigestive periods, basal acid secretion is approximately 10% of maximum and exhibits a circadian rhythm, with the output during the evening being significantly higher than that in the morning. The stimulation of gastric acid release in response to a meal is divided into three phases. The cephalic phase accounts for approximately 30% of gastric acid secretion, and the gastric and intestinal phases produce 60 and 10% of gastric acid secretion, respectively. Vagal innervation can increase gastric acid secretion directly by stimulating parietal cells via acetylcholine as well as indirectly by stimulating the release of gastrin via GRP. The cephalic phase release of gastric acid can be inhibited by low stomach pH. Because the pH of gastric acid secretion is about 2.0, acid release is impeded until food proteins reach the stomach and buffer the acid, thus causing the pH to climb above 3.0. This allows the cephalic phase to have its most significant impact on gastric acid secretion.

The gastric phase begins when distention of the stomach wall stimulates mechanoreceptors. This action elicits vagovagal and intramural reflexes that stimulate both gastrin release and acid secretion. The vagovagal reflex stimulates acid secretion by the same means as the cephalic phase. Furthermore, distention of the mucosa around oxyntic glands increases acid release by a local reflex mechanism. As mentioned previously, the release of gastrin is inhibited by a low gastric intraluminal pH; however, without regard to intraluminal pH, distention will still result in acid release by reflex and local mechanisms. Meanwhile, the intestinal phase of gastric acid secretion is relatively minor and not exactly clear. Duodenal luminal distention increases acid secretion by way of a hormone named entero-oxyntin. Furthermore, the uptake of amino acids into duodenal mucosal cells appears to be associated with increased acid release.

Pepsin

Pepsin is an endopeptidase and is manufactured and stored in an inactive pepsinogen proenzyme or zymogen form that has a molecular weight of approximately 42,500 daltons. There are two primary pepsinogen molecules, denoted as I and II. A third class of pepsinogen, called slow-moving protease because of its slow migration rate in an electrophoretic field, has also been identified. Pepsinogens are converted to active pepsins at a low pH by the loss of a portion of their NH_2-terminus amino acid sequence. They then function optimally at a pH below 3.5 and hydrolyze interior peptide bonds, especially those involving aromatic amino acids. The α-amylase derived from salivary secretions continues to digest complex carbohydrates in the stomach; however, it becomes inactivated in the highly acidic environment.

Intrinsic Factor

Intrinsic factor, which is a mucoprotein with a molecular weight of 55,000 daltons, is required for efficient absorption of vitamin B_{12} in the small intestine. Once vitamin B_{12} is released from polypeptides in foods (via gastric pepsin), it can combine with intrinsic factor. However, most of the vitamin B_{12} in the stomach will initially combine with R proteins because it has a greater affinity for R proteins. R Proteins are also secreted by gastric glands. The "R" denotes the rapid transit of those proteins in an electrophoretic field.

Gastric Emptying

Gastric emptying occurs as a result of intense peristaltic contractions in the antrum. For the most part, antral peristaltic contractions are weak and function as a mixing mechanism for food and gastric secretions. However, approximately 20% of the time when food is present, the peristaltic waves are about six times more intense than mixing waves, and the constricting rings propel food powerfully toward the pylorus. Each intense wave forces or pumps about 1 to 3 milliliters of chyme into the duodenum.

Release of gastric contents into the small intestine occurs intermittently and is regulated by several stimulatory and inhibitory factors that originate in both the stomach and small intestine. The degree of filling and the excitatory effect of gastrin on gastric peristalsis compete with duodenal signals such as enterogastric feedback reflexes and hormonal feedback. Generally, the greater the gastric distention, the more rapid the emptying. Furthermore, liquids seem to be emptied more rapidly than solids. Perhaps, the most rapidly emptied substance is an isotopic saline solution. Its emptying rate decreases as the solution is modified to a more hypotonic or hypertonic concentration. The presence of fat substances in the duodenum slows gastric emptying by stimulating the release of CCK, which inhibits emptying. Acid in the duodenum also decreases gastric emptying by a neural reflex mechanism.

Small Intestine

In the small intestine, chyme is mixed with pancreatic secretions and bile by way of segmentation or mixing contractions of circular smooth muscle and sleeve contractions of longitudinal smooth muscle. Meanwhile, peristaltic waves serve to propel food analward through the small intestine. The low pH of entering chyme is quickly neutralized by bicarbonate and H_2O secretions of both the pancreas as well as the Brunner glands, which are located in the mucosa of the first few centimeters of the duodenum. Cells in the crypts of Lieberkühn secrete approximately 1800 milliliters of fluid per day. The composition of this fluid is similar to extracellular fluid, with a slightly alkaline pH. The fluid provides a medium for nutrient absorption and is subsequently reabsorbed by enterocytes. Those cells are particularly sensitive to toxins such as those produced by *Vibrio cholerae*. Once small water-soluble substances, such as amino acids, monosaccharides, and certain vitamins and minerals, traverse the enterocyte lining, they can enter the circulation by entering the capillary within the center of the villus.

Pancreatic Digestive Juice

Pancreatic acini and associated duct cells secrete a juice that is clear, colorless, alkaline, and isotonic. It contains both organic and inorganic components, which ultimately reach the duodenum via the pancreatic duct and subsequently the common bile duct. Total pancreatic juice secretion for an adult is approximately 1 to 2 liters daily.

Protein, mostly in the form of enzymes, is a main component of pancreatic digestive juice (**TABLE 2.1**).

Digestive enzymes are produced and stored as inactive zymogen molecules to prevent autolysis of acini cells. Activation of digestive zymogen enzymes takes place in the duodenum and is initiated by the brush border enzyme enterokinase (enteropeptidase). Enterokinase activates trypsinogen by cleaving an NH_2-terminal portion of the molecule. Trypsin, the active form of trypsinogen, is then able to activate other digestive zymogens, including trypsinogen. Meanwhile, trypsin inhibitor and colipase are not necessarily digestive enzymes. Trypsin inhibitor appears to be active in pancreatic acini secretory vesicles. Its purpose is to protect pancreatic parenchyma by binding to trypsin molecules formed in premature autocatalysis. Procolipase, once activated, is a cofactor for lipase activity. In addition, other proteins, such as immunoglobulins, kallikrein, lysosomal enzymes, alkaline phosphatase, and albumin, are part of pancreatic secretions, although in relatively small quantities.

Pancreatic secretions include an inorganic component composed of water, sodium, potassium, chloride, calcium, and magnesium, plus bicarbonate (HCO_3^-). Calcium and magnesium are present in concentrations approximating 25 to 35% of their plasma concentrations. The large production of bicarbonate in ductal epithelium is attributed to intracellular conversion of CO_2 and H_2O via the enzyme carbonic anhydrase. The release of bicarbonate into the duct lumen uses a HCO_3^-/Cl^- antiport mechanism.

Pancreatic Juice Delivery

Basal secretion of the aqueous component of pancreatic juice, which is largely H_2O and bicarbonate, is about 2 to 3% of the maximal rate, whereas the basal secretion of the enzymatic component is approximately 10 to 15% of maximal. Although the mechanisms responsible for basal secretions are

TABLE 2.1 Pancreatic Digestive Enzymes

Proteolytic	Lipolytic	Amylolytic	Nucleases	Others
Trypsinogen	Lipase	α-Amylase	Deoxyribonuclease	Procolipase
Chymotrypsinogen	Prophospholipase A_1		Ribonuclease	Trypsin inhibitor
Proelastase	Prophospholipase A_2			
Procarboxypeptidase A	Esterase			
Procarboxypeptidase B				

undetermined, the mechanisms involved in stimulated secretion are well understood. The release of the aqueous portion of pancreatic secretion is largely related to duodenal intraluminal pH, whereas the enzymatic component is attributed primarily to the presence of fat and protein. Therefore, stimuli are strongest during the intestinal phase of digestion; however, secretion will also occur to a lesser extent during the cephalic and gastric phases.

During the cephalic phase, vagal efferents to the pancreas release acetylcholine at both ductule and acinar cells, with a stronger response being evoked within acinar cells. The result is a relatively low volume of pancreatic juice with a relatively high concentration of enzymes. Subsequently, distention of the stomach stimulates pancreatic secretion via a vagovagal reflex. The contributions of the cephalic and gastric phases to total pancreatic juice production may be approximately 20% and between 5 and 10%, respectively.

The intestinal phase accounts for as much as 70 to 80% of pancreatic secretory response because the presence of protein and fat in an acidic chyme mixture elicits the release of secretin and CCK. In addition, products of protein and fat digestion, as well as acid, stimulate pancreatic enzyme release as they interact with duodenal wall receptors. This results in a vagovagal reflex with acetylcholine being released at the synapses with both ductule and acinar cells. Acetylcholine and CCK, both independently and combined, have little stimulatory impact on ductule cells; however, they can potentiate the effects of secretin.

The Gallbladder and Bile Storage and Release

As much as 1200 milliliters of bile is secreted by the liver daily. Bile is produced almost continually in hepatocytes, which are epithelial cells arranged in plates in liver lobules. Bile is secreted into tiny bile canaliculi ("little canals") that run between the hepatocyte plates and drain into a series of larger ducts and then into the hepatic duct and then the common bile duct. Bile flowing through the common bile duct can then either be released into the duodenum or drain into the cystic duct.

During fasting periods, as much as half of the hepatic bile enters the gallbladder, while the remaining bile continues through to the small intestine. More than 90% of the bile acids (bile salts) emptied into the small intestine are reabsorbed in the distal ileum. Via the portal vein, they are returned to the liver and resecreted into bile, where again approximately half will drain into the gallbladder. As fasting becomes more protracted, bile storage in the gallbladder is increased. The recirculation of bile acids is called enterohepatic circulation. A single bile acid molecule may make as many as 18 circuits before being eliminated in the feces.

Bile Composition

Bile is a watery composite of substances such as bile acids, bilirubin, cholesterol, fatty acids, phospholipids, electrolytes, and bicarbonate (**TABLE 2.2**). During interdigestive periods, bile is routed into the cystic duct for storage in the gallbladder. Although the maximal volume of the gallbladder is approximately 20 to 60 milliliters, the equivalent of 450 milliliters can be stored within the gallbladder due to the concentrating efforts of its wall mucosal cells. Bile is normally concentrated 5-fold; however, mucosal efforts can produce a stored bile solution that is concentrated 12- to 20-fold. Water, sodium, chloride, and other electrolytes are absorbed by the mucosal cells, thereby concentrating the remaining substances, as shown in Table 2.2. Even though bile acids and other components are concentrated in the gallbladder, the stored solution is still isotonic, and the pH is lowered.

TABLE 2.2 Concentration Differences: Hepatic and Gallbladder Bile		
	Hepatic Bile[a]	**Gallbladder Bile**[b]
Bile salts (mEq/l)	30	300
Bilirubin (mg/100 ml)	100	1,000
Cholesterol (mg/100 ml)	100	600
Na^+ (mEq/l)	145	300
K^+ (mEq/l)	5	12
Ca^{2+} (mEq/l)	5	23
Cl^- (mEq/l)	100	10
HCO_3^- (mEq/l)	28	10

[a]pH 7.4, [b]pH 6.5

Bile is important not only because it supplies several substances essential for lipid digestion but also because it provides an avenue for the elimination of some substances that are inappropriate for urinary excretion. In general, these substances are organic and relatively large (molecular weight > 300). Also, their hydrophobicity results in their binding to plasma albumin, which decreases their filtration into the renal tubular system. The most significant of those substances is bilirubin, which is a metabolite of hemoglobin produced by reticuloendothelial cells of tissue such as the spleen. Bilirubin is released into the blood and binds with albumin. Hepatocytes remove bilirubin and conjugate it to glucuronic acid, forming bilirubin glucuronide, which is then added to bile. Because cholesterol circulates within lipoprotein complexes and is not filtered by the kidneys, its presence in bile may also be interpreted as an excretory mechanism for that substance.

In addition to entering the body in foods, water forms the basis of digestive secretions. Thus, digestion occurs within a water-based medium. Bile acids act as detergents to solubilize small lipid droplets in the watery medium. With the assistance of colipase, the coating of lipid droplets with bile acids allows the interaction of pancreatic lipase and cholesterol esterase with their substrates.

Gallbladder Contraction

When stimulated, such as in the presence of a meal, the smooth muscle within the wall of the gallbladder contracts and bile is propelled toward the small intestine. The most potent stimulus for emptying of the gallbladder during intradigestive periods is CCK. The emptying of the gallbladder can also be stimulated by cholinergic nerve fibers from both the vagal nerve and the enteric nervous system. It is likely that vagal discharges actually initiate gallbladder contraction and that combined stimuli maintain gallbladder contraction during digestion. This would discourage retrograde flow of bile back into the gallbladder as well as the draining of bile coming from the liver during periods of digestion. The gallbladder releases about two-thirds of its bile within the first hour of digestion. CCK also evokes relaxation of the sphincter of Oddi, thus allowing bile to flow into the duodenum.

Digestive Enzymes of the Small Intestine

Enterocytes not only provide the entry site for nutrient absorption but they also play an integral part in nutrient digestion. Several carbohydrate-digesting enzymes, including disaccharidases (e.g., lactase,

maltase, sucrase) and α-1-6 dextrinase, as well as enterokinase, are associated with the brush border. Furthermore, proteases specific for short-chain peptides are located within enterocytes and play a significant role in finalizing protein digestion.

Small Intestine Absorption

Several transport proteins are located on the luminal surface, as well as the basolateral surfaces, of enterocytes and facilitate absorptive operations. For example, the absorption of glucose first involves a Na^+-dependent transport system, which translocates glucose and sodium inside the enterocyte. Glucose can then cross the basolateral membrane by facilitative diffusion. Meanwhile, sodium is actively pumped across the basolateral membrane by a Na^+-K^+ ATPase pump. The continual absorption of glucose through enterocytes is dependent on an electrochemical gradient for sodium.

In contrast, lipid-soluble substances, such as cholesterol esters, triglycerides, and lipid-soluble vitamins are primarily incorporated into chylomicron lipoproteins within enterocytes, which then enter the lacteal in the central region of the villi. The small intestine absorbs the bulk of the nutrients, while some absorption also occurs in the stomach and colon.

Large Intestine

The large intestine, or colon, engages in two primary operations. First, it absorbs water and electrolytes from the entering content, a function that occurs predominantly in the proximal half. Second, it stores fecal matter until defecation, a function that occurs in the distal half. The large intestine can absorb as much as 5 to 7 liters of fluid and electrolytes in a day, if so challenged. Despite lacking villi, the mucosa of the large intestine is amply supplied with crypts of Lieberkühn, whose cells secrete copious amounts of mucus.

The large intestine is inhabited by more than 400 different species of bacteria. Some bacteria produce nutrients that can be absorbed, including vitamin K, biotin, and short-chain fatty acids (e.g., acetic, propionic, and butyric acids). The composition of feces is approximately 30% bacteria, 10 to 20% fat, 10 to 20% inorganic matter, 2 to 3% protein, and 30% undigested fibers and dried components of digestive juices, such as bilirubin and its metabolites. The coloring of feces is primarily attributable to the presence of stercobilin and urobilin, which are metabolites of bilirubin. Meanwhile, the odorous characteristics of feces are due to the presence of bacterial by-products, such as indoles, skatole, mercaptans, and hydrogen sulfide and are highly individualized based on diet and colonic bacterial profile.

Probiotics

The term **probiotic** literally translates as "for life" and is most commonly used to describe the bacteria in our digestive tract that are supportive of health. The digestive tract is home to trillions of bacteria, which fall into two general camps: those that promote health (probiotics) and those that seem to be problematic when it comes to optimal health. What seems to be very important is the balance between the two. Ideally, we want more of the health-promoting bacteria and less of the other type. Probiotic bacteria include lactic acid bacteria and Bifidobacteria; those are available in some food, such as dairy and soy yogurts, and as dietary supplements.

Probiotics promote optimal digestion and absorption of nutrients and promote a healthy digestive tract. Research supports the notion that regular consumption of probiotics may help with some intestinal conditions, such as irritable bowel syndrome and inflammatory bowel disease and help lower the risk of colon cancer.

What is more, the positive effects of probiotics might not be limited to the digestive tract. Research suggests that regular consumption of probiotics supports healthier blood cholesterol and blood pressure levels as well as supporting optimal immune system actions and playing a potential role in weight control.

Prebiotics

Nondigestible carbohydrates and other dietary substances that encourage the growth of beneficial bacteria (e.g., *Lactobacillus* bacteria) and decrease deleterious pathogens (e.g., *Escherichia coli*) in the gut are prebiotics. Resistant starches, oligofructose, and other oligosaccharides are examples of prebiotics. There are many products today that are sold as prebiotics in a supplement form. Besides the beneficial impact on promotion of favorable intestine microflora, the fermentation resulting from the bacteria upon the carbohydrates results in short-chain fatty acids. The short-chain fatty acids produce an environment more favorable to beneficial bacteria. Prebiotics are discussed in greater detail in Chapter 4 on health benefits of fiber and structural carbohydrates.

SPECIAL FEATURE 2.3

Bariatric Surgery

Bariatric surgery has become more frequent as a weight loss method. However, its use is restricted to the morbidly obese. Normally individuals with a BMI of 35 to 40 or greater, depending on the presence of other diseases, are good candidates for surgery. Prior to having such procedures, normally, other methods of calorie restriction and exercise should have been attempted. Lifelong changes in lifestyle are the likely outcomes of several of those procedures. There are four basic surgical procedures used: 1) gastric banding (lap-banding); 2) gastroplasty, 3) gastric sleeve, and 4) gastric bypass (Roux-En-Y) are the most common. (**FIGURE 1**).

With **gastric banding**, a silicon band is placed around the top portion of the stomach that leaves a small stomach pouch. The band has saline in it and this can be used to either enlarge or reduce the opening to the rest of the stomach. A pouch under the abdominal skin can have saline either injected or removed to alter the volume of the opening. The idea of having a pouch is that a feeling of fullness or satiety will be enhanced, resulting in decreased food intake. **Gastroplasty** requires that the upper portion of the stomach be stapled but leave a small opening to the distal stomach. The main difference between this procedure and gastric banding is that the opening to the distal stomach can be adjusted with the saline infusion within the silicon band. The opening to the distal stomach in gastroplasty is normally fixed in size compared with the banding technique. A variant of this surgery is the **gastric sleeve** procedure where a different portion of the stomach is stapled. Food travels from the esophagus, through the stomach or sleeve, and the small intestine.

Gastric bypass is a more involved procedure that facilitates weight loss not only on the smaller stomach size but on creating an environment for malabsorption of nutrients. A more common name for this procedure is **Roux-En-Y bypass**. Here, the upper part of the stomach is stapled and an opening is created that will feed into the small intestine, thereby eliminating food from entering the distal part of the stomach. Often, the entire duodenum is bypassed, depending on the type of bypass surgery. The procedure does result in more significant side effects. Dumping syndrome after eating is common. Micronutrients are often malabsorbed and require a lifelong monitoring of status of nutrients such as vitamin B_{12}, folic acid, potassium, magnesium, iron, and copper. Initially vomiting, rapid heartbeat, and other issues cause behavioral modification in the subject to decrease the volume of food. The pouch may increase somewhat over time as many patients tend to consume large amounts of liquid instead of solid food.

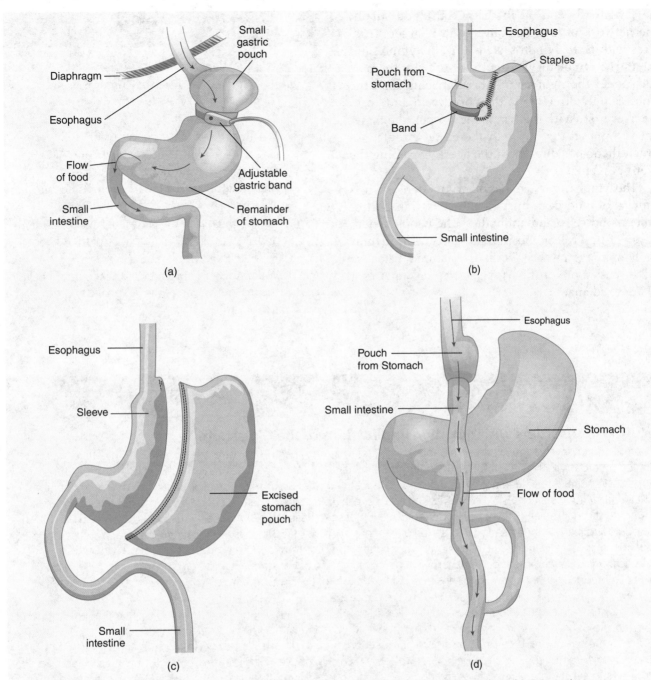

FIGURE 1 Various bariatric surgeries used for weight reduction. (a) Gastric or lap banding (b) Gastroplasty (c) Gastric sleeve d) Roux-En-Y.

Bariatric surgery can lead to significant reductions in weight, (up to 40% weight loss from initial weight) and also decrease adiposity. Additionally, diseases associated with obesity, such as arthritis, Type II diabetes, and heart disease may be attenuated with the weight loss.

▶ Lymphatic System

Absorption of certain nutrients occurs via the lymphatic system. In particular, lipid breakdown products and other fat-soluble vitamins are packaged into small lipids and proteins containing components of *chylomicrons* (See Chapter 5). Special lymphatic structures, or *lacteal capillaries,* are found within the villi of the small intestine. Later, they converge within the submucosa of the small intestine to form lacteals. The lacteals are important because chylomicrons are too large to enter the blood capillaries that eventually end up in the portal blood supply. The network of lacteals converge into larger structures within the lymph system and the lymph fluid enters the circulatory system through the thoracic duct under the right arm. Other nutrients enter the blood supply directly via the portal vein and go to the liver first. With the lymphatic system, the material is emptied directly into the blood circulation, which then goes directly to the heart, bypassing the liver upon entry.

The lymphatic system has other functions, such as removal of fluid from interstitial tissues, transport of white blood cells, and antibodies. The lymph system plays a critical role in the immune system. The thymus is a lymph organ where T cells are matured. Later, we will discuss more of the lymph system on water as it relates to edema.

● BEFORE YOU GO ON . . .

1. What are the three phases of digestion?
2. What is the relationship of R proteins and intrinsic factor in the stomach? Where are R proteins produced?
3. What is the role of the pancreas and gallbladder secretions in digestion?
4. Does the small intestine have any DIRECT enzymatic role in the breakdown of nutrients prior to absorption?
5. What is the role of the large intestine in digestion and absorption? What accounts for the color of fecal material?
6. With respect to digestion and absorption, what is the major function of the lymphatic system?

⚕ CLINICAL INSIGHT

Nutrition Disorders with Nutrition Implications of the GI System

Many nutrition interventions or diet therapies are linked to a wide spectrum of diseases of the gastrointestinal tract, including organs such as the liver, gall bladder, and pancreas that influence digestion and absorption. Some of those diseases require enteral feedings to help provide adequate nutritional support. The esophagus can develop conditions that lead to significant digestive problems. **Barrett's syndrome**, a precancerous condition and esophageal cancer, often results in removal of the esophagus and resection of the remaining esophageal tissue with the stomach. Nutrition support and lifetime modification of the type of feedings are essential. Gastroesophageal reflux disease, discussed already, is due to lower pressure of the lower esophageal sphincter muscle. Often, another condition with clinical implications is development of hiatal hernias, whereby a portion of the stomach moves to the thoracic cavity through the diaphragm. This can also lead to sensations of heartburn that may respond to dietary intervention. Esophagitis or inflammation of the esophagus can result from these diseases.

The stomach can develop various pathologies that impact the well-being of nutrition and require nutrition support. Gastric and peptic ulcers are common and diet intervention (along with some pharmacologic therapies) can alleviate many of the symptoms. Ulcers may also occur in the duodenum of the small intestine. In the stomach, many of the ulcers are caused by the organism *Helicobacter pylori*, which can induce inflammation of the gastric mucosa and lead to ulceration. Antibiotics are useful in treating this but, historically, nutrition support has been used to alleviate many of the symptoms. Cancer of the stomach is perhaps the one medical condition that requires significant medical nutrition therapy because, many times, portions of the affected stomach are surgically removed. Dumping syndrome is a common postoperative disorder that also needs to be kept in check via medial nutrition therapy.

Disorders/diseases of both the small and large intestines often require medical nutrition therapy. Flatulence is a common problem due to swallowing air while eating, bacterial fermentation of carbohydrates, or even decreased gastric motility, which may contribute to the problem. A common disorder among westerners is constipation, which can be minimized with appropriate lifestyle adjustments. A low-fiber diet may contribute to constipation and increasing dietary fiber is often used to alleviate constipation along with enhanced hydration. However, it is important to rule out other possible etiologies, such as neuromuscular disorders, interactions with other medications, and other diseases. Diarrhea, which often has a multitude of etiologies, often needs monitoring in order to prevent dehydration and significant loss of electrolytes. Inflammatory diseases or conditions, infections, medications, or increased osmotic pressure due to overconsumption of sugary foods can lead to diarrhea. On the other hand, malabsorption of nutrients, such as fat, leads to **steatorrhea**, or fatty stools.

Crohn's disease affects the distal part of the ileum and parts of the large intestine. **Ulcerative colitis** is most likely contained in the distal large intestine. Both of these diseases are **inflammatory bowel disease (IBD)**. Diarrhea and fever are common to both disorders and malnutrition is common. Crohn's disease is more difficult to manage and is lifelong compared with ulcerative colitis.

There are also a number of brush border diseases that affect the ability of nutrients to be absorbed from food. A good example is lactose intolerance, which leads to diarrhea due to increased osmotic pressure created by undigested lactose; and increased flatulence due to fermentation by bacteria.

Celiac sprue is another common gastrointestinal disorder. **Gluten-sensitive enteropathy** and **tropical sprue** are the two types. The former has gained wide attention in the development of gluten-free diets by eliminating certain grains such as wheat products from the diet. Tropical sprue appears to be geographically restricted and likely due to infectious agents compared with gluten-sensitive enteropathy. In both cases, diarrhea is common and loss of electrolytes and dehydration must be carefully monitored.

In addition to the issues above, there are a number of liver, gallbladder, and pancreatic disorders that have far-reaching nutrition implications. **Hepatitis**, whether viral (acute) or chronic, are serious diseases. Viruses A and E are infectious and common when there are fecal contaminants to food or liquids consumed. The other forms are spread by exchange of body fluids. Chronic hepatitis may be of an autoimmune origin or due to medicines or toxins. Nonalcoholic fatty liver disease may be classified into either **nonalcoholic fatty liver disease** or **nonalcoholic steatohepatitis**. Both of those disorders are characterized by the appearance of lipid droplets in the hepatocytes. Nonalcoholic fatty liver disease may be due to genetic anomalies, obesity, or diabetes. This can lead to cirrhosis, fibrosis, and liver cancer. Nonalcoholic steatohepatitis is similar in presentation but has much more fibrosis tissue. It is common that nonalcoholic fatty liver disease leads to nonalcoholic steatohepatitis.

The most common liver disease in the United States is **alcoholic liver disease**. In the metabolism of alcohol, acetaldehyde is produced as a byproduct, which results in significant toxicity to hepatocytes (See Chapter 5). Fat accumulation, inflammation, and, finally, liver cirrhosis are the stages of this disease. Regardless of what liver disease a person acquires, the most significant nutritional consequence is malnutrition. Diagnosing the disease and putting into place a Medical Nutrition Therapy plan is essential. Algorithms are available to help the dietitian develop a nutrition plan based on the liver disease.

The major gallbladder disease of nutrition consequence is **cholestasis**. Little or no bile is secreted. This is due to an obstruction. There are several types of cholestasis: **cholelithiasis**, **cholecystitis**, and **cholangitis**. Production of gall stones leads to cholelthiasis. Inflammation of the gallbladder is cholecystitis, and inflammation of the bile ducts is cholangitis.

Regarding the pancreas (exocrine), **pancreatitis** is the most common disorder. Chronic or severe pain may be present and can be severe enough to lead to vomiting. Medical Nutrition Therapy will depend on whether the condition is acute or chronic.

▶ Here's What You Have Learned

1. The digestive tract is a 6.5- to 8.5-meter (22- to 28-foot) tube that extends from the mouth to the anus, and the lumen is considered to be outside of the body. The wall of the digestive tract has several distinct layers composed of enterocytes, smooth muscle cells, neurons, and lymphatic cells

2. Several paracrine, endocrine, and exocrine tissues and organs support digestive activities, including the salivary glands, pancreas, liver, and gallbladder. The gastrointestinal system as a whole produces several liters of digestive juices daily

3. The three general phases of digestion are the cephalic, gastric, and intestinal phases. The cephalic phase occurs in the presence of the thought, smell, and taste of food. The gastric and intestinal phases are the result of distention of the stomach wall and mechanical and chemical events in the intestines

4. Digestion is a complex synergy of the physical actions of chewing, mixing, and moving and the chemical actions of saliva, enzymes, and emulsifiers. Digestion enables complex food systems and molecules to be simplified and reduced in size, allowing for efficient absorption

5. Absorption refers to the movement of nutrients from the digestive tract into the blood or lymphatic circulations, whereas the concept of bioavailability also includes the uptake and utilization of a nutrient by cells or tissue

6. Perceptions of hunger and satiety involve multiple hormonal and neurologic signals, including cholecystokinin, neuropeptide Y, ghrelin, insulin, and leptin. Despite a growing understanding of those signals, regulation of feeding is not enough to limit excessive weight gain

7. The pancreas produces and secretes more protein (protein per gram of tissue) than any other

organ. Digestive enzymes are produced and stored as inactive zymogen molecules to prevent digestion of the cells that produce them. En route to the small intestine, digestive enzymes mix with bile derived from the gallbladder and liver in the common bile duct

8. Bile is a watery composite of substances such as bile acids, bilirubin, cholesterol, fatty acids, phospholipids, electrolytes, and bicarbonate. During interdigestive periods, bile flow from the liver is routed primarily through the cystic duct into the gallbladder for concentration and storage. The remaining bile flows to the small intestine

9. The large intestine absorbs water and electrolytes from the entering content, which happens predominantly in the proximal half, and stores fecal matter until defecation, which occurs in the distal half

10. Different types of bacteria are found along the length of the digestive tract, depending on the environmental conditions of the segment and the properties of the bacterial species, with the highest concentration found in the colon. Many bacteria are considered supportive of human health in some manner and are referred to as probiotic. Some plant substances promote beneficial bacteria and decrease the growth of deleterious pathogens. These compounds are referred to as prebiotics

11. The lymphatic system is important in the absorption of lipids

12. Diseases of many types affect components of the gastrointestinal system. For many of these diseases, nutrition support is critical to the outcome and course of these diseases

▶ Suggested Reading

Blackshaw LA. New insights in the neural regulation of the lower oesophageal sphincter. *Eur Rev Med Pharmacol Sci.* 2008;12 (suppl 1):33–39.

Chandra R, Liddle RA. Neural and hormonal regulation of pancreatic secretion. *Curr Opin Gastroenterol.* 2009;25(5):441–446.

Ischia J, Patel O, Shulkes A, Baldwin GS. Gastrin-releasing peptide: different forms, different functions. *Biofactors.* 2009;35(1):69–75.

Magni P, Dozio E, Ruscica M, et al. Feeding behavior in mammals including humans. *Ann N Y Acad Sci.* 2009;1163:221–232.

Neary NM, Goldstone AP, Bloom SR. Appetite regulation: from the gut to the hypothalamus. *Clin Endocrinol (Oxford).* 2004;60(2):153–160.

Parahitiyawa NB, Scully C, Leung WK, Yam WC, Jin LJ, Samaranayake LP. Exploring the oral bacterial flora: current status and future directions. *Oral Dis.* 2010;16(2):136–145.

Saulnier DM, Kolida S, Gibson GR. Microbiology of the human intestinal tract and approaches for its dietary modulation. *Curr Pharm Des.* 2009;15(13):1403–1414.

Schubert ML. Gastric secretion. *Curr Opin Gastroenterol.* 2008; 24(6):659–664.

Wynne K, Stanley S, Bloom S. The gut and regulation of body weight. *J Clin Endocrinol Metab.* 2004;89(6):2576–2582.

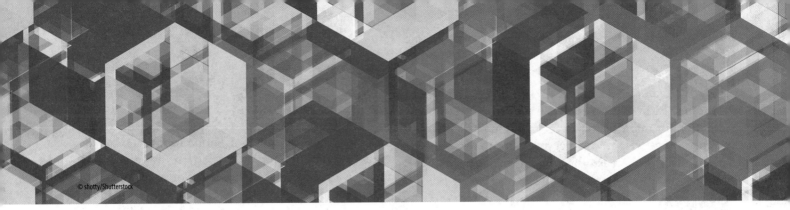

CHAPTER 3
Carbohydrates: Energy, Metabolism, and More

← HERE'S WHERE YOU HAVE BEEN

1. Digestion is a complex synergy of the physical actions of chewing, mixing, and moving and the chemical actions of saliva, enzymes, and emulsifiers.
2. Absorption refers to the movement of nutrients from the digestive tract into the blood or lymphatic circulations, whereas the concept of bioavailability also includes the uptake and use of a nutrient by cells or tissues.
3. Perceptions of hunger and satiety involve multiple hormonal and neurologic signals, including cholecystokinin, neuropeptide Y, ghrelin, obestatin, insulin, and leptin.
4. Different types of bacteria are found along the length of the digestive tract, depending on the environmental conditions of the segment and the properties of the bacterial species, with the highest concentration found in the colon.

HERE'S WHERE YOU ARE GOING →

1. Carbohydrates are a class of nutrients that includes sugars, starches, fibers, and related molecules, such as glycosaminoglycans, amino sugars, and more.
2. Key differences in covalent bonding make some carbohydrates more digestible than others.
3. Carbohydrates are absorbed as monosaccharides that circulate to tissue and are taken up by special glucose transporters.
4. Circulating glucose and stored glycogen are principal energy sources for most cells and tissue and are mandatory for others, such as red blood cells as well as the brain under normal conditions.
5. Carbohydrate metabolism is regulated by hormones such as insulin, epinephrine, glucagon, and cortisol.

▶ Introduction

How much carbohydrate and what type to eat is a consideration for many people as they plan their diet. For instance, some weight loss diet programs may restrict carbohydrates, whereas others may provide carbohydrates as more than 50% of total energy. Meanwhile, endurance athletes may derive a large portion of their total energy consumption from carbohydrates to optimize performance and recovery. Regardless, if an adult derives 50% of his or her dietary energy from carbohydrate, that would approximate half to total body carbohydrate content as a typical adult might have 350–500 grams total.

Although both myths and truths abound in relation to how much carbohydrate we need, it remains the greatest contributor to human energy intake, both in developed and underdeveloped countries worldwide. Moreover, the importance of carbohydrate is not limited simply to supplying energy. For instance, most dietary **fibers** are classified as carbohydrates. Although dietary fiber does indeed provide a limited amount of energy to the body, its role in digestive operations and disease prevention is much more significant. Meanwhile, carbohydrates, such as glycosaminoglycans, play structural roles, especially in connective tissue.

Because carbohydrate can be used for energy by all cells or be assimilated into energy stores or converted to other molecules, humans have several overlapping carbohydrate metabolic pathways, which also integrate with those for other nutrients, such as fatty acids and amino acids. This chapter describes and details the different types of carbohydrates and their properties, food sources, digestion, and metabolism.

▶ Carbohydrate Types and Characteristics

The term *carbohydrate* was coined long ago as scientists observed a consistent pattern in the chemical formula of most carbohydrates. Not only were they composed of only carbon, hydrogen, and oxygen, but also the ratio of carbon to water was typically one to one ($C:H_2O$). Thus, *carbohydrate* literally means "carbon with water." To create energy-providing carbohydrates from the non-energy-providing molecules H_2O and carbon dioxide (CO_2) is a talent bestowed only on plants and a select few microorganisms. In photosynthesis, plants couple H_2O and CO_2 by harnessing solar energy. Along with carbohydrates, molecular oxygen (O_2) is also a product of this reaction:

$$H_2O + CO_2 \xrightarrow{\text{Photosynthesis}} C_6H_{12}O_6 + O_2$$

Chemically, carbohydrates are defined as polyhydroxy aldehydes and ketones and their derivatives. Carbohydrates can vary from simpler three- to seven-carbon, single-unit molecules to very complex branching polymers. Although hundreds of different carbohydrates exist in nature, this text takes the simplest approach and groups them into just a few broad categories, namely, sugars (monosaccharides and disaccharides), oligosaccharides, and polysaccharides (**FIGURE 3.1**).

Monosaccharides

The **monosaccharides** that are relevant to human nutrition may be classified based on carbon number and may include the trioses, tetroses, pentoses, and hexoses. Both aldoses (aldehydes) and ketoses (ketones) are present (**FIGURE 3.2**). The six-carbon hexoses are the

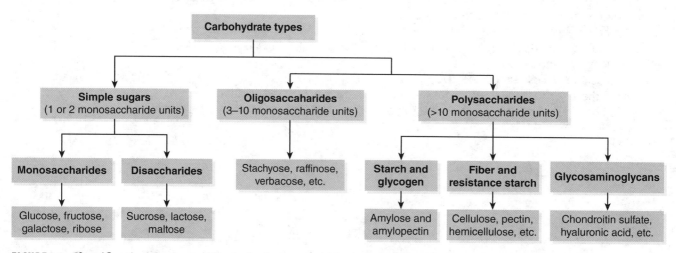

FIGURE 3.1 Classification System of Carbohydrates. Carbohydrates subclassified as sugars, oligosaccharides, and polysaccharides.

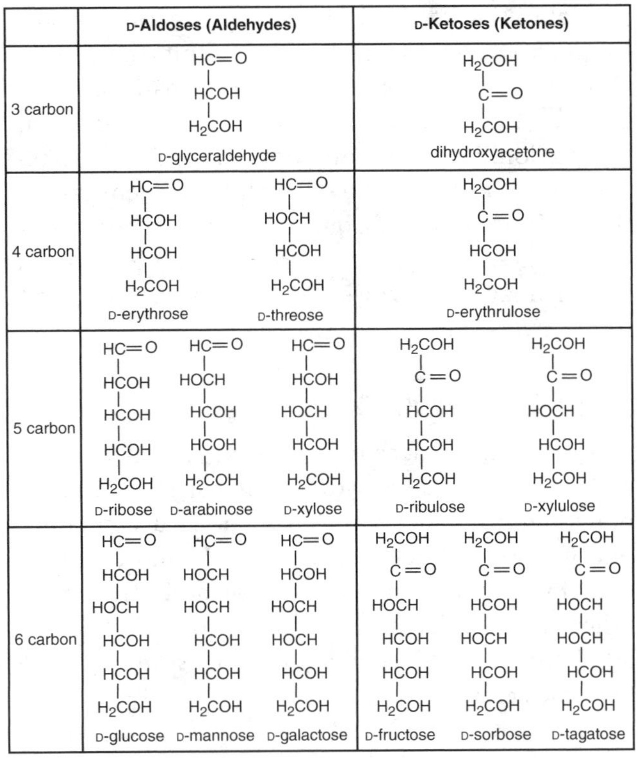

FIGURE 3.2 D-Aldoses and D-Ketones. Structures range from three to six carbons.

most common form of monosaccharides in the human diet. Those include glucose, galactose, and fructose. Glucose is the principal carbohydrate found in human circulation and is often referred to as blood sugar.

Three-carbon trioses, such as glyceraldehyde and dihydroxyacetone, are generally found as intermediary products of metabolic pathways (e.g., glycolysis). Four-carbon tetroses include erythrose, threose, and erythrulose. Five-carbon pentoses include the aldoses (xylose, ribose, and arabinose) and the ketoses (xylulose and ribulose). Of specific interest is ribose, which is a component of the nucleic acids (DNA and RNA); its alcohol derivative, ribitol, is found as a component of the water-soluble vitamin riboflavin. Also, **high-energy phosphate** compounds, such as adenosine triphosphate (ATP), adenosine diphosphate (ADP), and adenosine monophosphate (AMP), as well as dinucleotides, such as nicotinamide adenine dinucleotide (NAD) and nicotinamide adenine dinucleotide phosphate (NADP), all contain ribose as part of their chemical makeup. The other pentoses, especially xylose, are common in some fiber types, such as hemicellulose. **FIGURE 3.3** presents several of the more common monosaccharides.

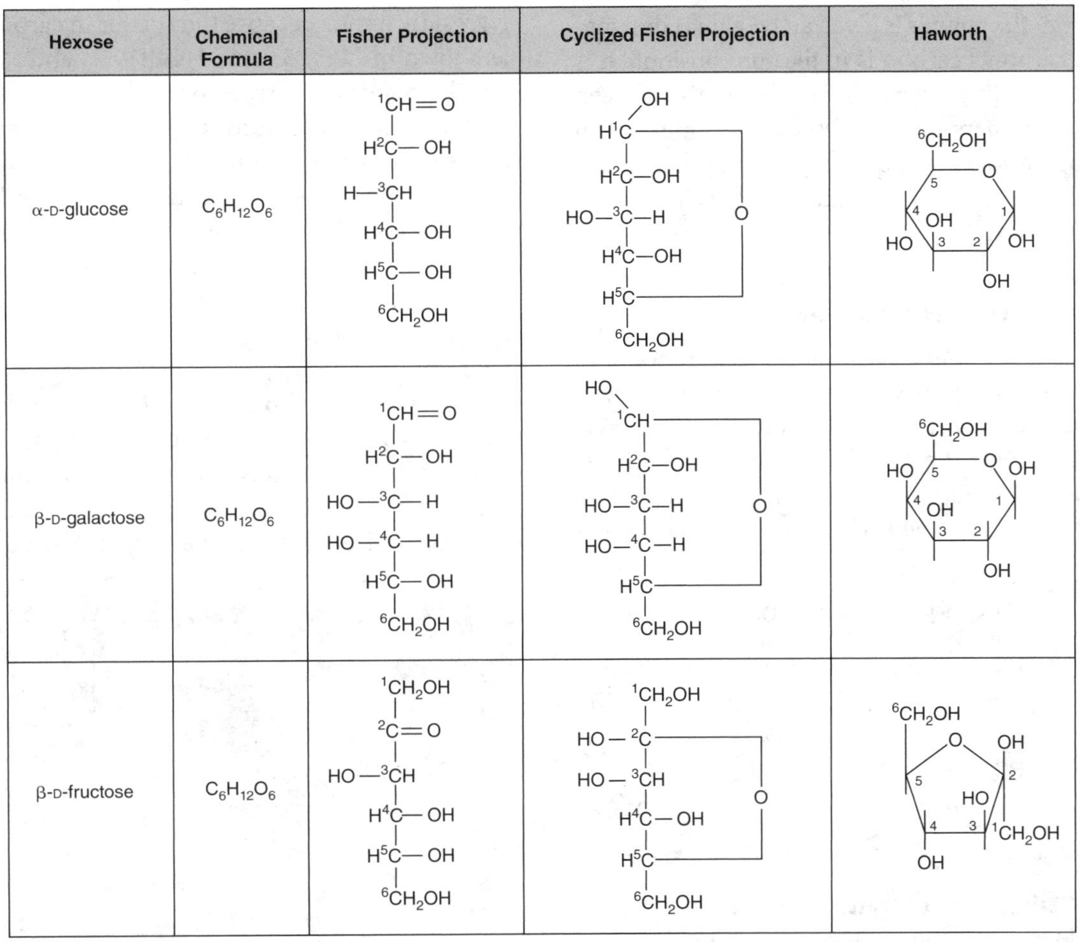

FIGURE 3.3 Basic Structures of Nutritionally Significant Monosaccharides. Note that different naming conventions and corresponding structures are presented.

Monosaccharide Structures

Although it is common to represent monosaccharides as straight-chain structures, in an aqueous environment there is a reaction between the aldehyde group (COOH) of carbon 1 and the hydroxyl group (OH) of carbon 5 (see Figure 3.3). That produces a hemiacetal group that allows for a cyclic structure, which naturally occurs almost all of the time. Many carbohydrates have the same chemical formula but vary in structure, making them isomers. For instance, **glucose**, **fructose**, **galactose**, and mannose have different structures but the same formula: $C_6H_{12}O_6$.

Monosaccharide epimers have differences in their configuration around only one carbon. A good example of this is the difference between glucose and galactose: their composition and molecular weights are the same, but the OH (hydroxyl) group on carbon 4 of the two compounds is different (**FIGURE 3.4**). In contrast, galactose and mannose are not epimers because they have differences in their OH positioning at two carbons. Another example of monosaccharide epimers is compounds with a difference in configuration around the carbonyl carbon; those are referred to as anomers. If the OH group around the carbonyl carbon is in the "down" position in a monosaccharide in the cyclic configuration, the epimer is given an α (alpha) designation. If the carbonyl carbon is in the "up" position, it is designated the β (beta) version. The difference between the α and β epimers becomes especially important in the bonding between monosaccharides and has a profound effect on the ability of human-produced enzymes to digest those carbohydrates.

Monosaccharide D and L Series

When looking at a monosaccharide as a straight chain, the position of the hydroxyl group on the asymmetric carbon farthest away from the carbonyl group (C=O) is used to designate the D and L isomer series. Specifically, if the OH group is on the right side, the monosaccharide is classified within the D series, as shown in Figure 3.4. If the OH group is on the left side, the monosaccharide is classified within the L series. One of the most important distinctions in nutrition between the D and L series is that the D isomers are the predominant naturally occurring form, whereas the L series isomers tend to result from chemical synthesis. Those types of isomers are often referred to as enantiomers, because the D and L molecules look like mirror images. Enzymes called racemases are able to interconvert between the two series.

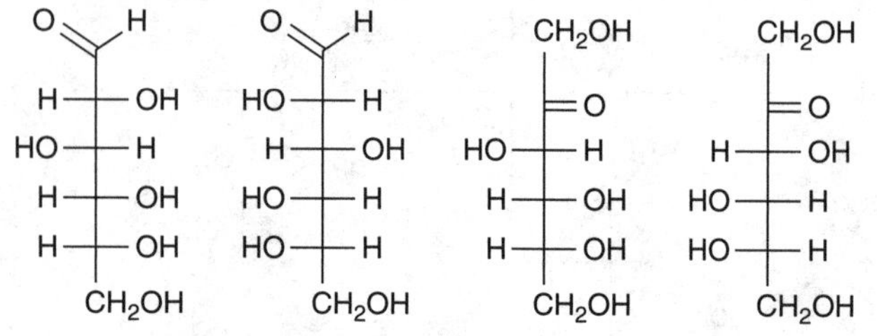

Monosaccharide Derivatives

Although monosaccharides are an important food and circulating carbohydrate, almost all of the carbohydrate present within cells—or as a component of cellular structure—is in the form of more complex carbohydrates and monosaccharide derivatives. Some other monosaccharide derivatives present within cells are amino sugars, acetyl amino sugars, uronic acids, glyconic acids, and sugar alcohols.

Disaccharides

Disaccharides are composed of two monosaccharides covalently linked by acetal (also known as *glyco*sidic bonds because they occur in carbohydrates), as shown in **TABLE 3.1** and **FIGURES 3.5** and **3.6**. The glycosidic bonds are formed between hydroxyl groups of adjacent monosaccharides, typically between carbon 1 and either carbon 4 or 6 in the polymer. Thus, specific bond designations, such as α1-4, α1-6, and β1-4, are used to describe the bond and explain the necessary specificity of disaccharidase enzymes.

The three most common disaccharides are sucrose, lactose, and maltose. **Sucrose**, which is composed of fructose and glucose, is commonly referred to as "cane sugar," "beet sugar," or "table sugar." **Lactose**, or "milk sugar," is composed of glucose and galactose; this sugar contributes energy to mammalian milk, aids in the absorption of calcium, and supports the growth of beneficial bacteria in the large intestine. **Maltose**

FIGURE 3.4 Carbohydrate D and L Isomers. Note the differences in the OH positions between the D and L isomers.

TABLE 3.1 Most Prevalent Food Disaccharides and Their Monosaccharide Building Blocks

Disaccharide	Monosaccharide
Lactose	Glucose + galactose
Sucrose	Glucose + fructose
Maltose	Glucose + glucose

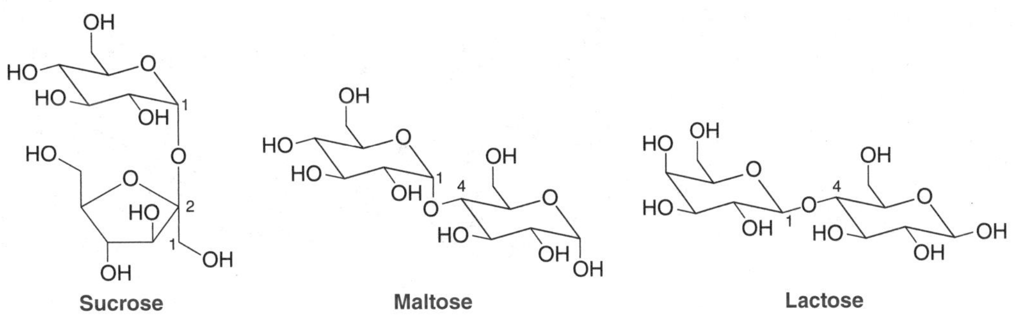

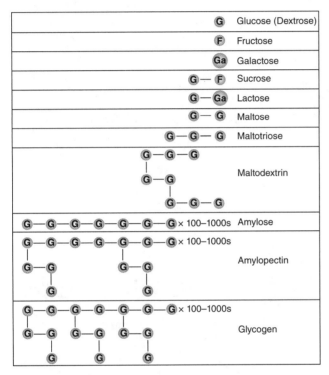

FIGURE 3.5 Common Disaccharides. Sucrose is consumed in the greatest amount of the above disaccharides. Lactose is the second most common disaccharide in diets.

FIGURE 3.6 Overview of Carbohydrate and Monosaccharide Building Blocks. Note that the monosaccharides are the basic building blocks that compose disaccharides, and the more complex carbohydrates in this schematic.

is composed of two glucose units. Maltose is found only for a brief time in the life of a plant, usually in the seed; however, it is also an intermediate product of the digestion of more complex carbohydrates (starch) in the gut as well as the partial hydrolysis of starch in ingredient processing and production of some foods, such as beer and malt liquors.

Of the disaccharides mentioned previously, only lactose is derived from animals. The remaining two disaccharides are derived from plants. The term *sugar* is often applied to monosaccharides and disaccharides. Those carbohydrates have a sweet taste, with

fructose being the sweetest. **TABLE 3.2** presents the relative sweetness of the sugars, along with high-intensity sweeteners, such as stevia and sucralose.

Polysaccharides

Polysaccharides are composed of repeating monosaccharide units, most commonly glucose (see Figure 3.6). Although their length may vary, they are rather long, and the covalent bonds in the primary structure are found between carbons 1 and 4. For branched polysaccharides, a bond is typically found between carbons 1 and 6 if hexoses are the monosaccharides involved. Those bond types are depicted in **FIGURE 3.7**. The position of the bonds, known as either the α or β configuration, determines the properties and digestive fate of those compounds because of the ability of digestive enzymes to recognize only a particular configuration. There are several types of polysaccharides, which are simplified here into several categories: oligosaccharides, starch, glycogen, glycosaminoglycans, and fiber (see Figure 3.1).

Oligosaccharides

Oligosaccharides are composed of 3 to 10 monosaccharides linked by glycosidic bonds between the OH groups of adjacent monomeric units (see Figure 3.7). Stachyose, verbascose, and raffinose are oligosaccharides whose metabolic fate is somewhat different from other oligosaccharides in that they are primarily fermented by bacteria in the colon. This property has resulted in their claim to fame as flatulence producers. Legumes (beans) have appreciable levels of those oligosaccharides.

Plant Starch

One of the most common polysaccharides on the planet is starch, which serves primarily as a storage form of carbohydrate in plants. Starch can be one long

TABLE 3.2 Sweetness of Sugars and Alternative Sweeteners

Type of Sweetener	Relative Sweetness Compared with Sucrose (Table Sugar)	Typical Dietary Sources
Sugars		
Lactose	0.2	Dairy
Maltose	0.4	Sprouted seeds
Glucose	0.7–0.8	Corn syrup, fruits
Sucrose	1.0	Table sugar, fruits
Fructose	1.4	Fruits, honey
HFCS[a]	1.2–1.6	Soft drinks, beverages
Sugar alcohols		
Sorbitol	60	Dietetic candies, sugarless gum
Mannitol	70	Dietetic candies
Erythritol	70	Sugarless candies, supplements, sweetener
Xylitol	90	Sugarless gum
High-Intensity Sweeteners		
Stevia	300	Sweetener used in tabletop packs and in foods and supplements
Aspartame (NutraSweet)	180	Diet soft drinks and fruit drinks, powdered sweetener
Acesulfame Potassium (AceK)	200	Sugarless gum, diet drink mixes, powdered sweetener, gelatins and puddings
Saccharin	300	Diet soft drinks, powdered sweetener
Sucralose	600	Beverages, baked goods, candies, breakfast, and protein bars

[a]HFCS, high-fructose corn syrup.

chain or it can be branched. Starch is referred to as a homopolysaccharide because it contains only glucose monomers linked via α1-4 and α1-6 glycosidic linkages. Starch is also referred to as a glucan because it only yields glucose when it is broken down.

Amylose is a straight-chain glucose polymer with α1-4 linkages (see Figure 3.7). It is present as a helical coil and forms hydrated micelles. Meanwhile, **amylopectin** is a branched-chain polymer, as shown in Figure 3.7. The α1-6 branches occur approximately

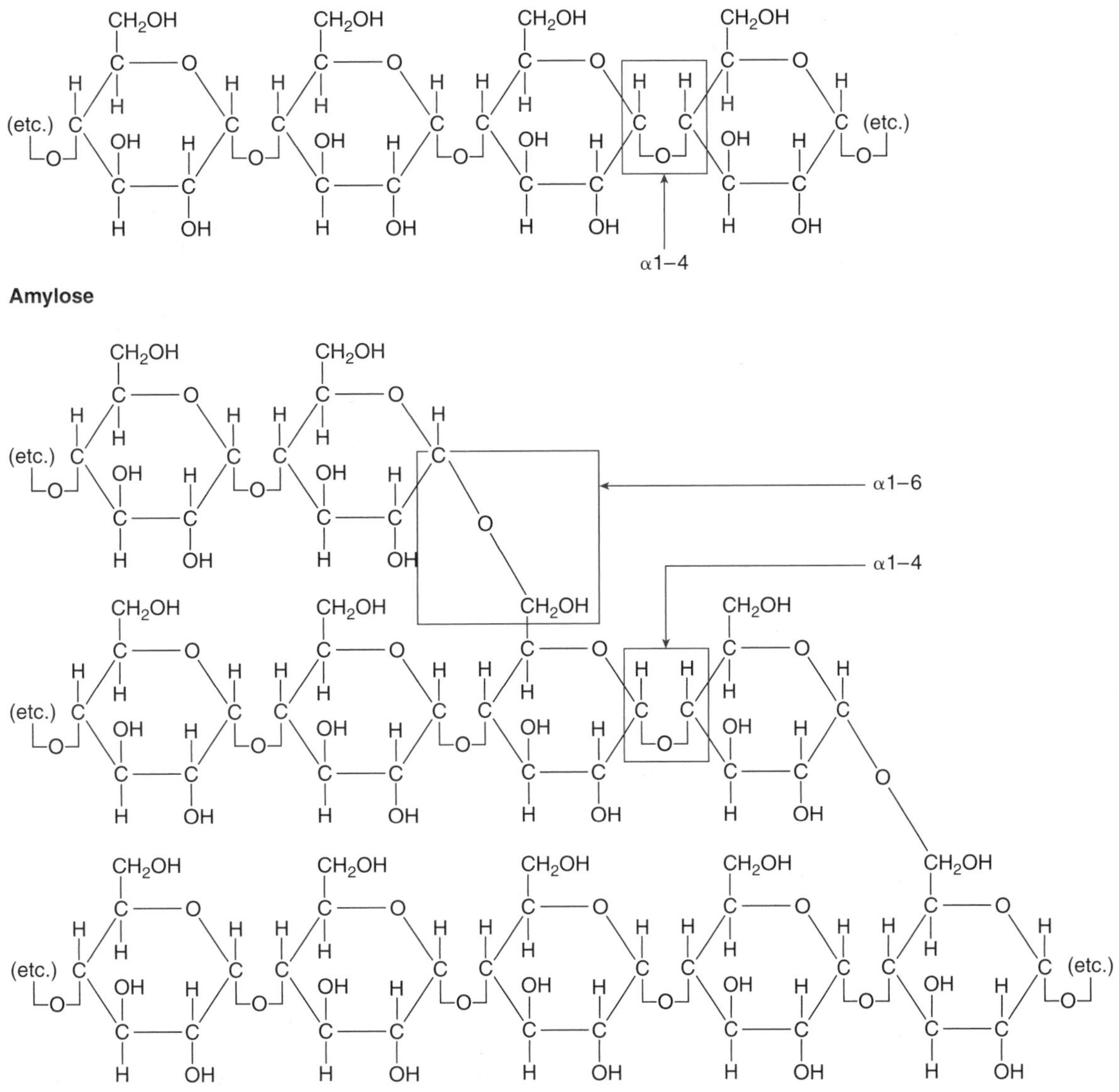

FIGURE 3.7 Structure of Common Starches. α1-4 and α1-6 links between glucose of starch components such as amylopectin.

every 24 to 30 glucose monomers. All other bonds between glucose monomers are α1-4 links; however, because of branching, amylopectin does not coil effectively and tends to form colloidal suspensions in water.

Animal Glycogen

Glycogen in animal tissue is also a homopolysaccharide. It is often referred to as "animal starch" because it contains repeating glucose units. However, glycogen differs from starch in that the branching occurs every 8 to 12 residues. Glycogen is a large branched polymer consisting of D-glucose linked by α1-4 bonds in straight portions and α1-6 linkages at branch points (**FIGURE 3.8**). Glycogen from animal flesh is not a significant source of dietary carbohydrate because it is depleted shortly after slaughter.

However, it is very important as a carbohydrate storage form, particularly in the liver and muscle tissue. The glycogen concentration is 1 to 2% of skeletal muscle, and it can reach up to 8 to 10% of the weight of the liver. Meanwhile, adipose tissue is less than 1% glycogen by weight.

Glycosaminoglycans

Another class of polysaccharides is the **glycosaminoglycans**, which are sometimes called mucopolysaccharides. Glycosaminoglycans are characterized by their content of amino sugars and uronic acids, which occur in combination with proteins in body secretions and structures. Those polysaccharides are responsible for the viscosity of body mucous secretions. They are components of extracellular amorphous ground

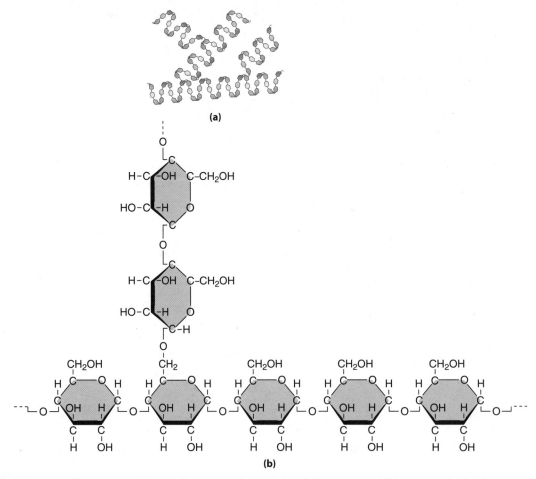

FIGURE 3.8 Animal Starch, Glycogen. (a) Three-dimensional structure of glycogen and (b) α1-4 and α1-6 linkages between glucose residues in glycogen.

substances surrounding collagen and elastin fibers and cells of connective tissues and bone. Those molecules hold onto large amounts of water and occupy space, which allows for some cushioning and lubrication. Some examples of glycosaminoglycans are hyaluronic acid and chondroitin sulfate.

Dietary Fiber

Dietary fiber is plant material, both polysaccharide and lignin, that is resistant to human digestive enzymes. Another descriptor used for those molecules is nonstarch polysaccharides (NSPs); however, this categorization would not include lignin. Dietary fiber has long been classified as either soluble or insoluble, based on its propensity to dissolve in water. Soluble fibers include pectin (pectic substances), gums, and mucilages. Insoluble fibers are composed of cellulose, hemicellulose, lignin, and modified cellulose. In addition, some fibers have been grouped together as functional fibers based on whether they have been isolated, extracted, or manufactured and potentially promote health when

consumed regularly and at efficacious levels. More recently, the classification of fibers has shifted to either dietary fiber or functional fiber, as described in Chapter 4.

● BEFORE YOU GO ON . . .

1. What are the key differences between monosaccharides, disaccharides, and polysaccharides?
2. Which monosaccharides are found in the different disaccharides, oligosaccharides, and starch?
3. How does plant starch differ from animal glycogen, and why is this important?
4. What is the nature of the links (chemical bonds) between monosaccharides in disaccharides and polysaccharides, and why is this significant?
5. What are glycosaminoglycans, and where are they found in the human body and in other life forms?

▶ Carbohydrate Intake, Food Sources, and Recommendations

Carbohydrate consumption has become one of the principal dietary issues for many people, ranging from athletes to people trying to lose weight or to control blood sugar levels. Carbohydrate in the form of glucose serves as the most basic energy source for all cells in the body. Foods high in carbohydrates include breads, pastas, potatoes, rice, and fruits. Legumes are also a good source of carbohydrate. Legumes are plants that have a single row of seeds in their pods. The foods commonly called legumes, such as peas, green beans, lima beans, pinto beans, black-eyed peas, garbanzo beans (chick peas), lentils, and soybeans, are often the seeds of legume plants. Dairy foods and vegetables are also good sources of carbohydrates, whereas meats, eggs, and plant oils are not.

Carbohydrate Consumption

During preagricultural times, carbohydrate intake largely came by way of fruits, vegetables, leaves, and tubers. Today, industrial processing has increased the consumption of cereal grains, especially milled grains, as well as refined sugar cane through the mass production of sucrose (table sugar). Within many developed countries, the 20th century heralded changes in the types of carbohydrates consumed as well as carbohydrate's contribution to total energy intake. In the United States, carbohydrate consumption was approximately 500 grams daily at the beginning of the 20th century; it declined to 374 grams in the 1960s largely because of a decrease in consumption of cereal grains. From there, carbohydrate consumption increased steadily during the last four decades of the 20th century to about the same level as seen nearly 100 years earlier. However, much of the carbohydrate that returned to the diet was in the form of refined carbohydrates, such as sugary products, and thus, was lacking fiber and many other beneficial nutrients. Today, the caloric contribution of carbohydrate to the adult diet is roughly 50% and is derived from a variety of foods. **TABLE 3.3** lists the general carbohydrate content (by weight) of select foods.

Monosaccharides and Disaccharides

Glucose is found in some foods in a free form, especially in ripening fruits and vegetables, although the majority of the glucose in the human diet is derived from the digestion of disaccharides and starch.

TABLE 3.3 Carbohydrate Content of Select Foods[a]	
Food	**Carbohydrate (%)**
Table sugar	>98[b]
Ice cream, cake, pie	20–40
Fruits–vegetables	5–20
Nuts	10–15
Peanut butter	~20
Milk	5
Cheese	2–5
Shellfish (e.g., crab, lobster)	<1
Fish	<1
Butter	0
Oil	0

[a]Percentage based on weight.
[b]Most remaining mass is moisture.

Galactose is also found free in some foods, but to a relatively small degree. Most of the galactose in the human diet is derived from the digestion of the disaccharide lactose, which is found in milk and dairy foods. Fructose is found naturally in fruits and honey and is also derived from the disaccharide sucrose.

Fruits may be somewhat deceiving; according to Table 3.3, their carbohydrate content is roughly 5 to 20%. However, because water makes up most of the remaining weight, carbohydrate is the major nonwater content of fruits. Cereal grains and products such as rice, oats, pastas, and breads also have a relatively high carbohydrate content, whereas animal foods, such as meats, fish, and poultry (and eggs) contain very little. Animal flesh (skeletal muscle) does contain a little carbohydrate, primarily as glycogen; however, this is lost during the processing of the meat. Milk and some dairy products (e.g., yogurt, ice cream) are the only significant animal-derived sources of carbohydrate.

Ripened fruits contain mostly monosaccharides and disaccharides, namely, fructose and glucose, as well as some sucrose. For example, a medium apple contains about 8 grams of fructose and 3 grams of both glucose and sucrose. Meanwhile, a medium banana contains between 5 and 6 grams of both fructose and glucose and 2 grams of sucrose. One tablespoon of honey contains 8 grams of fructose and 7 grams of glucose and less than 1 gram of sucrose, galactose, and maltose combined.

Added Sugars and Caloric Sweeteners

Caloric sweeteners and added sugars are used synonymously and will be considered as such on food labels with the next FDA labeling mandates. First and foremost, as recipe ingredients, they are used as a sweetener although there can be secondary roles. Specific examples of added sugars that can be listed as an ingredient include brown sugar, corn sweetener, corn syrup, dextrose, fructose, glucose, **high-fructose corn syrup (HFCS)**, honey, invert sugar, lactose, malt syrup, maltose, molasses, raw sugar, sucrose, trehalose, and turbinado sugar (sugar in the raw). Naturally occurring sugars, such as those in fruit or milk, are not added sugars. The U.S. Department of Agriculture (USDA) estimated that the consumption of caloric sweeteners at 153 pounds per adult at the turn of the 21st century. Added sugar can be considered the number one food additive; it is found in many foods, such as pizza, bread, hot dogs, boxed mixed rice, soup, crackers, spaghetti sauce, lunch meat, canned vegetables, fruit drinks, flavored yogurt, ketchup, salad dressing, mayonnaise, and some peanut butters. Carbonated sodas provided more than one-fifth (22%) of the added sugars in the American food supply in 2000, compared with 16% in 1970. Fructose is also provided in the human diet in the form of the popular food sweetening agent HFCS, which tends to be more than 60% fructose. As dietary consumption of fructose has increased over the past several decades there is growing concern that higher consumption of fructose might be partly responsible for the increasing incidence of obesity worldwide.

Cereal Grains

Grains are among the richest sources of starch, as are legumes. In cereal grains, most of the starch is found within the endosperm compartment, as depicted in **FIGURE 3.9**. Approximately 15 to 20% of the starch in the American diet is attributed to amylose. Amylopectin constitutes approximately 80 to 85% of the starch in the American diet. As mentioned previously, the level of consumption of cereal grains decreased in the 20th century.

Fiber

The amount of fiber present within the human diet can vary geographically as well as by gender. In some

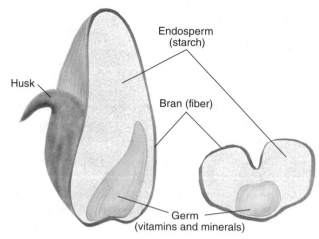

FIGURE 3.9 Structure of a Grain of Wheat. Some of the major nutrients found in different regions are indicated.

developed countries, such as the United States, fiber consumption is relatively lower than in other societies. The mean dietary fiber intake of all individuals 2 years and older, excluding breastfed children, was 16 grams per day. Intakes of males and females were 18 and 15 grams per day, respectively, which is well below recommendations. Americans consume a diet in which less than one-half of their carbohydrate intake comes from fruits, vegetables, and whole grains.

Carbohydrate Recommendations

As part of the Dietary Reference Intakes (DRIs), the Acceptable Macronutrient Distribution Range (AMDR) for carbohydrate intake in the United States and Canada is 45 to 65% of total energy. The range allows for different people to plan their dietary carbohydrate level based on different lifestyles and ability to metabolize food carbohydrates. Individuals are also advised to derive more of the carbohydrate they consume from more nutrient-dense sources, such as whole grain products, legumes, lower-fat dairy foods, and fruits and vegetables. Those foods provide vitamins, minerals, fiber, and **phytochemicals** that promote health and wellness.

The DRI for carbohydrate energy has been set at 130 grams per day for all people older than 1 year. This would provide 520 calories of energy, which is important to the central nervous system, red blood cells, and other tissue dependent on glucose as its primary energy source. The DRI for carbohydrate energy would be adequate to prevent **ketosis** in most people. It is important to note that the DRI recommendation does not take into consideration exercise and the additional calorie needs of working muscle.

The Dietary Guidelines for Americans 2015–2020 recommend that people consume less than 10% of calories per day from added sugars. The World Health Organization (WHO) has recently lowered its added sugar ceiling recommendation from 10 to 5%. Meanwhile, the American Heart Association (AHA) recommends limiting the amount of added sugars consumed to no more than half of daily discretionary calorie allowance. For most American women, that's no more than 100 calories per day, or about 6 teaspoons of sugar. For men, it's 150 calories per day, or about 9 teaspoons.

Dietary Fiber

The current Adequate Intake (AI) recommendation for total fiber intake for adults who are 50 years old and younger is 38 grams per day for men and 25 grams per day for women. For adults older than 50 years, the recommendation is 30 grams per day for men and 21 grams per day for women, or 14 grams per 1000 calories consumed. Meanwhile, WHO recommends 25 to 40 grams of fiber daily for adults. The Dietary Guidelines for American 2015–2020 set a goal of 14 grams/1000 calories, which ranges from 25 to 34 grams for adults with attention to achieving goals largely through fiber-dense foods, such as vegetables, fruits, whole grains, legumes, etc.

◆ BEFORE YOU GO ON . . .

1. How has the intake of carbohydrate changed over the last 100 years, and what are the current trends?

2. Which foods provide different types of carbohydrates, and how much carbohydrate do they contain?

3. What is the current recommended limit for added sugar, and what types of foods contain it?

4. What is the AMDR for carbohydrate intake in the United States and Canada, and how could it be applied to different people?

5. How does the average intake of fiber by American adults compare with recommendations, and what impact might that have on health?

▶ Carbohydrate Digestion and Absorption

The objective of carbohydrate digestion is to liberate monosaccharides from disaccharides and more complex polymers. This activity begins in the mouth because salivary secretions contain an amylase enzyme. The digestive impact of salivary amylase is short-lived, yet significant. After oral contents are swallowed, they traverse the esophagus and depot in the stomach. The optimal pH range for amylase activity is approximately 6.6 to 6.8. Therefore, once the swallowed contents are thoroughly mixed with the highly acidic gastric juice, amylase activity ceases. Virtually no carbohydrate digestion occurs in the gastric juice. Although some acid hydrolysis of sucrose may occur, it is not considered physiologically significant. Carbohydrate digestion picks up in the small and large intestines, with most of the monosaccharides being absorbed in the small intestine. **FIGURE 3.10** provides an overview of the carbohydrate digestion events taking place in the different parts of the digestive tract.

Starch and Disaccharides

The major carbohydrate digestive enzyme in the small intestine is α-amylase, which is secreted by acinar cells of the pancreas. Both salivary and pancreatic amylase hydrolyze the α1-4 glycosidic linkages, such that the starch consumed in a diet, is converted sequentially to maltose, maltotrioses, α-dextrins, and some trace glucose. With respect to branched starch, a mixture of dextrins is generated, averaging six glucose residues per molecule and containing α1-6 linkages. These linkages are hydrolyzed by a brush border enzyme, referred to as α-dextrinase or isomaltase.

The reaction that breaks down starch into α-dextrins, maltose, and maltotrioses occurs in the intestinal lumen. The remainder of carbohydrate digestion is believed to occur along the intestinal surface. When the sugars are hydrolyzed to monosaccharides, the products are, therefore, in close proximity to the transport proteins. Enterocytes lining the villi of the small intestine contain disaccharidases, namely **maltase**, **lactase**, and **sucrase**, as well as α-dextrinase. Those enzymes are associated with microvilli plasma membranes, as shown in **FIGURE 3.11**.

Disaccharidases may not always be present in sufficient amounts to handle the digestion of disaccharides in the gut. This leads to an accumulation of the undigested disaccharide and the potential for disaccharide intolerance, with symptoms including diarrhea resulting from the increased osmotic pressure in the lumen of the gut. Furthermore, bacterial fermentation of the disaccharides can result in common symptoms, such as flatulence, nausea, and bloating. This is the case with lactose intolerance (see **SPECIAL FEATURE 3.1**).

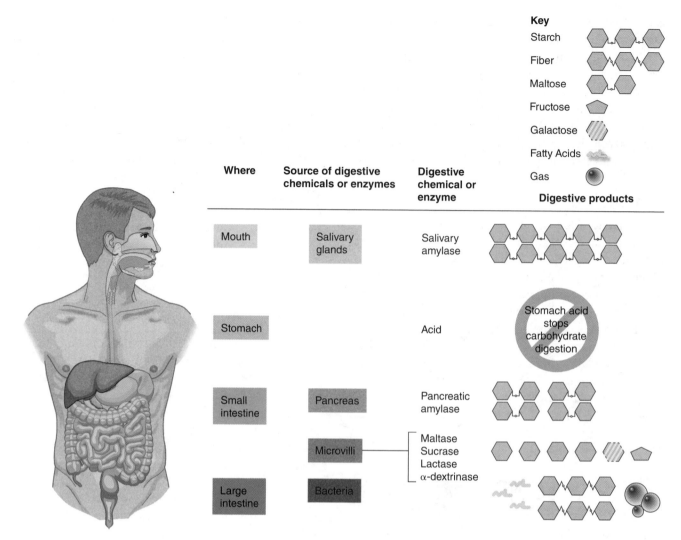

FIGURE 3.10 Carbohydrate Digestion. Key events involved in carbohydrate digestion in different parts of the digestive tract.

Absorption of Monosaccharides

The absorptive cells of the small intestinal lining absorb some hexoses at a greater rate than others. Galactose and glucose are known to be actively absorbed against a concentration gradient, whereas others, such as fructose, are not (see Figure 3.11). Apparently, the basic requirement for active transport is based on the presence of the six-carbon structure and an intact OH group at position 2. Oxygen and sodium are required, and selective metabolic inhibitors can block the active transport. Absorption takes place against a concentration gradient, and the transport is selective, with some sugars transported at a greater rate than others. With glucose transport serving as the reference standard (1.0), the rate of galactose transport appears to be slightly greater (1.1), whereas the transport rates of fructose (0.4), mannose (0.2), xylose (0.15), and arabinose (0.10) are lower.

Glucose and galactose seem to compete with one another for absorption aboard a common transporter called SGLT1 (**S**odium/**Gl**ucose co**T**ransporter 1). As mentioned, both of those monosaccharides are absorbed by active transport, as will be discussed soon. However, fructose is absorbed by facilitative diffusion utilizing **Glucose Transporter 5 (GLUT5)**. Thus, fructose needs to bind to a membrane protein carrier, as well as move down a concentration gradient. Mannose, xylose, and arabinose are also absorbed by passive diffusion.

SGLT1, sodium, and energy in the form of ATP are required for active transport of glucose and galactose. The sodium-gradient hypothesis states that glucose or galactose will associate with SGLT1 on the microvilli membrane, which also has a binding site for sodium (see Figure 3.11). The energy released by sodium moving down its concentration gradient into the cell is sufficient to also move glucose into the cell against its concentration gradient. Sodium is subsequently pumped out of the cell by ATPase to maintain the gradient. Two sodium ions are required for each monosaccharide transported.

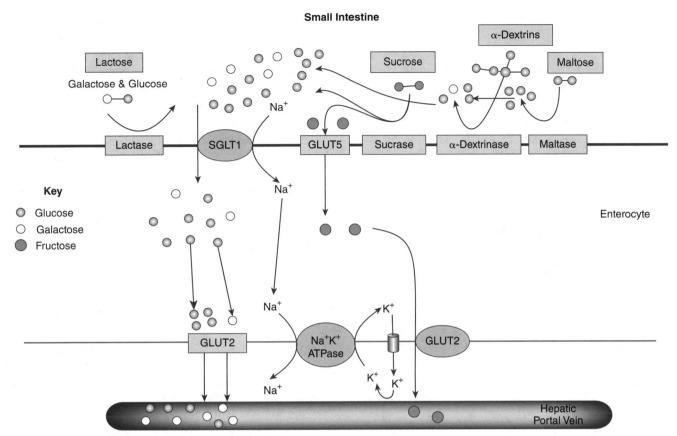

FIGURE 3.11 Absorption of Glucose and Galactose Across the Small Intestinal Mucosa. Both glucose and galactose bind to a transmembrane protein (SGLT1) that also binds to sodium. The energy from sodium moving down its concentration gradient is sufficient to transport glucose into the cell against its concentration gradient. Sodium is then pumped out of the cell by adenosine triphosphatase (ATPase).

SPECIAL FEATURE 3.1

Lactose Intolerance

Any medical situation that damages the intestinal mucosa by preventing cell proliferation of the enterocytes, such as protein energy malnutrition or celiac disease, can produce a brush border enzyme deficiency. The most well-known and widespread disaccharidase deficiency condition is lactase deficiency, which produces lactose intolerance. Lactase deficiency has been reported in approximately 55% of Mexican-American males, 74% of adult Mexicans from rural Mexico, 45% of Greeks, 56% of Cretans, 66% of Greek Cypriots, 68.8% of Jewish individuals living in North America, 50% of Indian adults and 20% of Indian children, 45% of African-American children, and 80% of Alaskan Eskimos. Caucasians and those of Scandinavian descent normally have a lower prevalence of lactose intolerance than Asian adults. Based on those estimates, one can argue that there are more individuals who are lactose intolerant than lactose tolerant.

Lactase begins to be synthesized in fetal life and is at its maximal activity at birth. At the time of weaning, lactase activity may have dropped to about 90% of the level of activity at birth. The decline in lactase activity is not a function of lactose in the diet, as was once popularly believed. It is more likely a genetically controlled event. Individuals who are tolerant are thought to have inherited the gene as a dominant gene from a genetic mutation. Those individuals who have the enzyme are descendants of some African and Middle Eastern tribes and Northern Europeans. Also, the genetic adaptation is thought to be related to the development of dairy farming in these regions.

Despite the problem of lactose intolerance, milk consumption need not be discouraged in susceptible populations. In most studies, 250 milliliters (approximately 1 cup) of milk, which normally contains 12 grams of lactose, does not cause adverse effects. Furthermore, recent research studies collapsing data from several studies suggest that almost all lactose intolerant people tend to tolerate 12 g of lactose in one meal or snack and approximately 18 g of lactose over the entire day. The drinking of milk by children should not be discouraged unless it causes severe diarrhea. Dairy products in which the lactose is prehydrolyzed or in which *Lactobacillus acidophilus* was added during processing to hydrolyze the lactose are available. Lactase enzyme tablets can also be added to milk to help digest the lactose. Fermented foods, such as yogurt, have bacteria that can digest lactose. Foods, such as cottage cheese and aged cheddar cheese, contain low levels of lactose and are not likely to produce problems.

Once inside the cell, 15% of the monosaccharides leak back out through the brush border, 25% diffuse through the basolateral membrane, and 60% leave on the serosal side through a carrier mechanism; all of those mechanisms are independent of sodium. Because of those multiple exit avenues, monosaccharides such as glucose and galactose do not accumulate within enterocytes at significant levels. Most of the absorption of monosaccharides occurs in the upper portion of the small intestine. The trioses and tetrasaccharides are absorbed through passive diffusion.

⬢ BEFORE YOU GO ON . . .

1. Where are the primary locations of carbohydrate digestion and absorption?
2. What are the key carbohydrate digestion enzymes, and where are they produced?
3. What are the key mechanisms involved in the absorption of monosaccharides?
4. What is the cause of lactose intolerance?
5. What makes fructose different from glucose and galactose with regard to the mechanism of absorption?

▶ Carbohydrate Circulation and Cellular Uptake

All cells can use glucose for energy purposes. This means that glucose must have a means of crossing the plasma membrane. Also, because carbohydrate can be used as an immediate source of energy, stored as glycogen or fat, or used to make certain amino acids or other molecules, several factors must direct its use inside of cells. This section provides an overview of the major metabolic pathways involved in carbohydrate metabolism.

Blood Glucose Regulation

Glucose must continually circulate in the blood in order to serve as a fuel resource for cells. A blood glucose concentration of 70 to 110 milligrams per 100 milliliters is typical in a fasting state. This would equate to roughly 5 grams of glucose in circulation given a total blood volume of 5.5 liters. However, the level of circulating glucose can increase after eating a meal or decrease during fasting based on changes in supply and demand. Several hormones are employed to control blood glucose levels, with the most significant being insulin, glucagon, epinephrine, and cortisol.

Insulin promotes cellular events that work to lower blood glucose level when it is elevated (**hyperglycemia**). Meanwhile, glucagon, epinephrine, and cortisol coordinate tissue operations in an attempt to raise blood glucose level when it declines (**hypoglycemia**), such as during fasting and times of increased glucose demand (e.g., exercise, stress). By and large, those hormones and other factors control blood glucose levels by regulating metabolic pathways involved in glycogen production and breakdown, glucose use for energy and glucose production from other energy molecules. The term **euglycemia** is used to denote the achievement and maintenance of an optimal fasting blood glucose level despite changing nutrition and metabolic states.

Glycemic Index

Glycemic index has become an important concept in general nutrition. Simply put, **glycemic response** refers to the degree and duration to which blood glucose level is elevated after consuming a portion of food that would provide 50 grams of digestible (available) carbohydrates and measured (the area under the curve [AUC]) for the next 2 hours following the meal (**FIGURE 3.12**). The **glycemic index** of a food is simply the comparison of its glycemic response to a food standard based on studies of healthy people. Glucose and white bread are used as the standards. For instance, if a food raises blood glucose level to 50% of the rise caused by glucose, the glycemic index of that food is 50. **TABLE 3.4** lists the glycemic index of several foods.

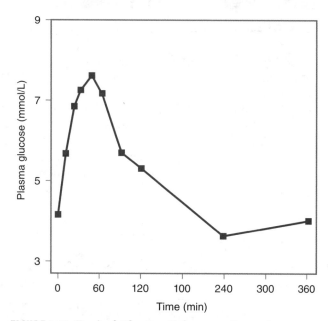

FIGURE 3.12 Typical Glucose Tolerance Curve to Measure Glycemic Response. The area under the curve (AUC) represents the rise and subsequent lowering of blood glucose levels by insulin and tissue processing after consuming a 50-gram glucose source.

TABLE 3.4 Glycemic Index and Glycemic Load Levels

Level	Glycemic Index	Glycemic Load	Glycemic Load/Day
Low	≤55	≤10	<80
Medium	56–69	11–19	80–120
High	≥70	≥20	>120

Food	Glycemic Index	Glycemic Load	Food	Glycemic Index	Glycemic Load
All-bran cereal	42	8	Peanuts	14	1
Apple juice	40	11	Pears	38	4
Apples	38	6	Pineapple	59	7
Bananas	52	12	Pinto beans	39	10
Beets	64	5	Popcorn	72	8
Buckwheat	54	16	Potatoes (new)	57	12
Cantaloupe	65	4	Potatoes (Russet, baked)	85	26
Carrots	47	3	Rice, white	64	23
Cheerios cereal	74	15	Rice, wild	57	18
Corn Flakes cereal	81	21	Sourdough wheat bread	54	15
Couscous	65	23	Spaghetti	42	20
Fettuccini	40	18	Strawberries	40	1
Grapes	46	8	Sucrose (table sugar)	68	7
Green peas	48	3	Shredded Wheat cereal	67	13
Kidney beans	28	7	Sweet corn	54	9
Life cereal	66	16	Sweet potatoes	61	17
Linguine	52	23	Watermelon	72	4
Macaroni	47	23	Whole wheat flour bread	71	9
Navy beans	38	12	White wheat flour bread	70	10

Because there are obvious differences between white bread and pure glucose, glycemic indexes determined for foods using those different standards can vary. The glycemic index scale is 0 to 100 when using glucose as the standard; this scale is more common because it is easier to understand and apply. Meanwhile, when white bread is used as the standard, the scale can be a little less user-friendly, because some foods, such as baked potatoes, rice cakes, and many breakfast cereals, will have a glycemic index exceeding 100.

The glycemic index of a food is influenced by several factors, including carbohydrate type and other nutrients that can influence rate of digestion or absorption. Because only half of the monosaccharide units in lactose and sucrose are glucose, whereas all of the monosaccharides in starch are glucose, this suggests that "starchy" foods, such as a baked potato, might have a higher glycemic index than milk and dairy foods and many "sugary" foods, such as candies. Fruits and honey with high fructose content only have a moderate impact on blood glucose. Meanwhile, the level of protein, fat, and fiber in a food can lower the glycemic index of a food by slowing the rate of digestion and absorption of monosaccharides. If monosaccharides are absorbed more slowly, there is more opportunity for the liver to remove them before they reach the general circulation. This helps explain why whole wheat bread can have a lower glycemic index than white bread.

Glycemic Load

The concept of glycemic index is simple to grasp; however, it is not always easy to apply to how people tend to eat. One issue with glycemic index is that the amount of food used to determine it is not the amount typically consumed by people. For instance, boiled carrots have a glycemic index of about 90; however, it would take over 10 cups of carrots to achieve the 50 grams of carbohydrate needed for the glycemic index test. For this and other reasons, a second glycemic measure more appropriate for the real world, called **glycemic load**, is used.

Glycemic load is basically glycemic index normalized to serving standards. A food's glycemic load is derived by multiplying a food's glycemic index by the amount of digestible carbohydrate in a serving and then dividing by 100. For instance, carrots have a glycemic index of 90, which, multiplied by 4 (the grams of digestible carbohydrate in 1 cup) and divided by 100, gives one a glycemic load of roughly 4. See Table 3.4 for a listing of the glycemic loads of common foods relative to their glycemic index.

Foods with a higher glycemic index (and, more applicably, glycemic load) may be undesirable food choices for people with chronic hyperglycemia (e.g., diabetes mellitus). First, the higher glycemic index food can worsen a hyperglycemic state. Second, further elevation of circulating glucose could lead to an increase in the level of circulating insulin (**hyperinsulinemia**). For many hyperglycemic people, insulin may already be circulating at normal or elevated levels relative to the blood glucose concentration. Chronic hyperinsulinemia is associated with elevated blood lipids (hypercholesterolemia and hypertriglyceridemia), blood pressure, and body fat.

Glucose Transport into Cells

Glucose moves across human cell plasma membranes by facilitative diffusion via **glucose transport proteins (GLUT)**. At least six glucose transport proteins have been described in detail at this time, each varying in its operational properties as well as the types of cells in which it is expressed (**TABLE 3.5**). GLUT1 is the most widely expressed isoform and provides most cells with their basal glucose requirements. GLUT1 is expressed in higher amounts in epithelial cells and the endothelium of barrier tissue such as the blood–brain barrier. GLUT2 is produced in higher amounts in hepatocytes, pancreatic β-cells, and the basolateral membranes of intestinal and renal epithelial cells. This glucose transport protein is a high-K_m isoform, meaning that it is most active when more glucose is available, such as during hyperglycemia. Meanwhile, GLUT3 is responsible for glucose transport in neurons and has a relatively low K_m to ensure glucose supply, even during hypoglycemia.

GLUT4 is expressed in insulin-sensitive cells, such as adipocytes and cardiac and skeletal muscle cells, and is primarily responsible for reducing elevated blood glucose levels (**FIGURE 3.13**). Here, insulin binds to its receptor and sets in play a series of phosphorylation steps that lead to the translocation of GLUT4 to the plasma membrane. GLUT5 is a fructose transporter expressed in greater amounts in spermatozoa and the apical membrane of intestinal enterocytes and, to a lesser degree, skeletal muscle. GLUT7 is a glucose transporter found on the endoplasmic reticulum membrane; it transports free glucose into the cytosol after the action of glucose-6-phosphatase upon glucose-6-phosphate. This is of particular importance to hepatocytes during glycogen breakdown because it allows for glucose liberation (from phosphate) for subsequent release into circulation.

Glucose is the principal energy source of the brain. Delivery of glucose to brain tissue requires transport

TABLE 3.5 Major Glucose Transport (GLUT) Proteins in Tissue

Protein	Tissue	Properties/Characteristics
GLUT1	Most cells	Low K_m (1–2 mM) Ensures glucose uptake during hypoglycemia
GLUT2	Pancreatic β-cells, renal tubular cells, small intestinal basolateral epithelial cells that transport glucose, liver cells, hypothalamus	High K_m (15–20 mM)
GLUT3	Expressed mostly in neurons, placenta, testes	Low K_m (1 mM) Very high affinity Probable main glucose transporter in neurons
GLUT4	Skeletal muscle fibers, adipose tissue, cardiac muscle cells	High K_m (5 mM) Insulin regulated to help regulate hyperglycemia
GLUT5	Mucosal surface of small intestine cells, hepatocytes, sperm, skeletal muscle fibers	Low K_m (1–2 mM) Fructose transporter
GLUT7	Hepatocytes	Transports glucose out of the endoplasmic reticulum after final step in gluconeogenesis

across the endothelial cells of the blood–brain barrier and then into neurons and glial cells (collectively referred to as glia). GLUT1 has been determined to be in higher concentration in the brain, with variations in the degree of glycosylation in neurons and in the blood–brain barrier. GLUT3 is also concentrated in

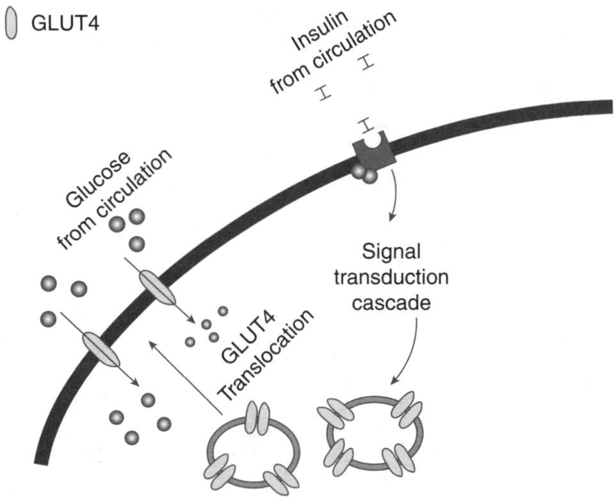

FIGURE 3.13 Insulin Interaction with Insulin Receptors and Translocation of GLUT4 to Cell Plasma Membranes to Bring Glucose into Cells. The binding of insulin to its receptor results in a series of phosphorylation of signaling factors that ultimately leads to the translocation of GLUT4 to the plasma membrane.

neurons, and GLUT5 in microglia. GLUT2, GLUT4, and GLUT7 have also been detected in the brain, but at lower concentrations.

Glucose transport across the plasma membrane of muscle (skeletal and cardiac) has additional considerations beyond the presence of insulin and the mobilization of GLUT4 transporters. Glucose transport is increased by alterations in the metabolic condition of muscle cells. In the heart, glucose transport can be increased by more powerful contractions, increased levels of circulating epinephrine and growth hormone, and intracellular AMP and ADP. Meanwhile, skeletal muscle contraction leads to an augmentation in glucose transport that is independent of insulin. This is important because insulin release is dampened during moderate to intense exercise. Muscle cell contractile activities result in an increase in intracellular Ca^{2+} content, which has been suggested to be associated with the translocation of GLUT4 from the intracellular pool to the plasma membrane.

Monosaccharide Activation

Free monosaccharides are found in low concentration in cells because they are quickly utilized or assimilated into stores. For a monosaccharide to be metabolized within a cell, it must be phosphorylated (i.e., have a phosphate attached). For example, glucose-6-phosphate is created in the first step of glycolysis from free glucose entering a cell. Not only does this serve to activate the monosaccharide but it also "locks" the monosaccharides within certain cells, such as hepatocytes. Glucose-6-phosphate is readily active and tends not to accumulate within a cell.

● BEFORE YOU GO ON . . .

1. What is glycemic index, and how is it measured?
2. How does glycemic load differ from glycemic index? How can both be applied to people and populations?
3. What are glucose transport proteins, and which cell types produce different isoforms?
4. What are the steps involved in GLUT4 movement to cell membranes?
5. What is the purpose of activating monosaccharides upon entering cells?

▶ Major Hormones in Carbohydrate Metabolism

The metabolism of carbohydrate is regulated by individual hormone levels and their relative ratios. Among the most significant hormones are insulin, which tends to elicit an anabolic effect on carbohydrates,

thus increasing cellular uptake and building stores; and glucagon, epinephrine, and cortisol, which tend to have the opposite effect (**TABLE 3.6**).

Insulin

Insulin is a polypeptide produced in β-cells of pancreatic islets, and it consists of two chains (A and B) linked by disulfide bonds (**FIGURE 3.14**). The A chain consists of 21 amino acids, the B chain consists of 30 amino acids, and the disulfide bonds arising from cysteine residues are located at A7–B7 and A20–B19. A disulfide bond also exists between cysteine residues from A6 and A11. Although there is some variation in the insulin amino acid sequence between mammalian species, the positioning of the three disulfide bonds seems invariant.

Insulin Production

Insulin is synthesized (via protein translation) as preproinsulin, which has a molecular weight of 11,500. Post-translational modification begins with the cleavage of the 23-amino acid pre- or leader sequence, resulting in proinsulin, which has a molecular weight of approximately 9000. The cleaved leader sequence is necessary for guiding pre-proinsulin into the endoplasmic reticulum during synthesis. Cleavage of the leader group also allows for the appropriate conformation for the formation of disulfide linkages.

TABLE 3.6 Actions of Insulin, Glucagon, Cortisol, and Epinephrine in Carbohydrate Metabolism

Hormone	Actions
Insulin	Increases the uptake of glucose by skeletal muscle and adipocytes Increases the synthesis of glycogen in skeletal muscle and liver hepatocytes Increases fatty acid synthesis from excessive dietary carbohydrate Decreases fat breakdown and mobilization from adipose tissue
Glucagon	Increases glycogen breakdown in liver Increases liver glycogen-derived glucose release into blood Increases glucose manufacturing in liver Increases fat breakdown and mobilization from adipocytes
Epinephrine (adrenalin)	Increases glycogen breakdown in liver hepatocytes and skeletal muscle Increases liver glycogen-derived glucose release into blood Increases fat breakdown and mobilization from adipocytes
Cortisol (stress hormone)	Increases skeletal muscle protein breakdown to amino acids (alanine and glutamine can circulate to the liver and be used for gluconeogenesis) Increases gluconeogenesis and liver glucose release into blood Increases fat breakdown and mobilization from fat tissue Increases glycogen content in liver

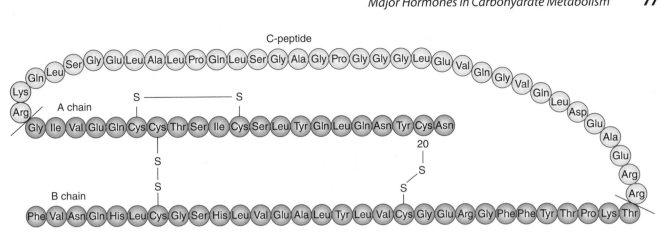

FIGURE 3.14 The Insulin Molecule. Amino acid sequence of insulin A and B chains and location of disulfide bonds.

Proinsulin then moves to the Golgi apparatus. In the Golgi apparatus, proinsulin begins conversion to mature insulin, or simply insulin, which involves the removal of a stretch of amino acids in the central portion of the proinsulin polypeptide. The removed amino acid sequence is called C peptide, and the remaining, once flanking, amino acid sequences are the A chain and B chain, which are secured by disulfide bonds. This process continues after vesicles bud from the Golgi apparatus and traverse the cytoplasm toward the plasma membrane and conversion of proinsulin to insulin is typically about 95% complete. Upon stimulus, the secretory vesicles will fuse with the plasma membrane to release insulin into the intercellular space (**FIGURE 3.15**).

Insulin Secretion

Insulin and proinsulin combine with zinc within secretory granules and form hexamer structures. The secretory vesicles then fuse with the plasma membranes of β-cells, releasing insulin, proinsulin, and C peptide into the extra-cellular space. Those molecules are then free to diffuse into the blood. Proinsulin has less than 5% of the bioactivity of insulin, and C peptide has none. The half-life of insulin is 3 to 5 minutes, whereas the half-life of proinsulin is much longer. Insulin is metabolized primarily in the liver, kidneys, and placenta. About 50% of circulating insulin is removed in a single pass through the liver.

On a daily basis, the adult pancreas secretes about 40 to 50 units of insulin, which represents about 15 to 20% of that which is available in secretory vesicles. A unit is equal to 45.5 micrograms of crystalline insulin. The release of insulin is an energy-dependent process, and the strongest stimulus is an elevation in plasma glucose concentration. The

threshold concentration for secretion is about 80 to 100 milligrams per 100 milliliters, and a maximal response occurs when blood glucose concentration is approximately 300 to 500 milligrams per 100 milliliters of blood.

Secretion of insulin via rising glucose levels can be influenced by several factors. For instance, α-adrenergic agonists such as norepinephrine via autonomic innervation and circulating epinephrine can dampen glucose stimulation of insulin release, which can be important for controlling blood glucose levels during more strenuous exercise and stressful events. In addition, insulin secretion is increased by chronic exposure to growth hormone, estrogens, and progestins. Thus, it is not surprising to find insulin secretion elevated during the last trimester of pregnancy. In addition, insulin release is promoted by certain amino acids and peptides and the mechanism of action is likely through incretin release. Incretins are hormones that cause insulin release by the pancreas. This aligns with the notion that insulin is a general feeding, anabolic hormone as even low carbohydrate, high protein foods can evoke a respectable elevation in circulating insulin. Furthermore, the combination of protein with moderate carbohydrate meals can lead to incremental insulin release. Perhaps, the most interesting and significant fact is the ability of whey protein, the principle protein in human milk, to do so.

Insulin-Mediated Glucose Uptake

Insulin promotes the lowering of blood glucose concentration by several means. In adipose tissue and skeletal muscle, which collectively constitute approximately 50 to 60% of the tissue in the adult body, insulin increases the number of glucose transporters at the plasma membrane face. Those transporters, particularly

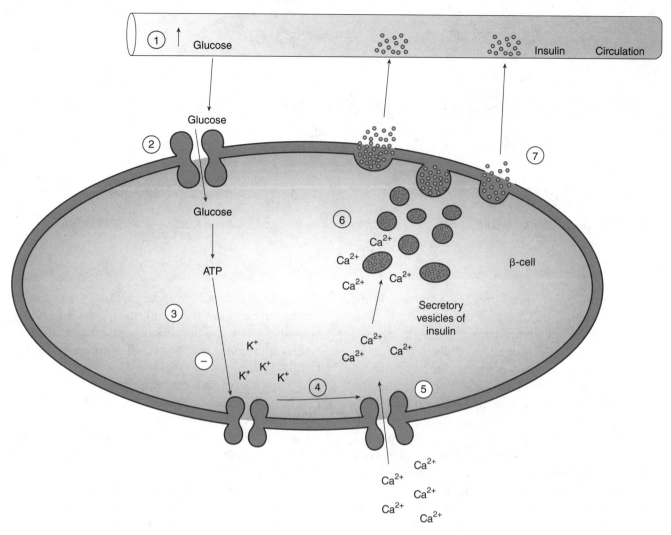

1. Blood glucose levels increase (e.g., meal)
2. Glucose uptake via GluT2
3. ATP formation through glucose utilization inactivates potassium channels
4. β-cell membrane becomes depolarized due to accumulation of potassium ions
5. Calcium channel opens and calcium diffuses into cell
6. Calcium promotes fusing of insulin secretory vesicles with plasma membrane
7. Insulin diffuses into circulation

FIGURE 3.15 Release of Insulin from Pancreatic β-Cells via Fusion of Secretory Vesicles with Plasma Membrane.
The numbers in the diagram correspond to events listed in the bottom of the figure.

GLUT4, are assumed to be mobilized from an inactive intracellular pool (see Figure 3.13). Increased glucose entry into hepatocytes appears to occur by increasing the activity of glucokinase. Once glucose enters hepatocytes (via GLUT1), it is quickly phosphorylated by glucokinase, thus maintaining a concentration gradient that favors further influx of free glucose from circulation. Similarly, the activity of skeletal muscle hexokinase II, which also catalyzes the phosphorylation of glucose, is increased due to insulin.

The actions of insulin on increased glucose entry are somewhat special to certain cell types, such as adipocytes, skeletal and cardiac myocytes, and hepatocytes (see Table 3.6). Most other cells in the body demonstrate a more consistent uptake of glucose from circulation based on their metabolic needs and glucose availability. This is explained by the variety of glucose transporter proteins. Insulin also promotes the uptake of certain amino acids into cells, especially muscle cells.

Metabolic Roles of Insulin

Insulin not only increases the uptake of glucose and amino acids into certain types of cells, but also strongly influences energy nutrient metabolic pathways within cells as well. Insulin promotes increased activities of glycolysis, the pentose phosphate pathway, glycogen formation (glycogenesis), and fatty acid synthesis (lipogenesis). Insulin inhibits glucose formation via glycogen breakdown (glycogenolysis) and the conversion from noncarbohydrate molecules (gluconeogenesis). Furthermore, insulin inhibits fat breakdown (lipolysis) and fatty acid oxidation in adipocytes and hepatocytes, while at the same time supporting protein synthesis in skeletal muscle and other tissue. Generally, insulin influences the associated pathways by either activating or deactivating key enzymes or influencing events of transcription or translation or both. In those ways, insulin is believed to influence either the quantity or activity of at least 50 different enzymes.

The net effect of insulin is to decrease the circulatory concentration of glucose. In that sense, insulin stands alone, and its general actions are opposed by several hormones, such as glucagon, epinephrine, and cortisol. The net effect of insulin is also to promote storage of diet-derived (exogenous) energy. Because the liver receives portal blood that has drained from the pancreas, it is exposed to insulin concentrations that can be three to ten times greater than in the systemic circulation. The liver binds and removes a significant amount of insulin on this pass. The liver is also more sensitive to insulin, presumably because it also has greater receptor concentrations than other tissue.

Insulin Receptors

Insulin acts by first binding with an insulin receptor on the plasma membrane (see Figure 3.13), and its indirect actions can arise within seconds to minutes (nutrient transport, activation or inhibition of enzymes, RNA transcription) or hours (protein and DNA synthesis and cell growth). The insulin receptor is a heterodimer transmembrane glycoprotein. Its cytoplasmic region has tyrosine kinase activity and an autophosphorylation site. The insulin receptor gene is located on chromosome 19. Insulin receptors undergo constant turnover because their half-life is only 7 to 12 hours. Most human cells synthesize insulin receptors, with the average concentration being approximately 20,000 receptors per cell. That is because insulin not only governs metabolic activity but is also involved in cell growth and reproduction.

Once insulin binds to a receptor, there is a conformational change, the receptor is internalized, and one or more signals are produced. The internalization of receptors is important to regulate receptor concentration, which, in turn, helps regulate cell turnover and metabolic activities. In hyperinsulinemic situations, such as in obesity, there is reduced production of insulin receptors. Fewer receptors are produced, resulting in fewer receptors on the plasma membrane, and thus, those cells become less sensitive to insulin. This results in hyperglycemia and is often the case in obesity-related type 2 diabetes mellitus.

Insulin elicits a second messenger action that culminates in a variety of intracellular events. Those events begin with the activity of tyrosine kinase, which results in an increase in tyrosine phosphorylation in both the receptor itself as well as in key intracellular proteins. That generally activates key enzymes, such as guanosine triphosphatases (GTPases), lipid kinases, and protein kinases, which mediate much of insulin's metabolic impact.

Glucagon

Glucagon is produced by α-cells of pancreatic islets. It is a single-chain polypeptide consisting of 29 amino acids. Like insulin, glucagon is also synthesized in a larger prohormone form. Glucagon circulates in the plasma unbound and has a half-life of about 5 minutes. The liver is the primary site of glucagon inactivation. Because pancreatic endocrine secretions drain into the hepatic portal vein, much of the secreted glucagon is actually metabolized without ever reaching the systemic circulation. Glucagon secretion is associated with hypoglycemia, and inhibition of secretion is associated with hyperglycemia. The exact inhibitory mechanisms are unclear. It could be a more direct inhibition via increased glucose reception, or a more indirect inhibition via insulin or insulin-related events, or a combination of those or associated events. Other stimulators may include some amino acids, particularly glucogenic amino acids such as alanine, serine, glycine, cysteine, and threonine. Those amino acids are important sources of glucose via gluconeogenesis. This also means that a protein-containing meal can, in theory, stimulate glucagon release, concomitant to stimulating insulin release.

Whereas the influence of insulin is diverse, glucagon focuses its actions mainly on the liver and adipose tissue (see Table 3.6). The binding of glucagon to glucagon receptors on the plasma membrane of hepatocytes results in an increase in intracellular cAMP. The activation of phosphorylase by cAMP promotes glycogen degradation while also inhibiting glycogen synthesis. Furthermore, glucagon promotes the conversion of noncarbohydrate molecules to glucose in hepatocytes. In adipose tissue glucagon promotes lipolysis principally by activating the enzyme hormone-sensitive lipase. As with hepatocytes, the binding of glucagon to receptors on the plasma membrane of adipocytes initiates a second messenger cascade that begins with the activation of adenyl cyclase through a G-protein-linked mechanism and produces increased cAMP levels, as discussed later in this chapter.

Skeletal muscle cells do not make glucagon receptors. Thus, glycogenolysis in skeletal muscle is not influenced by glucagon; it is primarily influenced by epinephrine and, to a lesser degree, norepinephrine. In general, glucagon is gluconeogenic, glycogenolytic, and ketogenic in hepatocytes and lipolytic in adipocytes.

Insulin-to-Glucagon Molar Ratios

Because many aspects of energy nutrient metabolism promoted by either insulin or glucagon are antagonistic in nature, the molar ratio of those two hormones is the dominating factor in determining net metabolic activity. For instance, in hepatocytes and skeletal muscle, the synthesis of glycogen can and will occur concurrent with the breakdown of glycogen. However, the algebraic net effect is dictated largely by the relative influences of insulin and glucagon and, to a lesser degree, other hormones, such as epinephrine and cortisol. An insulin-to-glucagon ratio of 2.3:1 may be expected from the consumption of a balanced meal. Meanwhile, the infusion of arginine increases the secretion of both hormones, but more so for insulin, which results in a ratio approximating 3:1. Conversely, if a glucose solution is infused into circulation, a ratio of 25:1 can be expected.

Epinephrine

Epinephrine (adrenalin) is produced in the adrenal glands (adrenal medulla) from the amino acid tyrosine, which itself can be synthesized from the essential amino acid phenylalanine. Intermediates of the synthesis of epinephrine include dopa, dopamine, and norepinephrine (noradrenaline). Epinephrine, norepinephrine, and dopamine are important molecules in the response to stress. They are synthesized in chromaffin cells and stored in secretory granules. Epinephrine is the principal catecholamine synthesized in chromaffin cells of the adrenal medulla, constituting 80% of the total catecholamine production.

The conversion of dopamine to norepinephrine is catalyzed by the copper-containing enzyme dopamine

β-hydroxylase (DBH). DBH requires ascorbate (an electron donor) and copper at the active site. Meanwhile, phenylethanolamine-N-methyltransferase (PNMT) catalyzes the production of epinephrine from norepinephrine (**FIGURE 3.16**). Synthesis of PNMT is induced by glucocorticoid hormones that reach the medulla, via a portal vein, from the adrenal cortex.

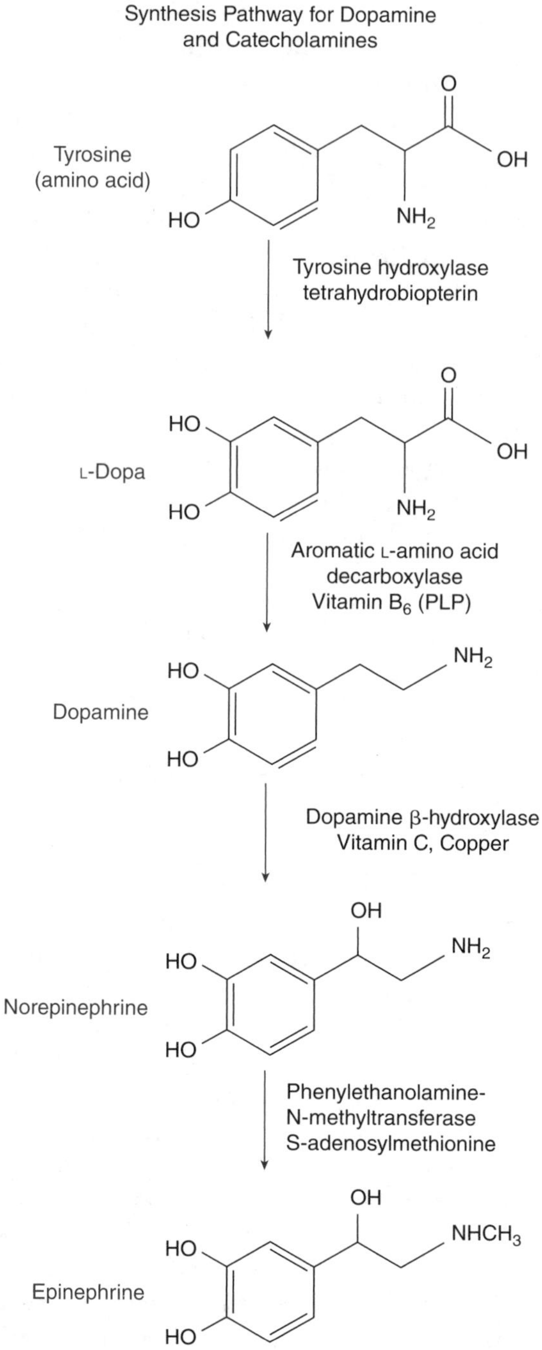

FIGURE 3.16 Steps Involved in the Production of Epinephrine and Norepinephrine. The amino acid tyrosine is an amino acid that is the parent compound. Note that several reactions require nutrients such as Vitamin B_6, Vitamin C, and copper.

The incorporation of catecholamines into secretory granules is an ATP-dependent transport mechanism. The granules also contain ATP-Mg^{2+}, Ca^{2+}, and DBH. Once inside the granule, epinephrine complexes with ATP in a 4:1 ratio. Secretory granules fuse with the plasma membrane upon appropriate neural stimulation. β-Adrenergic and cholinergic agents stimulate fusion, whereas α-adrenergic agents inhibit it. Catecholamines circulate loosely bound to albumin and have a half-life of about 10 to 30 seconds. Catecholamines are metabolized by catechol-*O*-methyltransferase (COMT) and monoamine oxidase (MAO), which are found in many tissues.

The effects of epinephrine are mediated via its reception by two classes of receptors. Both α and β receptors are subdivided into α_1 and α_2 and β_1 and β_2 respectively. This classification system is based on binding affinity of the different receptors for catecholamines. When epinephrine binds to β_1 on cardiac tissue, the force and rate of contraction are increased. Furthermore, the binding of epinephrine to β_2 receptors elicits smooth muscle relaxation and thus, vasodilation in skeletal muscle and the liver. Meanwhile, the interaction with α_1 receptors results in contraction in some smooth muscle.

The effects of epinephrine include the breakdown of glycogen in skeletal muscle and the liver and fat breakdown in adipose tissue (see Table 3.6). This serves to make fuel available for skeletal muscle and the heart during times of increased activity.

Cortisol

Cortisol is produced in the adrenal cortex and is the principal glucocorticoid in humans. It is derived from cholesterol and circulates in the blood bound predominantly to corticosteroid-binding globulin (CBG), which is produced in the liver and, to a minor degree, loosely associated with albumin. The binding of cortisol to a plasma protein allows for a longer half-life (60 to 90 minutes) than the polypeptide hormones discussed previously. Cortisol is principally removed and metabolized by the liver.

Cortisol has widespread effects in the human body, and greater secretion is associated with stress and fasting, whereby it mediates adaptive processes. Cortisol then plays a significant role in carbohydrate, protein, fat, and nucleic acid metabolism. Cortisol and its structural analogues (e.g., hydrocortisone) are also used clinically as anti-inflammatory agents because they inhibit the migration of polymorphonuclear leukocytes, monocytes, and lymphocytes at the site of inflammation.

In the liver, the effects of cortisol are largely anabolic (see Table 3.6). Cortisol promotes gluconeogenesis in hepatocytes by binding to intracellular receptors and inducing the production of a number of enzymes involved in gluconeogenesis as well as amino acid transamination. Additionally, glucose-6-phosphatase activity is increased, allowing for more glucose to leave the liver to serve as fuel for other tissue. Cortisol also promotes glycogen synthesis in the liver. This effect most likely occurs to maintain at least basal levels of glycogen stores during times when it could easily become exhausted (i.e., extended fasting, stress). However, it should be noted that during hypoglycemia, the impact of glucagon will supersede cortisol, and the net effect will be a breakdown of liver glycogen.

In peripheral tissue, cortisol-induced activity appears to antagonize insulin activity. Thus, cortisol works to reduce glucose and amino acid uptake in peripheral tissue, such as skeletal muscle, to preserve circulating glucose for other tissue with obligate demands, such as red blood cells and the brain. Meanwhile, protein and nucleic acid synthesis are inhibited and protein breakdown is promoted by cortisol in more sensitive tissue (i.e., skeletal muscle and connective tissue in the skin). Free amino acids in skeletal muscle, especially alanine, become resources for gluconeogenesis in the liver via the alanine–glucose cycle.

Cortisol also promotes lipolysis in adipose tissue, thereby allowing free fatty acids to be mobilized to serve as fuel for tissue throughout the body. Meanwhile, cortisol promotes an increase in total white blood cell count in circulation. However, this is a net effect, because although monocytes and polymorphonuclear leukocytes are increased, eosinophils, basophils, and lymphocytes are decreased.

● BEFORE YOU GO ON . . .

1. What cells in what tissue produce insulin, and how and when is it released from those cells?

2. What role does insulin play in the metabolism of energy nutrients? Is it generally anabolic or catabolic?

3. Where is glucagon produced, and what roles does it play in carbohydrate and fat metabolism?

4. Which cells produce cortisol; when is it released into circulation; and how does it affect carbohydrate, fat, and protein metabolism?

5. How is epinephrine produced, and what is its role in carbohydrate and fat metabolism?

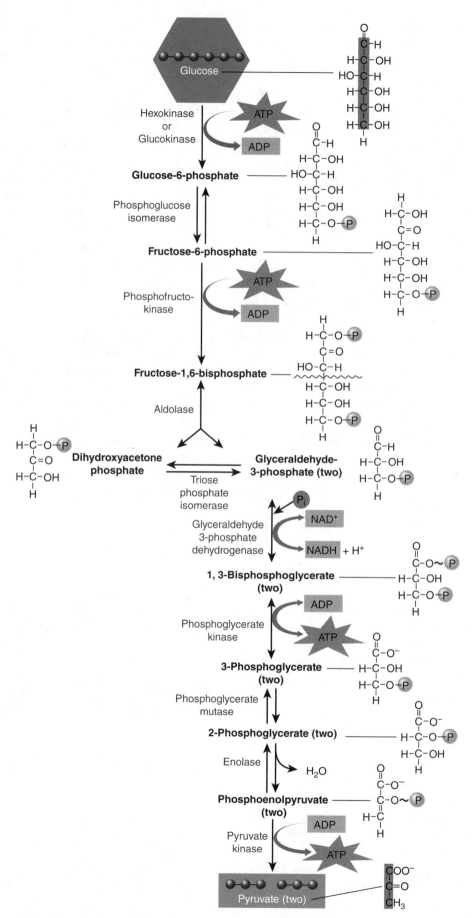

FIGURE 3.17 Steps and Key Regulation of Glycolysis. A key metabolic pathway in how cells catabolize glucose.

▶ Major Metabolic Pathways for Carbohydrate

The flux of glucose and other carbohydrates through metabolic pathways is regulated in several ways. First, hormonal influences, such as insulin and glucagon, can alter the activity of key enzymes by phosphorylation and dephosphorylation. Second, hormonal influences can either induce or repress transcription or translation or both of key enzymes. Third, intermediates and products of the metabolic reactions as well as other substances can elicit allosteric influences on the flux of metabolic pathways.

Most cells use more than one fuel source; red blood cells are the only true obligate glucose users. The brain is limited in its energy substrates, and under normal metabolic conditions, derives nearly all of its energy from glucose as well. However, the brain can adapt to use more ketone bodies during starvation to spare blood glucose for other tissue. Conversely, tissues, such as muscle, liver, and kidney, are more omnivorous in their energy substrates. Here, substrate availability and hormonal influences are the greatest influential factors.

Glycolysis

Glycolysis is a series of 10 reactions that convert one six-carbon glucose molecule to two three-carbon pyruvate molecules (**FIGURE 3.17**). The net ATP yield of glycolysis is two ATP molecules, with the potential for two more via the glycerol phosphate shuttle, which allows for the reducing equivalents of the NADH generated in the cytosol to be transferred to mitochondrial $FADH_2$. Glycolysis also allows entry points for the catabolism of other monosaccharides, such as fructose and galactose.

Glucose flux through glycolysis is regulated by several key enzymes, as described next.

Hexokinase and Glucokinase

The first influential enzymes in glucose metabolism in cells are hexokinase in all tissue and glucokinase in hepatocytes. Both enzymes phosphorylate glucose to produce glucose-6-phosphate. Hexokinase has a relatively low K_m, which allows it to operate despite a relatively low availability of glucose. However, hexokinase is inhibited by its product, glucose-6-phosphate. Those regulations ensure glucose entry into all cells for glycolysis but allow it to proceed based on cell need.

In contrast, glucokinase, which is produced in hepatocytes as induced by insulin, has a relatively high K_m and is not inhibited by its product. Glucokinase allows for large quantities of glucose to enter hepatocytes during hyperglycemic states, such as a fed state. This makes sense, because the liver is a major metabolizing site for glucose during a fed state and approximately 50% of glucose is converted to energy in the liver, with the remaining carbohydrate converted to glycogen and fatty acids. Because both absorbed glucose from the digestive tract and insulin secreted from the pancreas perfuse the liver before entering the general, or systemic, circulation, a large portion of the absorbed glucose is transported into hepatocytes and never reaches the general circulation. This is a major point of control for blood glucose levels.

Phosphofructokinase

The activity of phosphofructokinase 1 (PFK1), which catalyzes the conversion of fructose-6-phosphate to fructose-1, 6-bisphosphate, is regulated by several factors (**FIGURE 3.18**). In the liver, one of the

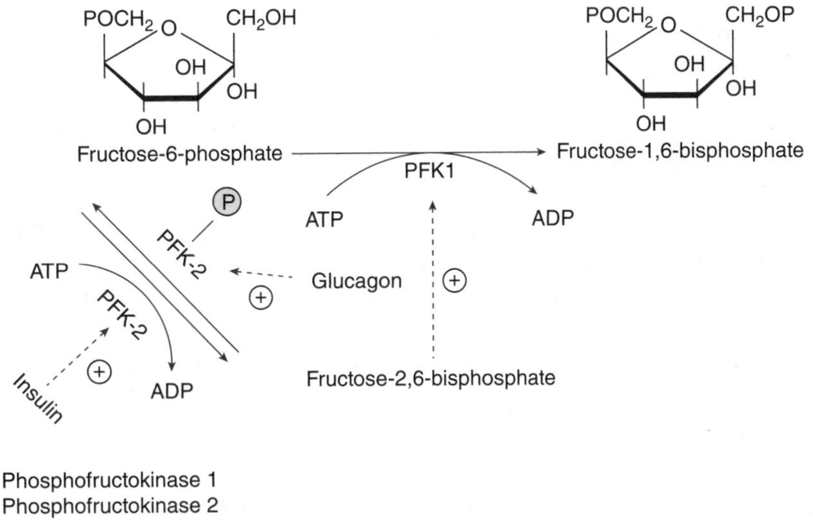

PFK1 = Phosphofructokinase 1
PFK2 = Phosphofructokinase 2

FIGURE 3.18 Activity of Phosphofructokinase 1 (PFK1). PFK1, which catalyzes the conversion of fructose-6-phosphate to fructose-1,6-bisphosphate, is regulated by several factors.

predominant factors is the activity of phosphofructokinase 2 (PFK2), an enzyme that catalyzes two opposite reactions, depending on whether it is phosphorylated. PFK2 is phosphorylated when glucagon levels are elevated. Increased intracellular cAMP activates protein kinase A, which phosphorylates PFK2. Conversely, the phosphate group is removed, via intracellular phosphatases, when insulin levels are elevated.

The nonphosphorylated form of PFK2 catalyzes the conversion of fructose-6-phosphate to fructose-2, 6-bisphosphate, which has an activating effect on PFK1. This makes sense because elevations of both circulating insulin and hepatocyte intracellular fructose-6-phosphate occur in a fed state. The phosphorylated form of PFK2 catalyzes the conversion of fructose-2, 6-bisphosphate back to fructose-6-phosphate, thus removing the activating influence of fructose-2, 6-bisphosphate on PFK1.

As glycolysis continues, the six-carbon fructose-1, 6-bisphosphate molecule is split into two three-carbon molecules: dihydroxyacetone phosphate and glyceral-dehyde-3-phosphate (see Figure 3.18). Dihydroxyacetone can then be converted to glyceraldehyde-3-phosphate. Therefore, two glyceraldehyde-3-phosphate molecules can result from one molecule of fructose-1, 6-bisphosphate. The conversion of glyceraldehyde3-phosphate to 1, 3-bisphosphoglycerate reduces NAD^+ to NADH. Therefore, two NADH molecules can be created in glycolysis from a single glucose molecule. In the next reaction, the phosphate at the number 1 position of 1, 3-bisphosphoglycerate is transferred to ADP to form ATP. This reaction can potentially happen twice for every glucose molecule that enters glycolysis. This reaction is catalyzed by phosphoglycerate kinase and produces two phosphoglycerate molecules, which are subsequently converted to phosphoenolpyruvate (PEP) by enolase.

Pyruvate Kinase

In the last reaction of glycolysis, PEP is converted to pyruvate by pyruvate kinase, which is activated by insulin. The binding of insulin to insulin receptors increases phosphatase activity, which dephosphorylates, and thus activates, pyruvate kinase. Conversely, the increased intracellular cAMP levels activate protein kinase A, which phosphorylates and deactivates pyruvate kinase. Increased cAMP can result from the binding of glucagon to glucagon receptors.

Fate of Pyruvate

Pyruvate is situated at a metabolic crossroad (**FIGURE 3.19**). Depending on the type of cell and hormonal and metabolic influences, pyruvate can either be converted to the amino acid alanine or to lactate in the cytosol or enter mitochondria and be converted to acetyl CoA or oxaloacetate. The conversion of pyruvate to lactate is a reduction reaction, and in the process, NADH is oxidized to NAD^+ (**FIGURE 3.20**). This negates the NADH created in glycolysis. This reaction is catalyzed in both directions by lactate dehydrogenase (LDH), which itself has five isoforms. LDH is composed of four subunits of either the heart (H) or muscle (M) type (i.e., MMMM, MMMH, MMHH, MHHH, HHHH), and different tissues express different forms. Lactate is produced in larger amounts in muscle and erythrocytes and can diffuse into the blood and serve as a gluconeogenic precursor in the liver or as an energy source for other cells.

Pyruvate in the mitochondria can be converted to acetyl CoA. Pyruvate dehydrogenase catalyzes this reaction, and NAD^+ is reduced to NADH in the process. NADH can then transfer electrons to the electron transport chain. Pyruvate dehydrogenase exists in either a phosphorylated (inactive) or dephosphorylated (active) form. The products of pyruvate dehydrogenase—acetyl CoA and NADH—activate the kinase that phosphorylates and inactivates pyruvate dehydrogenase. Conversely, CoASH (uncombined coenzyme A), NAD^+, and ADP inactivate the kinase, which keeps pyruvate dehydrogenase in an active state. Therefore, pyruvate dehydrogenase activity is controlled hormonally as well as by the metabolic state within the cell.

Glycogen Turnover

Like other bidirectional metabolic events, glycogen metabolism can be viewed as the algebraic net product of opposing operations: glycogen synthesis and glycogenolysis. It is possible, and often a reality, for those two mechanisms to operate at the same time. Thus, the governing factor becomes the relative influences of all the factors related to those operations. Some of the influences, such as metabolic products and intracellular factors (e.g., AMP, Ca^{2+}) may primarily exert their influence on only one of the two pathways, whereas others, such as hormones, can exert their influence on both pathways. For example, AMP increases glycogen degradative operations only, whereas epinephrine and glucagon both activate mechanisms involved in glycogen breakdown as well as inactivate mechanisms involved in glycogen synthesis.

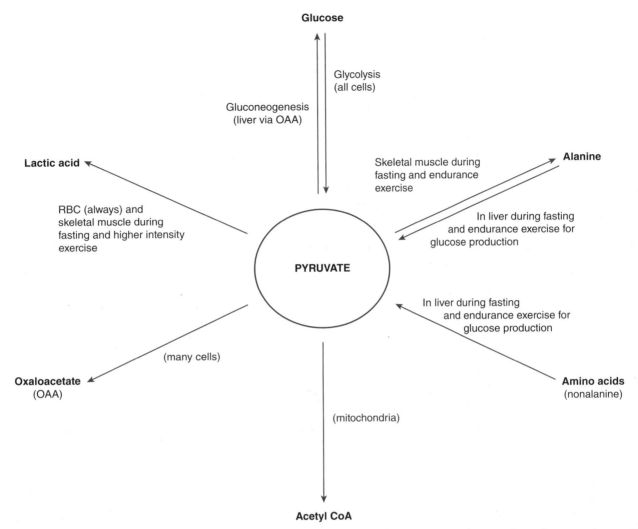

FIGURE 3.19 Pyruvate Sits at the Crossroads of Several Metabolic Pathways. Depending on the cell type and metabolic scenario, pyruvate can be used for fuel in mitochondria (via conversion to acetyl CoA), converted to lactate for exportation from a cell (e.g., red blood cell [RBC], skeletal muscle), or used to make glucose (in the liver) and the amino acid alanine (in skeletal muscle).

Glycogen contains more branching than plant starch, with points of branching occurring every 8 to 10 residues (see Figure 3.8). One glucose unit with an exposed anomeric carbon is located at the reducing end of each glycogen molecule, and this monomer is attached to the protein glycogenin. This glucose unit functions as perhaps the anchoring and initiating point for the glycogen molecule, and it is believed that this glucose molecule is not readily available. The straight-chain oligosaccharide that extends from the reducing glucose monomer is the glycogen primer. The glucose monomers at the ends of the initial straight chain as well as branch chains are called nonreducing units; those serve as points of attachment for new monomers during synthesis and as points of removal during glycogen breakdown.

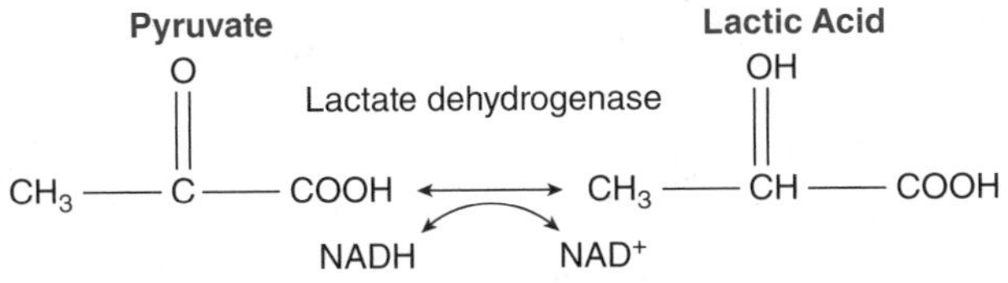

Glycogen Synthesis

Glycogen is found in several types of tissue, with the highest concentration being in hepatocytes of the liver and muscle cells (especially type II muscle fibers). The building block for glycogen is uridine diphosphate glucose (UDP-glucose), which is formed from glucose-1-phosphate, which itself is synthesized from

FIGURE 3.20 The Conversion of Pyruvate to Lactate. The conversion of pyruvate to lactate is a reduction reaction. In the process, NADH is oxidized to NAD^+.

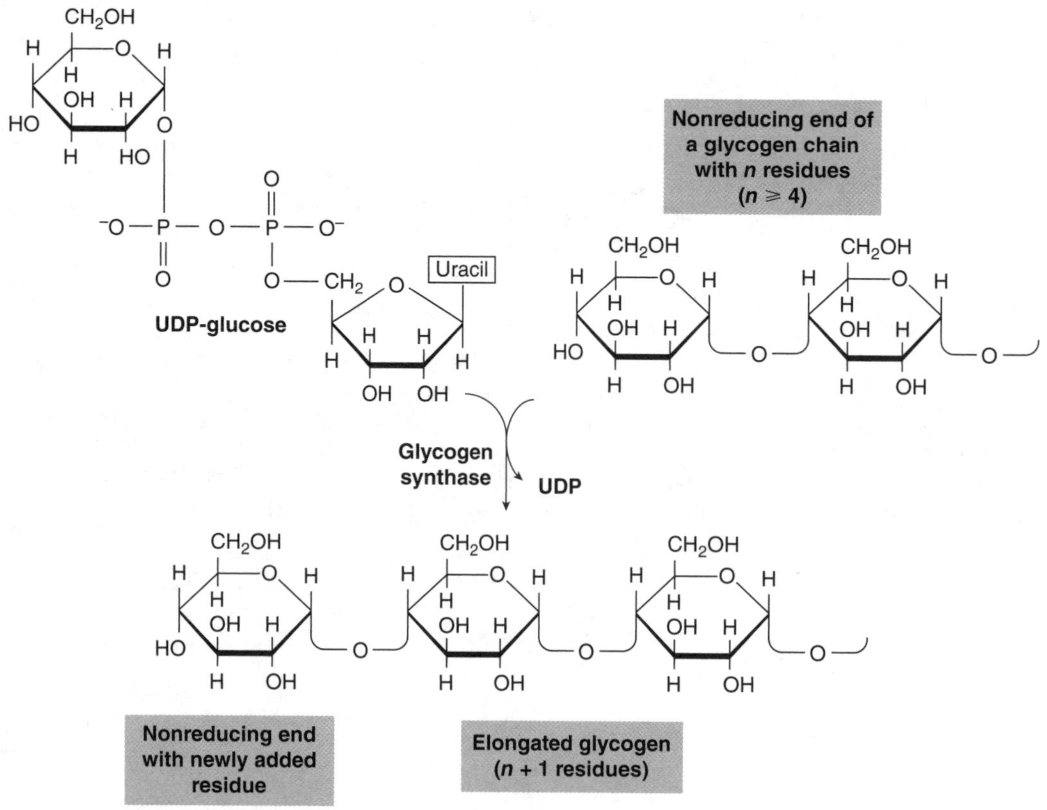

FIGURE 3.21 Glycogen Synthesis. The building block for glycogen is uridine diphosphate glucose (UDP-glucose), which is attached to the nonreducing end of a glycogen chain by glycogen synthase.

glucose-6-phosphate (**FIGURE 3.21**). Insulin activates glycogen synthase, which is the key regulatory enzyme in this process. When a growing straight chain contains 11 or more glucose monomers, another enzyme, called branching enzyme or glucosyl 4:6 transferase, relocates an oligomer of about 6 to 8 monomers and reattaches it via an α1-6 linkage at what becomes a branch point.

Glycogen Degradation

Glycogen degradation (glycogenolysis) is catalyzed by the active phosphorylase (phosphorylase a) enzyme (**FIGURE 3.22**). This enzyme is activated by epinephrine and increased intracellular AMP levels in muscle cells. The increased presence of AMP is mostly associated with muscle cell contraction and the hydrolysis of ATP to ADP. As a means of regenerating ATP, a phosphate from one ADP can be transferred to another ADP via adenylate kinase, producing ATP and AMP. Meanwhile, glucagon and epinephrine both participate in the activation of phosphorylase in hepatocytes. As mentioned earlier, both epinephrine and glucagon elicit a second messenger cascade that culminates in an increased intracellular concentration of cAMP. In a chain of events,

cAMP activates cAMP-dependent protein kinase, which, in turn, activates phosphylase kinase by converting it from inactive phosphorylase kinase b to the phosphorylated active phosphorylase kinase a form. Phosphorylase kinase a then can (1) activate phosphorylase (phosphorylase a), which can break down glycogen, and (2) inactivate glycogen synthase to inhibit counterproductive glycogen synthesis.

Phosphorylase a, with the assistance of vitamin B_6, detaches glucose monomers from glycogen, forming glucose-1-phosphate, which is subsequently converted to glucose-6-phosphate by phosphoglucomutase. Phosphorylase a can liberate about 90% of glucose residues from glycogen as it splits the α1-4 links (straight chain). Glucose-6-phosphate in hepatocytes can be dephosphorylated by glucose-6-phosphatase in the endoplasmic reticulum. Glucose is transported out of the endoplasmic reticulum by GLUT7 and can diffuse from the hepatocyte via GLUT2 and enter circulation. A debranching enzyme is responsible for the liberation of glucose units at branch points (approximately 10% of total glucose). The product of this activity is free glucose that can be transported out of the cell in the liver, again by GLUT2.

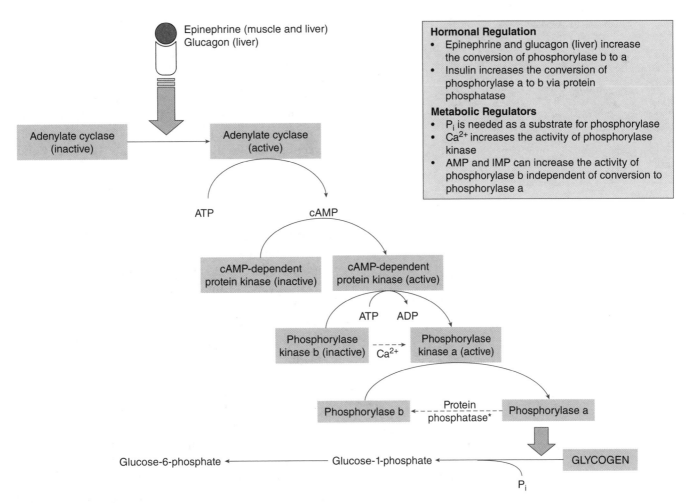

FIGURE 3.22 Glycogenolysis. Glycogen degradation, or glycogenolysis, begins with activation of phosphorylase. Phosphorylase activity is increased by the binding of epinephrine to receptors in skeletal muscle and liver cells (hepatocytes) and glucagon in the liver. The activation involves a cascade of steps. Phosphate (Pi), Ca^{2+}, adenosine monophosphate (AMP), and inosine monophosphate (IMP) all can increase the activity of phosphorylase, either directly or by increasing the activity of phosphorylase kinase. Active phosphorylase kinase also inactivates glycogen synthase (not shown) to minimize counterproductive glycogen synthesis.

Pentose Phosphate Pathway

The primary importance of the **pentose phosphate pathway** (**FIGURE 3.23**) is the reduction of NADP⁺ to NADPH, which can be used to reduce equivalents for the synthesis of certain molecules (i.e., fatty acids), **glutathione** reduction, or other reactions. Also, this reaction pathway allows for the creation of ribulose-5-phosphate, which may be isomerized to ribose-5-phosphate and used in nucleotide biosynthesis. The reactions of the pentose phosphate pathway can be described as either oxidative or nonoxidative. The oxidative reactions include the conversion of glucose-6-phosphate to phosphogluconolactone via glucose-6-dehydrogenase and the conversion of 6-phosphogluconate to ribulose-5-phosphate. Both reactions reduce NADP⁺ to NADPH, and the latter reaction also produces CO_2. The nonoxidative reactions

allow for the regeneration of the glycolytic intermediates glyceraldehyde-3-phosphate and fructose-6-phosphate.

Krebs Cycle (Citric Acid Cycle)

The Krebs cycle or citric acid cycle (**FIGURE 3.24**), which occurs in the mitochondrial matrix, consists of eight key sequential reactions whereby the final reaction produces the reactant for the first reaction that forms citric acid, the first product and reactant in the second reaction in the pathway. Therefore, this pathway is considered cyclic. In the reaction, acetyl CoA, which can be derived from a variety of sources, condenses with oxaloacetate, forming citrate. Citrate synthase is the catalyzing enzyme, and its activity is inhibited by its product. Aconitase catalyzes the conversion of citrate to isocitrate and has bidirectional activity but favors citrate formation. Isocitrate dehydrogenase then converts

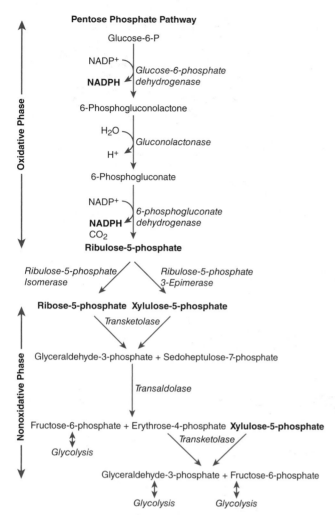

FIGURE 3.23 The Pentose Phosphate Pathway. This pathway is a principal means of reducing NADP⁺ to NADPH, which can be used for reducing equivalents for the synthesis of certain molecules (i.e., fatty acids), glutathione reduction, or other reactions and for creating ribose-5-phosphate, as well as being used in nucleotide biosynthesis.

isocitrate to α-ketoglutarate in the first oxidative reaction of the Krebs cycle. NAD⁺ is reduced to NADH, and CO_2 is produced. The next reaction is also oxidative, because α-ketoglutarate is converted to succinyl CoA by α-ketoglutarate dehydrogenase. Here again, NAD⁺ is reduced to NADH and CO_2 is produced.

In the next reaction, the energy liberated by the cleavage of the high-energy thioester bond of succinyl CoA to form succinate and coenzyme A is sufficient to phosphorylate GDP (guanosine diphosphate), forming GTP (guanosine triphosphate). Next, succinate is converted to fumarate by succinate dehydrogenase in the third oxidizing reaction of the Krebs cycle. However, here FAD is reduced to $FADH_2$. Then fumarate catalyzes the conversion of fumarate to malate. Malate is subsequently converted to oxaloacetate in the fourth oxidizing reaction, one that reduces NAD⁺ to NADH. This is

an equilibrium reaction that favors malate. The products of the Krebs cycle are three NADH, one $FADH_2$, and three CO_2 molecules. Thus, 12 ATP molecules can be generated from each citrate molecule formed in the initial reaction. So, in total, the complete oxidation of glucose can yield 36 to 38 ATP. Four total ATP are generated in substrate-level phosphorylation (2 each in glycolysis and the Krebs cycle), while 10 NADH and 2 $FADH_2$ are generated via glycolysis in the cyptoplasm and the conversion of pyruvate to acetyl CoA and the Krebs cycle in mitochondria. NADH and $FADH_2$ generated in the mitochondria yield 3 and 2 ATP via the electron transport chain, respectively, while NADH generated in the cytoplasm will yield either 2 or 3 ATP, depending on how it enters the mitochondria.

The events of the Krebs cycle are influenced primarily by the redox state of NAD⁺:NADH, the cellular level of intermediates, and the energy level (ADP:ATP) of a cell. For instance, if the ratio of NADH to NAD⁺ is high, the activities of isocitrate dehydrogenase, α-ketoglutarate dehydrogenase, and malate dehydrogenase slow down due to relative lack of a reactant. A high NADH:NAD⁺ ratio dictates that the reversible malate dehydrogenase catalyzes in the direction of malate, thus reducing the concentration of oxaloacetate, a reactant in the first reaction. Also, inhibition of isocitrate dehydrogenase by increased NADH:NAD⁺ ratio results in the accumulation of isocitrate, which is converted back to citrate by aconitase. Citrate inhibits citrate synthase, and thus citrate accumulates in the mitochondria. This will be important later when fatty acid synthesis is discussed.

Increased ADP:ATP ratio will speed up the Krebs cycle in general in two ways. Increased ADP indicates a need for cellular energy, and thus the electron transport chain will operate at a greater rate, thereby creating a higher NAD⁺:NADH ratio. Second, ADP allosterically increases isocitrate dehydrogenase activity.

Gluconeogenesis

Gluconeogenesis (**FIGURE 3.25**), the production of glucose from noncarbohydrate substrates, occurs mainly in the liver. The major precursors are lactate, glycerol, and certain amino acids. Gluconeogenesis uses several reversible reactions of glycolysis but must create chemical reaction bypasses around several unidirectional reactions in which the enzyme only catalyzes the reaction in the direction of glycolysis. Thus, gluconeogenesis cannot be viewed simply as the reversal of glycolysis.

Pyruvate cannot be made into phosphoenolpyruvate by a simple reversal of the reaction. The amino acid alanine and lactate are major gluconeogenic precursors,

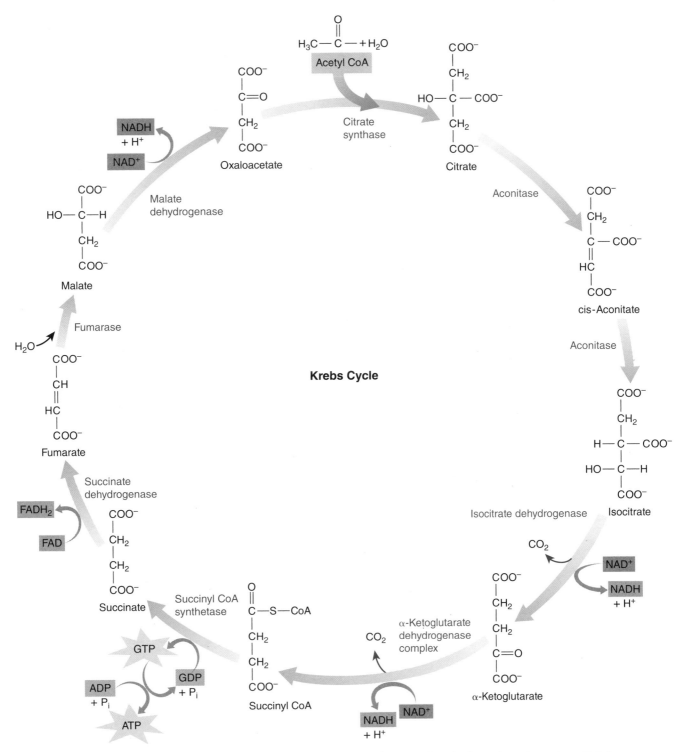

FIGURE 3.24 The Krebs Cycle. The Krebs (citric acid) cycle occurs in the mitochondrial matrix and consists of eight sequential reactions whereby the final reaction produces a potential reactant for the first reaction. NADH and $FADH^2$ can transfer electrons to the electron transfer chain to yield three and two ATP, respectively.

and both are converted to pyruvate in the liver. For pyruvate to be converted to phosphoenolpyruvate, pyruvate must first diffuse into the mitochondria and undergo conversion to oxaloacetate (OAA) and then malate. Pyruvate carboxylase catalyzes the conversion of pyruvate to OAA. Oxaloacetate is converted to malate by malate dehydrogenase. Malate can exit the mitochondria, but oxaloacetate cannot. Once the malate is in the cytoplasm, it is converted again to OAA by malate dehydrogenase. Finally, OAA is converted to phosphoenolpyruvate by the enzyme phosphoenolpyruvate carboxykinase (PEPCK).

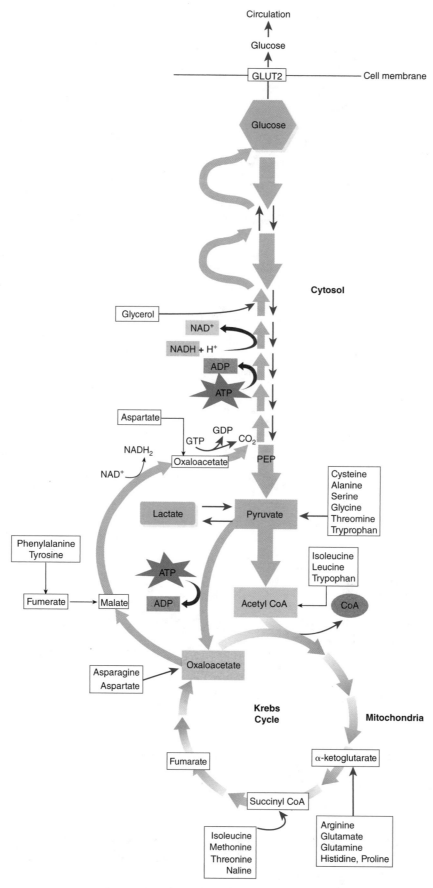

FIGURE 3.25 Gluconeogenesis. Gluconeogenesis, the production of glucose from noncarbohydrate substrates, occurs mainly in the liver. Lactate, glycerol, and alanine, as well as other amino acids, are major substrates in the liver. Glycerol is derived from fat breakdown in adipose tissue. Lactate is derived from RBCs and muscle during exercise. Most amino acids are derived from liver and muscle protein. PEP, phosphoenolpyruvate; CoA, coenzyme A.

Lipogenesis

Increased dietary carbohydrate intake may result in increased liver lipogenesis. Although insulin is released in response to carbohydrate intake and is well known for its lipogenic effects, some evidence suggests that glucose alone can enhance liver lipogenesis. Increased intake of carbohydrate can lead to gene expression of a variety of glycolytic and lipogenic pathways that play a role in converting glucose to fatty acids. Key enzymes that are upregulated in response to a high-carbohydrate diet include liver pyruvate kinase in glycolysis; acetyl-CoA carboxylase, the first enzyme in the biosynthesis of fatty acids; and fatty acid synthase, to name only a few. How does glucose upregulate those genes independent of insulin? The mechanism by which those events occur is due to the transcription protein **carbohydrate response element binding protein (ChREBP)**, which is activated by a high-carbohydrate diet. ChREBP was originally studied in the liver, because most glucose and lipid metabolism occurs in that organ, but other tissues also contain this protein, including adipose, intestine, kidney, and muscle tissue.

The promoters of enzymes involved in lipogenesis noted above have binding sites for ChREBP or response elements, which are nucleotide base pairs that bind ChREBP to DNA (**FIGURE 3.26**). This transcription protein is normally abundant in the cytosol in fasting conditions and is apparently unable to enter the cell nucleus due to the degree of phosphorylation. However, when glucose in the cytosol increases, a series of reactions occurs to partially dephosphorylated ChREBP, which allows it to translocate to the nucleus and bind to the promoters of the genes encoding those enzymes. Interestingly, it is not glucose itself, but rather a metabolite, xylulose-5-phosphate, that initiates the steps in dephosphorylating ChREBP. After upregulation of the target genes has occurred, ChREBP is phosphorylated by either cAMP or AMP-dependent kinases, which causes the ChREBP to disassociate from the gene promoters and exit the nucleus.

⬡ BEFORE YOU GO ON . . .

1. What are the impacts of insulin and glucagon on phosphofructosekinase 2 (PFK2) activity, and how is this activity mediated?

2. What is the role of uridine diphosphate glucose (UDP-glucose) in the synthesis of glycogen?

3. How do increased cAMP levels resulting from increased glucagon play a role in glycogen breakdown?

4. What are the two ways in which an increased ratio of ADP to ATP enhances activity in the Krebs cycle?

5. How is phosphoenolpyruvate in glycolysis made from pyruvate to generate more glucose in gluconeogenesis?

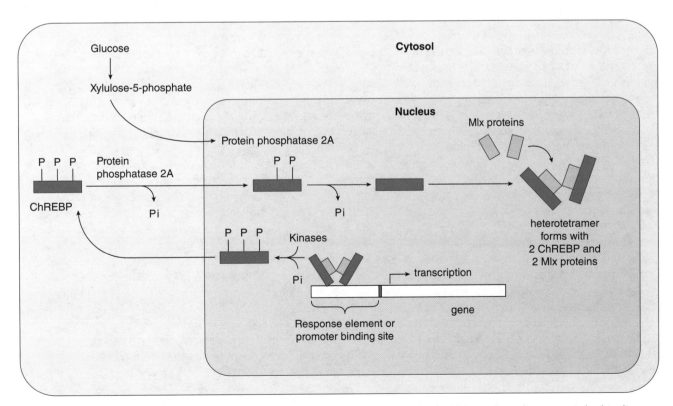

FIGURE 3.26 Carbohydrate Response Element Binding Protein (ChREBP). ChREBP regulates lipogenesis by binding to the promoters of genes to enhance transcription of genes involved with fat synthesis in response to glucose.

🩺 **CLINICAL INSIGHT**

Consumption of Sugar and Fructose—Are They Harmful to Your Health?

Nutritionists and dietitians are well aware of the concern pertaining to consumption of foods with high levels of sugar. This is especially concerning considering that many beverages on the market have natural sweeteners, such as sucrose and fructose. The Dietary Guidelines for Americans 2015 to 2020 recommend that sugar-sweetened beverages (soda) intake not exceed 10% of caloric intake. To implement this recommendation, the Guidelines suggest that water be consumed in place of sugar-sweetened beverages. Half of all Americans consumed at least one sugar-sweetened beverage per day according to the National Health and Nutrition Examination survey, 2011–2014. Approximately 6.5% of the total calorie intake came from such beverages with teens having the highest percentage of caloric intake and older adults having the lowest.

There has been much debate about fructose being potentially harmful to health as it relates to obesity, cardiovascular disease, and diabetes and is the sugar that should be targeted for diet reduction. In Western diets, much of the fructose consumption is linked to sucrose and/or high fructose corn syrup consumption. Animal studies, in particular, have shown a link between excess intake of those sugars and deleterious changes in risk factors for heart disease and diabetes, as well as increased body weight. With respect to body weight, evidence emerged that body weight increased as fructose availability increased in U.S. diets. The popular press started to discuss the negative implications of consuming diets high in fructose and sucrose.

Why have researchers focused specifically on fructose? Laboratory studies used rather high levels of this sugar in many studies, in fact, levels not likely to be equivalent to daily intake of Westerners. High levels of fructose consumed can induce fatty acid synthesis. That fructose did not stimulate insulin secretion compared with glucose, nor was there an increase any of the satiety hormones. Such findings have primarily been observed in rodent studies. There have been studies with humans that suggest humans and rodents do not respond in a similar manner when it comes to fructose intake. Much of the fructose consumed by humans can be converted to glucose compared with rodents as one example of a major difference.

Prospective cohort studies have not revealed an association between fructose intake and body weight, diabetes, and cardiac disease. However, when specific foods were evaluated, such as sugar-sweetened beverage intake, such associations became evident. The argument put forward is that excess energy intake from sugar-sweetened beverages is what is associated with those risk factors and not fructose intake per se. In studies in which calories are lowered by reduction in the intake of sugar-sweetened beverages, the risk factors for disease decreases accordingly with weight reduction.

There has been another argument independent of the increased calorie intake contributing to increased risk factors of heart disease, obesity, and diabetes. Individuals who consume sugar-sweetened beverages may have unhealthy lifestyles in general, which contributes to those risk factors. Dietary patterns may be less healthy; increased smoking and lack of exercise may be more predominant in those who choose to consume higher levels of sugar-sweetened beverages. There is yet another way of thinking about this: increased sugar-sweetened beverage consumption may be a marker of an unhealthy lifestyle due to other factors. Those other lifestyle factors are cited as having a greater impact on risk factors for diseases compared with increased sugar-sweetened beverages. Thus, perhaps the most important aspect of the Dietary Guidelines for Americans 2015 to 2020 is that it would reduce calorie input, especially when substituted with water.

Data from controlled trials that substituted an equal amount of calories for fructose with other carbohydrates revealed no difference in risk factors between the two groups. In fact, there was a slight improvement of glycemic control in fructose fed subjects. However, with any digestible carbohydrate recommendation and investigation, it is important to keep normal glucose turnover rate and potential in perspective. Digestible carbohydrate in any form will be problematic when intake exceeds carbohydrate absorption, disposal, and metabolism rates. Dietitians must always keep in mind that the human body is not capable of efficiently managing high loads of carbohydrate in a desirable manner if their client/patient is not physically active and/or conditioned to store and use more carbohydrate.

Human blood only has 5 grams of glucose (20 calories) at normal levels of 100 mg/100 ml with 5 l of total blood volume. Plus, the liver can store 75–100 grams and skeletal muscle 300–400 grams. Taken together, body carbohydrate stores approximate tissue glucose use in 24–36 hours. Expressed differently, the equivalent of total body carbohydrate is turned over in every 1–2 days for an inactive person. For instance, blood and the CNS will use at least half of the stores daily and the basic metabolism of other tissue, including skeletal muscle, will use the rest. However, liver and muscle glycogen stores will only be reduced during unfed/fasting or low carbohydrate intake states and physical activity, respectively. Thus, if neither of those metabolic scenarios exist, the primary "carbohydrate fuel tanks" of the human body do not move toward empty, thereby reducing the capability and capacity to dispose ingested carbohydrates. Its fate is to continue to circulate with incremental glucose entering from the digestive tract until it can be disposed of and metabolized, processed, or stored by tissue.

To emphasize the role of exercise in more efficient carbohydrate intake, disposal and use, athletes of most energy-demanding sports will use carbohydrate drinks (5–8%) and recommendations can be as high as 8–12 grams/kg/day. For a 160-lb runner, the high end of the recommendation is over 850 grams/day of carbohydrate. Those athletes will use a lot of carbohydrate during activity as well as adapt to store more carbohydrate in muscle tissue. For other athletes, such as a U.S. football lineman, complications for higher carbohydrate intake become apparent when caloric intake is excessive and fat mass increases. In this case, as with nonathletes, as the human body accumulates more and more body fat, it actually becomes less efficient at disposing and metabolizing blood glucose and some argue that this is to allow for the caloric excess (glucose) to spill into the urine and be removed from the body.

For years, Westerners have been told to decrease foods high in fat and, in particular, saturated fat, in order to improve health. What occurred; however, is that the level of obesity increased when fat intake decreased. Similarly, it may not be prudent to single out sugar and/or fructose, in particular, to be reduced in diets from a policy perspective given the unintended consequences of our experience with advocating a low-fat diet. Regardless, this subject is likely to remain controversial and emotional. As nutritionists and dietitians, the emphasis once again should be on caloric control and exercise. There never appears to be a magic bullet outside of adhering to a diet with variety, caloric balance, and a change in lifestyle.

▶ Here's What You Have Learned

1. Carbohydrates are a class of nutrients that include sugars, starches, fibers, and related molecules, such as glycosaminoglycans, amino sugars, and more. Carbohydrates provide energy for all cells and play structural and functional roles in cells and tissue

2. Fibers are special carbohydrates and related molecules that are not broken down by digestive enzymes. However, based on their metabolism by gut microflora and conversion to absorbable energy molecules, they can provide a small amount of energy

3. Carbohydrate contributes approximately 50% of the calories in the typical adult diet. Although some monosaccharides are available in the diet via fruits, most are derived from disaccharides and polysaccharides. Cereal grains, such as rice and wheat, as well as potatoes, make a significant contribution to carbohydrate intake, as do fruits and dairy foods

4. The Acceptable Macronutrient Distribution Range (AMDR) for carbohydrate intake in the United States and Canada is 45 to 65% of total energy. The broad range of AMDR is meant to provide individual guidance based on glucose tolerance and activity level. Meanwhile, it is recommended that the intake of added sugar not exceed 25% of calories, providing guidance for people to derive more than 75% of their carbohydrates from foods such as dairy products, grains, legumes, and fruits and vegetables

5. Circulating glucose and stored glycogen are principal energy sources for most cells and tissues and are mandatory for others, such as red blood cells and the brain. Red blood cells can only use glucose for fuel, and, in the process, generate lactate

6. Monosaccharides gain access to cells via glucose transport proteins, which vary based on their presence in different tissue and their K_m. GLUT4 is the glucose transporter in muscle and adipose tissue responsible for reducing much of circulating blood glucose after a meal

7. Carbohydrate metabolism is regulated by hormones, such as insulin, epinephrine, glucagon, and cortisol. In general, insulin is anabolic with regard to carbohydrate, whereas epinephrine is catabolic, leading to glycogen breakdown in the liver and muscle. Cortisol supports glycogen storage and gluconeogenesis simultaneously in the liver

8. Insulin is primarily anabolic, directing the uptake of glucose into muscle and adipose tissue cells during hyperglycemic states. That happens via stimulation of the translocation of GLUT4 from storage sites within those cells

9. Glucagon, cortisol, and epinephrine work to raise blood glucose levels by supporting gluconeogenesis in hepatocytes. Glucagon strongly promotes glycogen breakdown in the liver, whereas epinephrine promotes glycogen breakdown in both the liver and skeletal muscle

10. Glycogen is found in a variety of tissues but is most concentrated in the liver and muscle. Liver glycogen serves as a resource to preserve blood glucose levels during early fasting, whereas muscle glycogen serves as an immediate energy resource during intense physical activity, including strenuous exercise. Lactate derived from muscle glycogen metabolism can circulate to the liver and be converted to glucose, which, in turn, can enter the blood and serve as energy for muscle and other tissue

▶ Suggested Reading

Brand-Miller JC. Glycemic load and chronic disease. *Nutr Rev.* 2003;61(5 pt 2): S49–S55.

Campos FG, Logulla Waitzberg AG, Kiss DR, Waitzberg DL, Habr-Gama A, Gama-Rodrigues J. Diet and colorectal cancer: current evidence for etiology and prevention. *Nutr Hosp.* 2005;20(1):18–25.

Corgneau M, Scher J, Ritié-Pertusa L, et al. Recent Advances on Lactose Intolerance: Tolerance Thresholds and Currently Available Solutions. *Crit Rev Food Sci Nutr.* 2017: 57(15):3344–3356.

Dekker MJ, Su Q, Baker C, Rutledge AC, Adeli K. Fructose: a highly lipogenic nutrient implicated in insulin resistance, hepatic steatosis, and the metabolic syndrome. *Am J Physiol Endocrinol Metab.* 2010;299(5):E685–E694.

Eastwood M, Kritchevsky D. Dietary fiber: how did we get where we are? *Ann Rev Nutr.* 2005;25:1–8.

Erkkilä AT, Lichtenstein AH. Fiber and cardiovascular disease risk: how strong is the evidence? *J Cardiovasc Nurs.* 2006;21(1):3–8.

Institute of Medicine, Food and Nutrition Board. *Dietary Reference Intakes for Energy, Carbohydrate, Fiber, Fat, Fatty Acids, Cholesterol, Protein, and Amino Acids (Macronutrients).* Washington, DC: National Academies Press; 2002/2005.

Ishii S, Iizuka K, Miller BC, Uyeda K. Carbohydrate response element binding protein directly promotes lipogenic enzyme gene transcription. *Proc Natl Acad Sci U S A.* 2004;101(44): 15597–15602.

Khan TA, Sievenpiper JL. Controversies about sugars: results from systematic reviews and meta-analysis on obesity, cardiometabolic disease and diabetes. *Eur J Nutr* 2016;55(suppl 2):25–43.

Klein S. Clinical trial experience with fat-restricted vs. carbohydrate-restricted weight-loss diets. *Obes Res.* 2004;12(suppl 2):141S–144S.

Merchant AT, Vatanparast H, Barlas S, et al. Carbohydrate intake and overweight and obesity among healthy adults. *J Am Diet Assoc.* 2009;109(7):1165–1172.

Rosinger A, Herrick K, Ganche J, Park S. Sugar-sweetened beverage consumption among U.S. adults, 2011-2014. *NCHS Data Brief* 2017; 270:1–8.

Schaefer EJ, Gleason JA, Dansinger ML. Dietary fructose and glucose differentially affect lipid and glucose homeostasis. *J Nutr.* 2009; 139(6):1257S–1262S.

Seal CJ. Whole grains and CVD risk. *Proc Nutr Soc.* 2006;65(1): 24–34.

U.S. Department of Health and Human Services and U.S. Department of Agriculture. 2015–2020 Dietary Guidelines for Americans. 8th Edition. December 2015. Available at http://health.gov/dietaryguidelines/2015/guidelines/

Uyeda K, Repa JJ. Carbohydrate response element binding protein, ChREBP, a transcription factor coupling hepatic glucose utilization and lipid synthesis. *Cell Metab.* 2006;4(2):107–110.

Watson RT, Pessin JE. Intracellular organization of insulin signaling and GLUT4 translocation. *Recent Prog Horm Res.* 2001;56:175–193.

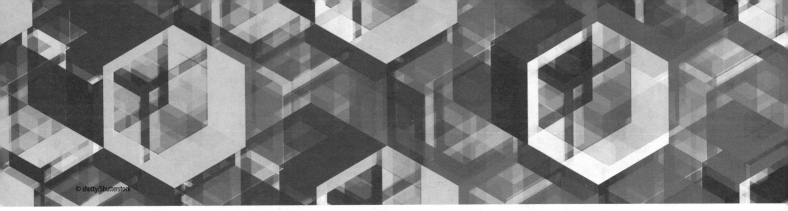

CHAPTER 4
Dietary Fiber: Digestion and Health

← HERE'S WHERE YOU HAVE BEEN

1. Carbohydrates are a class of nutrients that includes sugars, starches, fibers, and related molecules, such as glycosaminoglycans, amino sugars, and more.
2. Key differences in covalent bonding make some carbohydrates more digestible than others.
3. Carbohydrate metabolism is regulated by hormones, such as insulin, epinephrine, glucagon, and cortisol.
4. Absorption refers to the movement of nutrients from the digestive tract into the blood or lymphatic circulations, whereas the concept of bioavailability also includes the uptake and use of a nutrient by cells or tissue.
5. Circulating glucose and stored glycogen are principal energy sources for most cells and tissue and are mandatory for others, such as red blood cells as well as the brain, under normal conditions.

HERE'S WHERE YOU ARE GOING →

1. Dietary fiber is a class of plant structural material that is largely monosaccharide based and, due to the nature of its covalent bonds and three-dimensional structure, more resistant to digestion.
2. Fibers are special carbohydrates and related molecules that are categorized as dietary or functional fibers based on characteristics such as whether they are naturally occurring in a food or added as an ingredient.
3. Certain types of fiber can form a gel-like complex in the stomach and potentially support perceived hunger and satiety, thus potentially influencing energy intake and weight management.
4. Different types of bacteria are found along the length of the digestive tract, depending on the environmental conditions and the properties of the bacterial species, with the highest concentration found in the colon.
5. Certain fibers are metabolized by bacteria in the digestive tract, especially the large intestine, and can influence the microflora balance, which, in turn, can influence health.

▶ Introduction

Decades ago, dietary fiber was referred to as roughage. Later, it was called crude fiber and targeted for removal from animal feeds and grain-based ingredients for human consumption. In grain-based food production (e.g., breads, pastas, breakfast cereals, ready-to-mix powders, etc.), fibers were viewed as undesirable from a functional and final product sensory experience, and thus, grains were milled to remove most of the fiber. However, over the last several decades, the health benefits of different fibers have been identified and their intake is now broadly recommended. Furthermore, the definition of *fiber* continues to evolve, and new forms of dietary fiber are regularly becoming available in the food supply.

To complicate fiber as a nutrient classification, The U.S. Food and Drug Administration (FDA) published the final rule, titled Food Labeling: Revision of the Nutrition and Supplement Facts Labels (Final Rule) in the Federal Register on May 27, 2016. The compliance date for this regulation and thus label updates was initially set for July 26, 2018, but since extended, meaning that any product produced after this date must have the new Nutrition Facts format. As part of that communication, the FDA stated that fiber is nondigestible soluble and insoluble carbohydrates (with 3 or more monomeric units), and lignin that are intrinsic and intact in plants; isolated or synthetic nondigestible carbohydrates (with 3 or more monomeric units) was determined by the FDA to have physiologic effects that are beneficial to human health. The last part is interesting because it places the responsibility of reviewing the physiologic benefit of purported fiber ingredients and, in turn, whether they can labeled as fiber, on the FDA. While many of the fiber sources from intact plant ingredients and those involved in Health Claims were not initially reviewed, several functional fiber ingredients faced the scientific and nutraceutical scrutiny of the FDA.

▶ Dietary Fiber and Functional Fibers

The definition for *fiber* varies from country to country. The United States Food and Nutrition Board provides updated definitions and categorized fiber into dietary fiber and functional fiber based on the following distinctions:

1. Dietary fiber: Nondigestible carbohydrates and lignin that are intrinsic and intact in plants.
2. Functional fiber: Isolated, nondigestible carbohydrates that have beneficial physiologic effects in humans.
3. **Total fiber**: The sum of dietary fiber and functional fiber.

This classification system recognizes the diversity of carbohydrates in the human food supply that are not digested. It includes (1) plant cell wall and storage carbohydrates that predominate in foods, (2) carbohydrates contributed by animal foods, and (3) isolated and low-molecular-weight carbohydrates that occur naturally or have been synthesized or otherwise manufactured. This more modern definition and classification system allows for greater global conformity and affords ample flexibility to incorporate new fiber sources in the future, which is especially important as processing and manufacturing systems continue to advance. One interesting feature of classifying fiber as either dietary or functional fiber is that a form of fiber can be considered either dietary or functional, depending on whether it is naturally occurring or is used as a recipe ingredient with the intention of increasing the health benefits associated with the finished product.

Dietary Fiber

Dietary fiber is plant material, both polysaccharide and lignin, that is resistant to human digestive enzymes. Because it is resistant to digestion, carbohydrate building blocks (monosaccharides) are not absorbed across the wall of the small intestine. Another descriptor used for dietary fiber is nonstarch polysaccharides (NSPs). NSPs include cellulose, hemicellulose, pectin, gums, β-glucans, and other molecules, but not lignin. Lignin is not considered a polysaccharide or a carbohydrate. However, it is generally considered a fiber.

Dietary fiber sources typically provide other macronutrients as well, including nonfiber carbohydrates and protein. **TABLE 4.1** provides the percentage of the total weight of a number of foods that is attributable to fiber. For instance, isolated dietary fiber sources, such as cereal bran, include intact cells, starch, and protein. Naturally occurring resistant starch or resistant starch created during processing would also be considered dietary fiber. Legumes contain oligosaccharides (3 to 10 monosaccharide units), namely raffinose, stachyose, and verbacose, which are considered dietary fiber. Fructans, such as inulin found in onions, chicory, and Jerusalem artichokes, as well as methylcellulose, resistant maltodextrin, and polydextrose are all considered dietary fiber.

TABLE 4.1 Percentage of Fiber Content of Various Foods

Food	Fiber (% weight)
Almonds	12.0
Apples	2.5
Lima beans	19.0
String beans (green beans)	2.7
Broccoli	2.6
Carrots	2.8
Flour, whole wheat	10.7
Flour, white wheat	2.7
Oat flakes	13.0
Pears	3.0
Pecans	9.6
Popcorn	14.5
Strawberries	2.0
Walnuts	6.7
Wheat germ (crude)	13.2

Functional Fiber

Functional fiber is composed of isolated or extracted nondigestible carbohydrates that are recognized for their potentially beneficial effects in the human body. A variety of processing methods is used to isolate functional fibers from their natural sources, including chemical, enzymatic, and/or aqueous methods. Synthetically produced or isolated naturally occurring oligosaccharides and manufactured resistant starches are also categorized as functional fibers. Functional fiber is also the default classification for indigestible animal carbohydrates, such as chitin. This is because they are non-plant-based molecules, not because their health benefit has been firmly established. In contrast, sugar alcohols are not considered to be functional fiber,

although health benefits are often associated with this family of indigestible carbohydrates. Those carbohydrate forms are listed separately on food labels (e.g., the Nutrition Facts panel).

▶ Soluble and Insoluble Fiber

Dietary fiber was long classified as either *soluble* or *insoluble*, based on its propensity to dissolve in water. **Soluble fibers** include pectins, gums, and mucilages. **Insoluble fibers** are composed of cellulose, hemicellulose, lignin, and modified cellulose. **TABLE 4.2** lists the various fiber classifications and lists food sources for each type. Foods vary in their level of total fiber and the contribution of soluble and insoluble fibers. Foods that tend to be better sources of soluble fibers are fruits, legumes, oats, and some vegetables. Richer sources of insoluble fibers include cereals, grains, legumes, and vegetables, especially those with a mature cell wall.

Soluble fibers, such as pectin, are composed mostly of galactosyluronic acid that has been methylated. The units are connected by β1-4 linkages. The degree of methylation normally increases during the ripening of fruit and allows for gel-like properties. Gums and mucilages are similar to pectin in structure and properties, with hexose and pentose monomers making up those soluble fiber types. For instance, guar gum is a linear mannan with galactose side chains. Mucilages are produced by the secretory cells of plants to prevent excess transpiration. Gums are polysaccharides that are often synthesized by plants at the site of an injury and may function similarly to human scar tissue. Meanwhile, xanthan gum and gellan gums are produced by bacteria and are commonly employed as stabilizing and thickening ingredients in food recipes.

▶ Dietary Fiber Types and Characteristics

Dietary fiber types can differ in several ways, including the exclusivity or predominance of specific monosaccharides and the bonding between monomers. The following is an abbreviated review of the key characteristics of the different dietary fibers.

Cellulose

Cellulose is the main structural polysaccharide found within plant cell walls. Cellulose is the most abundant organic molecule on the earth and is easily recognizable in terms of its structure. Cellulose has repeating

TABLE 4.2 Fiber Types and Characteristics, Food Sources, and Bacterial Fermentability in the Gut

Fiber Type	Characteristics	Food Sources	Fermentability[a]
Soluble			
Pectins	Plant cell walls and middle lamella between cells; major fiber consumed	Fruits, especially citrus fruits, apples, bananas, and cherries; cabbage, apples, potatoes, beans	High
Gums	Plant exudates, bacterial fermentation product	Dried beans, oats, fruits, bran, vegetables, seaweed, bacterial fermentation	High
Mucilages	Synthesized by plant cells	Typically a food additive	High
Fructans (inulin, oligofructose, and fructo-oligosaccharides)	Oligosaccharide	Chicory root, bananas, onions, agave, garlic, asparagus, jícama, and leeks; food additives	High
Insoluble			
Cellulose	Structural framework of green plants and algae	Lettuce, green leaves, stems, seaweeds, most plant sources	Low
Hemicellulose	Structural component of cell walls and binds to cellulose and pectin	Most plant sources, whole grains, bran	Low
Lignin	Mature cell walls	Vegetables, wheat, and other cereal grains	Low

[a]High and Low denote the relative degree of bacterial fermentation.

glucose units, similar to amylose, but with the β1-4 linkage described earlier (**FIGURE 4.1**). It is synthesized on the plant cell wall by an enzyme complex called cellulose synthase. Almost as soon as nascent cellulose chains are formed, they assemble with other cellulose molecules and form microfibrils that strengthen the cell wall. Cellulose, along with certain other fibers (hemicellulose and pectin) and proteins, is found within the matrix between the cell wall layers. This organization is not unlike the human connective tissue matrix found within bone, tendons, and ligaments. Because cellulose can be consumed as naturally occurring in foods as well as an added ingredient to a manufactured food, it can be classified as either dietary or functional fiber. Much of the cellulose used in food and supplement manufacturing is derived from wood or cotton, and it is often added as an anticaking and/ or thickening agent.

Hemicellulose

Hemicellulose is quite different from cellulose and is classified as a dietary fiber. It is rather heterogeneous and is composed of many pentoses and hexoses covalently bonded in a β1-4 linkage with branching side chains. The monosaccharides found in hemicelluloses include xylose, glucose, mannose, and galactose. Those sugars are referred to as xylans, mannans, and galactans when they are in the form of polymers composing the hemicelluloses. Other monosaccharide subunits include arabinose and 4-O-methyl glucuronic acids. Hemicellulose is a structural polysaccharide and is also a component of plant cell walls. It is composed of a mixture of both straight-chain and highly branched polysaccharides containing pentoses, hexoses, and uronic acids. Hemicelluloses are different from cellulose in that they are not limited to glucose but also include those other

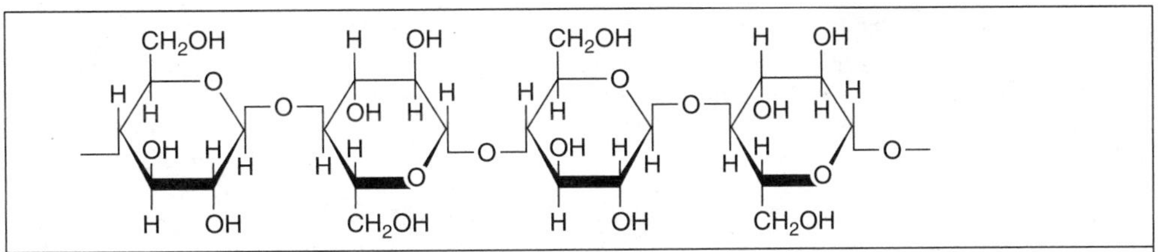

Cellulose is unbranched repeating β-D-glucose units.

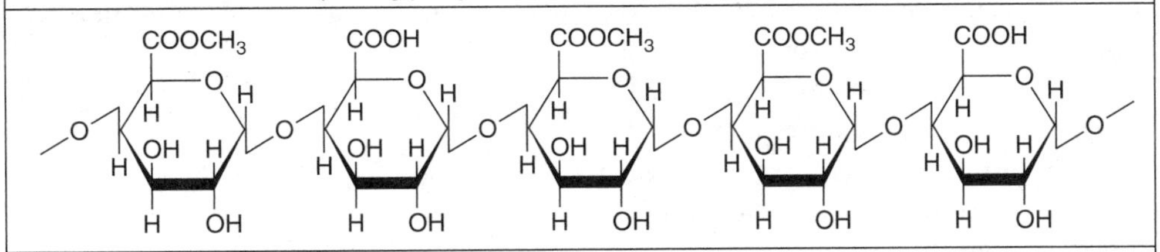

Pectin is a polymer of α-galacturonic acid with a variable number of methyl ester groups.

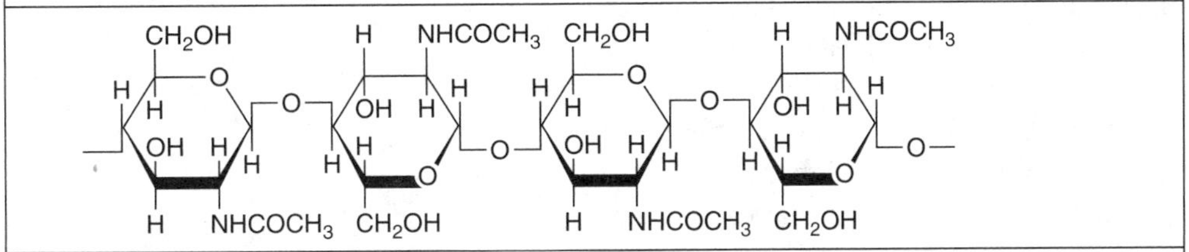

Chitin is an unbranched polymer of N-acetyl-D-glucosamine.

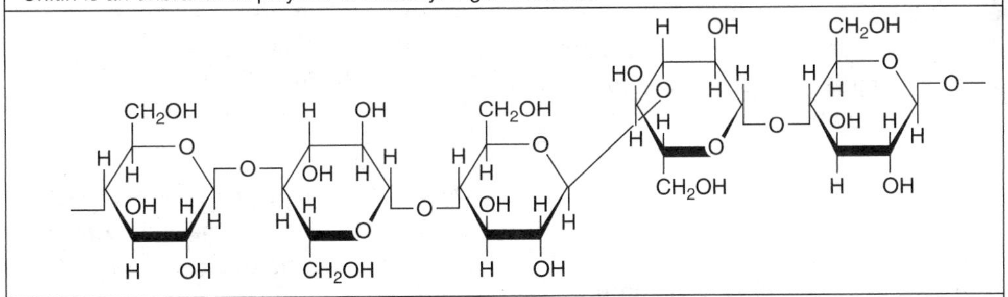

β-glucans consist of linear unbranched polysaccharides of β-D-glucose with one 1β-3 linkage for every three or four 1β-4 linkages.

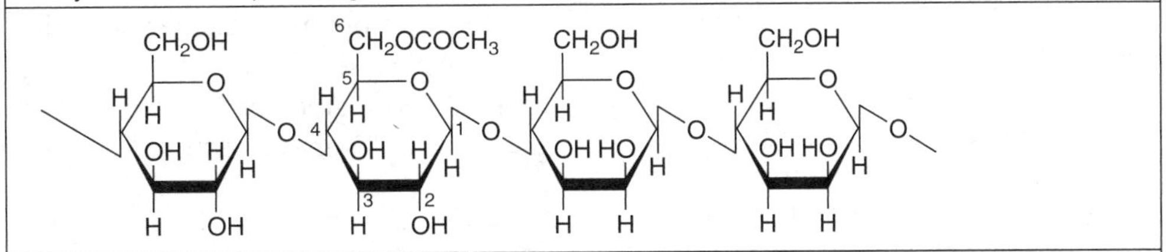

Glucomannan polysaccharide consists of glucose and mannose in a 5:8 proportion joined by 1β-4 linkages.

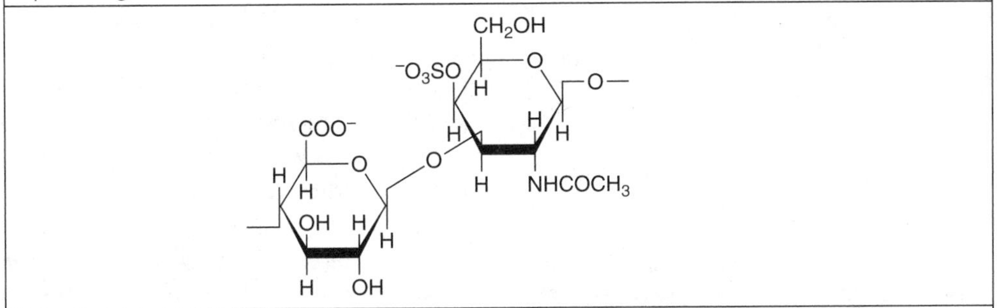

Chondroitin sulfate is composed of β-D-glucuronate linked to the number 3 carbon of N-acetylgalactosamine-4-sulfate.

FIGURE 4.1 Structural Characteristics of Certain Fibers. Fibers are composed of various repeating monosaccharides linked together by either α or β linkages between either carbons 1 and 4 or 1 and 3, depending on fiber type.

sugars. Xylose, arabinose, mannose, and galacturonic acid are found in relatively higher abundance and are more vulnerable to hydrolysis by bacterial degradation compared with other sugars.

Pectins

Pectins are homopolysaccharides that are composed of repeating galacturonic acid subunits connected by a β1-4 linkage. The carboxyl groups are often methylated, and their repeating subunits are sometimes referred to as methylgalactosyl uronic acid (see Figure 4.1). The carboxyl groups become methylated in a seemingly random manner as fruit ripens.

A pectin is a jelly-like material that acts as a cellular cement in plants. It is found in the cell wall as well as in the middle lamella between plant cells. Pectin is a major fiber component of the diet, and its amount in different plant sources varies. Pectin is found in higher amounts in legumes, apples, citrus fruits, apricots, beets, cabbage, and carrots. Pectin is often used in the food industry as a gelling or thickening agent or as a stabilizer in semi-solid foods such as yogurts, jellies, jams, and gelatins. Based on how pectins are either found or used, they can be classified as dietary or functional fiber.

Lignin

As discussed earlier, **lignin** is not a carbohydrate but is considered an insoluble dietary fiber. It is composed of aromatic, highly branched polymers of phenylpropanoid units from plant cell walls and provides plants with some of their "woody" characteristics. Lignins are highly complex and variable polymers that are associated with carbohydrate-based fibers. Although they have no specific organizational structure, they are composed of three major aromatic alcohols: coumaryl, coniferyl, and sinapyl (**FIGURE 4.2**). Those units are often modified, allowing for as many as 40 different lignin structures. Based on how lignins are either found or used, they can be classified as either dietary or functional fiber.

Gums

Gums are polysaccharides. They are most often found in the woody elements of plants or in seed coatings. Gums are derived from land-based plants, seaweeds, or bacterial fermentation. They have the ability to bind a lot of water and are thus used in the food industry as thickeners, gelling agents, emulsifiers, and stabilizers. Natural gums can be classified according to their origin or as uncharged or ionic polymers (polyelectrolytes). Sea-

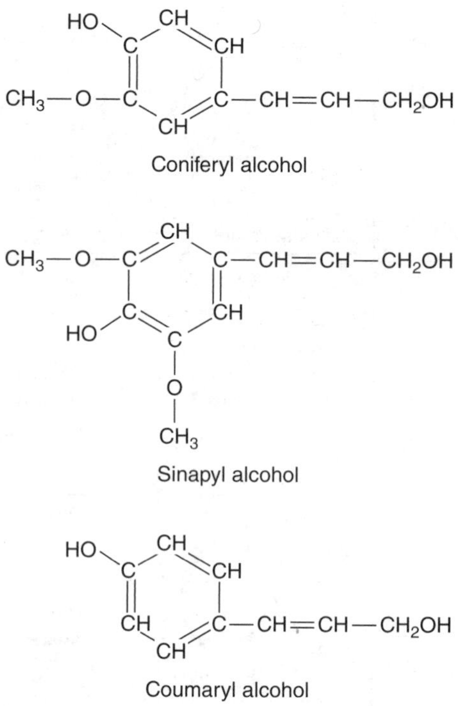

FIGURE 4.2 Structure of Common Phenolic Compounds of Lignin. Lignin is not considered a carbohydrate but is composed of polymers of the above major aromatic alcohols.

weed gums include carrageenan, agar, alginic acid, and sodium alginate. Nonmarine gums include gum arabic, gum ghatti, gum tragacanth, karaya gum, guar gum, locust bean gum, β-glucan, glucomannan, tara gum, and spruce gum. Many gums used in the food industry are derived from microbial fermentation. Because gums can be consumed as naturally occurring in foods as well as an added ingredient to a recipe-manufactured food, they can be classified as either dietary or functional fiber.

β-Glucans

β-Glucans are polysaccharides composed of D-glucose units linked by β-glycosidic bonds. They vary in molecular size and configuration as well as solubility and viscosity when in a fluid. The most active forms of β-glucans are those comprising D-glucose units with 1-3 links and with side chains of D-glucose attached at the 1-6 position (see Figure 4.1), which are referred to as β-1,3/1,6 glucan. Some β-glucans exist as single-strand chains, whereas the backbones of other β-1,3 glucans exist as double- or triple-stranded helical chains. In addition, proteins can be associated with specific configurations and are believed to support some of the unique attributes of some β-glucans.

β-glucans occur mostly as cellulose in plants such as cereal grains as well as in the cell wall of

Saccharomyces cerevisiae (Baker's yeast), some mushrooms, and bacteria. The bran component of barley and oats is one of the richest sources of β-glucans. Yeast is the source of much of the β-glucans used in dietary supplements and foods. It is also extracted from oats and barley and, to a lesser degree, rye and wheat. As discussed later in the chapter, β-glucans have been recognized for their potential health benefit, and specific health claims can be made on product packaging for foods containing β-glucans. Because β-glucans can be consumed as naturally occurring in foods as well as an added ingredient to a recipe-manufactured food, they can be classified as either dietary or functional fiber.

Chitin and Chitosan

Chitin is chemically related to pectin; however, chitin is not a plant polysaccharide. It is found within the animal kingdom, but not in humans. It is found in the shells or exoskeletons of insects and crustacea (e.g., crabs, lobsters) and the cell walls of fungi (see Figure 4.1). It is a β1-4 homopolymer of *N*-acetyl-glucosamine. Chitosan is structurally similar to chitin, but as a deacetylated form. Chitin and chitosan are mostly consumed as part of dietary supplements and can be classified as a functional fiber, pending proven physiologic benefits.

Fructans (Inulin, Oligofructose, and Fructo-oligosaccharides)

Fructans, as the name suggests, are fructose-based polymers of varying length. Inulin, oligofructose, and fructo-oligosaccharides (FOS) are commonly occurring fructans. Typically, the linkage between fructose monomers occurs at the β2-1 position with a glucose monomer at the end position. Fructans are generally indigestible by amylase and amylopectinase digestive enzymes; however, certain bacteria, including Bifidobacteria, produce β-fructosidase, which can hydrolyze the β-linkages between fructose molecules. Inulin, which typically contains dozens of fructose monomers, is becoming more prevalent in the commercial food chain as an added ingredient. FOS can be produced from the partial breakdown of larger inulin molecules or commercially synthesized from sucrose. Fructans are naturally occurring in foods such as agave, artichokes, asparagus, leeks, garlic, onions, yacon, jícama, and wheat. Naturally occurring fructans are classified as dietary fiber; manufactured fructans that are then added to foods can be classified as functional fiber, pending proof of health benefit.

Glycosaminoglycans

Another class of polysaccharides is the glycosaminoglycans (GAGs), which are sometimes called mucopolysaccharides. Glycosaminoglycans are characterized by the presence of amino sugars and uronic acids, which occur in combination with proteins in body secretions and structures. Those polysaccharides are responsible for the viscosity of body mucous secretions. They are components of extra-cellular amorphous ground substances surrounding collagen and elastin fibers and cells of connective tissues and bone. Those molecules hold onto large amounts of water and occupy space, which allows for some cushioning and lubrication. Also, in combination with glycoproteins and glycolipids, the glycosaminoglycans form the cell coat or carbohydrate-dense glycocalyx present in human and other animal tissue.

Examples of glycosaminoglycans include hyaluronic acid and chondroitin sulfate (see Figure 4.1). Hyaluronic acid is a component of the ground substance found in most connective tissue, including the synovial fluid of joints. It is a jelly-like substance composed of repeating disaccharides of β-glucuronic acid and *N*-acetyl-D-glucosamine. Hyaluronic acid can contain several thousand disaccharide residues and is unique among the other glycosaminoglycans in that it will not interact with proteins to form proteoglycans. Chondroitin sulfate is composed of repeating units of β-glucuronic acid and *N*-acetylgalactosamine-4-sulfate. This molecule has a relatively high viscosity and capability to bind water. It is the major organic component of the ground substance of cartilage and bone. Hyaluronic acid and chondroitin sulfate both have β1-3 linkages between uronic acid and acetylated amino sugars but are linked by β1-4 covalent bonds to other polysaccharide units. Unlike hyaluronic acid, chondroitin sulfate will bind to proteins to form proteoglycans.

Heparin is a naturally occurring anticoagulant and serves as another example of a glycosaminoglycan. It is produced by mast cells in connective tissue and is stored as granules within these cells. Mast cells are located around the inner portion of capillaries of connective tissue. Chemically, heparin is composed of variably sulfated repeating disaccharide units, including sulfated glucosamine and iduronic acid. It has an α1-4 linkage between the disaccharide repeating units. Heparin inhibits the action of thrombin upon fibrinogen and prevents the formation of fibrin threads and clots. Heparin also interferes with prothrombin activator, which converts prothrombin to thrombin. Larger glycosaminoglycans are used in dietary supplements and are recognized by some as functional fibers.

Oligosaccharides

Oligosaccharides are composed of 3 to 10 monosaccharides linked by glycosidic bonds between the OH groups of adjacent monomeric units. The metabolic fate of the oligosaccharides stachyose, verbascose, and raffinose is somewhat different from that of other oligosaccharides in that they are primarily fermented by bacteria in the colon. This property has resulted in their claim to fame as flatulence producers. Legumes (beans) have appreciable levels of those oligosaccharides. In beans, those carbohydrates comprise 2% to 4% of dry weight.

Those oligosaccharides are often referred to as the raffinose family of sugars and are galactosylsucrose derivatives. For example, raffinose is sucrose linked with galactose (**FIGURE 4.3**). Stachyose is raffinose bonded to a second galactose monomer. Verbascose, which is composed of five monosaccharides, is stachyose with a third galactose monomer bonded to it.

Stachyose and raffinose are found in most legumes, and those shorter links of monosaccharides are generally resistant to human carbohydrate digestive enzymes. Thus, like lactose, those carbohydrates stay intact in the intestinal lumen. Once in the colon, those carbohydrates are subject to bacterial fermentation. Similar by-products are produced, as with lactose digestion, as well as similar symptoms. Commercially available antigas products (e.g., Beano) are enzyme preparations that enhance digestion of those carbohydrates when consumed just prior to the legume-containing meal.

Polydextrose

Polydextrose is a polysaccharide that is produced by polymerization of glucose and sorbitol. Food manufacturers use polydextrose as a bulking agent in foods and to bolster fiber claims on labels. Because it imparts some sweetness, it can also be used to replace some sugar in foods. Polydextrose is not digested in the small intestine and is partially fermented in the colon; what is not digested is excreted in the feces. Based on its potentially beneficial effects in the large intestine, polydextrose could be considered a functional fiber, pending research validation.

Psyllium

Psyllium (also known as ispaghula husk) is the common term applied to several members of the plant genus *Plantago*, whose seeds are used commercially for the production of mucilage. More specifically, psyllium refers to the very viscous mucilage from the husk of psyllium seeds, which are small, dark, reddish-brown, odorless, and nearly tasteless. The husk is usually derived from *Plantago ovata*, known as blond or Indian plantago seed. It can also be obtained from *P. ramose*, which is also called Spanish or French psyllium seed. Recent interest in psyllium has arisen primarily due to its use as an ingredient in high-fiber breakfast cereals. Some believe that it can be effective in reducing blood cholesterol levels. Psyllium can be classified as a functional fiber.

Resistant Dextrins

Resistant dextrins are the indigestible components of starch breakdown resulting from heat-acid and enzymatic (amylase) treatment. Indigestible dextrins are also called resistant maltodextrins, not to be confused with nonresistant maltodextrin or simply, **maltodextrin**. Resistant maltodextrins have broad application in food manufacturing and are easily added to foods and promote desirable mouth-feel. Resistant dextrins consist of polymers of glucose containing α1-4 and α1-6 glucosidic bonds, as well as α1-2 and α1-3 linkages. The average molecular weight of resistant maltodextrins is 2,000 daltons. Resistant dextrins can potentially be classified as functional fibers, pending sufficient data on their physiologic benefits in humans.

Resistant Starches

Some naturally occurring starches are not completely hydrolyzed by amylases in the upper digestive tract and are referred to as enzyme-resistant starch, or simply, **resistant starch**. They are often considered a form of fiber because they move through the upper digestive system undigested and then are metabolized by bacteria in the colon in a manner similar to some fibers. Resistant starches tend to be classified as one of four types:

RS1: Physically inaccessible (yet digestible) resistant starch that can be found in seeds, legumes, or unprocessed grains.

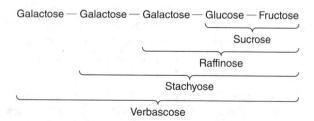

FIGURE 4.3 Structure of Raffinose, Stachyose, and Verbascose. The three compounds differ in the number of galactose units each has.

RS2: Naturally occurring semicrystalline granules that are present in foods such as uncooked potatoes and green bananas.

RS3: Resistant starches that are formed during cooking and cooling of foods such as legumes, cooked or chilled potatoes, and cornflakes. RS3 also includes retrograded high-amylose corn.

RS4: Starches that are specially processed to yield chemically modified resistant starches.

Resistant starches are either physically inaccessible, yet amylase-digestible, starches or they are not amylase-digestible starches based on their granular nature or chemical alteration. Interestingly, if RS2 granules are heated to over 100°C, their granularity is lost, and the starch gelatinizes or the granules swell, thereby increasing the availability of the starch to amylase. However, upon cooling, there is some recrystallization of the starch. This is called retrogradation, which is resistant to α-amylase hydrolysis.

Uncooked starch, such as that present in a banana (roughly 4 to 5 grams), is also resistant to hydrolysis for similar reasons relating to the crystalline structure. That implies that the metabolizable energy is decreased in those types of food sources. The undigested starch can be fermented in the colon by bacteria, and the short-chain fatty acids produced (e.g., acetate, butyrate) will be absorbed and contribute about 3 kilocalories per gram. The glycemic effect of starch is, therefore, lowered, which decreases insulin secretion. In addition to glycemic management, resistant starches may play a role in weight management as well.

⬣ BEFORE YOU GO ON . . .

1. What is the general definition for fiber?
2. What are the building blocks and dietary sources of different fiber types?
3. What is the difference between a dietary fiber and a functional fiber?
4. What are resistant starches?
5. What are some examples of fibers used in food manufacturing and for what purpose?

▶ Health Benefits of Fiber and Structural Carbohydrates

The physiologic effects of dietary fiber largely depend on the fiber's physical characteristics, namely, its molecular design and solubility. Whereas most of the physiologic interactions of dietary fibers were once thought to be limited to within the digestive tract, and thus outside of the human body, newer evidence suggests that derivatives of intestinal fiber metabolism can influence several internal operations. In turn, fiber intake can have a beneficial impact on general health and acute well-being and also play a role in risk reduction for certain chronic degenerative diseases, such as heart disease (**TABLE 4.3**).

The physical characteristics of dietary fiber can evoke different gastrointestinal responses,

SPECIAL FEATURE 4.1

Analysis of Fiber in Foods

Historically, there was a lot of confusion as to how much fiber was present in a particular food. This early misinformation was probably caused by the methods used to quantify fiber in food items. This feature discusses some of the key methods that have been used over time to estimate fiber content and the advantages and disadvantages of those methods when applied to fiber in the human diet. **TABLE 1** reviews each of those fiber analysis methods, noting which fiber components each estimates, as well as the method's relative accuracy. Some of the methods presented here are historic and may no longer be used in some studies, but they may be referred to in older literature. Also, some of the more current methods are used for food labeling purposes.

Crude Fiber Method

Much of the early fiber analysis work used the crude fiber method because that was the primary method used to determine the quantity of fiber for ruminant animals. The method is essentially a sequential extraction of the material to be analyzed with hot dilute acid followed by dilute alkali. The crude fiber method is good for analyzing fiber content for cattle, but not for humans. What is fiber to a human is not fiber to cattle, so this system underestimated the soluble and insoluble fiber content of foods for humans.

(continues)

SPECIAL FEATURE 4.1 (*continued*)

TABLE 1 Methods of Fiber Analysis

Method	Details	Accuracy
Crude	Analysis for cellulose, hemicellulose, and lignin	Underestimates fiber
Acid detergent	Good for cellulose and lignin; marginal for hemicellulose and pectin	Underestimates fiber
Neutral detergent	Good for cellulose, hemicellulose, and lignin, but not for soluble fibers	Underestimates fiber
Van Soest	Combination of acid and neutral detergent methods; not good for soluble fibers	Underestimates fiber
Southgate	A fractionation method of analysis; good for all fractionation fiber components, including insoluble and soluble; best reference method	Very time consuming
Enzymatic (Prosky)	Very good method for analyzing all components of fiber; does not break them down into individual fiber types; rapid	Overestimates fiber
AOAC[a] 2011.25	Separates fiber into insoluble, soluble, and total fiber	Most current and good for food labeling; slower than the enzymatic method

[a]Association of Official Analytic Chemist.
Data from AOAC 2011.25

Acid Detergent Method

Newer methods emerged once the limitations of the crude fiber method became apparent. The acid detergent method, so called because the analysis protocol involves boiling samples in sulfuric acid, was used to estimate the fiber component of cellulose and lignin. This method was developed for feeds and forages and was not very good for determining soluble fiber.

Neutral Detergent Method

The neutral detergent method involves boiling the material to be analyzed in sodium lauryl sulfate and EDTA-borate at a pH of 7.0. It adequately determined plant cell wall components, such as cellulose, lignin, and hemicellulose, but it was not good for determining the soluble components of dietary fiber. The neutral detergent method was modified for the analysis of human foods, because those foods are often high in starch and fat. The modification allowed for fat extraction followed by treatment with amylase to break down the starch.

Van Soest Method

In the years that followed, a newer method was developed that combined the acid detergent and the neutral fiber methods. Termed the Van Soest method, it provided an even better estimation of all insoluble fiber components than either the acid or neutral detergent methods. However, this methodology was also limited by its inability to quantify soluble fibers.

Southgate Fractionization System

A good method developed for the complete analysis of dietary fiber, both soluble and insoluble, is the Southgate fractionation system. This was the benchmark reference method or state-of-the-art method for years. It allowed for an accurate estimation of pectic substances, hemicellulose, cellulose, and lignin using a sequential extraction procedure. Nonfibrous material is removed first, followed by removal of pectic substances with hot water and a chelator. Hemicellulose is then extracted in several fractions by first adding dilute sodium hydroxide (NaOH) and nitrogen to precipitate the material. This step is then repeated, with alcohol added, to obtain a second component of hemicellulose. Finally, under the influence of strong sodium hydroxide and nitrogen, the final fraction of hemicellulose can be obtained (hemicellulose fractions A, B, and C). Cellulose is extracted by precipitation in 17.5% NaOH. Finally, lignin is extracted by the addition of 72% sulfuric acid. Although this method obtains accurate estimations of individual fiber components, it is time consuming and laborious. Laboratories wanting to analyze large numbers of food samples found this method relatively expensive and rather impractical.

Enzymatic Method
With respect to simply determining the total fiber content of a food sample, the greatest breakthrough came with the development of the enzymatic method, or Prosky method. In this method, enzymatic removal of protein and starch from fat-extracted food occurs first. Next, 95% ethanol is used to precipitate the soluble dietary fiber. Residual protein is then quantified, the sample is corrected for ash and protein content, and fiber is determined gravimetrically. Some soluble fibers may still be lost, but this system provides a good estimate of total dietary fiber. However, unlike the Southgate fractionation system, this method does not break down fiber into its individual components. In fact, it may actually overestimate fiber by not completely removing some of the nonfibrous material from a sample.

CODEX and AOAC Approaches
The CODEX Alimentarius Commission was established by the Food and Agriculture Organization of the World Health Organization (WHO), in part, to develop global food standards. Food labeling is often determined by the methods recommended by CODEX in combination with other organizations, such as the Association of Official Analytical Chemists (AOAC). The most current method of fiber analysis used for food labeling purposes is referred to as AOAC 2011.25. This method separates fiber into three categories: (1) insoluble dietary fiber, (2) soluble dietary fiber, and (3) total dietary fiber. Total dietary fiber is essentially the sum of insoluble dietary fiber plus soluble dietary fiber. Resistant starches are included in this approach and are found in the insoluble dietary fiber fraction. This method uses an enzymatic approach to simulate human digestion. Insoluble dietary fiber is determined gravimetrically following enzymatic digestion of a food component. The soluble fiber fraction is divided into two fractions: (1) soluble dietary fiber that is precipitated by the addition of ethanol and gravimetrically determined and (2) the soluble dietary fiber that does not precipitate. This latter fraction is determined using liquid chromatography. This method and others similar to it include some of the resistant starches along with oligosaccharides that are resistant to digestion.

TABLE 4.3 Functional Fibers: Benefits and Sources

Functional Fiber[a]	Potential Health Benefit(s)	Natural/Primary Sources
Cellulose	Laxation	Plant foods
Guar gum	Lowers blood lipid levels; decreases glycemic effect of food	Guar bean (legume)
Inulin, oligofructose, fructo-oligosaccharide	Prebiotic activity; promotes calcium absorption	Chicory root, Jerusalem artichoke—Fermented Synthesized from simple CHO
β-Glucan (beta glucan) and oat bran	Lowers blood lipid levels; attenuates blood glucose response	Oats and barley
Pectin	Lowers blood lipid levels; attenuates blood glucose response	Plant foods
Polydextrose	Laxation; prebiotic activity	Synthesized from dextrose (glucose)
Psyllium	Laxation; lowers blood lipid levels	Psyllium husk (plant)
Resistant dextrins	Lowers blood lipid levels	Corn and wheat
Resistant starch	Attenuates blood glucose response	Plant foods
Soluble corn fiber	Laxation	Corn

[a]Added (fortified).

TABLE 4.4 Physical Properties of Different Fiber Types	
Type	**Action**
Cellulose	Binds water, reduces colonic pressure, reduces fecal transit time
Hemicellulose	Binds water, increases stool bulk, may bind bile acids, reduces colonic pressure, reduces fecal transit time
Pectins, gums, mucilages	Slow gastric emptying, bind bile acids, may bind trace materials
Lignin	Binds water, may bind trace minerals, affects fecal steroids

depending on the segment of the digestive tract involved (**TABLE 4.4**).

Dietary fiber may:

- Promote gastric distention
- Influence gastric emptying and the intestinal motility rate
- Augment the amount of residue and the moisture content of digesta in the small intestine and feces in the colon
- Interact/bind with certain molecules
- Be fermented by bacteria in the lower digestive tract and influence the turnover of the types of bacteria species present. The bacterial population of the colon likely increases due to fiber fermentation and may contribute as much as 45% to fecal dry weight.

▶ Gastrointestinal Fermentation and Health

Fiber remains largely intact during transit through the upper gastrointestinal tract. However, the bacterial populations inhabiting the colon can metabolize several forms of fiber, which, in turn, can benefit the colon and other bodily systems in several ways, as described below. Amylase is not able to hydrolyze the β1-4 covalent bonds found in such fibers as cellulose; however, the microflora of the human colon are able to metabolize some fiber and produce short-chain fatty acids (e.g., acetic, propionic, and butyric acids) as metabolites. These short-chain fatty acids (sometimes called volatile fatty acids) are potential energy sources for colonic mucosal cells or can be absorbed

into the hepatic portal vein. Thus, the classic idea that fiber does not impart energy to the human diet is not entirely true, because the volatile fatty acid byproducts of fiber fermentation can be absorbed by the lumen of the colon and subsequently used for energy. In fact, food labels in the European Union (EU) factor 2 kilocalories (8.4 kilojoules) per gram of fiber. Hydrogen gas, carbon dioxide, and methane are also produced during bacterial metabolism of fibrous material.

Fiber is subject to bacterial degradation in the colon. Pectins, mucilages, and gums appear to be almost completely fermented, whereas cellulose is only partly degraded. Also, because of its unique molecular design, lignin goes virtually unfermented. The degradation of food fibers by intestinal bacteria may be related to the physical structure of the plant itself, because fibers derived from fruits and vegetables appear to be, in general, more fermentable than those from cereal grains.

A clinical estimation of bacterial fermentation of fibrous material can be made via the hydrogen breath test. Hydrogen gas produced by bacterial fermentation dissolves into the blood and circulates to the lungs, where it diffuses into alveoli and is subsequently exhaled. However, note that bacterial fermentation of other digestive residues, such as lactose, will also produce hydrogen gas. This fact must be considered if quantification of expired hydrogen gas is to be used as an indicator of fiber fermentation. The opposite is true as well: bacterial fermentation of fiber must be controlled if the hydrogen breath test is to be applied to estimate **lactose intolerance**.

▶ Reduced Glycemic Effect

Fiber is recognized for its potential impact on the rate of absorption of monosaccharides, which, in turn, can lower the glycemic effect of a food source. Much of these effects are associated with the ability of certain, largely soluble, fiber types, such as raw guar gum, high molecular weight beta glucan, and psyllium to form gels and increase the viscosity of content in the stomach (chyme) and slow its release into the small intestine. However, prehydrolyzed guar gum, often seen with food ingredients, loses much of it gel-forming properties and, in turn, its ability to slow gastric release and impact of glycemic response.

In the small intestine, the hydrated, gel-forming fiber can increase the viscosity of the contents and slow the interaction of digestible carbohydrate with digestive enzymes and, in turn, the rate of nutrient absorption. It has been suggested that a slowing of the rate of carbohydrate absorption may be beneficial to individuals with diabetes by potentially decreasing the glycemic index of foods and chronic hyperglycemia.

▶ Cholesterol Binding and Reduction of Lipids

Higher fiber intakes are inversely associated with heart disease risk. One of the most prominent explanations accounting for a significant amount of this benefit is that certain fibers may bind intestinal material, such as bile acids, cholesterol, and other less-desirable compounds. When more bile acids are complexed to fiber components, fewer bile acids are reabsorbed by the intestine; thus, the enterohepatic circulation of bile acids is decreased, and more bile acids are excreted in the feces (**FIGURE 4.4**). That is believed to result in the dedication of more hepatic cholesterol to the synthesis of new bile acids. Thus, less cholesterol may be available for incorporation into VLDL and export into circulation. As VLDL becomes LDL, the effect is a reduction in total cholesterol and LDL-cholesterol levels. Among the most potent soluble fibers are those that have greater gel-forming properties. Those fibers are namely psyllium, guar gum, and beta-glucan. Pectin and other

acidic polysaccharides also appear to bind bile acids well; however, the potential for lipid lowering is not as great as those soluble fibers noted to have greater gel-forming, viscous properties. Meanwhile, cellulose has little ability to bind bile acids.

▶ Fecal Bulking, Constipation, and Diverticulosis Support

The physical attributes of fiber contribute to perhaps its most renowned effect—the ability to alter the bulk and composition of feces as well as its transit time. Increased fecal bulk from a high dietary fiber intake is due to (1) the presence of nondegraded fiber residue, (2) an increase in fecal water, and (3) an increase in bacterial cell mass caused by fiber fermentation. Fecal bulking is influenced by fiber type.

The water-holding capacity, or hydration, of fiber is one of its more interesting physical properties. The capacity of a fiber to hold onto water is enhanced by the presence of sugar residues that have free polar groups, such as OH, COOH, SO_4, and C=O groups. Pectic substances, mucilages, and hemicellulose have high water-holding capacity. Cellulose and lignin

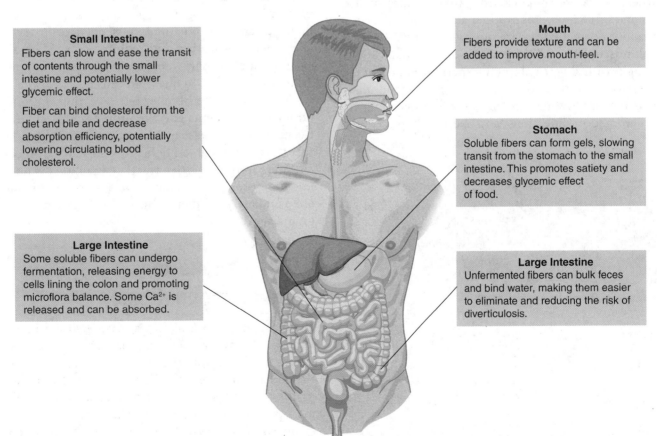

Small Intestine
Fibers can slow and ease the transit of contents through the small intestine and potentially lower glycemic effect.

Fiber can bind cholesterol from the diet and bile and decrease absorption efficiency, potentially lowering circulating blood cholesterol.

Large Intestine
Some soluble fibers can undergo fermentation, releasing energy to cells lining the colon and promoting microflora balance. Some Ca^{2+} is released and can be absorbed.

Mouth
Fibers provide texture and can be added to improve mouth-feel.

Stomach
Soluble fibers can form gels, slowing transit from the stomach to the small intestine. This promotes satiety and decreases glycemic effect of food.

Large Intestine
Unfermented fibers can bulk feces and bind water, making them easier to eliminate and reducing the risk of diverticulosis.

FIGURE 4.4 Processing of Fiber. Note the different physiologic impact of fibers among various organs.

also have a propensity to hold onto water. However, because soluble fibers tend to be more fermentable, the water is normally released into the colon and absorbed. Therefore, in a practical sense, it is the insoluble fibers that hold onto water throughout the total length of the intestinal tract and give the fecal mass greater water content.

In general, noncellulose polysaccharides, such as gums, mucilages, and pectin, are ineffective physical bulking agents largely because of their almost complete degradation via bacterial fermentation (see Table 4.2). Cellulose, hemicellulose, and lignin are more effective bulking agents. **TABLE 4.5** presents the influence of fiber on fecal mass.

A low-fiber diet increases transit time, and a high-fiber diet decreases transit time. In cultures that have high-fiber diets, 24 to 48 hours is the average transit time. In Western cultures, where the dietary fiber content is considerably less, it is not unusual for transit time to be as high as 72 hours or more. In some individuals, the transit time can be as long as 2 weeks! With respect to intestinal motility, a higher-fiber diet is a standard recommendation for the prevention and alleviation of constipation.

A common gastrointestinal disorder in Western societies is **diverticulosis**. This is a condition where there are outpocketings (diverticula) of the colon (**FIGURE 4.5**). Many older adults have diverticula, but normally they are not problematic. Routine colonoscopies usually detect those diverticula. Some people with diverticula may experience abdominal cramps. Bacteria and fecal matter may accumulate and become trapped in the diverticula, leading to inflammation, infections, and abdominal pain. This

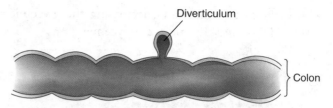

FIGURE 4.5 Diverticulum in the Colon. This GI disorder is more common among western populations and is thought to be related to a low-fiber diet.

condition, called **diverticulitis**, sometimes requires surgical intervention. The fact that people in Western societies have a higher incidence of diverticulosis compared with those in other parts of the world is thought to be linked to the low fiber content of the Western diet. Defecation by people consuming a low-fiber diet likely requires an increase in intra-abdominal pressure, which may lead to the development of diverticula. A high-fiber diet will reduce this condition by decreasing the pressure exerted during defecation.

▶ Mineral Binding

Cation exchange, or the mineral binding capacity of fiber, is also recognized as a physical property of fiber. It can have potential consequences in terms of nutrient absorption and requirements. Minerals, such as calcium, zinc, copper, iron, cadmium, and mercury, may bind to fiber and thus be less available for absorption. The number of free carboxyl groups on fiber components and the uronic acid content of the fibers will increase metal binding. Lignin also has this property. Soluble fibers are very efficient metal chelators in the digestive tract. Overall, this is not a nutrition problem if dietary levels of those minerals are adequate or if dietary fiber does not exceed 50 grams per day.

▶ Daily Intake and Recommendations

During preagricultural times, carbohydrate intake largely came by way of fruits, vegetables, leaves, and tubers. Today, industrial processing has increased the consumption of cereal grains, especially milled grains, as well as refined sugar cane through the mass production of sucrose (table sugar). With these changes, came a reduction in the level of fiber consumption.

TABLE 4.5 Changes in Fecal Bulk Due to Various Dietary Fiber Sources	
Food Item	Percentage Increase in Fecal Weight (%)
Bran	127
Cabbage	69
Carrots	59
Apple	40
Guar gum	20

The amount of fiber present within the human diet can vary geographically as well as by gender. In some developed countries, such as the United States, fiber consumption is relatively lower than in other societies. The average intake of fiber in the United States is only approximately 12 and 18 grams daily for women and men, respectively, which is well below recommendations. Americans consume a diet in which less than one-half of their carbohydrate intake comes from fruits, vegetables, and whole grains. Meanwhile, some African societies consume as much as 50 grams of fiber daily. Recent estimates of South American countries suggest below-recommendation intake levels as well.

As part of the DRIs, the AMDR for carbohydrate intake in the United States and Canada is 45% to 65% of total energy. The range allows for different people to plan their dietary carbohydrate level based on different lifestyles and ability to metabolize food carbohydrates. Individuals are also advised to derive more of the carbohydrate they consume from more nutrient-dense sources, such as whole grain products, legumes, lower-fat dairy foods, and fruits and vegetables. Those foods provide vitamins, minerals, fiber, and phytochemicals that promote health and wellness.

The current AI recommendation for total fiber intake for adults who are 50 years old and younger is 38 grams per day for men and 25 grams per day for women. For adults older than 50 years, the recommendation is 30 grams per day for men and 21 grams per day for women, or 14 grams per 1000 calories consumed. Meanwhile, WHO recommends 25 to 40 grams of fiber daily for adults.

● BEFORE YOU GO ON . . .

1. What are the general health benefits associated with dietary and functional fibers?
2. What is the mechanism(s) whereby fiber impacts cholesterol metabolism, potentially lowering blood lipids?
3. Which fiber types may have the biggest impact on cholesterol metabolism?
4. Can fiber impact satiety and potentially help people manage their energy intake and weight? If so, how, and with which fiber types?
5. What is the current AI for total dietary fiber in adults?

CLINICAL INSIGHT

Fiber Tolerance and Physiologic Assessment

Fiber remains a unique nutrient classification in that much of its benefit is based on the resistance to break down to smaller, absorbable nutrients. This renders fiber different from starches, proteins, and fats where the goal is to efficiently liberate smaller, absorbable subcomponent nutrients. Technically speaking, the digestive tract remains outside the human body, so in many ways, the role and benefits for fiber are external to the body and not cellular and tissue specific. Furthermore, based on the degree of digestibility, and, to some degree, the microbial content of the digestive tract, some signs and symptoms can result from the consumption of certain fibers, including abdominal distention, gas, flatulence, and loosening of stools. Clinicians can keep in mind that while fiber is generally promoted as part of a healthy, balanced diet, some individuality to tolerance of significant levels of ingested fiber can exist. Those potential experiential aspects can deter some people from purposely seeking higher fiber foods and dietitians should keep this in mind when trying to improve diet patterns.

Additionally, the typical response to fiber in the digestive tract presents an opportunity for food scientists to assess different polysaccharides for potential fiber designation. For a fiber to be a fiber, it should largely resist digestion in the upper digestive tract and thus blood glucose should not be elevated. In addition, there should be an elevation of gas production as content progresses through the small intestine into the large intestine or colon. This is especially true for soluble fibers experiencing more fermentation. Some of the gas production is measurable as hydrogen gas (H_2) in the breath, as some of the gas diffuses into the body and circulates to the lungs to be excreted in exhalation. Thus, glycemic response and hydrogen breath tests are common tools to assess fiber.

Recently, one polysaccharide, called IMO (iso-malto-oligosaccharide) was purported to be a functional fiber and was used in nutrition bars to improve sensory properties as well as increase fiber claim. When tested for 1) glucose and insulin response and 2) hydrogen breath, IMO dramatically increased glucose and insulin and failed to yield a proportionate response in exhaled hydrogen. Based on those results, IMO was no longer considered a fiber and either labels had to be changed or a different ingredient (fiber) had to be substituted.

▶ Here's What You Have Learned

1. Fibers are carbohydrates and related molecules that are not broken down by digestive enzymes. However, based on their metabolism by gut microflora and conversion to absorbable energy molecules, they can provide a small amount of energy.

2. Fibers are broadly categorized in the United States as being dietary fiber, functional fiber, or both.

3. Fibers have health benefits in the digestive tract by serving as probiotics and reducing the risk of intestinal disorders and supporting immune function and cardiovascular health.

4. In more recent years, food manufacturers have been fortifying foods with fibers such as resistant maltodextrin and inulin to support the achievement of fiber-intake goals.

5. Many functional fibers can support positive health benefits and impact the prevention and or treatment of disorders and diseases.

6. Certain functional fibers, such as β-glucans, pectins, and gums, can support the development of gums in the stomach, which can slow the transit of content from the stomach to the small intestine and, in turn, lower the glycemic impact of foods.

7. Certain fibers, such as cereal brans, are not fermented in the lower digestive tract and, in turn, add bulk to stool. This makes it easier to pass stools, thus reducing the risk of diverticulosis.

8. Fibers, especially soluble fibers, can bind cholesterol from food and bile salts in the upper digestive tract and reduce its absorption efficiency. In turn, this can support healthier blood cholesterol levels.

9. Fibers, especially soluble fibers, can bind calcium in the upper digestive tract and release it when fermented in the colon. Calcium is then available for absorption.

10. The average intake of fiber by American adults is only about 12 to 18 grams daily, which is well below the DRI recommendations of 25 to 38 grams daily.

▶ Suggested Reading

Campos FG, Logulla Waitzberg AG, Kiss DR, Waitzberg DL, Habr-Gama A, Gama-Rodrigues J. Diet and colorectal cancer: current evidence for etiology and prevention. *Nutr Hosp.* 2005;20(1):18–25.

Du H, van der A DL, Boshuizen HC, et al. Dietary fiber and subsequent changes in body weight and waist circumference in European men and women. *Am J Clin Nutr.* 2010;91(2):329–336.

Eastwood M, Kritchevsky D. Dietary fiber: how did we get where we are? *Annu Rev Nutr.* 2005;25:1–8.

Erkkilï AT, Lichtenstein AH. Fiber and cardiovascular disease risk: how strong is the evidence? *J Cardiovasc Nurs.* 2006; 21(1):3–8.

Flood-Obbagy JE, Rolls BJ. The effect of fruit in different forms on energy intake and satiety at a meal. *Appetite.* 2009;52(2): 416–422.

Institute of Medicine, Food and Nutrition Board. *Dietary Reference Intakes for Energy, Carbohydrate, Fiber, Fat, Fatty Acids, Cholesterol, Protein, and Amino Acids (Macronutrients).* Washington, DC: National Academies Press; 2002/2005.

King DE. Dietary fiber, inflammation, and cardiovascular disease. *Mol Nutr Food Res.* 2005;49(6):594–600.

Lambeau KV, McRorie JW Jr. Fiber supplements and clinically proven health benefits: How to recognize and recommend an effective fiber therapy. *J Am Assoc Nurse Pract.* 2017;29(4):216–223.

Latulippe ME, Meheust A, Augustin L, et al. ILSI Brazil International Workshop on Functional Foods: a narrative review of the scientific evidence in the area of carbohydrates, microbiome, and health. *Food Nutr Res.* 2013;57:1–18.

McCleary BV, DeVries JW, Rader JI, et al. Determination of insoluble, soluble, and total dietary fiber (CODEX definition) by enzymatic-gravimetric method and liquid chromatography: collaborative study. *J AOAC Int.* 2012;95(3):824–844.

McRorie JW Jr, McKeown NM. Understanding the physics of functional fibers in the gastrointestinal tract: an evidence-based approach to resolving enduring misconceptions about insoluble and soluble fiber. *J Acad Nutr Diet.* 2017;117(2):251–264.

Pereira MA, Ludwig DS. Dietary fiber and body-weight regulation. Observations and mechanisms. *Pediatr Clin North Am.* 2001;48(4):969–980.

Seal CJ. Whole grains and CVD risk. *Proc Nutr Soc.* 2006; 65(1):24–34.

Sierra M, Garcia JJ, Fernández N, et al. Effects of ispaghula husk and guar gum on postprandial glucose and insulin concentrations in healthy subjects. *Eur J Clin Nutr.* 2001;55(4):235–243.

Tucker LA, Thomas KS. Increasing total fiber intake reduces risk of weight and fat gains in women. *J Nutr.* 2009;139(3): 576–581.

U.S. Department of Health and Human Services and U.S. Department of Agriculture. *Dietary Guidelines for Americans, 2005.* HHS Publication No. HHS-ODPHP-2005-01-DGA-A. http://www.health.gov/dietaryguidelines/dga2005/document/pdf/DGA2005.pdf

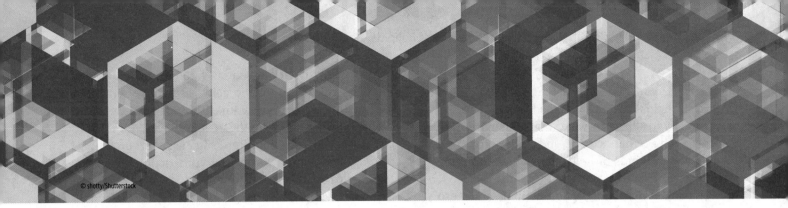

CHAPTER 5

Lipids: Fatty Acids, Triglycerides, Phospholipids, and Sterols

← HERE'S WHERE YOU HAVE BEEN

1. Carbohydrates as a major source of energy are utilized via glycolysis and the Krebs cycle.
2. Several transporters are known to aid in the intracellular uptake of glucose by cells.
3. Many hormones affect the rate of carbohydrate and glucose utilization, such as insulin, glucagon, and epinephrine, among others.
4. The end product of carbohydrate digestion and metabolism is adenosine triphosphate (ATP), as generated through the electron transport chain.
5. Over the years, fiber analysis has varied and has been refined to the point at which more accurate measurements of the fiber in food are possible.

HERE'S WHERE YOU ARE GOING →

1. Lipids may be divided into the major classes of fatty acids, triglycerides, phospholipids, and sterols.
2. There are two nomenclature systems for identifying fatty acids: the omega and delta systems.
3. Phospholipids and triglycerides are related to one another but have distinctive metabolic functions.
4. Molecular control of fat metabolism involve both nuclear receptor and non-nuclear receptor mechanisms.
5. All classes of fatty acids are building blocks of lipoproteins that can have a major impact on cardiovascular health.

▶ Introduction

Classically, lipids have been defined as substances that are generally insoluble in water but soluble in organic solvents, such as ether, acetone, and chloroform. A variety of different kinds of lipids are essential to human structure and function, including fatty acids, triglycerides (triacylglycerols), phospholipids, and **sterols** (e.g., cholesterol). All too often, lipids are viewed only from an energy perspective. For instance, fatty acids are oxidized to form ATP in almost all human cells and are the principal source of energy during periods of fasting. Furthermore, the storage of triglycerides can represent as much as 90,000 to 100,000 kilocalories of energy for an average adult male. Triglycerides (or, more commonly, fat) account for as much as one-third or more of the total energy consumed in many countries and are the focus of many efforts to reduce body weight. However, to view lipids only from an energy perspective would greatly understate their unique properties and physiologic significance.

Body fat has excellent insulating properties, thereby guarding against heat loss. Also, body fat deposits provide internal padding to protect visceral organs. The dietary essential fatty acids (EFAs)— linoleic acid and linolenic acid—are converted into local-acting eicosanoid factors. Those factors are fundamentally involved in the regulation of numerous cellular and tissue operations, such as blood pressure, platelet aggregation, bronchial constriction, chemotaxis, and inflammation. Diglycerides are the basis of phospholipids, which are the foundational component of cellular membranes and lipoproteins. Glycolipids and cholesterol are key components of cell membranes. Cholesterol also serves as the precursor molecule for a variety of steroid molecules, such as testosterone, dehydroepiandrosterone (DHEA), estrogens, cortisol, and aldosterone.

▶ General Properties and Nomenclature of Lipids

Fatty Acids

Fatty acids (**FIGURE 5.1**) are unique in a molecular sense in that they have a polar carboxyl end and a nonpolar methyl end. The two ends of a fatty acid are separated

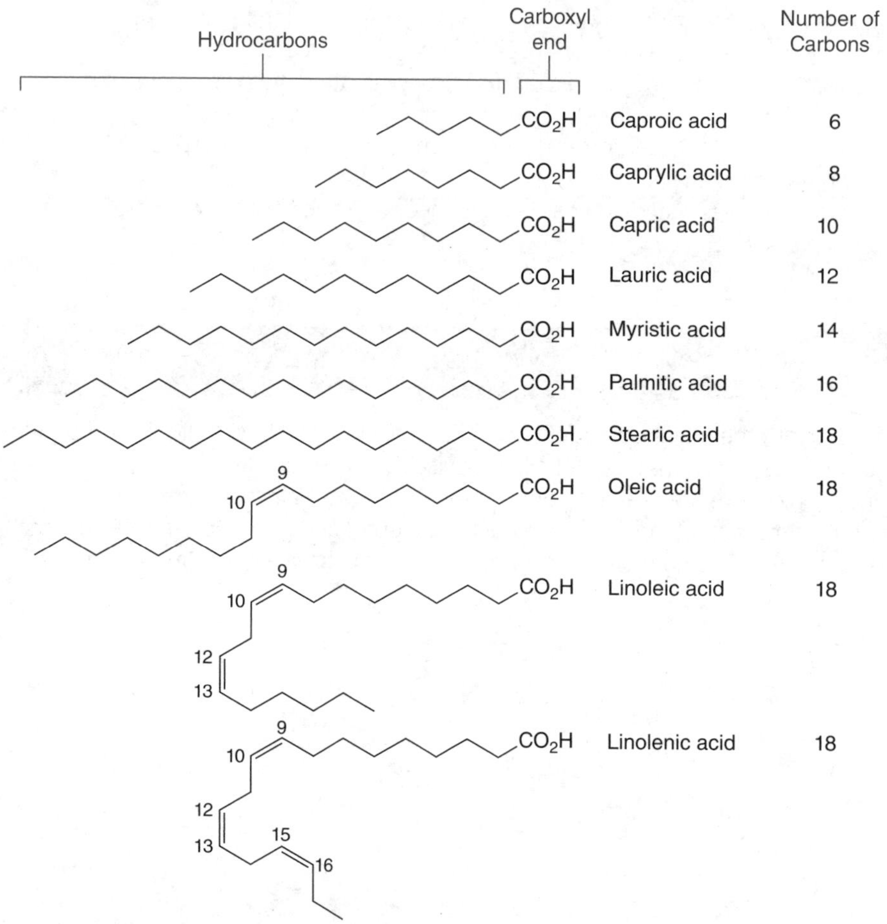

FIGURE 5.1 Fatty Acids. Capoic, caprylic, lauric, myristic, and stearic acids are all saturated. Oleic acid is monounsaturated. Linoleic and linolenic acids are polyunsaturated fatty acids.

by a hydrocarbon region of varying length. Fatty acids do not cyclize; therefore, they exist as chains of hydrocarbons. The carboxyl end has water-soluble properties, whereas the hydrocarbon tail, which includes the methyl end, is insoluble. Thus, shorter fatty acids tend to be more water soluble than longer fatty acids. For instance, fatty acids containing 6 carbons or fewer are very miscible in water (i.e., are capable of being mixed in water), whereas those with 10 or more carbons are not miscible. The fatty acids of relevance to human nutrition are monocarboxylic (one carboxyl group) and have an even number of carbons. Odd-chain-length fatty acids do occur in the diet as well as within human tissue, but to a significantly lesser degree. **TABLE 5.1** lists common fatty acids.

Fatty acid chain length is easily determined by counting the total number of carbon atoms. Acetic acid is the smallest fatty acid, having only 2 carbons, and arachidic acid is one of the longer fatty acids, consisting of 20 carbons. Fatty acids are often subclassified in terms of their length. Short-chain fatty acids contain 2 to 4 carbons, whereas medium-chain and long-chain fatty acids contain 6 to 12 and 14 to 26 carbons, respectively. However, there does seem to be some variation by scientists in the designation of fatty acids into those three categories.

Beyond length, fatty acids can vary in their degree of saturation. This quality refers to whether the hydrocarbon tail contains the maximal number of hydrogen atoms. Locations along the fatty acid hydrocarbon chain where a double covalent bond is present are sometimes referred to as **points of unsaturation**. The terms **saturated**, **monounsaturated**, and **polyunsaturated** are applied to fatty acids containing no double bonds, a single double bond, or more than one double bond, respectively. Figure 5.1 presents examples of saturated fatty acids (SFA), a monounsaturated fatty acid (MUFA), and polyunsaturated fatty acids (PUFA).

Identifying the position of double bonds can be accomplished by counting from either end of the fatty acid molecule. Starting at the carboxyl end and counting the carbons to the double bonds applies the delta (Δ) system. Counting from the methyl end is referred to as the omega (ω) system (ω is the last letter of the Greek alphabet; "n" is often used in substitution for "ω"). For instance, linoleic acid in Figure 5.1 can be identified as either $18:2^{\Delta 9,12}$ or $18:2\ \omega\text{-}6$. The "18" indicates the total number of carbon atoms, and the "2" following the colon indicates the total number of double bonds. Using the delta system, the first carbon of the two double bonds can be found at carbon 9 and carbon 12 when counting from the carboxylic end. When applying the omega system, and thus counting from the methyl end, only the position of the first carbon of the initial double bond is indicated because the ensuing double bond will occur following a methylene group.

TABLE 5.1 Common Fatty Acids

Saturated Fatty Acid	Nomenclature	Unsaturated Fatty Acid	Nomenclature
Acetic acid	2:0	Palmitoleic acid	16:1 ω-9
Butyric acid	4:0	Oleic acid	18:1 ω-9
Caproic acid	6:0	Linoleic acid	18:2 ω-3
Caprylic acid	8:0	Linolenic acid	18:3 ω-3
Capric acid	10:0	Arachidonic acid	20:4 ω-6
Lauric acid	12:0	Eicosapentaenoic acid (EPA)	20:5 ω-3
Myristic acid	14:0	Docosahexaenoic acid (DHA)	22:6 ω-3
Palmitic acid	16:0		
Stearic acid	18:0		
Arachidic acid	20:0		

Because the length of a fatty acid influences its solubility properties, the degree of unsaturation will also influence its solubility. The greater the number of double bonds, the greater the polarity of a fatty acid and thus its solubility in water. Melting point is also influenced by chain length and the number of double bonds in a manner similar to solubility. Thus, in general, the greater the chain length and the more saturated a fatty acid, the higher its melting point. All common **unsaturated fatty acids** are liquid at room temperature, except for oleic acid.

Fatty Acid Synthesis, Elongation, and Desaturation

Many human cells can synthesize fatty acids; however, the liver and, to a lesser degree, adipose tissue, are the primary sites of synthesis. Other tissues possessing a recognizable ability to synthesize fatty acids are the kidneys, mammary glands, lungs, and the brain. Acetyl coenzyme A (acetyl CoA), which is an intermediate of carbohydrate, amino acid, and ethanol metabolism, is the building block for cytosolic fatty acid synthesis. **Acetyl CoA carboxylase** and **fatty acid synthase** are the key regulatory enzymes involved. The latter enzyme is actually a complex system of several enzymatic and nonenzymatic protein subunits all coded by the same gene. The process of making fatty acids is referred to simply as **fatty acid synthesis** or **de novo lipogenesis**.

Fatty acid synthesis (**FIGURE 5.2**) is a series of cytosolic reactions beginning with the two-carbon acetyl CoA. In the preliminary reaction (see Figure 5.2a), bicarbonate (a source of CO_2) provides a carbon to acetyl CoA, resulting in malonyl CoA. Acetyl CoA carboxylase is a multienzyme complex that catalyzes the reaction, and ATP and biotin are necessary for the reaction to occur. The subsequent enzymes propagating fatty acid synthesis are complexed together and referred to collectively as fatty acid synthase (FAS). The next reaction (see Figure 5.2b) is the attachment of acetyl CoA and malonyl CoA to the condensing enzyme and acyl carrier protein (ACP) of the FAS complex. The next reaction in fatty acid synthesis (see Figure 5.2c) occurs when the acetyl group is transferred to a malonyl CoA on the ACP. CO_2 is removed in a subsequent reaction, and the remaining four-carbon molecule engages with further enzymes that comprise FAS.

The fatty acid synthase enzyme complex includes β-ketoacyl-ACP synthase, β-ketoacyl-ACP reductase, β-hydroxyacyl-ACP dehydratase, and enoyl-ACP reductase enzymes as well as ACP, which contains pantothenic acid in the form of 4′-phosphopantetheine. ACP takes over the role of CoA. Although those

proteins are complexed together in humans; as well as other mammals, birds, and yeast; they are independent proteins in bacteria and plants. Fatty acids under construction derive their carbons from malonyl CoA via acetyl CoA. The end product is the 16-carbon saturated fatty acid palmitate with the original "primer" acetyl CoA representing carbons 15 and 16. If the three-carbon fatty acid propionate is available, it, too, can be used as the primer in fatty acid synthesis. This process results in longer fatty acid chains of uneven numbers and is more predominant in ruminants because propionate is formed by microbes inhabiting their rumens.

Fatty acid synthesis is regulated at several levels. For instance, the expression of acetyl CoA carboxylase may be induced by insulin, and elevated levels of insulin and cytosolic citrate increase its activity. Long-chain acyl CoA, cAMP, and glucagon all decrease its activity. Citrate probably acts as an activator by forming an aggregate with an inactive acetyl CoA protein, thereby activating it. Many of the same influences on acetyl CoA carboxylase also exist for FAS. It has recently become clear that PUFA can actually decrease the expression of FAS complex enzymes. It appears that there may be a nuclear binding protein that selectively binds ω-3 and ω-6 PUFA. ω-3 PUFA are believed to be more potent at this task. The proteins complexed within FAS appear to be coded by a single gene; thus, transcription results in the formation of all components. Increasing levels of plasma free fatty acids (FFA) are associated with decreased lipogenesis, whereas high-carbohydrate diets, especially those high in sucrose, are associated with increased lipogenesis.

NADPH provides the reducing hydrogens for fatty acid synthesis. Most of the NADPH is derived from the pentose phosphate pathway (or hexose monophosphate shunt), which is explained in more detail below under "Pentose Phosphate Pathway." Cytosolic malic enzyme and isocitrate dehydrogenase are also sources of NADPH; however, the significance of the latter enzyme is believed to be minor.

Human cells can elongate and desaturate existing fatty acids. The cellular organelles responsible for **elongation** are either the endoplasmic reticulum or mitochondria, with the former being more significant. In the endoplasmic reticulum, the sequence of elongation reactions is similar to fatty acid synthesis, in which the source of the two-carbon unit is malonyl CoA and the reducing power is provided by NADPH. The fatty acid elongase system of enzymes catalyzes the reactions. Fatty acids that can act as primers for elongation include saturated fatty acids containing 10 carbons or more as well as unsaturated fatty acid. Elongation of stearic acid is elevated during the myelination of brain tissue, thereby providing

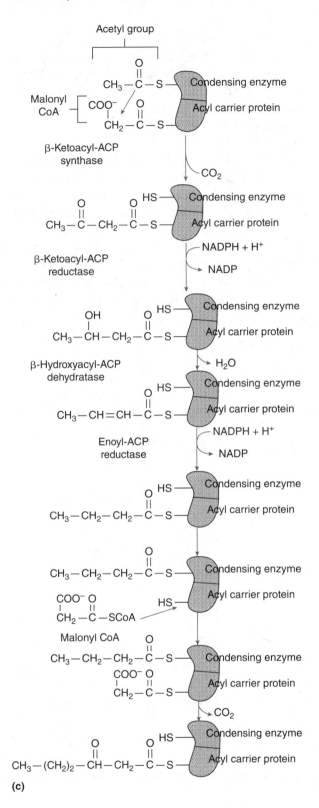

(a)

(b)

FIGURE 5.2 Fatty Acid Synthesis. (a) In the preliminary reaction (catalyzed by acetyl CoA carboxylase), carbon dioxide provides a carbon to acetyl CoA, resulting in malonyl CoA. (b) The next reaction is the attachment of acetyl CoA and malonyl CoA to the condensing enzyme and acyl carrier protein (ACP) of the fatty acid synthase (FAS) complex. (c) The next reaction occurs when a second acetyl group, associated with an ACP, is utilized and attached to malonyl CoA.

(c)

22- and 24-carbon fatty acids. Fatty acids of this length are found in sphingolipids (explained later in this chapter). Elongation of fatty acids appears to be depressed during caloric deprivation.

Double bonds may be added to fatty acids via desaturating enzymes. This occurs within the endoplasmic reticulum. Desaturating enzymes were named with the delta system in mind. Certain human cells express

Δ-5 desaturase, Δ-6 desaturase, and Δ-9 desaturase. For instance, **desaturation** of stearic acid (18:0) by Δ-9 desaturase results in oleic acid (18:1 ω-9). Because humans lack enzymes to desaturate beyond the ninth carbon of a fatty acid, the vital unsaturated fatty acids linoleic acid (18:2 ω-6) and linolenic acid (18:3 ω-3) are dietary essentials. These processes are discussed in greater detail below.

Pentose Phosphate Pathway

The primary importance of the pentose phosphate pathway (**FIGURE 5.3**) is the reduction of NADP⁺ to NADPH, which can be used for reducing equivalents for the synthesis of fatty acids (as well as for other compounds, such as glutathione). This reaction pathway also allows for the creation of ribulose-5-phosphate, which may be isomerized to ribose-5-phosphate and used in nucleotide biosynthesis. The reactions of the pentose phosphate pathway can be described as either oxidative or nonoxidative. The oxidative reactions include the conversion of glucose-6-phosphate to 6-phosphogluconate via glucose-6-phosphate dehydrogenase and the conversion of 6-phospho-glucolactone to 6-phosphogluconate by gluconolactone hydrolase to ribulose-5-phosphate. Those reactions reduce

NADP⁺ to NADPH. From that point on, the ribulose-5-phosphate can take several routes and enters nonoxidative reactions. Ribulose-5-phosphate may undergo a reaction with an isomerase to form ribose-5-phosphate, or it may react with an epimerase to form xylulose-5-phosphate. Those compounds enter a series of reactions that allow for the regeneration of the glycolytic intermediates glyceraldehyde-3-phosphate and sedoheptulose-7-phosphate. The enzyme transketolase is required, which needs magnesium and vitamin B_1 as cofactors. Next, transaldolase will convert glyceraldehyde-3-phosphate and sedoheptulose-7-phosphate to fructose-6-phosphate and erythrose-4-phosphate. Another set of transketolase reactions will convert erythrose-4-phosphate and xylulose-5-phosphate to glyceradehyde-3-phosphate and fructose-6-phosphate, which enters glycolysis.

cis vs *trans* Fatty Acids

The orientation of hydrogen atoms about a double bond influences the structure and thus the physical properties of a fatty acid. If the hydrogens associated with the carbons of a double bond are positioned on the same side, it is a **cis** arrangement. In contrast, if the hydrogens bonded to the carbons are on opposite sides of the double bond, it is a **trans** arrangement, and the fatty acid is called a *trans* fatty acid. Fatty acids with the same length and position of double bonds, yet differing in the orientation of their hydrogen atoms, have different chemical names. For instance, 18:1 ω-9 with a *cis* arrangement is called oleic acid, whereas 18:1 ω-9 with a *trans* arrangement is called elaidic acid.

Cis-configured double bonds tend to kink or bend a fatty acid chain, whereas *trans* fatty acids maintain a straighter chain similar to saturated fatty acids (**FIGURE 5.4**). That fact influences the physical properties of cellular membranes. Quite simply, an increased presence of *cis*-configured bonding creates a more fluid membrane. Conversely, an increased amount of saturated or *trans*-bonded fatty acids leads to a less-fluid membrane. The *cis* arrangement is by far the more prevalent arrangement of double bonds in fatty acids in foods and in the human body.

Trans fatty acids have received a great deal of publicity due to their potential negative health effects. *Trans* fatty acids also influence several metabolic operations by influencing the operation of several lipid enzymes. *Trans* isomers of 18:2 ω-6 decrease prostaglandin synthesis, thereby increasing the requirement for linoleic acid for prostaglandin functions. *Trans* isomers of 18:2 ω-6 (*cis*, *trans* and *trans, trans*) are devoid of essential fatty acid activity. Also, the *trans* isomer of 18:1 ω-9 (elaidic acid)

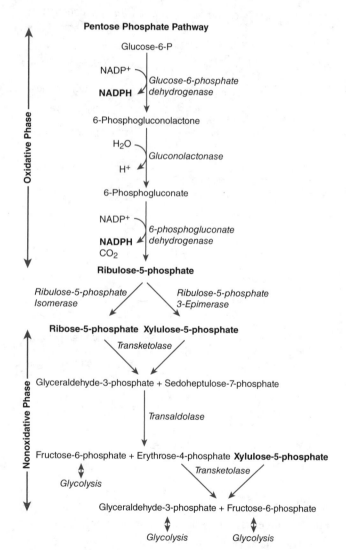

FIGURE 5.3 The Pentose Phosphate Pathway. The importance of this pathway is the conversion of NADP⁺ to NADPH. The NADPH can reduce other compounds in various biochemical reactions. Ribose-5-phosphate is also produced, which is needed for nucleotide biosynthesis.

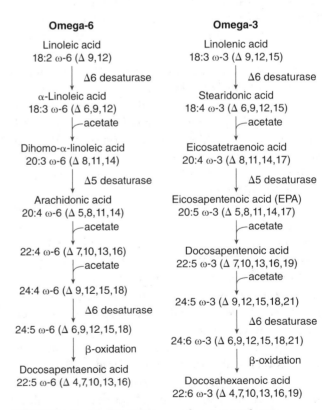

FIGURE 5.4 *cis* **Versus** *trans* **Configuration and the Effect on the Kinking or Bending of the Hydrocarbon Tail.** A *cis* configuration creates a more fluid membrane compared with the *trans* configuration.

may decrease the activity of Δ-6 desaturase and Δ-9 desaturase (see below). Studies involving human fibroblasts have shown that *trans* fatty acids impair the microsomal desaturation and chain elongation of both linoleic and linolenic acid (essential fatty acids) to their longer-chain metabolites, especially arachidonic acid and docosahexaenoic acid. The ramifications of those effects may be most significant during the gestational development of humans. *Trans* fatty acids appear to cross the placental barrier and are probably also secreted in human milk. Thus, it has been recommended that pregnant women decrease their *trans* fatty acid consumption.

Essential Fatty Acids

For decades, it was believed that dietary fatty acids served only to provide fuel and had no essential physiologic function. However, in the 1920s, research began to reveal the fact that fatty acids play an essential role because animals fed a fat-free diet demonstrated poor growth and impaired reproduction. Scientists suggested that fat contained an essential factor that, at the time, they called vitamin F; however, its structure and function were still unknown. Linoleic acid (18:2 ω-6 PUFA) was soon identified and suggested to be the sole **essential fatty acid (EFA)**. Some even referred to linoleic acid as vitamin F. However, in the 1970s, scientists began to further recognize the essentiality of ω-3 PUFA as well. Humans do not have Δ-12 desaturase and Δ-15 desaturase; therefore, 18-carbon ω-3 and ω-6 PUFA are by nature dietary essentials to man. The true essential fatty acids for humans are thus linoleic acid (18:2 ω-6) and linolenic acid (18:3

ω-3). Those fatty acids are presented in Figure 5.1.

Other longer-chain PUFA, such as arachidonic acid (AA; 20:4 ω-6), eicosapentaenoic acid (EPA; 20:5 ω-3), and docosahexaenoic acid (DHA; 22:6 ω-3), can be made from available linoleic and linolenic acids by a series of elongations and desaturations (**FIGURE 5.5**). To create 20:4 ω-6 from 18:2 ω-6 and 20:5 ω-3 from 18:3 ω-3 first requires the activity of Δ-6 desaturase, then elongation, and then Δ-5 desaturase. The formation of 22:6 ω-3 (DHA) is a little more involved. First 20:5 ω-3 is elongated to 22:5 ω-3 and then 24:5 ω-3, then Δ-6 desaturation occurs to yield 24:6 ω-3, followed by partial β-oxidation to 22:6 ω-3 (DHA). Alternatively, to seemingly go backward and create 20:5 ω-3 (EPA) from 22:6 ω-3 (DHA) requires peroxisomal and endoplasmic reticulum enzyme assistance. The endoplasmic reticulum membrane is the site of the desaturating enzymes, which can be found in various tissues and/or organs, such as the liver, intestinal mucosa, retina, and brain.

Interestingly, Δ-6 desaturase activity is known to be regulated by several hormonal and dietary factors. For instance, insulin and the presence of EFA tend to increase its activity, whereas glucose, epinephrine, and glucagon tend to decrease its enzymatic activity. Although ω-3 and ω-6 PUFA compete for the same

Omega-6	Omega-3
Linoleic acid	Linolenic acid
18:2 ω-6 (Δ 9,12)	18:3 ω-3 (Δ 9,12,15)
↓ Δ6 desaturase	↓ Δ6 desaturase
α-Linoleic acid	Stearidonic acid
18:3 ω-6 (Δ 6,9,12)	18:4 ω-3 (Δ 6,9,12,15)
⌐acetate	⌐acetate
Dihomo-α-linoleic acid	Eicosatetraenoic acid
20:3 ω-6 (Δ 8,11,14)	20:4 ω-3 (Δ 8,11,14,17)
↓ Δ5 desaturase	↓ Δ5 desaturase
Arachidonic acid	Eicosapentenoic acid (EPA)
20:4 ω-6 (Δ 5,8,11,14)	20:5 ω-3 (Δ 5,8,11,14,17)
⌐acetate	⌐acetate
22:4 ω-6 (Δ 7,10,13,16)	Docosapentenoic acid
	22:5 ω-3 (Δ 7,10,13,16,19)
⌐acetate	⌐acetate
24:4 ω-6 (Δ 9,12,15,18)	24:5 ω-3 (Δ 9,12,15,18,21)
↓ Δ6 desaturase	↓ Δ6 desaturase
24:5 ω-6 (Δ 6,9,12,15,18)	24:6 ω-3 (Δ 6,9,12,15,18,21)
↓ β-oxidation	↓ β-oxidation
Docosapentaenoic acid	Docosahexaenoic acid
22:5 ω-6 (Δ 4,7,10,13,16)	22:6 ω-3 (Δ 4,7,10,13,16,19)

FIGURE 5.5 Synthetic Pathways for ω-6 and ω-3 Polyunsaturated Fatty Acids. Numbers in parentheses indicate positions of double bonds from the carboxyl end of the fatty acid.

desaturating enzymes, both Δ-5 desaturase and Δ-6 desaturase prefer ω-3 over ω-6 PUFA. However, an increased ratio of ω-6 to ω-3 PUFA in the diet, as typical of the Western diet, will slow the conversion of linolenic acid to EPA and DHA. The activity of Δ-6 desaturase seems to decline relative to age. Premature infants are limited in their ability to produce EPA and DHA from linolenic acid, as are some hypertensive individuals and some diabetics. Individuals consuming a diet rich in DHA and EPA, typically from fish, tend to have higher levels of those fatty acids in plasma and tissue phospholipids and lesser amounts of arachidonic acid.

Linolenic acid is found mostly in triglycerides and cholesterol esters and in only small amounts in phospholipids. Conversely, EPA is found mostly in phospholipids and in cholesterol esters and only in smaller amounts in triglycerides. DHA is also found mostly in phospholipids. The cerebral cortex, retina, testis, and sperm contain higher concentrations of DHA.

It is believed that Paleolithic man consumed a diet with an essential fatty acid ratio (ω-6:ω-3) of approximately 1:1. Today, most developed societies consume a diet lower in ω-3 PUFA and higher in ω-6 PUFA. This is largely attributed to the domestication of animals and the increased consumption of vegetable oils. For instance, the wild game consumed by our human ancestors was very lean (3 to 4% total fat) and contained a respectable quantity of ω-3 PUFA. However, today's domesticated animals, such as cattle, contain much more fat, which is relatively high in saturated fatty acids and lower in ω-3 PUFA. A wild chicken egg, for instance, may have a ω-6:ω-3 PUFA ratio of 1.3:1. However, a domesticated chicken egg, as available in most supermarkets, may have a ratio of 19:1. Furthermore, selective hydrogenation of ω-3 PUFA in soybean oil, which is used in the production of many foods (e.g., snack foods), has further increased the ω-6:ω-3 PUFA ratio.

Canola, soy, and flaxseed are sources of linolenic acid in the diet. While linolenic acid from those sources can be converted to EPA and DHA, the efficiency and level that is converted in humans is limited in that this ω-3 PUFA is not likely to contribute to the total amount of EPA or DHA in tissues. As indicated above, a rate-limiting step in the conversion of linolenic acid to the longer chain ω-3 PUFA is the rate-limiting Δ-6 desaturase. This enzyme converts linolenic acid to stearidonic acid. From a practical perspective, increased levels of EPA and DHA need to come from dietary sources, particularly increased intake of fish, as the plant sources of linolenic acid contain little EPA and DHA. A concern is that the levels of fish production to meet the EPA and DHA are limited and, in fact, fish farms are actually

nearing their limit in terms of productivity. Furthermore, the use of fish in such large quantities is likely ecologically not well founded as this can lead to the extinction of certain fish species.

There is a growing consensus that there is a solution to the above problem. Increasing stearidonic acid in the diet does result in elevated EPA and DHA, in contrast to linolenic acid, although there is a discrepancy with respect to DHA. The conversion of EPA to DHA does depend on the rate-limiting Δ-6 desaturase. Unfortunately, the level of stearidonic acid is rather low in plant oils but is found in the borage and primrose family of plants. A solution to this issue can be the use of biotechnology to enhance its production in soybeans. The percent of stearidonic acid in such genetically modified soybeans is 15 to 20% in contrast to echium oil, which is 3.5% to 9.0%. Stearidonic enriched soybean oil fed to humans increased red blood cell EPA. Stearidonic enriched oils may be considered a major source of ω-3 PUFA intake and thus be a method of obtaining greater omega-3 fatty acids from plant-based foods.

Triglycerides

Triglycerides are sometimes referred to as triacylglycerols. This is the form of fat in both food and the body that has the greatest weight. Simply stated, a triglyceride is a chemical structure composed of a three-carbon compound referred to as glycerol. Each carbon of this glycerol backbone has a fatty acid attached to it (**FIGURE 5.6**). The three fatty acids present in glycerol likely will differ and most often reflect dietary fat intake. At times, there

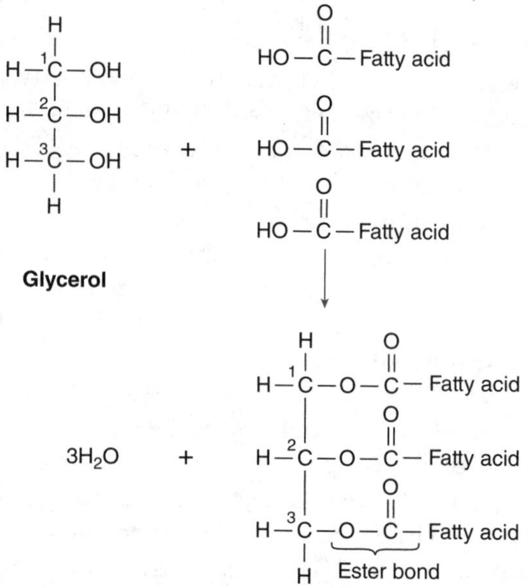

FIGURE 5.6 Structure of Triglycerides. Triglycerides have a glycerol backbone and three fatty acids joined by an ester bond.

may be only one fatty acid bonded to a carbon of glycerol, which is referred to as a monoglyceride or monoacylglycerol. Similarly, there could be only two fatty acids; this would be referred to as a diglyceride or diacylglycerol. The fatty acids are bonded to the glycerol via an ester bond. Water is released when the hydroxyl groups of glycerol and the fatty acids condense.

Whether triglycerides are solid or liquid at room temperature largely depends on the fatty acids that comprise them. Those with more saturated fatty acids are likely to be solid at room temperature, whereas those with either more unsaturated fatty acids or shorter-chain fatty acids may be liquid. For energy to be derived from triglyceride, the fatty acid must be removed from the glycerol backbone of the molecule.

Phospholipids

Phospholipids are lipid compounds that contain phosphatidic acid, which is composed of glycerol, two fatty acids, and a phosphate (PO_4) group (**FIGURE 5.7**). They are amphiphilic by nature, able to attract both water- and fat-soluble substances, therefore, making them ideal for cellular membranes and lipoprotein shells. Generally, phospholipids are unavailable as an energy source. The various phospholipids differ from each other by what is attached to the PO_4 group. The sn-1 or α-carbon is usually esterified to a saturated fatty acid, whereas the sn-2 or β-carbon usually is esterified to an unsaturated fatty acid, which can be an EFA or a derivative of an EFA. The sn-3 carbon is attached to a phosphate group, again, by an ester

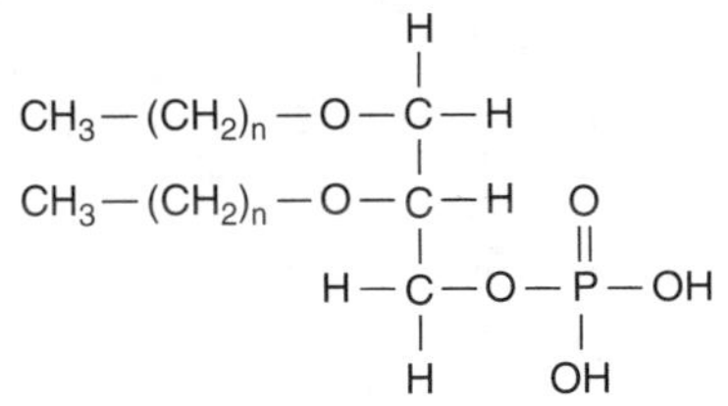

FIGURE 5.7 Phosphatidic Acid. This compound is the basic building block of phospholipids.

bond. Phosphatidylcholine (lecithin), phosphatidylethanolamine (cephaline), phosphatidylserine, and phosphatidylinositol are the most common types of phospholipids, as depicted in **FIGURE 5.8**. All of those phospholipids are found in abundance in the cell membranes of various tissues.

Plasmogens are compounds in which one of the fatty acids, usually at the sn-1 carbon of ethanolamine, is replaced by a long-chain ether group (**FIGURE 5.9a**). Another type of compound related to phospholipids is the sphingolipids (Figure 5.9b). Those compounds do not contain glycerol but instead contain sphingosine, an 18-carbon monounsaturated alcohol. Sphingomyelin is found in large amounts in the myelin sheath of nerve tissue. It contains phosphatidylcholine at the terminal carbon and a fatty acid at the sn-2 position. In a rare, inherited condition termed Niemann-Pick disease, individuals lack sphingomyelinase, which is the enzyme responsible for sphingomyelin cleavage. This disease is characterized by the deposition of sphingomyelin in almost every organ and tissue of the body and is usually fatal before the third year of life.

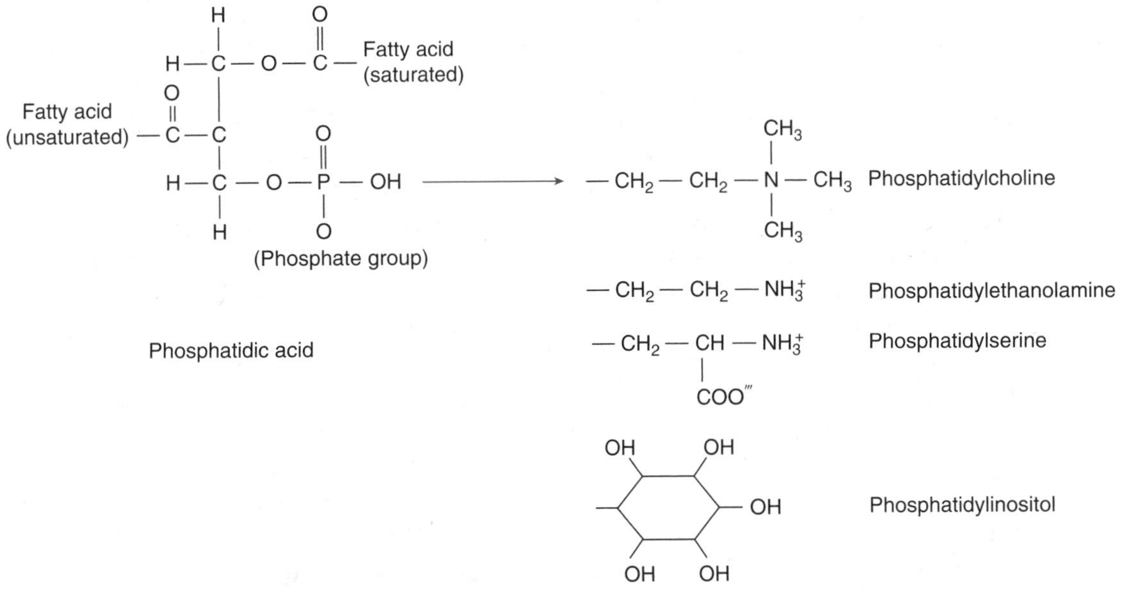

FIGURE 5.8 Different Phospholipids of Nutritional and Physiologic Relevance. The phosphatidic acid molecule has various groups attached to it as indicated on the right side of the figure.

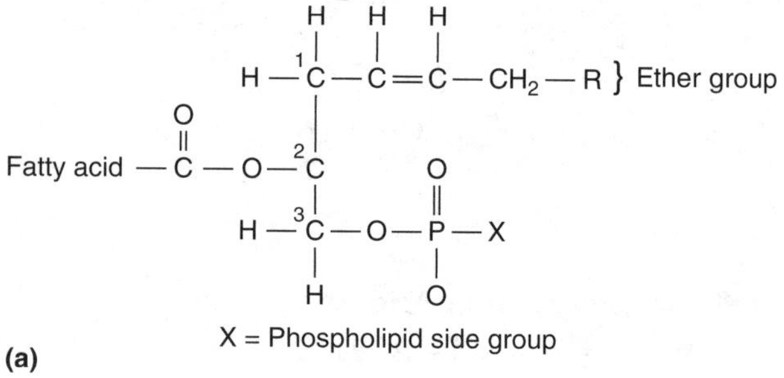

(a)

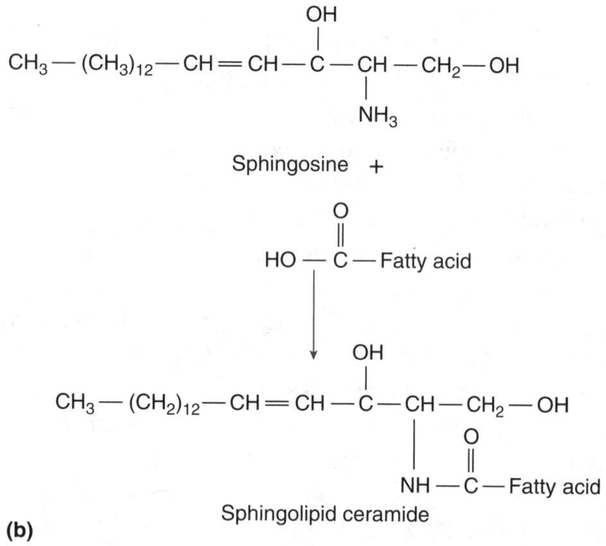

CH$_3$—(CH$_3$)$_{12}$—CH=CH—C—CH—CH$_2$—OH
with OH above C, and NH$_3$ below

Sphingosine +

HO—C—Fatty acid (with O double bond)

↓

CH$_3$—(CH$_2$)$_{12}$—CH=CH—C—CH—CH$_2$—OH
with OH above, and NH—C—Fatty acid below

Sphingolipid ceramide

(b)

FIGURE 5.9 Compounds Related to Phospholipids.
(a) The phospholipid plasmogen. Note that an ether group is on the sn-1 carbon instead of a fatty acid. (b) A sphingosine molecule binds to a fatty acid to form sphingolipid ceramide.

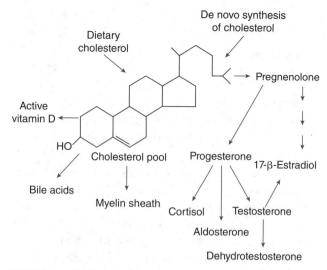

FIGURE 5.10 Biologically Important Cholesterol Derivatives. Dietary cholesterol and de novo synthesis of cholesterol forms the cholesterol pool. From that pool, active vitamin D, bile acids, and pregnenolone are formed. Once pregnenolone is formed, further reactions will lead to the synthesis of several hormones, including the sex hormones. Also, cholesterol is a vital component of the myelin sheath of nerve fibers.

Sterols

Steroid hormones are a class of lipid molecules that are derived from the basic sterol structure of cholesterol. Steroids include estrogens (17-β-estradiol), androgens (testosterone and dehydrotestosterone), DHEA (dehydroepiandrosterone), adrenocorticoid hormones (cortisol and aldosterone), and cholesterol itself. Vitamin D and bile salts are derived from cholesterol as well.

Because cholesterol is an amphipathic lipid, it is employed as a structural component of cell membranes and lipoprotein shells. It is also a component of myelin sheaths, which coat peripheral nerves. Cholesterol-based hormones tend to have intracellular receptors and exert much of their effect by influencing gene expression. **FIGURE 5.10** presents an overview of biologically important steroids.

In a typical adult human, about 700 to 1,000 milligrams of cholesterol is synthesized daily, and the liver and the intestines each synthesize approximately 10% of the total. Virtually all nucleated cells have the ability to synthesize cholesterol, a process that takes place within the endoplasmic reticulum and cytosol. Acetyl CoA is the source of all carbon atoms in cholesterol. In the initial reaction, two molecules of acetyl CoA condense to form acetoacetyl CoA, a reaction catalyzed by the enzyme cytosolic thiolase (**FIGURE 5.11**). Acetoacetyl CoA condenses with another molecule of acetyl CoA to form 3-hydroxy-3-methylglutaryl (HMG). This reaction is catalyzed by HMG CoA synthase. The next reaction is the rate-limiting step and the target of many drugs prescribed to lower blood cholesterol levels. HMG is converted to mevalonate in a two-stage reduction by HMG CoA reductase, an enzyme of the endoplasmic reticulum, using NADPH. Mevalonate is then activated by three ATPs in a series of kinase reactions to form mevalonate 3-phospho-5-pyrophosphate, which is subsequently decarboxylated to form the active isoprenoid unit isopentenyl pyrophosphate. Two isopentenyl pyrophosphate molecules will form farnesyl pyrophosphate. From this point on through a series of reactions, squalene and lanosterol are formed, ultimately leading to the production of cholesterol and cholesterol esters.

Cholesterol synthesis is influenced by several factors and primarily involves the regulation of HMG CoA reductase. Fasting seems to significantly reduce the activity of HMG CoA reductase. A negative feedback mechanism is applied by the intermediate mevalonate and the final product, cholesterol. Cholesterol synthesis is also influenced by dietary consumption of cholesterol. It seems that as the dietary level of cholesterol increases,

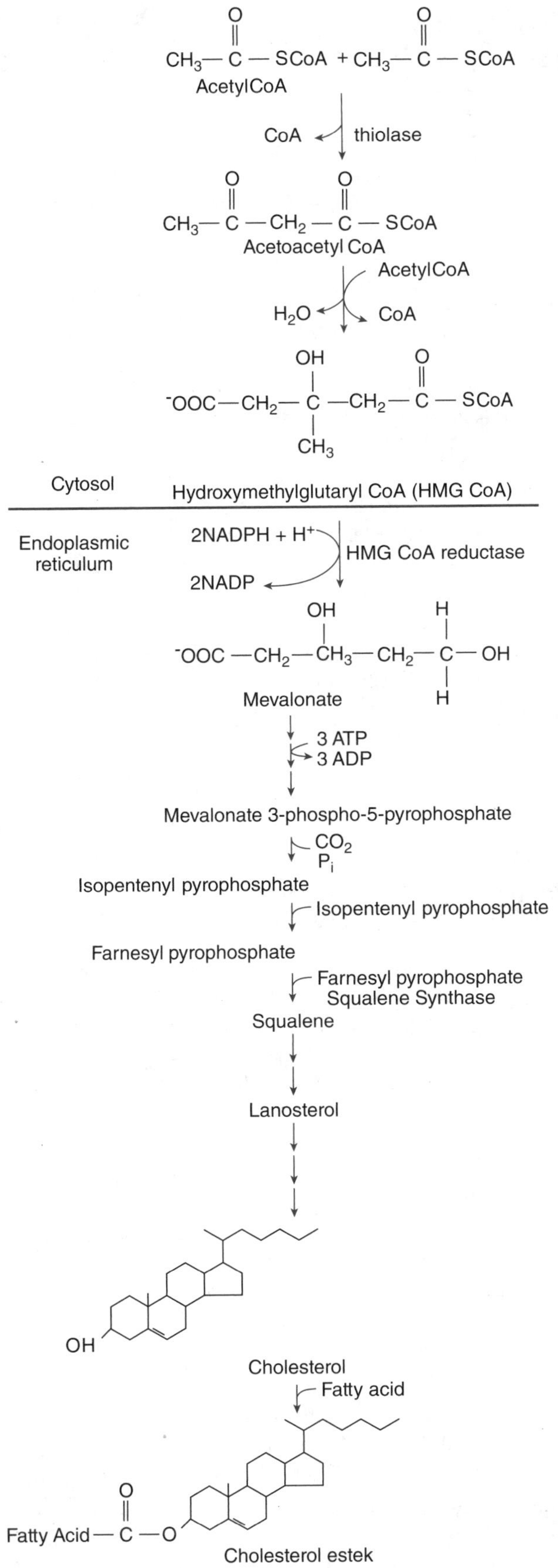

FIGURE 5.11 Cholesterol Synthesis. The starting material is acetyl CoA, with acetoacyl CoA forming HMG CoA. A number of reactions lead to the synthesis of cholesterol. HMG CoA reductase, which leads to the synthesis of mevalonate, is the rate-limiting enzyme for cholesterol biosynthesis.

the level of endogenous cholesterol production decreases. However, this effect mainly takes place in the liver.

● BEFORE YOU GO ON . . .

1. Outline the steps that occur in the synthesis of DHA from α-linolenic acid (18:3 ω-3), name the desaturases and chain lengths involved, and state where the double bonds occur.

2. Draw the initial steps in the pathway by which acetyl CoA initiates the synthesis of a fatty acid, including the key enzymes involved.

3. Is linolenic acid a good source of EPA and DHA? Explain your answer.

4. Distinguish among phospholipids, triglycerides, and sterols in terms of structure and general function.

5. What is a key regulatory aspect of cholesterol biosynthesis?

6. What is the purpose of the pentose phosphate pathway with respect to lipid metabolism?

▶ Molecular Control Mechanisms of Fat Metabolism

Nuclear Receptors

Much lipid metabolism is under the control of a super family of nuclear hormone receptors. Those receptors are transcription factors that mediate nuclear-acting hormones, such as glucocorticoids, mineralocorticoids, estrogens, progestins, androgens, thyroid hormones, vitamin D, and retinoic acid. One type of nuclear receptor that has profound effects on lipid metabolism is the class of peroxisome proliferator-activated receptors (PPARs), which belong to the steroid/thyroid/retinoid receptor super-family. PPARs were first shown to be activated by substances that induce peroxisomal proliferation. Those are termed **orphan receptors** because no known hormone specifically binds to those receptors. However, orphan receptors, such as the PPARs, are activated by a number of compounds.

The PPARs are important in the control of fatty acid oxidation and synthesis. Three subtypes have been identified thus far: PPARα, PPARδ, and PPARλ. PPARα was the first to be discovered and has been the most studied. Those receptors bind to promoter regions of genes that play a critical role in fat metabolism. Induction of this receptor results in the proliferation of peroxisomes, which are involved in the metabolism of longer-chain fatty acids. Subsequently, it was discovered that PPARα could induce enzymes associated

SPECIAL FEATURE 5.1

Fat Substitutes in Our Diet

Given the link established between heart disease and the fat we eat in the typical Western diet, the food industry has put considerable effort into making fat-free foods. This task is challenging because fat is one of the main reasons foods taste the way they do; fat has high levels of flavor compounds. Fat substitutes can be divided into three basic classes:

- Carbohydrate-based fat substitutes
- Protein-based substitutes
- Fat-based substitutes

Carbohydrate-based fat substitutes include compounds such as dextrins, maltodextrins, modified food starches, cellulose, and various gums. They are able to mimic fat's creaminess, bulk, and moistness. However, many of those carbohydrate-based substitutes cannot replace its cooking qualities. Whereas 1 gram of fat yields 9 calories, those carbohydrate-based substitutes only yield 1 to 4 kilocalories per gram (kcal/g). Carbohydrate-based fat substitutes are easy to digest, hold onto more water than fat, and provide good mouth-feel. However, fat-free products are not necessarily low-calorie foods because many products may have more carbohydrate added to make up for the difference in taste. In fact, the total number of calories may be similar. Many consumers purchase foods containing a fat substitute to lose weight, but later learn that the net calories in the modified product are similar to the original version. Many consumers may actually eat more of the food containing the fat replacer because of the misconception that it does not have as many calories.

Proteins used as fat substitutes may contain things such as modified egg whites and whey from milk. A negative aspect of this type of substitute is that a high cooking temperature can lead to protein breakdown. Simplesse is an example of a product with this problem. Because of the problems with potential breakdown in cooking, those fat replacers are most often used in frozen desserts. They contain approximately 4 kcal/g.

The last class of substitutes is fat replacers that are fat based. Olean, Salatrim, and Caprenin are some of those products made from lipids. Those replacers are nondigestible. Olean (or Olestra) remains the most widely used, although use has since waned. It does not contain calories and is not digested. It is mostly used in the processing of potato chips and other similar foods. Salatrim and Caprenin are substitutes that have been chemically altered so that they cannot be digested. They contain half the calories of fat (4 to 5 kcal/g). Those substitutes provide food products with the real fat taste and mouth-feel demanded by consumers but with less caloric absorption due to their impaired digestion.

Concerns have been raised by consumer advocate groups regarding the potential side effects of Olestra and its interaction with the absorption of some nutrients. Because it cannot be digested, Olestra can cause abdominal cramps and diarrhea. Olestra may also reduce the absorption of fat-soluble vitamins (vitamins A, D, E, and K). As a result of this concern, manufacturers promised the U.S. Food and Drug Administration (FDA) that they would provide notice to consumers on the product label and fortify food products with those fat-soluble vitamins. Fortification ensures that what little fat is left in the product is bound to those essential nutrients. The FDA, until recently, required labels that stated the following:

> This product contains Olestra. Olestra may cause abdominal cramping and loose stools. Olestra inhibits the absorption of some vitamins and other nutrients. Vitamins A, D, E, and K have been added.

The sentence about abdominal cramping is no longer required by the FDA, but the facts about soluble vitamins are. The FDA restricts the use of Olestra to a handful of snack foods, such as chips. Some people have no side effects from Olestra, especially if it is consumed in limited amounts. Salatrim is mainly used in chocolate chips, and Caprenin is a substitute for the cocoa butter used in candy bars. Despite the limitations of Olestra, Salatrim, and Caprenin, those fat replacers do allow consumers to enjoy the sensory attributes of fat without the caloric concerns.

with fatty acid catabolism, such as medium-chain acyl dehydrogenase and carnitine-palmitoyltransferase I. Furthermore, it was discovered that for those receptors to function, they had to be activated by the binding of particular compounds (not hormones, however). Many such agents, termed ligands, have been identified. In the case of PPARα, it was discovered that several naturally occurring fatty acids could activate this receptor. A large number of unrelated compounds have been discovered that activate PPARα, including various fatty acids, such

as oleate; eicosanoids; fibrates; peroxisome proliferators; and inhibitors of mitochondrial β-oxidation.

At the promoter level, however, it was determined that PPAR–ligand complexes cannot act by themselves. They need to interact with a retinoic acid receptor (RXR), which itself is first activated by a retinoic acid derivative, such as 9-*cis* retinoic acid. Together, the entire complex must bind to the promoter 5′ at specific recognition or response elements (nucleotide base pairs). Thus, PPARs function as a heterodimer with RXRs and are separated from each other by one base pair on the promoter regions of candidate enzyme genes (**FIGURE 5.12**).

PPARα has been identified in a variety of tissues, including liver, heart, and kidney. Other isoforms of PPARs were later discovered to exist. PPARγ has received a lot of interest and is found in appreciable amounts in fat cells. It is thought to be activated by such compounds as prostaglandins and a class of diabetic drugs termed thiazolidinediones. PPARγ, again with its heterodimeric partner RXR, stimulates fat synthesis. PPARγ appears to increase insulin sensitivity in adipose and skeletal muscle when a thiazolidinedione (a class of drugs for diabetics) is administered; however, the exact mechanism is unknown. PPARγ can increase the expression of phosphoenolpyruvate carboxykinase (PEPCK), which catalyzes the conversion of oxaloacetate to phosphoenolpyruvate, which is the rate-limiting enzyme in gluconeogenesis. It can also stimulate the peroxisomal acyl CoA oxidase gene. Fibroblasts that overexpress PPARγ using transfection techniques developed adipocyte-like characteristics once an appropriate ligand is added.

PPARδ has not had as many studies conducted on it as the other isoforms. It is widely distributed in tissues, and evidence from PPARδ knockout mice and other studies have suggested a diverse spectrum of functions in embryo implantation, early development, wound healing, and cancer development.

The PPARs present a newer piece of the puzzle of understanding how lipid metabolism is controlled at the molecular level. It would appear that PPARα favors fat catabolism and PPARγ favors fat synthesis. In some fashion, fatty acids, acting as ligands to those receptors, are acting as hormones. An entirely new area of research pursuing metabolic control mechanisms related to fat metabolism and adiposity has thus been opened up.

A second type of nuclear receptor that has profound effects on lipid metabolism is **liver X receptors (LXRs)**. The mechanism of action of LXRs is very similar to that of the PPARs. LXRs form heterodimeric partners with RXRs on the promoters of target genes. Like the PPARs, there is more than one isoform. Here we have LXRα and LXRβ. LXRβ appears to be expressed in a wide variety of tissues, whereas LXRα is expressed at relatively high levels in the liver, adipose tissue, the

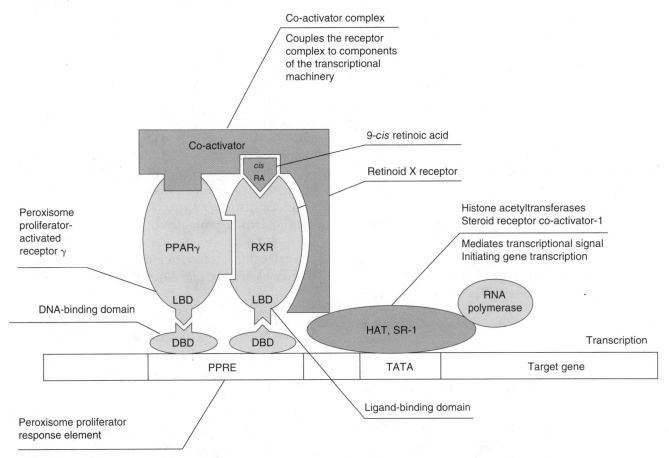

FIGURE 5.12 PPARγ and RXR Binding to a Gene Promoter to Initiate Transcription of mRNA. PPRE represents the nucleotide base sequences recognized by PPARγ and RXR as binding sites. TATA is the start site for mRNA transcription. RA denotes retinoic acid.

intestine, kidneys, and macrophages. Those receptors are activated by ligands that bind to them, similar to the PPARs and RXRs. The LXR ligands are likely to be oxysterols, or the breakdown products of cholesterol. Both LXR isoforms have a special role in promoting reverse cholesterol transport, preventing the development of atherosclerosis and having anti-inflammatory effects. LXRs activate transporters to transfer cholesterol to high-density lipoproteins (HDL), which are subsequently brought to the liver for breakdown. At the intestinal level, LXRs play a role in preventing the absorption of cholesterol. LXRs target three genes (ABCA1, ABCG5, and ABCG8) in the small intestine. Those three genes encode ATP-binding cassette (ABC) transporter proteins, which are proteins that limit cholesterol absorption. Those three transporter proteins are also present in liver cells and are targets of LXRs to facilitate the efflux of phospholipids and cholesterol from the liver into either the blood or the bile.

A third type of nuclear receptor that is involved with lipid metabolism is the **farnesoid X receptor (FXR)**. Like the others already discussed, this receptor requires a ligand to bind to it for activation and also requires heterodimerization with RXR. This receptor targets those genes involved in bile metabolism. Liver and intestine have high levels of this receptor. Bile acids and some of the secondary bile acids discussed later in this chapter act as ligands to this receptor to enhance activity. The FXR essentially suppresses bile synthesis; the mechanism by which this occurs is indirect. The FXR also suppresses the rate-limiting enzyme that converts cholesterol to bile acid, 7 α-hydroxylase . This is *not* a direct inhibition of the gene that encodes for this enzyme. Rather, FXR promotes the expression of a gene that is produced, known as **small heterodimer partner (SHP)**. SHP, in turn, inhibits the transcription of the mRNA for 7 α-hydroxylase. Another role for FXRs, through a complex series of reactions, is in modulating blood triglyceride levels. This is thought to involve PGC-1α, acting as a coactivator of FXR. It is currently thought that FXR, in conjunction with PGC-1α, may (1) reduce liver triglyceride synthesis, (2) increase very low-density lipoprotein (VLDL, a triglyceride-rich lipoprotein) clearance from the blood, and (3) promote fatty acid oxidation.

Non-Nuclear Receptors

Sterol regulatory element binding protein (SREBP) is not a nuclear receptor. It is often referred to as basic-helix-loop-helix leucine zipper transcription factor (**FIGURE 5.13**). Such transcription factors are composed of two α-helix proteins that dimerize. This dimerization is due to interactions between hydrophobic side chains of amino acids, most notably leucine. For each monomer, there is a short α-helix chain

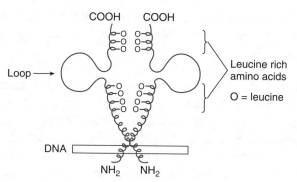

FIGURE 5.13 Structure of a Base-Helix-Loop-Helix Leucine Zipper Transcription Factor. The structure is rich in the amino acid leucine and consists of two peptides that dimerize and bind to the DNA of the promoter region of a gene.

connected by a loop to another longer α-helix chain. Upon dimerization, the two longer α-helix chains will directly bind to DNA and promote transcription.

SREBP is primarily involved in cholesterol metabolism but it is also involved in lipogenesis. Mammals have two forms of this protein: SREBP-1 and SREBP-2. There are two subtypes of SREBP-1: SREBP-1a and SREBP-1c. SREBP-1a and SREBP-1c are both involved in lipid biosynthesis, whereas SREBP-2 is involved in cholesterol biosynthesis. There appears to be a feedback inhibition regulating those proteins. As an example, when cellular cholesterol declines below a critical level, the enzymes involved in cholesterol biosynthesis are up-regulated. SREBP is located in the endoplasmic reticulum. Another protein located in the endoplasmic reticulum is **SREBP cleavage-activating protein (SCAP)**. SCAP responds to the level of cell cholesterol. When cell cholesterol levels decline, SCAP will escort SREBP from the endoplasmic reticulum to the Golgi apparatus, where a portion of SREBP is cleaved and translocated to the nucleus. The cleaved SREBP protein then binds to the promoters of genes encoding enzymes for cholesterol biosynthesis, such as HMG CoA reductase. All of those transcription factors upregulate genes that are biosynthetic for either lipids or cholesterol.

◆ BEFORE YOU GO ON . . .

1. What is an orphan receptor?
2. In general, what are PPARs, and how did they get their name?
3. Distinguish between the functions of PPARα and PPARγ.
4. What is the role of FXR in lipid metabolism and how does it function at the molecular level?
5. How do SREBP and SCAP regulate cholesterol biosynthesis?

► Dietary Lipids: Food Sources, Requirements, and Digestion

Food Sources

Although the diet provides lipids other than triglycerides and cholesterol, most attention is focused on those forms of lipids. Food triglycerides are often referred to as either fats or oils, with fats having a more solid consistency at room temperature and oils being more fluid. Food triglycerides contain a variety of fatty acid types (**TABLE 5.2**). As mentioned

TABLE 5.2 Approximate Fatty Acid Composition of Common Triglyceride Sources			
Triglyceride Source	SFA (%)	MUFA (%)	PUFA (%)
Beef fat	52	44	4
Butter fat	66	30	4
Canola oil	6	62	32
Coconut oil	87	6	2
Corn oil	13	25	62
Lard	41	47	12
Margarine	17	49	34
Olive oil	14	77	9
Palm kernel oil	81	11	2
Palm oil	49	37	9
Peanut oil	18	49	33
Safflower oil	10	13	77
Soybean oil	15	24	61
Sunflower oil	11	20	69
Vegetable shortening	28	44	28

SFA, saturated fatty acids; MUFA, monounsaturated fatty acids; PUFA, polyunsaturated fatty acids.

previously, it is the contributory proportions of different fatty acids in a triglyceride source that dictate its phase, either liquid or solid, at a given temperature. Again, longer-chain fatty acids with a lesser degree of unsaturation allow for a more solidified triglyceride source.

Oil is a natural component of plants and their seeds. It became available after the invention of the continuous screw press (trade named Expeller) and the steam-vacuum deodorization process developed by D. Wesson. Later, solvent extraction methods were developed, which further increased the availability of vegetable oils. Common oils include sunflower, safflower, corn, olive, coconut, and palm oil. In contrast, butter is made from the fat in milk, lard is hog fat, and tallow is the fat of cattle or sheep. Because plants are cholesterol free, the cholesterol intake of humans is solely attributable to the consumption of animal foods or of foods that use animal products in their recipe. Cholesterol is found in animal tissue primarily in the form of cholesterol esters; a smaller proportion is free cholesterol. **TABLES 5.3** and **5.4** provide lists of foods and their triglyceride and cholesterol content by percentage and weight, respectively.

A triglyceride that contains the same fatty acid esterified at all three positions on glycerol is called a simple triglyceride. Examples are tripalmitate and tributyrate. However, it is more common to find more than one type of fatty acid in the same triglyceride. Those molecules are called mixed triglycerides. A fat source that contains a greater percentage of saturated fatty acids is often referred to as a saturated fat, despite the presence of other types of fatty acids. The same applies for MUFA and PUFA as well. Often, food fat is expressed as a ratio of PUFA to SFA, or more simply, the P/S ratio. Animal foods have a lower P/S ratio, whereas most oils have a higher P/S ratio. Notable exceptions are tropical plant oils (coconut, palm, and palm kernel oils), which have a lower P/S ratio due to a relatively high content of medium-chain-length saturated fatty acids. Even though they are solid at room temperature, they are considered oils because they still have much lower melting points than animal fats.

The most prevalent saturated fatty acids in the Western diet are palmitic acid (16:0) and stearic acid (18:0), and the most prevalent unsaturated fatty acids are oleic acid (18:1 ω-9) and linoleic acid (18:2 ω-6). Collectively, those four fatty acids account for over 90% of the fatty acids in the typical American diet. Most of the fatty acids consumed by Americans have an even number of carbons, which generally ranges between 14 and 26 carbons. A notable exception is

TABLE 5.3   Approximate Fat and Cholesterol Content of Various Foods, by Percentage

Food	Fat (%)	Cholesterol	Food	Fat (%)	Cholesterol
Animal products					
Beef (4 oz)	32	<1	Hamburger (4 oz)	13	<1
Bologna (1 piece)	29	1	Lamb chops (2.5 oz)	36	1
Butter (1 pat)	82	2	Mackerel (4 oz)	6	Trace
Chicken, white meat (3 oz)	4	<1	Margarine (1 pat)	82	—
Cheese, cheddar (1 cup)	32	1	Milk, whole (1 cup)	3	<1
Cheese, cottage (4%) [1 cup]	4	<1	Milk, skim (1 cup)	Trace	Trace
Codfish (4 oz)	<1	Trace	Pork chops (2.5 oz)	21	—
Egg, whole (1 each)	12	4	Pork sausage (1 piece)	46	—
Egg, white (1 each)	<1	Trace	Salmon (4 oz)	4	Trace
Halibut (4 oz)	3	Trace			
Plant products					
Avocado (1 each)	13	—	Leafy vegetables (½ cup)	<1	—
Bread, white (1 piece)	4	<1	Legumes (½ cup)	<1	—
Cereals and grains (1 cup)	1–2	—	Margarine (1 tbsp)	82	—
Crackers (4 pieces)	1	—	Root vegetables (½ cup)	<1	—
Fruits (1 each)	<1	—			

butyric acid (4:0), found in dairy foods. Quite simply, foods contain very few odd-chain-length fatty acids. For instance, less than 0.5% of the total fatty acids in olive oil contain an odd number of carbons. Lard contains less than 1% of its fatty acids as odd-chain-length fatty acids.

The major sources of the essential fatty acids are PUFA-rich vegetable oils and marine oils. Linoleic acid is particularly high in sunflower, corn, safflower, and soybean oils. Canola, linseed, and soybean oils all contain respectable amounts of linolenic acid; however, only linseed oil contains more linolenic acid than linoleic acid (**TABLE 5.5**). It is estimated that soybean oil contributes as much as two-thirds of the oil used to make shortening by manufacturers in the United States and as much as 84% of the fat used in margarines. However, selective hydrogenation

processing reduces more of the linolenic acid than the linoleic acid, further increasing the linoleic to linolenic acid ratio of the oil. Linolenic acid is especially concentrated in marine oils. Therefore, the consumption of fish is the primary source of this essential fatty acid.

Human milk contains both ω-3 and ω-6 PUFA, which is probably indicative of their essentiality for growth and development. Maternal dietary fat composition can affect the EFA content of the milk. For instance, lactating mothers who consume fish have a higher DHA content in their breast milk than lactating vegetarian mothers.

Concern has been expressed recently regarding dietary *trans* fatty acids and their impact on human health. *Trans* fatty acids can be found in most natural fat sources, although their prevalence is generally

TABLE 5.4 Approximate Fat and Cholesterol Content of Various Foods, by Weight

Food	Fat (g)	Cholesterol (mg)	Food	Fat (g)	Cholesterol (mg)
Animal products					
Beef (4 oz)	9	101	Hamburger (4 oz)	14	58
Bologna (1 piece)	7	13	Lamb chops (2.5 oz)	18	84
Butter (1 pat)	4	11	Mackerel (4 oz)	16	78
Chicken, white meat (3 oz)	3	41	Margarine (1 pat)	3	—
Cheese, cheddar (1 cup)	44	139	Milk, whole (1 cup)	8	33
Cheese, cottage (4%) (1 cup)	10	31	Milk, skim (1 cup)	Trace	Trace
Codfish (4 oz)	7	35	Pork chops (2.5 oz)	8	18
Egg, whole (1 each)	5	213	Pork sausage (1 piece)	6	11
Egg, white (1 each)	—	Trace	Salmon (4 oz)	23	Trace
Halibut (4 oz)	9	131			
Plant products					
Avocado (1 each)	27	—	Leafy vegetables (1/2 cup)	<1	—
Bread, white (1 piece)	1	Trace	Legumes (1/2 cup)	<1	—
Cereals and grains (1 cup)	1	—	Margarine (1 Tbsp)	6	—
Crackers (4 pieces)	2	—	Root vegetables (1/2 cup)	<1	—
Fruits (1 each)	<1	—			

low. Beef, butter, and milk triglycerides may contain 2 to 8% *trans* fatty acids. *Trans* fatty acids are created by microbes in the rumen and then absorbed and circulated to mammary glands and other tissue. Additionally, *trans* fatty acids can be created during the processing of oils (e.g., margarine and other hydrogenated oils). Salad oils may contain 8 to 17% *trans* fatty acids, and shortenings contain 14 to 60%. Typically, approximately one-half of the *trans* fatty acids in the Western diet are derived from animal sources. (*Trans* fatty acids may constitute 3 to 7% of the total fatty acids consumed in Western diets.) The remaining one-half of the *trans* fatty acids are derived from processed oils, either consumed plain or used in recipes (e.g., snack foods). The substitution of hydrogenated oils for tropical oils by many food manufacturers has further increased the consumption of *trans* fatty acids. However, many food companies are eliminating *trans* fat from their food products in response to this health concern.

TABLE 5.5 Linoleic and Linolenic Acid Composition of Common Oils (Percentage of Total Fatty Acids)

Oil	Linoleic Acid (%)	Linolenic Acid (%)
Canola oil	22	10
Corn oil	54	1
Cotton seed oil	54	1
Linseed oil	16	54
Olive oil	10	1
Palm oil	10	1
Peanut oil	32	—
Safflower oil	76	0.5
Soybean oil	54	7
Sunflower oil	68	1

Dietary Lipid Requirements

Efficient cholesterol synthesis in hepatocytes, and, to a lesser degree in other tissue, eliminates the dietary need for cholesterol. Similarly, the ability to make and modify fatty acids nearly eliminates the absolute need for fat in the human diet. However, because they are needed to make eicosanoids, ω-3 and ω-6 PUFA are indeed dietary essentials. It has been estimated that as long as humans receive 2 to 3% of their fat from a variety of natural sources, they will meet their minimal EFA requirements. The optimal intake for linolenic acid is estimated to be 800 to 1,100 milligrams per day, and that of EPA and DHA to be 300 to 400 milligrams per day.

EFA deficiencies result in several anatomic and physiologic anomalies. For instance, 18:2 ω-6 is critical to dermal integrity as a component of O-linoleoyl-ceramides. These molecules help form the lipid bilayers that fill the intercellular spaces in the outer epidermis (stratum corneum). When there is an EFA deficiency, 18:2 ω-6 is replaced by 18:1 ω-9, which decreases epidermal water barrier integrity and also results in cell hyperproliferation. Some of the growth and other anomalies associated with EFA deficiencies may be related to eicosanoid involvement in pituitary and hypothalamic hormone release.

Digestion of Lipids

Fat digestion begins in the mouth with the secretion of lingual lipase, which is a component of the secretion derived from a salivary gland at the base of the tongue. Lingual lipase activity increases as the food-and-saliva mixture enters the stomach and the pH becomes more acidic. Furthermore, this enzyme does not require the emulsifying effect of bile to penetrate fat droplets. Thus, the contribution of lingual lipase to total fat digestion is significant, yet still quantitatively minor in comparison with small-intestinal digestion. There are gastric and intestinal mucosa-secreted lipases as well; however, collectively, those lipases contribute

SPECIAL FEATURE 5.2

The Trend of Fat Consumption in the United States

Despite the dramatic increase in the incidence of obesity in the population, Americans have not increased the amount of fat consumed in their diets. Quite the contrary, over the past 20 years, Americans have actually decreased the percentage of calories in their diets that come from consuming fat. In 1977–1978, the intake of dietary fat represented approximately 40% of our caloric intake. This percentage decreased to 36% in 1985–1986, 34% in 1989–1991, and 33% in 1994–1996. Equally as surprising is that saturated fat, long demonized as proatherogenic, changed from 13% of caloric intake in 1985–1986 to 11% in 1994–1996. The trend of lower fat and saturated fat intakes as a percent of total calories has continued to more recent surveys since 2000. Recently, the American Heart Association recommended saturated fat to not exceed 5–6% of the calories consumed and that consumption of trans fats be reduced.

However, percentages do not tell the entire story, because more calories may often be consumed. Someone who consumes 3,000 calories a day and obtains 30% of his or her calories from fat would translate this into 100 grams of fat per day. However, if another person consumed 40% of his or her calories from fat on a 2,000-calorie daily diet, this would be less than 90 grams of fat per day. In terms of absolute quantity, the amount of gram fat intake decreased between 1977 and 1991. After 1991, the intake in grams increased slightly but still remained below earlier levels. In summary, Americans have achieved an overall decrease in dietary fat over the past 20 years, in part, by consuming a variety of lower-fat foods and fat-modified products.

SPECIAL FEATURE 5.3

Does linoleic acid increase the incidence of obesity?

Public health groups have long advocated increased intake of polyunsaturated fats, but decreased saturated fat, to decrease a number of diseases prevalent in western diets, in particular, cardiovascular disease. Additionally, oleic acid has been advocated with evidence to support a decreased incidence of cardiovascular disease and certain cancers with increased intake. However, the major PUFA intake in western societies is linoleic acid (ω-6). As noted in this chapter, it is metabolized to arachidonic acid. As already reviewed, increased intake of omega-3 fatty acids has been recommended; but the sources of these fatty acids compared with the omega-6 fatty acids in western diets is limited.

Recently, concern has developed as possible negative health effects of intake of linoleic acid. Much data that assessed increased dietary linoleic acid as protective against heart disease ignored the fact that omega-3 fatty acids also increased over time as the food supply changed. The omega-3 fatty acids could have been the component that afforded the cardiovascular health benefits. The change in overall agricultural practices have increased the quantity of linoleic acid in our diet based on the composition of plant foods used, as well as the grains fed to animals, that also lead to an increase in this fatty acid.

Is linoleic acid harmful to human health? Arachidonic acid is a metabolite of linoleic acid. Arachidonic acid can be converted into proinflammatory compounds via the cyclooxygenase and lipoxygenase pathways. One compound that can lead to increased oxidative stress that is a metabolite of arachidonic acid is 20-hydroxy-5, 8, 11, 14-eicisatetrenoic acid. This compound is also associated with greater adiposity. Other metabolites are known to increase PPARγ, which favors fatty acid synthesis and differentiation of adipocytes. Human studies on whether increased linoleic acid in humans can lead to increased inflammation has led to contradictory results. An argument has been made that perhaps the ratio of ω-6: ω-3 is more critical than the absolute amount of linoleic acid. A rodent study did report that increased ratios lead to pro-inflammatory chemicals; such as tumor necrosis factor α; interleukins 1β, 3 and 17; which are involved with obesity development.

That linoleic acid is associated with weight gain is gaining traction. Some research suggests that genetic predisposition may interact with greater intakes of linoleic acid to increase obesity. Additionally, there is evidence that some of the metabolites of linoleic acid (anandamide and 2-arachidonyl) can stimulate appetite in rodents and humans as well as stimulating liver fatty acid synthesis. The leading opinion is that there is a connection between increased linoleic acid intake and inflammation and increased adiposity. Adiposity, however, can also lead to inflammation, leading one to speculate about whether one condition leads to another. Experts suggest that until more definitive evidence is forthcoming, a "safe" approach may be to advocate a Mediterranean-type diet higher in monounsaturated fatty acids.

---

very little to overall lipid digestion. Gastric lipase is usually more active in the duodenum. The simplest approach to lipid digestion is to discuss the process in three phases: **intraluminal phase**, **mucosal phase**, and **secretory phase**.

Intraluminal Phase

The most active site of lipid digestion is the upper jejunum. Emulsification of lipids by bile salts is a prerequisite prior to enzymatic hydrolysis. The process begins by mechanical action in the stomach to form a coarse emulsion of chyme. Chyme then mixes with pancreatic secretions in the small intestine as the stomach empties. The release of lecithin from the bile and the production of monoglycerides from earlier digestion facilitate the emulsification process. The polar nature of those compounds allows for the formation of micelles within the aqueous environment of the small intestine (**FIGURE 5.14**). As emulsification proceeds, the pancreatic lipases hydrolyze the lipid. This releases polar lipids and further enhances the emulsification process and the formation of micelles.

Three types of pancreatic lipases and one coenzyme are active in the small intestine. The release of the

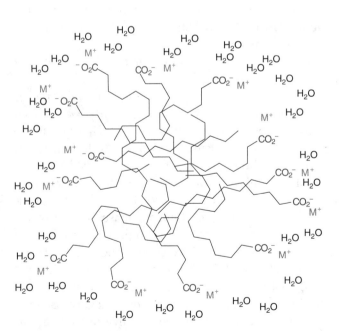

FIGURE 5.14 Micelle Formation with Phospholipids (e.g., lecithin), Bile Salts, Glycerides, and Cholesterol. Lecithin from the bile and monoglycerides produced by digestion allow for emulsification to occur. Micelles are formed due to the polar nature of those compounds that allow them to be miscible in an aqueous environment. M = Mineral (eg. Na^+, Ca^{2+}).

pancreatic lipases is under the control of the hormone cholecystokinin (CCK), produced by the intestinal mucosal cells. This hormone not only controls pancreatic secretion but also facilitates the release of bile from the gallbladder by stimulating the gallbladder to contract. CCK also produces a relaxation of the sphincter muscle at the neck of the gallbladder as well as relaxation of the sphincter of Oddi.

Pancreatic lipase is responsible for most of the triglyceride hydrolysis and cleaves the fatty acids preferentially at sn-1 and secondarily at sn-3. Fewer than half of the triglycerides are completely hydrolyzed to fatty acids and glycerol; most of the fatty acids liberated will have more than 10 carbons. The enzyme acts on the surface of micelles that have the triglycerides exposed. The pancreatic coenzyme colipase promotes the formation of a lipase-colipase bile salt complex that allows for hydrolysis. Colipase is composed of about 100 amino acids and has distinct hydrophobic properties. It has been speculated that colipase associates strongly with pancreatic lipase molecules while, at the same time, anchoring itself to lipid globules. As a result of lipase activity, monoglycerides, fatty acids; and glycerol are released into the aqueous environment of the intestinal lumen and are continually solubilized by the bile salts. Those products are brought into contact with the surface of the microvilli.

Cholesterol esterase is another pancreatic enzyme. Cholesterol esters in the small intestine constitute about 15% of the total cholesterol. The esterified form cannot be absorbed intact, so it must be hydrolyzed. If the ester linkage is not broken, the cholesterol ester passes into the colon.

Another pancreatic lipid-digesting enzyme is phospholipase, which hydrolyzes fatty acids from phospholipids. In actuality, the role of phospholipase is rather minor, because the average Western diet contains only about 2 grams of phospholipids daily. Most of this is phosphatidylcholine (lecithin), which is poorly absorbed. There are actually two forms of phospholipase: A_1 and A_2. Phospholipase A_2 hydrolyzes the sn-2 fatty acid of lecithin to produce lysolecithin and a free fatty acid. Lysolecithin and fatty acids are readily absorbed. Within mucosal enterocytes, some of the lysolecithin is re-esterified with a fatty acid by the enzyme lysophosphatidylcholine acyl-transferase. The phospholipid is needed for chylomicron formation. The remaining lysolecithin has the sn-1 fatty acid removed by phospholipase A_1 within the mucosal cell.

Bile is a major factor in lipid digestion. Bile is a complex composite. Along with its emulsifying factors, namely bile salts, phospholipids, and cholesterol; bile also contains bilirubin, which is a breakdown product of hemoglobin. When bile is secreted by the liver and is deposited into the gallbladder between meals, it is concentrated about five- to tenfold or even more. Bile salts should be considered an excretory mechanism for the elimination of cholesterol.

Cholic acid and chenodeoxycholic acid are formed from cholesterol and are the primary bile salts. Cholesterol has a hydroxyl (OH) group on carbon 3. In hepatocytes, cholesterol is hydroxylated at carbon 7 to produce 7α-hydroxycholesterol; NADPH + H$^+$ and two CoA molecules will convert this to chenodeoxycholic acid. Further hydroxylation at carbon 12 yields cholic acid. The hydroxylation of the bile acids makes them more "detergent" like. After those compounds have been formed, another enzyme conjugates the bile acids with an amino acid. Conjugation with glycine forms glycocholic (or glycochenodeoxycholic) acid, whereas conjugation of bile salts to taurine forms taurocholic (or taurochenodeoxycholic) acids. Once those bile acids are secreted into the small intestine, they may be further modified in the ileum or colon by intestinal bacteria. For instance, glycocholic acid may be deconjugated of the glycine and dehydroxylated at carbon 7 to produce deoxycholic acid (**FIGURE 5.15**). Chenodeoxycholic acid may have the same reaction to produce lithocholic acid. Collectively, those two derivative bile acids are referred to as secondary bile acids. The primary and secondary bile acids are absorbed by the ileum and colon and are passed into the portal circulation for recirculation via an energy-dependent process. The bile acids return to the liver to be recycled again. Approximately 94% of the bile acids secreted into the intestine are reabsorbed; this process is referred to as the enterohepatic circulation. In the blood, the bile acids are normally complexed to albumin. Of the approximately 18 grams of bile acids secreted each day, less than one-half of a gram is lost via the feces.

Mucosal Phase

The micelle allows the lipid breakdown products to diffuse to the surface of the intestinal epithelium. Absorption of micelle-associated substances occurs through the partitioning from the micelle into the aqueous phase followed by uptake by the plasma membrane. The free fatty acids and monoglycerides are transported across the microvillus membrane by a passive process due to the lipid solubility of those products in the membrane. Glycerol is absorbed by a carrier-mediated mechanism. Most of the absorption occurs in the first half of the intestine.

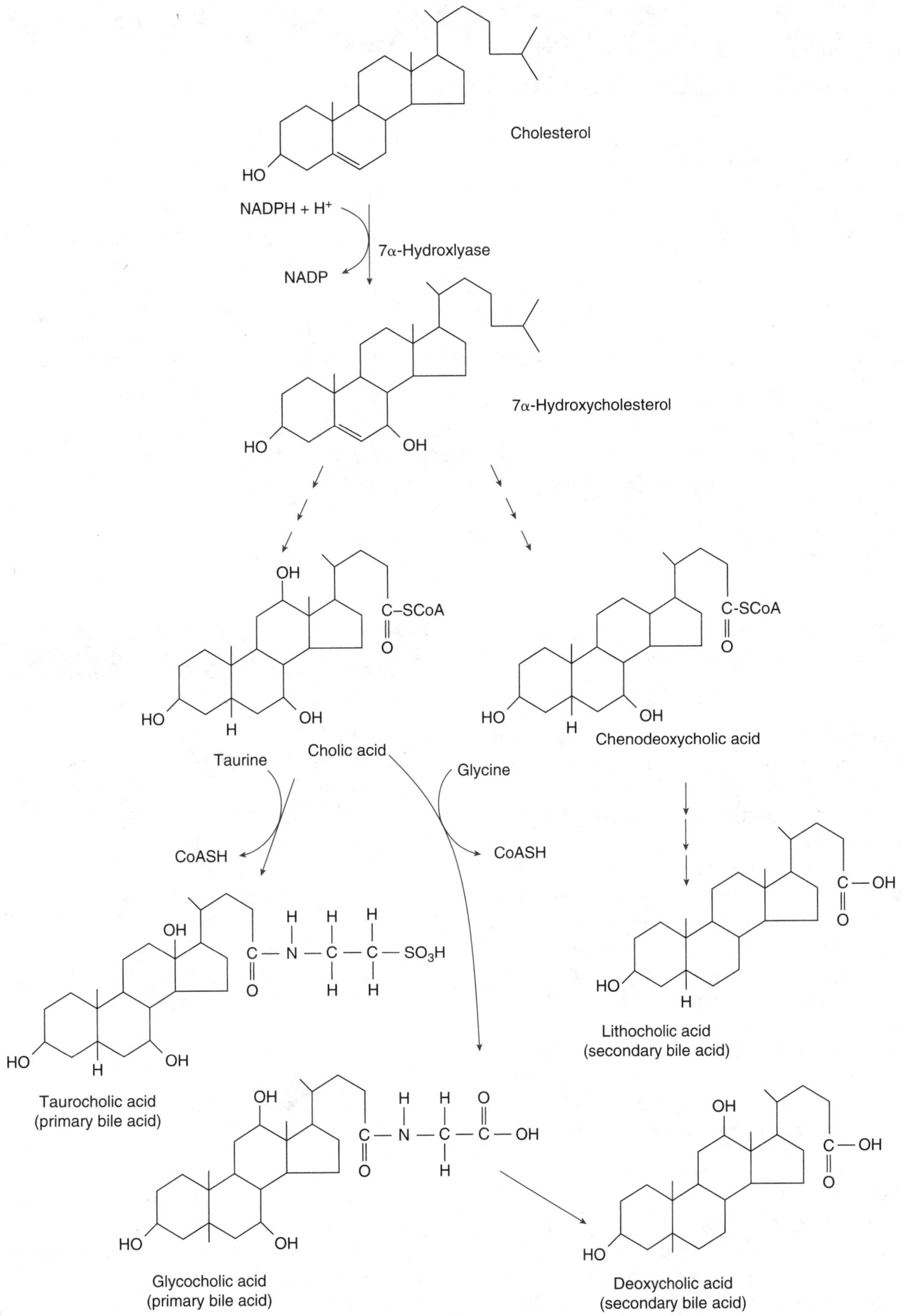

FIGURE 5.15 Conversion of Cholesterol to Primary and Secondary Bile Acids. The primary bile acids produced are taurocholic and glycocholic acids. The secondary bile acids are deoxycholic and lithocholic acids.

Proteins Involved with Dietary Cholesterol Intestinal Absorption and Biliary Reabsorption

Nutrition students are well aware that dietary cholesterol is packaged into chylomicrons in the small intestine for absorption and that the liver is a site of cholesterol and bile acid biosynthesis. However, one unresolved question has been how cholesterol is absorbed by the small intestine. Recently, a protein on the brush border of the small intestine enterocyte has been identified that is responsible for this absorption. Called **Niemann-Pick C1-Like 1 (NPC1L1)**, this protein is key to dietary cholesterol absorption and biliary cholesterol reabsorption. NPC1L1 is a transmembrane protein, traversing the cell membrane several times between the cell cytosol and gut lumen. The amino end of this protein is in the gut lumen, and the carboxyl end is in the cytosol of the enterocyte. The ileum and jejunum are the primary sites where this protein is expressed in the greatest amount. In the liver, structures referred to as hepatic canaliculi collect the bile and cholesterol that are produced by the liver. NPC1L1 is involved in transporting cholesterol from the hepatic canaliculi back into the hepatocyte. This is thought to protect the liver from excessive loss of liver cholesterol, serving as a "counterbalance" for overall liver cholesterol homeostasis.

In the small intestine, a portion of NPC1L1 binds cholesterol on the gut lumen side of the cell membrane. After the cholesterol is bound to NPC1L1, it is transferred to the cell membrane that is adjacent to the NPC1L1 protein, and that portion of the cell membrane becomes cholesterol enriched. This portion of the membrane is referred to as the **NPC1L1-flotillan-cholesterol membrane microdomain**. This structure undergoes endocytosis and triglycerides are released into the cell cytosol for subsequent incorporation into chylomicrons and eventual entry into the portal blood supply for delivery to the liver.

A low-molecular-weight protein in the mucosal cell cytoplasm called fatty acid binding protein (FABP) functions to transport longer-chain fatty acids (>12 carbons) to the smooth endoplasmic reticulum, where triglycerides can be resynthesized. The longer-chain fatty acids and monoglycerides are resynthesized into triglycerides and exit via the lymphatic system as chylomicrons. With respect to cholesterol, some of it may be re-esterified by acyl-CoA cholesterol acyltransferase (ACAT). Cholesterol is re-esterified primarily to unsaturated fatty acids. The resynthesized triglycerides are incorporated into a lipoprotein by the addition of phospholipids, cholesterol, cholesterol esters, and apoprotein B. Chylomicrons then migrate to the Golgi apparatus, where glycoproteins may be added. Those fatty acids with 10 carbons or fewer are transported unesterified and leave the mucosa through the portal blood system. Those may be bound to albumin or are free fatty acids, but both forms are deposited in the liver. No free fatty acids are found within the lymph.

Secretory Phase

The secretory phase is relatively simple. Formed chylomicrons are discharged, via exocytosis, through the lateral portion of the mucosal cells into the extracellular space and enter the lacteal, a blind-ended lymph vessel. As mentioned previously, the shorter-chain fatty acids leave directly through the portal vein.

1. What are the most common fatty acids in the Western diet?

2. Discuss some of the key hormones and bile salts involved in the intraluminal phase of lipid digestion.

3. Distinguish between primary and secondary bile salts, and explain how they interrelate.

4. What are the functions of phospholipase A_1 and phospholipase A_2 and where within the intestine do those two enzymes function?

5. What is your opinion on the relationship of linoleic acid with obesity?

▶ Lipid Metabolism

Fatty Acid Oxidation

Fatty acids are a major source of energy for humans. Most cells, with the notable exceptions of erythrocytes and the cells of the brain, use fatty acids. Fatty acids primarily undergo oxidation in the mitochondria and to a lesser degree in peroxisomes. β-oxidation reduces even-chain-length fatty acids to acetyl CoA and odd-chain-length fatty acids to propionyl CoA. β-oxidation involves four sequential steps catalyzed by enzymes. The products of β-oxidation are FADH$_2$ and NADH + H$^+$ and acetyl CoA. The latter product is available to either condense with oxaloacetate to form citrate and engage in the Krebs cycle or to form ketone bodies in the liver. Unsaturated fatty acids, which may account for as much as half of the fatty acids humans oxidize, require additional enzymes.

Before a fatty acid can be oxidized, it must first be available in the cytosol. Fatty acids can either be liberated from intracellular pools, such as triglycerides in lipid droplets, or they can diffuse across the plasma membrane from the extra-cellular fluid (i.e., circulation). Circulatory fatty acids are primarily derived from triglycerides hydrolyzed in lipoproteins (such as VLDL and chylomicrons) by lipoprotein lipase, or they are loosely bound to albumin. Once in the cytosol, fatty acids are found associated with a FABP or Z protein, which may help guide the fatty acid toward mitochondria.

Cytosolic long-chain fatty acids are activated in the cytosol by the attachment of coenzyme A via long-chain acyl CoA synthetase. This enzyme is associated with the outer mitochondrial membrane. The fatty acid–coenzyme A complex is called acyl CoA. This reaction requires energy, which is provided as ATP, is split into AMP and pyrophosphate (PP$_i$). The latter complex is cleaved into two phosphate (Pi) molecules by pyrophosphatase, thus regenerating the intracellular phosphate pool. Because AMP and two P$_i$ are produced in the production of acyl CoA, the equivalent of two ATP is required before fatty acid oxidation can begin. Shorter-chain-length fatty acids also undergo activation, but not until they are inside mitochondria.

Although shorter-chain fatty acids can diffuse across the inner membrane of the mitochondria, longer-chain fatty acids, in the form of acyl CoA, must be transported across the inner membrane. This requires the assistance of carnitine transport systems. To begin, acyl CoA diffuses through the porous outer mitochondria membrane, and carnitine is attached to acyl CoA by the actions of carnitine palmitoyltransferase I (CPTI) [sometimes called carnitine acyl transferase I]. CPTI is an integral protein located in the outer mitochondrial membrane whose catalytic site is exposed on the intermembrane side of this membrane (**FIGURE 5.16**). This enzyme is inhibited by malonyl CoA, an intermediate of fatty acid synthesis.

Acyl carnitine is then transported across the inner membrane by carnitine acylcarnitine translocase, a symport protein. What this means is that this

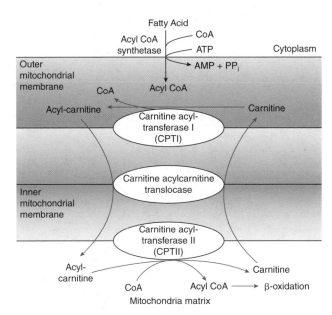

FIGURE 5.16 Carnitine Acyltransferase System Associated with the Mitochondrial Inner Membrane. Note that this mechanism is used to transport fatty acids in the mitochondria for β-oxidation.

protein transports one carnitine molecule out of the mitochondrial matrix for every carnitine acylcarnitine molecule it transfers into the matrix. Once inside the inner membrane, carnitine is split from the transferred fatty acid, which is reactivated with coenzyme A. This reaction is catalyzed by carnitine palmitoyltransferase II (CPTII).

Mitochondria contain three almost identical FAD-dependent acyl CoA dehydrogenase enzymes that act on short-chain, medium-chain, and long-chain fatty acids. FAD is reduced to FADH$_2$ in a reaction that produces trans-Δ^2-enoyl CoA, which is hydrated to form L-3-hydroxyacyl CoA. L-3-Hydroxyacyl CoA is then oxidized by NAD$^+$ forming NADH + H$^+$ and the product 3-ketoacyl CoA. Thiolase then splits 3-ketoacyl CoA to acetyl CoA and a fatty acyl CoA. The fatty acyl CoA is two carbons shorter than the fatty acyl CoA that began β-oxidation. Thus, if the original fatty acyl CoA was palmitoyl CoA, it becomes myristoyl CoA. For each "turn" of β-oxidation, or liberation of acetyl CoA, one FADH$_2$ and one NADH are generated. They are the equivalent of five total ATP molecules (**FIGURE 5.17**).

Ketone Body Production

Ketone bodies (acetoacetate, β-3-hydroxybutyrate, and acetone) are generally misunderstood and considered detrimental to human health. Although they can present a health concern, it should be understood

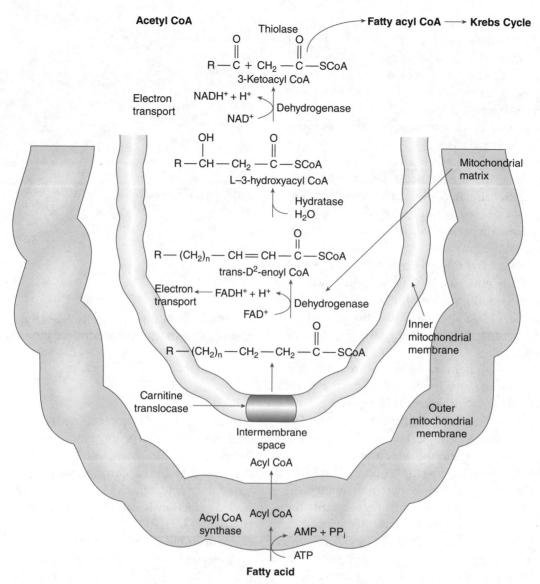

FIGURE 5.17 Fatty Acid Oxidation. Once the acyl CoA is transported into the mitochondria, as detailed in Figure 5.16, the fatty acid can be degraded for the generation of ATP via the electron transport and eventually enter the Krebs cycle.

that this concern may only arise under atypical metabolic scenarios, such as uncontrolled diabetes, and sometimes during pregnancy. The two primary sources of **ketone body** production are fatty acid oxidation and conversion of amino acids (leucine, isoleucine, lysine, phenylalanine, tyrosine, and tryptophan). Alcohol oxidation can also result in ketone body formation. **FIGURE 5.18** illustrates the formation of ketone bodies.

Ketone bodies are formed in the liver to a limited degree daily. The most significant precursors for ketogenesis are fatty acids. During uncontrolled diabetes and starvation, the rate of ketone body production can increase significantly to reach levels that may have health consequences. Although ketone bodies are produced in the liver, hepatocytes do not use them as an energy source. Instead, ketone bodies diffuse out of

the liver and circulate to other tissue, such as the heart, skeletal muscle, and the kidneys, and are combusted as fuel. During starvation, the brain can adapt to use more and more ketone bodies as an energy source. As much as 50% of the brain's energy demands may be met by ketone bodies after several weeks of starvation. Because an adult brain may use 140 to 150 grams of glucose daily, reducing its glucose demands will slow the rate of body protein catabolism to serve gluconeogenesis.

Fatty acids, made available by hormone-sensitive lipase (HSL) catabolism of adipocyte triglycerides, are oxidized in liver mitochondria to acetyl CoA. During periods when gluconeogenic operations are increased, such as starvation, oxaloacetate is used as a glucose precursor, thereby decreasing its availability to condense with acetyl CoA to form citrate. This increases the flux of acetyl CoA through acetoacetyl CoA thiokinase in

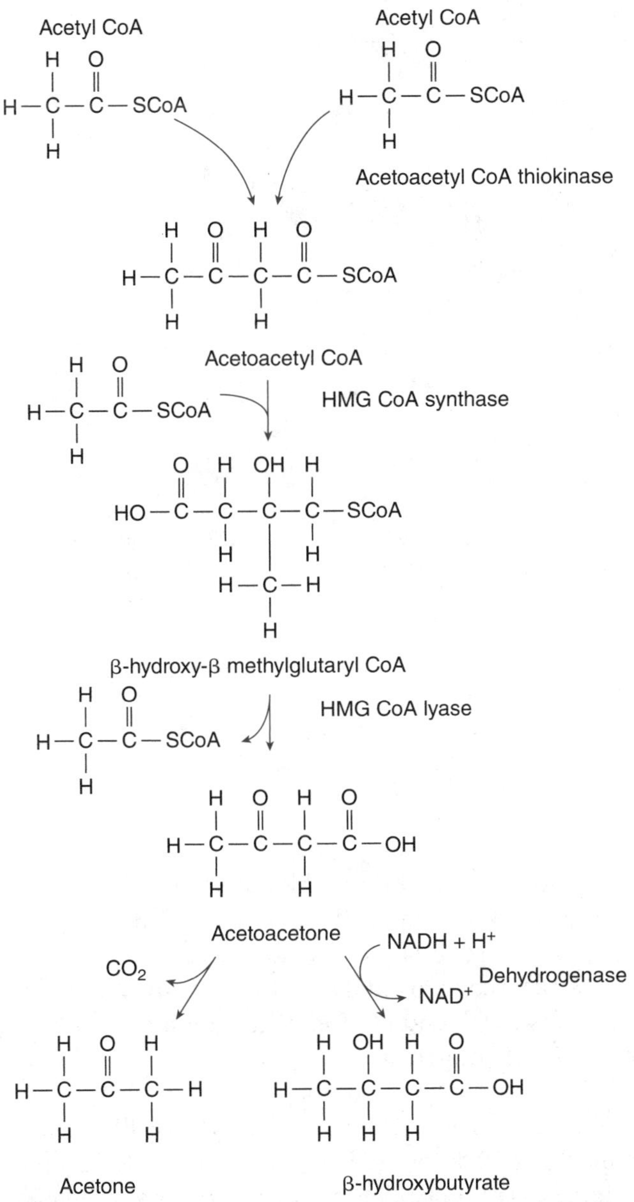

FIGURE 5.18 Ketone Body Formation from Acetyl CoA.
Acetoacetate, β-3-hydroxybutyrate, and acetone are the ketone bodies produced. They are produced by fatty acid oxidation or by the conversion of certain amino acids. Ketone bodies can be used as a source of energy by the heart, skeletal muscle, and kidneys; and in starvation, the brain.

the direction of ketogenesis. Acetoacetyl CoA thiokinase condenses two molecules of acetyl CoA to form acetoacetyl CoA. Acetoacetyl CoA can then condense with a third acetyl CoA, via HMG CoA synthase, to form hydroxy-3-methylglutaryl CoA (HMG CoA), which is then cleaved by lyase to form **acetoacetate** and acetyl CoA. Acetoacetate can undergo reduction by NADH to form **β-hydroxybutyrate**. **Acetone** can be formed by a nonenzymatic decarboxylation of acetoacetate. Acetone production is relatively small, and much of what is created is volatilized in the lungs and expired.

Eicosanoids

Essential fatty acids are precursors for **eicosanoids**, a large group of physiologically and pharmacologically active compounds that include prostaglandins (PGs), thromboxanes (TXs), and leukotrienes (LTs). However, not all of the physiologic properties associated with ω-3 and ω-6 PUFA are related to their conversion to eicosanoids.

Eicosanoids are derived from three 20-carbon PUFA, namely 20:3 ω-6 (dihomo-γ-linolenic acid, DGLA, or γ-linolenic acid), 20:4 ω-6 (arachidonic acid, arachidate, or AA), and 20:5 ω-3 (eicosapentanoic acid, or EPA) (**FIGURE 5.19**). The preliminary enzymes that initiate their conversion to eicosanoids are **lipoxygenase** and **cyclooxygenase**. However, AA can undergo a variety of enzymatic processing by the cytochrome P450 system in the endoplasmic reticulum to form metabolites with interesting biologic properties. That occurs mainly in the liver and kidney. For instance, epoxygenase metabolites of AA have renal vasoconstricting properties and are involved in ion transport. Also, free radical-mediated peroxidation of AA leads to the creation of a series of prostaglandin-like compounds called **isoprostanes**, which may have potent vasoconstrictive properties. Free radicals may attack AA as part of lipoproteins or cellular membranes creating those derivatives. Measurement of isoprostane levels in the urine and plasma has been suggested as a reliable indicator of **in vivo** lipid peroxidation. Enhanced urinary isoprostane levels have been identified in smokers.

EFAs are primarily stored as fatty acids esterified to phospholipids at the sn-2 position of glycerol. Liberation of the EFA from this location is accomplished by cleavage via phospholipase A$_2$. This enzyme can be inhibited by certain steroid drugs used as anti-inflammatory agents. The EFA composition of the diet can influence the concentration of the various EFAs and derivatives in membrane phospholipids. Thus, dietary fat composition can influence eicosanoid function by manipulating the pool of available eicosanoid precursors.

Different prostaglandin, leukotriene, and thromboxane structures can be derived from different EFAs or derivatives and are designated within series or groups. Series 1, 2, and 3 eicosanoids (i.e., PGE$_1$, PGI$_2$, PGI$_3$) are derived from 20:3 ω-6 (DGLA), 20:4 ω-6 (AA), and 20-5 ω-3 (EPA), respectively, where the subscript number identifies the series. Arachidonic acid is also the precursor for series 4 leukotrienes (leukotrienes and lipoxins), and 20:5 ω-3 (EPA) is also a precursor for series 5 leukotrienes. One notable exception is that the series 3 leukotrienes are derived from

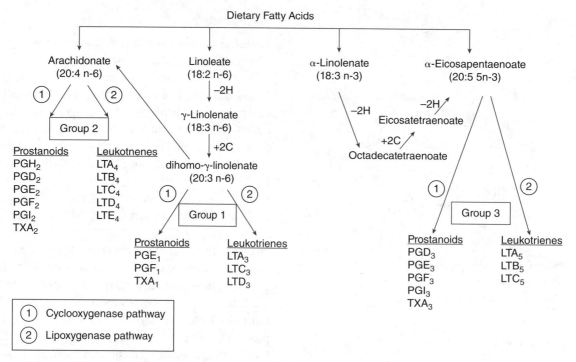

FIGURE 5.19 Eicosanoid Formation Pathways. The prostanoids are formed through the cyclooxygenase reaction, which is indicated by (1), and the lipoxygenase reaction, which is indicated by (2).

DGLA, not EPA. Furthermore, DGLA is converted to AA, where some can end up as series 2 eicosanoids and series 4 leukotrienes, respectively. A limited amount of ω-linolenate may also be converted to EPA. In several situations, eicosanoids derived from 20:4 ω-6 work in opposition to those derived from 20:5 ω-3.

Prostaglandins may be derived from each of the above three groups via the cyclooxygenase pathway. Thromboxanes, which have significant effects on blood platelet function, are also synthesized via this pathway. Leukotrienes are synthesized by the lipoxygenase pathway. The involvement of those enzymes is indicated in Figure 5.19. The cyclooxygenase pathway involves the consumption of two molecules of molecular oxygen and is catalyzed by prostaglandin-endoperoxide (prostaglandin G/H) synthases. The pathway really involves the activities of two separate enzymes: cyclooxygenase and peroxidase. Aspirin and nonsteroidal anti-inflammatory drugs can inhibit cyclooxygenase activity. The end product of the cyclooxygenase activity associated with AA is prostaglandin PGH_2, which is converted to either PGD_2, PGE_2, or PGF_2, as well as to TXA_2 and PGI_2.

The production of these eicosanoids depends on the needs of the cell type. For instance, PGD_2 is a major AA metabolite produced in the brain (involved in sleep and thermoregulation), platelets, mast cells, uterus, skin, skeletal muscle, and renal medulla. PGE_2

formation occurs in the blood vessels, intestines, prostate, uterus, and fallopian tubes. Thromboxane A synthase, a primary eicosanoid-converting enzyme in platelets, converts PGH_2 to TXA_2. TXA_2 is a potent vasoconstrictor and platelet aggregation agent that is critical in hemorrhagic response. Overproduction of TXA_2 has been suggested as a pivotal factor in myocardial infarction associated with atheromas. TXA_2 has a half-life of 30 seconds. PGI_2, with a half-life of a few minutes, is produced in the aorta and has vasodilative and platelet antiaggregative effects. In contrast, greater production of TXA_3 via increased consumption of ω-3 fatty acids results in a weaker physiologic product in which less platelet aggregation occurs. Thus, increased intake of ω-3 fatty acids compared with ω-6 fatty acid intake will tilt the balance away from platelet aggregation and toward vasodilation because PGI_3 is similar in potency to PGI_2.

The various prostaglandins differ only slightly in their molecular composition. For instance, E designates that there is a C=O group at carbon 9, whereas F indicates that the OH group is at carbon 9.

Lipoproteins
Types of Lipoproteins

Within the blood, triglycerides and cholesterol esters are transported within a phospholipid, cholesterol, and protein shell. Those transport vesicles, called lipoproteins, are produced primarily within hepatocytes and enterocytes. The core of the typical lipoprotein is composed of cholesterol, which is almost entirely esterified, and triglycerides. Some diglycerides and monoglycerides may be present as well.

Phospholipids contribute most of the molecules found as part of the outer shell. Their polar phosphate group is oriented toward the outer, aqueous environment of the blood, and their two fatty acids are oriented toward the hydrophobic core. Also in the shell are specialized proteins (apoproteins or apolipoproteins). Although some of the significance of those proteins is that they enhance the miscible properties of lipoproteins, perhaps, more important, are their other properties. As described in greater detail below, apoproteins have enzymatic and receptor-associated activities.

The composition of lipoproteins differs, depending on their type, origin, and physiologic function. The four basic types are chylomicrons, very-low-density lipoproteins (VLDL), low-density lipoproteins (LDL), and high-density lipoproteins (HDL). There are often intermediate types, such as intermediate-density lipoprotein (IDL), and various subtypes of HDL (1, 2, C, and Apo E rich). **FIGURE 5.20** provides a good summary of the chemical and physical characteristics of those basic lipoprotein types.

Chylomicrons are produced in the small intestine, where their primary function is to absorb diet-derived triglycerides and cholesterol and transport them in the blood. VLDL are produced in the liver and transport both endogenously produced triglycerides and cholesterol as well as that derived from chylomicrons to peripheral tissues. LDL are formed as a metabolic product from VLDL. The change is the result of successive hydrolysis of VLDL core triglycerides by lipoprotein lipase. Fatty acids are translocated into peripheral tissue, whereas glycerol dissolves into circulation. With the removal of triglycerides from their core, VLDL become more dense and the relative mass of cholesterol in the core increases. VLDL become IDL and then cholesterol-rich LDL. Cholesterol from LDL is delivered to selective cell types. HDL may be produced both in the small intestine and the liver. However, about 80% of the HDL is of hepatic origin. The exchange of apoproteins between certain lipoproteins occurs within the framework of lipoprotein metabolism, as discussed below.

Lipoproteins differ in their densities, with chylomicrons being the least dense but the largest in diameter (see Figure 5.20). The opposite is true of HDL. The various classes of lipoproteins may be separated by a variety of means, including ultracentrifugation,

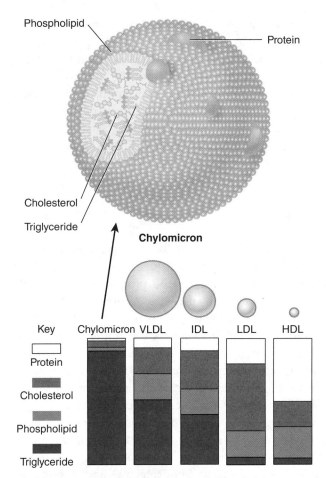

FIGURE 5.20 Lipoprotein Characteristics and Composition. The phosphate component of phospholipids and the apoproteins are found in the outer shell of lipoproteins as they are polar and allow for their solubility in an aqueous environment. Cholesterol and fatty acids are found inside the particles where there is a nonpolar environment.

various types of chromatography, electrophoresis, and chemical precipitation techniques. Sequential ultracentrifugation is often used, whereby the plasma is layered with a salt, such as sodium chloride (NaCl), sodium bromide (NaBr), or potassium bromide (KBr), at a particular density. For example, if KBr is the salt of choice and its density is 1.006 g/ml, VLDL will float to the top because it is less dense than the salt solution. If the lipoproteins beneath the salt layer are carefully removed and again layered with KBr or another substance with a slightly higher density, flotation of LDL will occur. Electrophoresis is an older method used to separate the lipoproteins. Because this approach separates proteins based on mass or size, HDL will migrate the furthest and the chylomicrons will often remain at the origin.

Using gel permeation chromatography, the lipoproteins are placed on top of a column (usually

1 meter in length) and traverse a collection of agarose beads with varying pore sizes. Smaller particles, such as HDL, will move through the beads more rapidly and thus will be released from the other end of the column first. Conversely, larger lipoproteins, such as chylomicrons and VLDL, will navigate the column more slowly and thus will be eluted last.

The apoprotein portions of lipoproteins have several types and designations. HDL has apoproteins A-I and A-II. Chylomicrons also have some apoprotein A-II. LDL has apoprotein B-100. Chylomicrons contain a protein closely related to B-100, called B-48, which is smaller than B-100. B-48 is synthesized in the small intestine, and B-100 is synthesized in the liver; however, both apoproteins are expressed from the same gene. B-48 is the product of posttranslational modification of B-100. Apoproteins C-I, C-II, and C-III are smaller polypeptides found in VLDL, HDL, and chylomicrons. An arginine-rich apoprotein, designated Apo E, is found scattered among the VLDL, chylomicrons, and HDL. As alluded to earlier, some of those apoproteins are activators of certain key enzymes or may serve as binding sites for cell membrane receptors. For instance, lipoprotein lipase requires apoprotein C-II as an activator or cofactor.

Two other types of lipoproteins that can lead to various diseases are lipoprotein(a) and apolipoprotein E. Lipoprotein(a) is a derivative of LDL that has a glycoprotein referred to as apolipoprotein(a). Studies have suggested that elevated levels of this lipoprotein increases the risk of cardiovascular disease. Apolipoprotein E, as previously discussed, is a component of HDL, LDL, and VLDL. There are various isoforms: ApoE2, ApoE3, and ApoE4. The ApoE4 isoform has been linked to increased risk of various diseases. The presence of Apo4 has a genetic basis with ¼ of white people likely to have this isoform. The presence of this isoform is known to increase the risk of cardiovascular disease and may be due to its proinflammatory and oxidative stress properties. Elevated levels of ApoE in the brain has also been linked to Alzheimer's disease and some forms of cognitive impairment.

Metabolism of Lipoproteins

Chylomicrons are formed in the small intestine, and the enzyme lipoprotein lipase plays an important role in hydrolysis of their core triglycerides (**FIGURE 5.21**). Lipoprotein lipase is located attached to the endothelial lining of tissue capillaries, primarily muscle, adipocytes, and lactating mammary glands, and secondarily in the spleen, lungs, renal medulla, aorta, and diaphragm. Lipoprotein lipase has a specific phospholipid binding site that anchors chylomicrons to the enzyme. The actions of lipoprotein lipase reduce the quantity of triglycerides in circulating chylomicrons by 90%. The remaining triglyceride ultimately enters the liver as chylomicron remnants are transported into hepatocytes.

Apoprotein A and B-48 are present in just-released or nascent chylomicrons. As they circulate, chylomicrons must pick up apoproteins C-II and E. Apoproteins A and C-II eventually dissociate from chylomicrons and associate with HDL as chylomicrons become smaller through the successive hydrolysis of the triglycerides. The chylomicron remnant is taken up by the liver by an apoprotein E receptor-mediated site (see Figure 5.21).

The liver is the site of origin for VLDL; however, it should be noted that very small amounts of VLDL-like particles are released from the small intestine in between meals (**FIGURE 5.22**). VLDL transport triglycerides and cholesterol from the liver to extrahepatic tissue. VLDL are initially constructed within the smooth endoplasmic reticulum. Apoprotein B-100, which is synthesized by ribosomal complexes in the rough endoplasmic reticulum, is incorporated into VLDL within the smooth endoplasmic reticulum. Apoprotein B-100 is perhaps the largest protein in the human body. The smooth endoplasmic reticulum is also the site of triglyceride formation, using phosphatidic acid as the base. Semideveloped VLDL particles are then passed to the Golgi apparatus, where more lipids and carbohydrate residues are added. This formation is very similar to the synthesis of chylomicrons. VLDL and chylomicrons are released from their synthesizing cell into the extracellular fluid by reverse pinocytosis. In the liver, VLDL gain access to the blood by entering sinusoids, or channels flowing between rows of hepatocytes. Chylomicrons, however, must enter a lacteal, located in the center of a villus, and navigate the lymphatic circulation, eventually gaining access to the general circulation via the thoracic duct.

In some individuals, the ability to synthesize apoprotein B is genetically obstructed. This results in the inability to synthesize both chylomicrons and VLDL. Large fat droplets are observed in the liver and small intestine in those individuals. This condition is referred to as abetalipoproteinemia.

Although traces of apoproteins C and E can be found in nascent VLDL, by and large, VLDL do not receive those apoproteins until they encounter HDL in the bloodstream. VLDL breakdown occurs in a manner similar to chylomicron breakdown. Triglycerides are digested by the actions of lipoprotein lipase, and

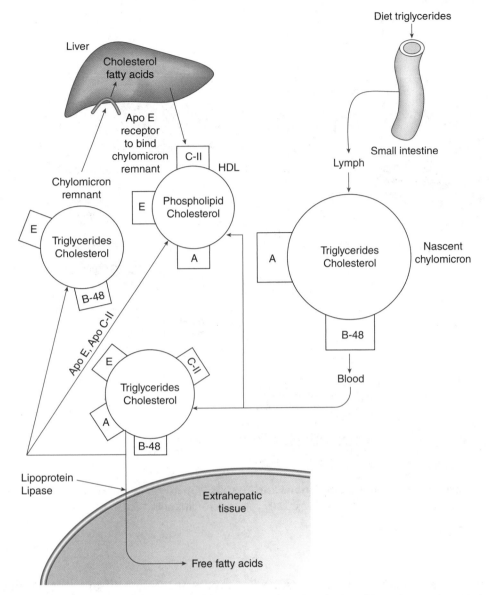

FIGURE 5.21 Metabolism of Chylomicrons. Chylomicrons are produced in the small intestine, and once absorbed, the triglycerides are delivered to the endothelial lining of blood vessels of various tissues that contain lipoprotein lipase. Lipoprotein lipase hydrolyzes triglycerides to liberate free fatty acids for the cells.

VLDL shrink in size and change in composition. VLDL becomes IDL and then LDL. In the process, apoprotein C is transferred back to HDL, thereby generally limiting further triglyceride removal (see Figure 5.22).

Specific binding sites for apoprotein B-100 exist in various tissues or organs, such as liver, arterial smooth muscle, fibroblasts, and lymphocytes. The liver removes about 70% of circulating LDL; the remaining 30% is removed by all the other tissues combined. The receptor is referred to as the LDL (B-100, E) receptor, because not only will it recognize apoprotein B-100-rich LDL but also apoprotein E-rich lipoproteins. The entire complex binds to the receptor and is engulfed by pinocytosis.

Apoprotein B-100 is broken down by lysosomes. Cholesteryl esters are hydrolyzed, but later are re-esterified. The buildup of cholesterol in the cell inhibits the key cholesterol-producing regulatory enzyme, 3-hydroxyl-3-methylglutaryl CoA reductase (HMG CoA reductase). However, the oversupply of cholesterol by this process also inhibits the synthesis of LDL receptors. If too much cholesterol accumulates in the cells, the receptor synthesis decreases, and LDL-cholesterol cannot enter the cell. This results in a buildup of cholesterol within the blood, increasing the risk of heart disease. Figure 5.22 reviews the metabolism of VLDL and LDL.

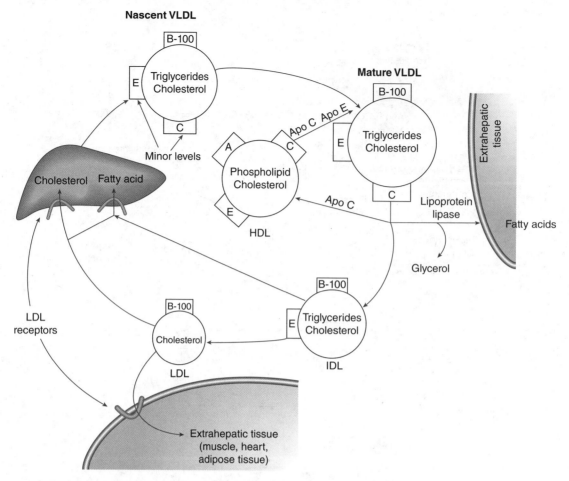

FIGURE 5.22 Metabolism of VLDL and LDL in Organs and Tissues. A major feature of lipoprotein metabolism is the interplay with the various lipoprotein types, particularly the apoproteins and the relative levels of cholesterol and triglycerides.

HDL is synthesized by both the small intestine and the liver (**FIGURE 5.23**). Intestinal HDL lacks apoprotein C and E, but has apoprotein A. Apoprotein C and E are synthesized only in the liver and later transferred to intestinal HDL by interaction with hepatic HDL. The initially synthesized lipoprotein by either tissue (nascent HDL) contains phospholipid bilayers composed of apoproteins and free cholesterol and is disc shaped. It is often called discoidal HDL. The plasma enzyme lecithin-cholesterol acyltransferase (LCAT) binds with the surface of HDL. This enzyme is activated by apoprotein A-I and converts HDL shell phospholipid and free cholesterol into cholesterol esters and lysolecithin. Cholesterol esters enter the HDL core, whereas lysolecithin is transferred to plasma albumin. The result is a more spherically shaped HDL particle. LCAT esterifies cholesterol from other lipoproteins and extrahepatic tissue as well. SR-B1 is called a scavenger receptor that internalizes cholesteryl esters from HDL. HDL is

eventually removed from circulation by HDL SR-B1 receptors in the liver. The presence of apoprotein A-I on HDL greatly enhances its removal.

Cholesteryl ester transfer protein, or apoprotein D, is another component of HDL. It transfers the esterified cholesterol on HDL to the other lipoproteins. Thus, the cholesterol endowed to HDL can be transported to the liver and removed via a HDL receptor, or it can be transferred to other lipoproteins (i.e., chylomicron remnants and LDL) that themselves are subject to removal from the circulation. The removal of cholesterol from extrahepatic tissue by HDL and its delivery to the liver has been called **reverse cholesterol transport**.

As HDL acquires more cholesterol esters in its core, its size and density change. The uptake of cholesterol by HDL_3 increases its diameter approximately twofold, and its density decreases from between 1.125 and 1.210 grams per milliliter to between 1.063 and 1.125 grams per milliliter, forming HDL_2. The

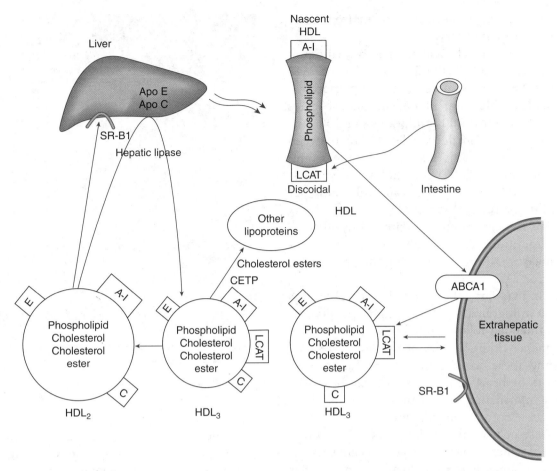

FIGURE 5.23 HDL Metabolism. Note that A-I is added by the intestine to the nascent HDL and Apo E and Apo C originate from the liver and then are added to the nascent HDL. SR-B1, scavenger receptor family (transports lipids); ABCA1, ATP-binding cassette transporter family (transports cholesterol and phospholipids to HDL); LCAT, lecithin acyltransferase (forms cholesterol esters by transferring fatty acid from C-2 of phosphatidylcholine to free cholesterol); CETP (Apo D), cholesteryl ester transfer protein (transfers cholesteryl ester from HDL to other lipoproteins).

hydrolyzation of HDL phospholipid and triglyceride by **hepatic lipase** allows HDL_2 to reduce its size and regain some of its density, thereby regaining some of its HDL_3 qualities. HDL_3 then reenters circulation. HDL_2 concentrations are inversely related to the incidence of coronary artery disease.

▶ The Health Implications and Interpretation of Lipoprotein-Cholesterol and Triglyceride Levels

The ability to control plasma cholesterol levels, in particular LDL-cholesterol levels, is partly genetic because it relates to the density of apoprotein B-100 receptors on hepatocyte membranes. A decreased ability to produce those receptors could be the result of a genetic anomaly or of decreased mRNA synthesis of the apoprotein B-100 transcript. The result is elevated plasma cholesterol levels, a strong risk factor for heart disease. A decreased level of HDL-cholesterol, especially HDL_2, is also a risk factor for heart disease. Other factors that increase the risk of heart disease are cigarette smoking, **hypertension**, diabetes, obesity, decreased physical activity levels, and male gender.

Serum cholesterol levels demonstrate a linear relationship with the percentage of arterial intimal surface covered with raised lesions, but the relationship with coronary heart disease risk ratio is curvilinear. How can this discrepancy be resolved? The key lies in the fact that a critical percent area of the surface of blood vessels must be covered with raised lesions before a statistical effect is observed. When 60% or more of the surface area of blood vessels is covered with lesions, a linear response with respect to mortality from coronary heart disease is observed.

Defining, from a clinical perspective, who is at risk for heart disease has undergone revision over the years. One scheme uses a screening approach in which desirable total blood cholesterol levels are defined as below 200 milligrams per 100 milliliters of plasma, borderline levels are between 200 and 239 milligrams per 100 milliliters, and high blood cholesterol (hypercholesterolemia) is defined as levels greater than 240 milligrams per 100 milliliters. Total blood cholesterol represents the sum of the cholesterol distributed in all lipoprotein fractions. This should be an overnight fasting measure, thereby removing the presence of chylomicrons.

If an individual's total blood cholesterol level is below 200 milligrams per 100 milliliters of plasma, the recommended follow-up is simply to repeat the measurement within 5 years. If the levels are borderline and there are not two other heart disease risk factors or heart disease present, the provision of dietary information and an annual recheck of the serum level is recommended. However, if coronary heart disease or two other risk factors for heart disease (one of which may be male gender) are present, a lipoprotein analysis is recommended, and further clinical action should be guided by the LDL-cholesterol level. An LDL-cholesterol level defined as optimal is a level below 100 milligrams per 100 milliliters plasma, near optimal is 100 to 130 milligrams per 100 milliliters plasma, borderline high is between 130 and 159 milligrams per 100 milliliters, high- risk is 160 to 189 milligrams per 100 milliliters, and very high is greater than 189 milligrams per 100 milliliters. A special note is that some health organizations have recommended that LDL-cholesterol be less than 70 milligrams per milliliter if a person has heart diseases or who has had a heart attack. **TABLE 5.6** presents a typical blood lipid profile.

Dietary treatment is recommended for those with levels of LDL-cholesterol greater than 160 milligrams per 100 milliliters, or, if two other risk factors are present, greater than 130 milligrams per 100 milliliters. In addition to dietary modifications, drug treatment is recommended if LDL-cholesterol levels are 190 milligrams per 100 milliliters or greater with no evidence of coronary heart disease. If two heart disease risk factors are already present or there is evidence of coronary heart disease, drug therapy concomitant with nutrition modification is the recommended course of treatment when LDL-cholesterol levels exceed 160 milligrams per 100 milliliters.

TABLE 5.6 Typical Blood Lipid Profile for an Adult

Lipid	Result	Normal Range
Triglycerides (TG)	137 mg/dL	0–210 mg/dL
Cholesterol	163 mg/dL	50–200 mg/dL
HDL	42 mg/dL	30–90 mg/dL
VLDL	27 mg/dL	5–40 mg/dL
LDL	94 mg/dL	50–140 mg/dL
Chol:HDL	3.9 (ratio)	3.7–6.7 (ratio)
LDL:HDL	2.2 (ratio)	3.3– 4.4 (ratio)

HDL, high-density lipoprotein; VLDL, very-low-density lipoprotein; LDL, low-density lipoprotein; Chol, cholesterol.

Older classes of drugs used to treat blood cholesterol, such as bile-sequestering agents (e.g., cholestyramine and colestipol) may still be used today. Those block the uptake of bile acids by the gut, thereby interfering with the enterohepatic circulation. This forces the liver to replace the lost bile acids through conversion of more hepatic cholesterol into the primary bile acids, thus decreasing the available cholesterol for VLDL synthesis. This effect, in theory at least, also leads to upregulation of mRNA transcripts for the apoprotein B-100 receptors on the cell membranes. Similarly, the class of drugs that inhibits HMG CoA reductase (e.g., lovastatin) directly lowers hepatocyte levels of cholesterol and thereby relieves the inhibition of mRNA synthesis for apoprotein B-100. Those drugs, in particular, have been very effective; their use may decrease blood cholesterol levels by as much as a third compared with approximately a 10% reduction through dietary means. Some early evidence suggests that delayed onset of coronary heart disease is possible with those newer agents.

Another blood lipid receiving much attention in relation to risk is plasma triglyceride levels. Triglyceride levels less than 150 milligrams per 100 milliliters is desirable, 150 to 199 milligrams per 100 milliliters is borderline high, 200 to 499 milligrams per 100 milliliters is high, and greater than 499 milligrams per 100 milliliters is very high.

Weight loss and dietary measures are the first line of defense to lower blood triglycerides. Niacin containing drugs in very large doses are medications that have been historically used in treating high triglyceride levels, but the side effects of patients feeling flushed and presence of mental impairment have been cause for concern. Drugs such as Lopid have been effective in the past. More recently, pharmacologic grade fish oils high in EPA and DHA have been shown to be highly effective in lowering plasma triglyceride levels while at the same time increasing HDL-cholesterol levels.

▶ Alcohol

While alcohol is not considered a lipid, it is discussed here. Alcohol is absorbed by the gastrointestinal tract, including the stomach, and enters the blood stream and subsequently enters the liver for metabolism. At this point, alcohol can be converted to acetaldehyde via the enzyme alcohol dehydrogenase. Acetaldehyde is a toxic compound. Acetaldehyde is further metabolized by another enzyme, aldehyde dehydrogenase 2, which converts acetaldehyde to *acetic acid* and eventually to acetyl CoA. Acetyl CoA can be metabolized by the body for energy or it can enter a fat cell where it is used for lipid biosynthesis. Some individuals who lack aldehyde dehydrogenase 2 are unable to metabolize ethanol. Those individuals cannot consume alcohol without having major mental impairment and damage to their organs (**FIGURE 5.24**).

Acetaldehyde is the compound that leads to tissue damage where it may cause damage to liver mitochondria and lead to inflammation or hepatitis. Hepatitis may lead to secondary effects such as abdominal fluid accumulation, jaundice, and neurologic problems caused by liver failure. Those events may cause hardening and scarring of the liver or **cirrhosis**. Cirrhosis is serious, irreversible, and often fatal. Liver cirrhosis from alcohol abuse is one of the ten leading causes of death in the United States. Between 10–15% of alcoholics have liver cirrhosis by the time they die. Women that consume the same amount of alcohol as men are more likely to have liver disease.

In the brain acetaldehyde may interfere with enzymes involved with neurotransmitter synthesis in such a way that slightly different compounds are produced, which then react with acetaldehyde to produce morphine like compounds. This could be an explanation as to why alcohol may become

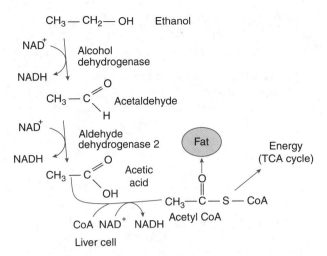

FIGURE 5.24. Metabolism of alcohol by the liver. Ethanol can be converted to Acetyl CoA and used either for energy or fat biosynthesis. The intermediate product, acetaldehyde, is toxic. Some individuals lack the enzyme aldehyde dehydrogenase 2 in which the acetaldehyde cannot be metabolized. Intake of alcohol by those individuals can result in mental impairment and organ damage.

addictive. Alcohol may also lead to the development of **fatty liver**, which can cause inflammation. However, if alcohol consumption ceases, fatty liver can be reversed.

● BEFORE YOU GO ON . . .

1. What is the role of coenzyme A in the initiation of fatty acid oxidation?

2. How do longer-chain fatty acids get into the mitochondria for oxidation?

3. Discuss how fatty acids lead to prostaglandin and thromboxane production and how ω-3 versus ω-6 fatty acids may alter the physiologic impact of the resulting products.

4. Characterize each of the four lipoproteins fully in terms of chemical composition and functions. In addition to the four major lipoproteins, what roles do lipoprotein(a) and apoprotein E have with human health and disease?

5. Discuss the optimal and suboptimal levels of LDL-cholesterol level in conjunction with other heart disease risk factors.

6. Excess alcohol intake may be harmful to one's health. Explain the metabolism of alcohol in relation to what diseases it may cause as a result of the breakdown products.

⚕ *CLINICAL INSIGHT*

Determination of risk for a cardiac event

In 2013, the American College of Cardiology and American Heart Association published guidelines to assess the risk of developing atherosclerotic cardiovascular disease (ASCVD) events. The group was charged with evaluating and updating guidelines on blood cholesterol, blood pressure and overweight/obesity issues as they relate to risk for ASCVD. The group evaluated the literature from large cohort studies such as the Framingham Heart Study to develop equations to determine the 10-year risk of developing an ASCVD event. The group was able to develop two sets of equations for this goal: one for non-Hispanic, African-American men and women and one for non-Hispanic white men and women 40 to 79 years old.

An ASCVD event was defined as a nonfatal myocardial infarction or coronary heart disease death, or fatal or nonfatal stroke. Evidence for developing predictive equations for Hispanics and Asian Americans was not developed as the evidence of specific risks for heart disease was weak, but it was recommended that the non-Hispanic white men and women equations be used for these two groups.

Various risk factors were considered in the equations to develop a risk calculator. Some of those calculators may differ slightly on which variables to include by some groups. The most common variables used to predict a 10-year likelihood of an ASCVD event are race, gender, age, systolic blood pressure, total cholesterol levels, HDL-cholesterol levels, current smoking status, and presence of diabetes. Some calculators include diastolic blood pressure, family history of heart disease, the presence of atherosclerotic heart disease or blood vessel disease, and whether triglyceride levels are above 150 milligrams per 100 milliliters of plasma. The percent chance of developing heart disease is predicted from those variables. In some calculators, the results indicate whether there is a need for statin treatment or other modifiable factors to lower the risk. A search engine with the key words "heart disease risk calculator" can be entered. Calculators used by the National Heart, Lung, Blood Institute and the American Heart Association can be found in this manner.

▶ Here's What You Have Learned

1. Fatty acids can be named in one of two ways: (1) the omega system, in which the carbon number from the methyl end of the fatty acid where the first double bond occurs is used to designate the fatty acid family, and (2) the delta system, in which the carbon number from the carboxyl end of the fatty acid is used to designate the fatty acid family.

2. Acetyl CoA carboxylase and fatty acid synthase are the key regulatory enzymes involved in fatty acid synthesis.

3. Human cells can elongate fatty acids with elongase enzymes and can create new double bonds through the presence of desaturase enzymes.

4. Reducing equivalents are essential for fatty acid synthesis and are generated via the pentose phosphate pathway.

5. The *cis* and *trans* forms of unsaturated fatty acids can affect physiologic function. The *cis* form is the form that is most common in food and living organisms.

6. Although we can obtain most of the fatty acids from our diet, there are some that we cannot make ourselves; those are termed essential fatty acids. Most important are the ω-3 fatty acids such as EPA and DHA, which offer health benefits above those offered by ω-6 fatty acids.

7. Phospholipids are lipid compounds that contain phosphatidic acid, which is composed of glycerol, two fatty acids, and a phosphate group. They are able to attract both water-soluble and fat-soluble substances, therefore, making them ideal for cellular membranes and lipoprotein shells.

8. Triglycerides and phospholipids are structurally similar except that in triglycerides, the third carbon of glycerol has a fatty acid, whereas in phospholipids, the carbon has phosphatidic acid.

9. Cholesterol synthesis starts with acetyl CoA through a variety of biochemical reactions. A significant rate-limiting aspect of cholesterol biosynthesis is the enzyme 3-hydroxy-3-methylglutaryl (HMG) reductase, which results in decreased cholesterol synthesis if inhibited, and vice versa.

10. Lipid metabolism is under the control of a superfamily of nuclear hormone receptors. One type of receptor is the class of peroxisome proliferator-activated receptors (PPARs), which

belong to the steroid/thyroid/retinoid receptor superfamily. Those receptors can influence both the synthesis and oxidation of fatty acids.

11. Liver X receptors (LRXs) play a significant role in cholesterol metabolism. LXRs activate transporters to transfer cholesterol to HDL. They also prevent cholesterol absorption at the intestinal level.

12. Farnesoid X receptor (FRX) targets genes involved with bile metabolism. It suppresses bile synthesis by inhibiting the rate-limiting enzyme that converts cholesterol to bile acid, 7 α-hydroxylase. It does this indirectly by promoting the expression of small heterodimer partner (SHP), which suppresses the transcription of 7 α-hydroxylase.

13. A nonnuclear receptor, sterol regulatory element binding protein (SREBP), regulates genes involved in the biosynthesis of lipid and cholesterol. It is considered a basic-helix-loop-helix leucine zipper transcription factor.

14. The most prevalent saturated fatty acids in the Western diet are palmitic acid (16:0) and stearic acid (18:0), and the most prevalent unsaturated fatty acids are oleic acid (18:1 ω-9) and linoleic acid (18:2 ω-6).

15. The requirement for fat is related to essential fatty acids. It has been estimated that as long as humans receive 2 to 3% of their fat from a variety of natural sources, they will meet their minimal EFA requirements. The optimal intake for linolenic acid is estimated to be 800 to 1,100 milligrams per day and that of EPA and DHA to be 300 to 400 milligrams per day.

16. Fat digestion is complex. Many enzymes, hormones, and organs are involved in the emulsification of fat—from lingual, gastric, and pancreatic lipases to bile salts. Fat digestion is often divided into intraluminal, mucosal, and secretory phases. The actual digestion takes place in the lumen of the small intestine, and the mucosal phase occurs in the enterocytes, where the lipid breakdown products are packaged for eventual absorption, including the synthesis of chylomicrons that are secreted into the lymph system.

17. Fatty acid oxidation takes place in the mitochondria of cells. Here, the end product of fatty acid breakdown feeds into the Krebs cycle. In some cases, where there is limited carbohydrate in the diet, the acetyl CoA is unable to be fully metabolized and uses another pathway to form ketone bodies, which are excreted in the urine.

18. Essential fatty acids are precursors for eicosanoids, a large group of physiologically and pharmacologically active compounds that include prostaglandins, thromboxanes, and leukotrienes. The function of those products and their potency are largely affected by the family of fatty acids, such as ω-3 vs ω-6 fatty acids; the former yields compounds that have better health benefits to humans.

19. The transport of lipids from the intestine to the liver and between the liver and other organs depends on various types of lipoproteins: chylomicrons, very-low-density lipoproteins, low-density lipoproteins, and high-density lipoproteins. Lipoproteins are not static substances in the blood; there is a dynamic state of change whereby components of lipoproteins, particularly the protein or apoprotein portions, are exchanged between the different types.

20. Dietary lipids are found in chylomicrons, and very-low-density lipoproteins transport lipids synthesized by the liver. Low-density lipoproteins are remnants of VLDL; their major function is the deposition of cholesterol to other organs and blood vessels. High-density lipoproteins are involved in reverse cholesterol transport back to the liver.

21. Lipoprotein(a) and ApoE can lead to cardiovascular disease. Additionally, ApoE has been implicated in Alzheimer's disease development.

22. Recommended levels of LDL-cholesterol are dependent on other risk factors for heart disease. Triglyceride levels are also components of risk for heart disease.

▶ Suggested Reading

Alberts B, Johnson A, Lewis J, Raff M, Roberts K, Walter P. *The Molecular Biology of the Cell*. 5th ed. London: Garland Press, Taylor and Francis; 2007.

Banz WJ, Davis JE, Clough RW, Cheatwood JL. Stearidonic acid: is there a role in the prevention and management of type2 diabetes mellitus? *J Nutr.* 2012;142(3):635S–640S.

Christophe AB, Stephanie DeVriese S, eds. *Fat Digestion and Absorption*. Champaign, IL: AOCA Press; 2000.

Deckelbaum RJ, Torrejon C. The omega-3 fatty acid nutritional landscape: health benefits and sources. *J Nutr.* 2012;142(3):587S–591S.

Edwards PA, Kast HR, Anisfeld AM. BAREing it all: the adoption of LXR and FXR and their roles in lipid homeostasis. *J Lipid Res.* 2002;43(1):2–12.

Engler MM, Engler MB. Omega-3 fatty acids: role in cardiovascular health and disease. *J Cardiovasc Nurs.* 2006;21(1):17–24.

Fürnsinn C, Willson TM, Brunmair B. Peroxisome proliferator-activated receptor-delta, a regulator of oxidative capacity, fuel switching and cholesterol transport. *Diabetologia.* 2007;50(1):8–17.

Goff DC, Lloyd-Jones DM, Bennett G, et al. 2013 ACC/AHA guideline on the assessment of cardiovascular risk: a report of the American College of Cardiology/American Heart Association Task Force on Practice Guidelines. *J Am Coll Cardiol.* 2014; 63(25 pt B):2935–2959.

Hall JE, Guyton AC. *Textbook of Medical Physiology.* 11th ed. St. Louis, MO: Elsevier; 2005.

Harris WS, Kris-Etherton PM, Harris KA. Intakes of long-chain omega-3 fatty acid associated with reduced risk for death from coronary heart disease in healthy adults. *Curr Atheroscler Rep.* 2008;10:503–509.

Jakobsson T, Treuter E, Gustafsson JÅ, Steffensen KR. Liver X receptor biology and pharmacology: new pathways, challenges and opportunities. *Trends Pharmacol Sci.* 2012;33(7):394–404.

Jeon T, Osborne TF. SREBPs: metabolic integrators in physiology and metabolism. *Trends Endocrinol Metab.* 2012;23(2):65–72.

König A, Bouzan C, Cohen JT, et al. A quantitative analysis of fish consumption and coronary heart disease mortality. *Am J Prev Med.* 2005;29(4):335–346.

Kris-Etherton PM, Taylor DS, Yu-Poth S, et al. Polyunsaturated fatty acids in the food chain in the United States. *Am J Clin Nutr.* 2000;71(1 suppl):179S–188S.

Landow MV. *Trends in Dietary Fats Research.* New York: Nova Biomedical Books; 2006.

Lenihan-Geels G, Bishop KS, Ferguson LR. Alternative sources of omega-3 fats: can we find a sustainable substitute for fish? *Nutrients.* 2013;5(4):1301–1315.

Madrazo JA, Kelly DP. The PPAR trio: regulators of myocardial energy metabolism in health and disease. *J Mol Cell Cardiol.* 2008;44(6):968–975.

Michael DR, Ashlin TG, Buckley ML, Ramji DP. Liver X receptors, atherosclerosis and inflammation. *Curr Atheroscler Rep.* 2012;14:284–293.

Murray RK, Rodwell VW, Granner DK. *Harper's Illustrated Biochemistry.* 27th ed. New York: McGraw-Hill; 2006.

National Cholesterol Education Program (NCEP) Expert Panel on Detection, Evaluation, and Treatment of High Blood Cholesterol in Adults (Adult Treatment Panel III). Third report of the National Cholesterol Education Program (NCEP) Expert Panel on Detection, Evaluation, and Treatment of High Blood Cholesterol in Adults (Adult Treatment Panel III) final report. *Circulation.* 2002;106(25):3143–3421.

Naughton SS, Mathai ML, Hryciw DH, McAinch AJ. Linoleic acid and pathogenesis of obesity. *Prostaglandins Other Lipid Mediat.* 2016;125:90–99.

Ory DS. Nuclear receptor signaling in the control of cholesterol homeostasis: have the orphan receptors found a home? *Circ Res.* 2004;95(7):660–670.

Russo GL. Dietary n-6 and n-3 polyunsaturated fatty acids: from biochemistry to clinical implications in cardiovascular prevention. *Biochem Pharmacol.* 2009;77(6):937–946.

Sato R. Sterol metabolism and SREBP activation. *Arch Biochem Biophys.* 2010;501(2):177–181.

Wang LJ, Song BL. Niemann-Pick C1-Like 1 and cholesterol uptake. *Biochem Biophys Acta.* 2012;1821(7):964–972.

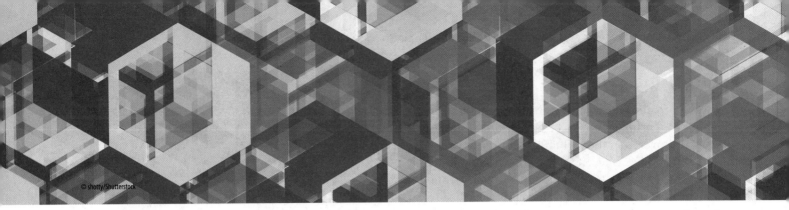

CHAPTER 6

Proteins and Amino Acids: Function, Quantity, and Quality

← HERE'S WHERE YOU HAVE BEEN

1. Carbohydrates and fats primarily provide energy for the body.
2. Glycolysis and the Krebs cycle are ways in which glucose is metabolized, and fatty acids use the Krebs cycle during oxidation.
3. The electron transport chain is the site of ultimate ATP production to harness energy from carbohydrates and fats.
4. Carbohydrates and fats provide health benefits beyond energy. For instance, fiber is a carbohydrate that has a myriad of positive health effects. Essential fatty acids also have many positive health effects.
5. Carbohydrates and fats have unique digestive and absorptive mechanisms.

HERE'S WHERE YOU ARE GOING →

1. Amino acids are the key forms in which nitrogen is delivered to the body for protein synthesis. However, amino acids have other functions besides being a component of protein; they may also serve as precursors to other biologically significant compounds.
2. Protein digestion involves a set of enzymes that are specific in recognizing amino acids in which a bond will cleave. Absorption of end products of protein digestion, amino acids, and peptides depends on several mechanisms.
3. Amino acids are metabolized by several different pathways that involve the removal or transfer of the nitrogen group to a carbon skeleton to form another amino acid. The urea cycle is a key metabolic pathway involved in nitrogen excretion.
4. The requirement for protein may be greater, depending on methods used to determine nitrogen requirements.
5. A variety of methods are used to assess protein quality, each with its own advantages and disadvantages.

▶ Introduction

The word *protein* is derived from the Greek *proteos*, which means "primary" or "to take place first." Protein was first discovered in the early 19th century, at which time scientists described it as a nitrogen-containing part of food essential to life. Whereas the elemental composition of the other energy nutrients is limited to carbon, oxygen, and hydrogen, protein also contains nitrogen (N) as well as sulfur (S). About one-half of the dry weight of a typical human cell is attributable to protein. Some of the most significant roles for proteins are as structural components, contractile filaments, antibodies for immune responses, transporters, neurotransmitters, hormones, and enzymes.

▶ Amino Acids

Proteins are composed of amino acids, many of which also have significant biologic functions or are used to make other important molecules, such as neurotransmitters and hormones. Although approximately 140 types of amino acids are known to exist in nature, a much smaller number of amino acids are commonly found as constituents of proteins. Only 20 amino acids are genetically coded via mRNA. Human proteins also contain modifications of a few of those amino acids (e.g., hydroxylated amino acids); however, the modifications take place after the protein is initially synthesized. Said another way, they are post-translational modifications of amino acids. **TABLE 6.1** presents the amino acids found in human proteins along with other amino acids found in the human body that are not part of proteins.

A common characteristic of amino acids found in proteins is that they have an asymmetric or alpha (α) carbon, which has attached to it an amino group, a carboxyl group, and a hydrogen atom. The fourth entity attached to the asymmetric carbon is unique from one amino acid to the next (**FIGURE 6.1**). This feature has been called the R group, or side group. Glycine is the simplest of the amino acids because its side group is merely a hydrogen atom.

Amino acids have the potential to present both d and l isomeric forms, with the l form occurring in nature. This is the reverse of carbohydrates, for which the d isomer is the type of isomer found naturally. Amino acids are linked together by peptide bonds formed covalently between adjacent hydroxyl and amine groups (**FIGURE 6.2**).

Amino acids (**FIGURE 6.3**) can be classified based on the type of side group they possess. The aliphatic amino acids have straight carbon chains, aromatic

TABLE 6.1 Amino Acids Found in the Human Body

Essential Amino Acids Found in Protein	Nonessential Amino Acids Found in Protein[a]	Nonessential Amino Acids Not Found in Protein
Tryptophan	Glycine	Ornithine
Valine	Aspartic acid	Taurine
Threonine	Asparagine	γ-aminobutyric acid (GABA)
Isoleucine	Proline	Beta-Alanine
Lysine	Glutamine	
Leucine	Glutamic acid	
Phenylalanine	Arginine	
Methionine	Cysteine	
Histidine	Tyrosine	
	Serine	
	Alanine	

[a]This list could also include post-translational derivatives of nonessential amino acids, such as hydroxyproline, hydroxylysine, homocysteine, and 3-methyl histidine.

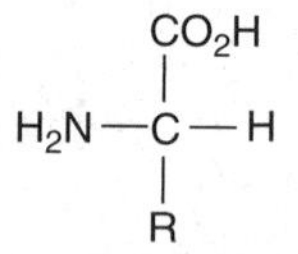

$$H_2N - \underset{\underset{R}{|}}{\overset{\overset{CO_2H}{|}}{C}} - H$$

FIGURE 6.1. General Amino Acid Structure. Amino acids have an amino group, carboxyl group, hydrogen, and a side chain (R).

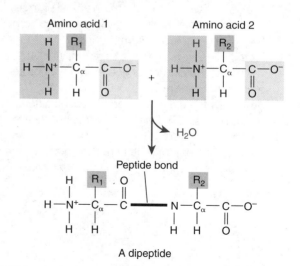

FIGURE 6.2. Peptide Bonds. A peptide bond forms from a reaction of an amino group with a carboxyl group between adjacent amino acids.

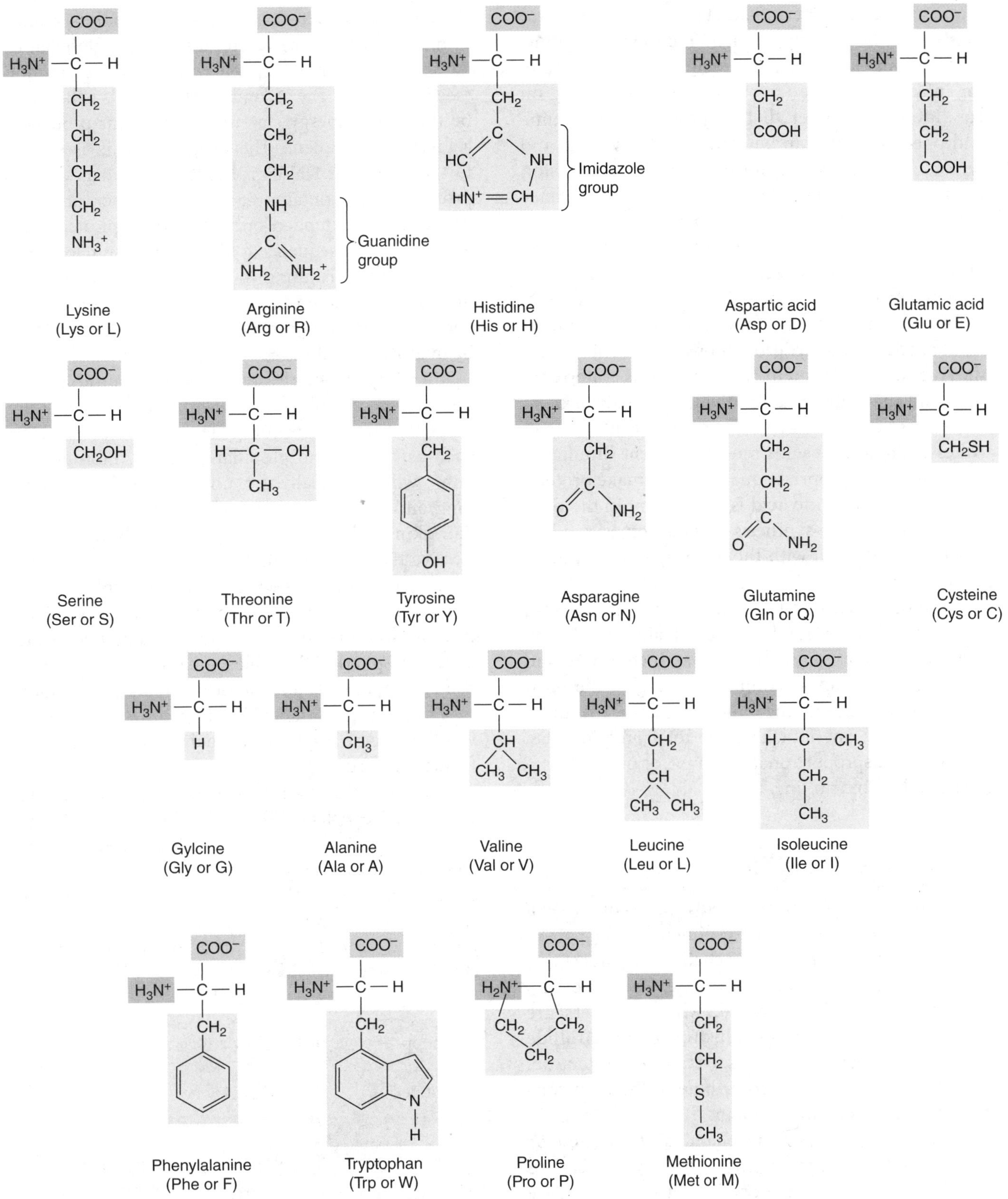

FIGURE 6.3. Amino Acids. Chemical structure of all amino acids.

amino acids have a ring structure, and acidic amino acids and basic amino acids are normally classified separately due to their extreme pH within aqueous solutions. Sulfur-containing amino acids (cysteine and methionine) may be recognized as one class, and the imino acid proline and its derivative hydroxyproline constitute another class.

Human cells are unable to synthesize eight to nine amino acids, either at all or in adequate amounts to meet the body's needs for growth and maintenance.

Those amino acids, termed dietary **essential amino acids**, are lysine, tryptophan, methionine, valine, phenylalanine, leucine, isoleucine, threonine, and, for infants, histidine (see Table 6.1). Depending on conditions and other dietary proteins, methionine and phenylalanine can be converted to cysteine and tyrosine, respectively. However, if the conversion is impaired, the latter amino acids become dietary essentials as well.

Often, the term **limiting** is used in discussion of the essential amino acid content of various foods. That refers to a state in which one of the essential amino acids present in a food is found in an amount insufficient to support growth or maintenance if it is the sole source of protein. The lack of this amino acid will limit the ability of an individual to make protein regardless of the amount of other amino acids present. All essential amino acids must be present simultaneously, and in appropriate quantities, to make protein. If one essential amino acid is not present in the right amount, the whole synthesis process comes to a halt at a level associated with the quantity of the limiting amino acid.

The occurrence of particular amino acids within proteins is neither random nor equally distributed. Alanine is quite common, whereas methionine and tryptophan are not as common. Collagen, the most abundant protein in the human body, constituting approximately one-fourth of the total protein mass, contains a disproportionate amount of glycine, proline, and hydroxyproline.

▶ Protein Structures

The sequencing of amino acids that comprise a protein determines the three-dimensional **protein structure**. It is really the side chains that impart this character. Some side chains are large, whereas others are small; some are charged, whereas others are neutral; and some can form hydrogen and disulfide bonds with other amino acids to stabilize a structure. Those characteristics all contribute to the final conformational design of a protein.

The main polypeptide chain, as translated or synthesized, is termed the **primary structure** (**FIGURE 6.4**). The R groups of adjacent amino acids are located on opposite sides (*trans*) of the straight chain and do not interact.

The secondary structure of a protein is determined by the number and sequence of amino acids. The secondary structure refers to chemical interactions among the amino acids forming the primary structure via hydrogen bonds and disulfide linkages. The hydrogen

bonding occurs between the C=O and H−N groups of different amino acids. Spiral (α-helix), globular, or flat sheet arrangements (β-pleated sheets) are common (see Figure 6.4). The secondary structure is believed to be the lowest energy state for a particular protein in a given environment. The protein α-helix is similar to the α-helix of DNA in that it is right handed. The protein α-helix contains 3.6 amino acids per turn, with the R groups extended outward. The β-pleated sheet has the peptide sequence folding in a hairpin loop and doubling back, running in an antiparallel manner. R groups alternate between the inside and outside of the backbone, and antiparallel chains are linked together by hydrogen bonding.

Tertiary structures of proteins are produced by the coiling of molecules and bonding within molecules that determine the general shape of proteins, such as fibrous and globular proteins. Fibrous proteins, which typically are not soluble in water, are long and tough fibers. Examples are the keratin of hair, skin, and nails; the collagens and elastins of connective tissue; the fibrin of blood; and the actin and myosin proteins composing muscle. Globular proteins, which are relatively compact and fairly soluble in most solvents, are polypeptide chains folded into compact spheres. Examples include most enzymes, protein hormones, and blood proteins. The solubility of proteins is largely based on how they coil and whether the hydrophobic or hydrophilic portions are facing outward.

Finally, the quaternary structure of proteins involves two or more polypeptide chains interacting to form functional entities. Insulin, hemoglobin, and immunoglobulins are examples.

Amino acid links can vary tremendously in length. The system outlined in the following table can be applied for different terms associated with amino acid links of varying length.

Dipeptide	Linkage of 2 amino acids
Peptide	Linkage of between 3 and 10 amino acids
Polypeptide	Linkage of more than 10 amino acids and typically fewer than 100 amino acids
Proteins	Very long linkages of amino acids (> 100) or more than one linkage complexed together (some scientists label amino acid links of more than 50 as proteins)

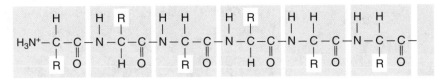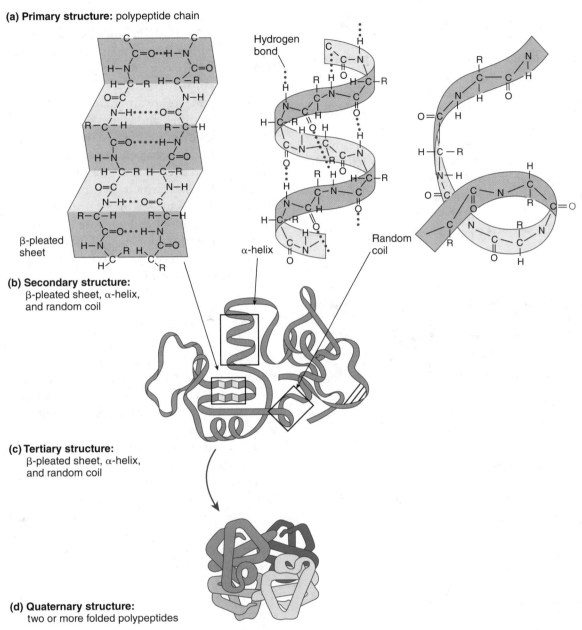

(a) Primary structure: polypeptide chain

Hydrogen bond

β-pleated sheet

α-helix

Random coil

(b) Secondary structure:
β-pleated sheet, α-helix, and random coil

(c) Tertiary structure:
β-pleated sheet, α-helix, and random coil

(d) Quaternary structure:
two or more folded polypeptides

FIGURE 6.4. Basic Protein Structures. (a) Primary, (b) secondary, (c) tertiary, and (d) quaternary structures of proteins.

Data from Tropp, B. E. Biochemistry: Concepts and Applications. Brooks/Cole Publishing Company, 1997.

Protein mass is often expressed in dalton units. Daltons are an arbitrary unit of mass equal to one-twelfth the mass of carbon 12, or 1.657×10^{-24} grams. Amino acids average around 110 daltons while Titan, the largest protein in the human body, is estimated at 3–3.7 megadaltons (3,000,000 daltons). Based on average weights a polypeptide would weigh approximately 1.1-10.1 kilodaltons and protein would be greater than 10.1 kilodaltons. Daltons of a protein can be calculated from its molecular weight.

● **BEFORE YOU GO ON . . .**

1. What are the four entities that constitute an amino acid?
2. List the basic, acid, neutral, and sulfur-containing amino acids.
3. Distinguish between the secondary, tertiary, and quarternary structures of amino acids.

▸ Dietary Protein and Protein Digestion and Absorption

Food Protein

All organisms contain protein but the protein content of organisms varies. In general, foods of animal origin have a greater protein content than plants and plant-derived foods (**TABLE 6.2**). This is largely due to the skeletal muscle of animals or protein requirements before (e.g., egg) or after birth (e.g., milk). The protein content of skeletal muscle or animal flesh is approximately 22%. Water-packed tuna derives more than 80% of its energy from protein. Approximately 65% of the protein that Americans eat is derived from animal sources. In comparison, many African and Asian societies derive only about 20% of their protein from animals. Below is a general overview of different types of proteins and their protein content based on portion size:

Meat Protein

Animal meat proteins are very similar to human skeletal muscle proteins and include myosin, actin, troponins, and other proteins. Typically, animal meat is more than 80% protein on a dry weight basis. In addition to protein, meats deliver iron, selenium, and vitamin B$_{12}$. Meats are among the best food sources of creatine, carnosine, and beta-alanine. However, meats are often a contributor of fat to the diet. Chicken tends to store more fat beneath the skin (subcutaneously) whereas cows have adipose tissue *marbled* throughout their muscle tissue, which is visually obvious. Removing the skin of a chicken breast or thigh would greatly lower the fat content and increase the protein content (as a percentage of total energy). Beef can be trimmed of visible fat to lower its fat content. However, fat in food provides flavoring.

Fish Protein

Fish proteins are very similar to mammalian meat proteins with a few striking differences. For instance, microscopically, the striated appearance of fish myofibrils is similar to mammals and contains the same proteins. However the skeletal muscle of fish is organized with shorter fibers and arranged between connective tissue sheets. Fish is generally a lean protein source containing relatively little fat. For instance, water-packed tuna derives more than 80% of its energy from protein. While being a leaner protein option is true for many fish, consumers need to check the food label, as some fish are fatty or perhaps canned in oils which can increase the nonprotein calories of a fish source.

Milk Protein

Milk proteins include casein and serum proteins or whey. Casein proteins account for roughly 78% of milk's nitrogen-based mass and whey is 17%. The remaining nitrogen compounds found in milk are mostly amino acids and peptides. Casein is a family of spherical phosphoproteins while whey consists largely of β-lactoglobulin, lactalbumin, immunoglobulins, and other albumins. The most abundant whey protein is β-lactoglobulin, which is rich in the amino acids lysine, leucine, glutamic acid, and aspartic acid while the immunoglobulins are largely immunoglobulin M (IgM), IgA, and IgG. Whey and casein proteins are among the most common proteins in protein

TABLE 6.2 Approximate Protein Content of Various Foods	
Food	**Protein (g)**
Beef (3 oz)	25
Pork (3 oz)	23
Cod, poached (3.2 oz)	21
Oysters (3.2 oz)	17
Milk (1 cup)	8
Cheddar Cheese (1 oz)	7
Egg (1 large)	6
Peanut butter (2 tbsp)	8
Potato (1 large)	7
Bread (1 slice)	2
Banana (1 medium)	1
Carrots, sliced (2 cups)	1
Apple (1)	Trace
Sugar; oil	0

supplements with sourcing as whey protein concentrate (WPC; 80% protein dry weight) and whey protein isolate (WPI; 90% protein dry weight). Whey tends to be digested and absorbed faster than other proteins, including slower digesting casein proteins. The main difference is that whey is more acid stable than casein, which results in whey moving from the stomach to the small intestine quickly while casein forms a gel and slows the transit time dramatically.

Egg Protein

There are at least eight main proteins in egg whites, including ovalbumin, conalbumin, ovomucoid, avidin, flavoprotein-apoprotein, "proteinase inhibitor," ovomucin, and globulins. Protein collectively accounts for about 11–12% of liquid egg white. Meanwhile, much of the egg yolk proteins are found in the form of emulsifying lipoproteins due to the high lipid content of the yolk. Egg yolk is rich in fat and consequently egg white has higher protein concentration (gram for gram) than a whole egg or the yolk. To highlight the difference, a whole egg will have 6 g protein (24 kcals) and about 75 kcals total, so a whole egg is roughly 33% protein while at the same time, one egg white will have 3–4 grams of protein, which accounts for > 90% of its 15–16 kcals.

Wheat Protein

The four main protein fractions in wheat are albumin, globulin, gliadin, and glutenin. When gliadin and glutenin, as part of flour, are mixed with water, they form gluten, which provides the structural network that allows bread to rise. Gluten proteins are rich in glutamine and relatively low in lysine, methionine, and tryptophan. Gluten-free products have appeared on the market in high amounts during the last decade. Some individuals have a sensitivity and/or allergic reaction to gluten in the intestine that results in diarrhea and malabsorption issues (gluten-sensitive enteropathy). Whether gluten is responsible for other health conditions is debatable and controversial.

Soy Protein

Soy proteins are complex multiprotein globulins in general and soy protein is a good source of all essential amino acids except methionine and tryptophan. Soy protein isolate (SPI) is used commercially in drinks mixed with fruit and water, coffee whiteners, liquid whipped toppings, and sour cream dressings. Soy proteins are often found associated with *isoflavone* molecules, such as *genestein* and *daidzein*, which might have health-promoting properties and are considered *nutraceuticals* (Soy protein isolate is used in some protein supplements and is a more cost-effective protein ingredient than WPI.

Protein Quantity

The most common methods for determining the nitrogen content of a food or nutrition product is to first assess the nitrogen content and then apply a conversion factor for grams of nitrogen to estimate grams of protein. Although certain other molecules contain nitrogen, such as nucleic acids and some vitamins, their contribution to the nitrogen content of a food is relatively small. In general, protein is 16% nitrogen and thus the amount of protein in a food can be estimated by multiplying grams of nitrogen by 6.25. Vice versa, the nitrogen content of a food can be estimated by multiplying total protein by 0.16.

Example of estimating grams of protein from grams of nitrogen:

$$12 \text{ g of nitrogen} \times 6.25 = 75 \text{ g of protein}$$

Example of estimating grams of nitrogen from grams of protein:

$$80 \text{ g of protein} \times 0.16 = 12.8 \text{ g of nitrogen}$$

However, one important consideration is that different food protein sources can have different nitrogen conversions and that 6.25 is a general factor and applicable to meats, fish, and eggs, which were long the greatest contributor of protein to the adult diet. A more accurate conversion factor for milk proteins (e.g., casein and whey) is 6.38, while soy is 5.7, rice 5.95, legumes and nuts 5.3, and most grains roughly 5.80. The primary difference in the nitrogen conversion factor for different food protein sources is the proportion of different amino acids and the concentration of nitrogen (nitrogen atoms in the molecule, see Figure 6.3). For instance, glutamine has two nitrogen atoms; arginine has four; and highly revered BCAAs (leucine, isoleucine, and valine) only have one atom of nitrogen. In addition, the nitrogen content in food protein sources is influenced by the presence of nonprotein sources, including nitrates and betaine in plants and amino acid-derived molecules in meats, including carnitine and creatine.

Protein Digestion and Absorption

Compared with carbohydrate and lipid digestion, protein digestion is a little more complex in that a variety of enzymes and tissues are involved in the breakdown of protein into end products (**FIGURE 6.5**).

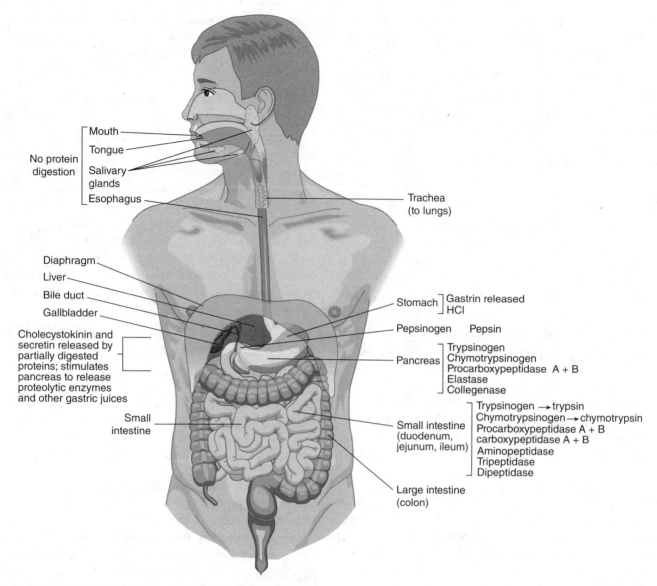

FIGURE 6.5. Digestion of Proteins Based on Anatomic Locations. Note the various biochemical compounds that digest proteins and their origins within the gastrointestinal tract.

The regulation of the hormones associated with protein digestion is also more involved than is the case with carbohydrate and fat digestion.

The stomach is the first major organ involved in protein digestion. Parietal cells secrete a fluid rich in hydrochloric acid (HCl) that has a pH of 0.8 to 0.9, which, when mixed with other components of gastric juices, allows for a very acidic environment (pH 1.5 to 2.5) during digestion. With regard to protein digestion, the acidity of stomach juices has two primary functions. First, it activates pepsin from its zymogen form as well as creating a favorable pH for its proteolytic activity. Second, the acidity of stomach juice allows for the denaturing of proteins. **Denaturing** is the straightening and uncoiling of proteins, thereby allowing greater access to proteolytic enzymes. HCl may also directly hydrolyze proteins, but the extent is probably not significant.

Pepsin is a key enzyme that begins the process of protein hydrolysis after HCl has uncoiled or linearized the proteins to some extent. The mucosal chief cells secrete pepsin in the zymogen form, pepsinogen. HCl stimulates the conversion of pepsinogen to pepsin by the loss of a portion of the NH$_2$-terminus amino acid sequence. The optimal pH for enzyme activity of pepsin is less than 3.5. When the pH rises above 5.0, the activity of pepsin declines rapidly. Pepsin, as is the case with other digestive proteolytic enzymes, cleaves proteins and peptides at specific peptide bonds. Pepsin stimulates hydrolysis at peptide bonds involving the carboxyl group of the aromatic amino acids, such as phenylalanine, tryptophan, and tyrosine. Some evidence suggests that it may cleave where leucine and acidic amino acids are found (**TABLE 6.3**).

Some individuals lack the ability to secrete HCl (a condition termed achlorhydria) or have decreased

TABLE 6.3 Protein Digestive Enzymes

Enzyme	Organ of Origin	Endo or Exo Peptidase	Amino Acids at Site of Hydrolysis
Pepsin	Stomach	Endo	Arginine, phenylalanine, tryptophan, tyrosine
Trypsin	Pancreas	Endo	Arginine, lysine
Chymotrypsin	Pancreas	Endo	Phenylalanine, tryptophan, tyrosine
Carboxypeptidase A	Pancreas	Exo	Phenylalanine, tryptophan, tyrosine, and aliphatic amino acids
Carboxypeptidase B	Pancreas	Exo	Arginine, lysine
Aminopeptidase	Small Intestine	Exo	All amino acids

secretion (hypochlorhydria). Those problems are especially prevalent among the elderly, resulting in decreased protein hydrolysis and digestion that may have clinical consequences and require special dietary measures.

When the partially broken down protein products enter the small intestine, the pancreatic proteolytic enzymes (namely, trypsin, chymotrypsin, and carboxypeptidases A and B) are the major enzymes that result in further digestion. However, all are secreted from the pancreas in inactive zymogen forms. Trypsinogen, chymotrypsinogen, and procarboxypeptidase A and B are the zymogen forms of trypsin, chymotrypsin, and carboxypeptidases A and B, respectively. The mucosal intestinal cells secrete the enzyme enterokinase, which cleaves a hexapeptide from trypsinogen to form active trypsin. Once formed, trypsin can also perform the hexapeptide cleavage of trypsinogen, yielding more trypsin. The activation of trypsin is a critical step in protein digestion because trypsin also converts the other inactive pancreatic enzymes to the active forms. Trypsin acts on the peptide linkages involving the carboxyl groups of arginine and lysine. It is an endopeptidase because it cleaves proteins and peptides internal to the chain.

The pancreatic enzyme chymotrypsinogen, in the presence of trypsin, will cleave a peptide fragment to produce active chymotrypsin. Similar to trypsin, chymotrypsin will degrade proteases, denatured proteins, peptones, and large polypeptides as its substrate to produce smaller polypeptides, peptides, and some individual amino acids. Chymotrypsinogen is an endopeptidase and is specific for linkages involving the carboxyl ends of phenylalanine, tyrosine, and tryptophan.

Carboxypeptidase has two forms, A and B. Carboxypeptidase A contains zinc and hydrolyzes the carboxyl terminal residues that possess aromatic and aliphatic linkages. The B form acts on terminal arginine or lysine residues. Both carboxypeptidase forms are considered exopeptidases in that they cleave amino acids at the carboxyl end of the polypeptide. Inactive forms (procarboxypeptidase) reaching the small intestine are activated by trypsin as well.

The pancreas also synthesizes and releases a substance known as trypsin inhibitor. This compound prevents the autoactivation of the inactive trypsinogen molecules in secretory vesicles in the pancreas, thus preventing autodigestion of the pancreas. However, because of pathologic conditions of the pancreatic parenchyma or the obstruction of pancreatic exocrine ducts, large quantities of pancreatic secretions may pool and overwhelm the limited quantity of trypsin inhibitor. Within a few hours, the pancreas then sustains autodigestive damage, resulting in inflammation or acute pancreatitis.

The final hydrolysis of the peptides produced by those series of reactions via pancreatic enzymes occurs at the surface of the microvilli membranes of the intestinal mucosal cells. The aminopeptidases take the peptides and yield individual amino acids and oligopeptides (three or four amino acid fragments). Aminopeptidase is considered an exopeptidase. Thus, the net result of luminal digestion in the small intestine is short oligopeptide fragments, dipeptides, and amino acids.

The absorbed form of protein is primarily individual amino acids. However, dipeptides, small oligopeptides, and polypeptides; and possibly intact or nearly intact proteins can be taken into enterocytes along with amino acids. With regard to whole proteins, this event is insignificant in adults, adolescents, and children. However, during infancy, it has physiologic significance. Although some absorption may occur between cells (transcellular), most occurs by enterocyte pinocytosis. This is particularly important for infants because the fetus does not synthesize antibodies. Gamma globulins in the colostrum may be absorbed by the small intestine of the newborn in order to convey passive immunity from the mother during the neonatal period. This occurs within the first few hours of birth. The subsequent consumption of more mature breast milk proteins eventually limits this activity. Breast milk lactoferrin in infants may also be absorbed by pinocytosis. This protein binds iron in breast milk and is thought to promote iron uptake by the infant.

Free amino acids may occur, primarily in the ileum of the small intestine, but more absorption can take place in the upper part of the small intestine. Over the years, knowledge as to how amino acid transport occurs has evolved. Many nutritionists are familiar with a basic scheme that is similar to the absorption that occurs with monosaccharides. According to this classic model, absorption occurs via an energy-dependent, carrier-mediated mechanism. There are several transport carriers for amino acids, all of which have the following elements in common:

- Transport is against a concentration gradient
- The carrier is specific for l isomers; it will not absorb d isomers
- Energy in the form of ATP is required
- Sodium and vitamin B_6 are required
- Carboxyl, amino, and α-H groups are required

Separate amino acid carriers are present in the microvilli membrane. Those carriers transport four groups of amino acids:

1. *Neutral:*
   a. Aromatic amino acids: tyrosine, tryptophan, histidine, and phenylalanine
   b. Aliphatic amino acids: examples are alanine, serine, threonine, valine, leucine, isoleucine, and glycine
   c. Other neutral amino acids: methionine, glutamine, asparagine, and cysteine
   The common feature among those amino acids is the existence of nonpolar side groups. However, each amino acid has a different binding affinity to the carrier that follows Michaelis-Menton kinetics, similar to those of enzymes. Those amino acids with greater affinities, such as methionine, can inhibit those amino acids with lower affinities, such as threonine.

2. *Basic amino acids:* Specific for lysine, arginine, and ornithine
3. *Dicarboxylic acids:* Glutamic and aspartic acids
4. *Imino acids:* Proline and hydroxyproline. Glycine may also use this carrier in addition to the neutral carrier, as may other amino acids, such as taurine and γ-aminobutyric acid. Proline and hydroxyproline can also be absorbed by the neutral carrier system, but this activity may be insignificant due to competitive inhibition with other amino acids.

In all of these systems, there is a coupling with sodium for absorption (**FIGURE 6.6**), similar to that detailed for glucose and galactose monosaccharide absorption. The Na^+–K^+ pump is maintained by an ATPase enzyme, whereby the concentration of Na^+ is greater outside of the mucosal cell. Na^+ binds to the membrane carrier, as does the amino acid, and the complex transverses the membrane such that sodium goes down its concentration gradient. The energy requirement is for maintaining the ion gradient. Amino acids need to exit the enterocyte to the blood, again by a sodium-dependent, carrier-mediated mechanism.

A more nuanced version of how amino acids are transported arises from the specific protein carriers that have been cloned. Some transport systems involve one protein, whereas others involve more than one protein subunit in the mucosal membrane. Therefore, the interactions of amino acid transporters may be monomeric or heterodimeric. Transporters are also found on the apical part of the mucosal cells and on the basolateral portion of the cells. The

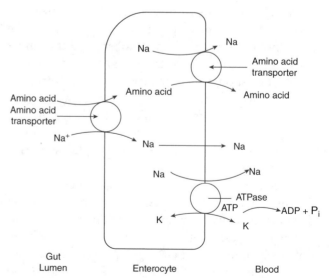

FIGURE 6.6. Active Absorption of Amino Acids in Enterocytes. Note the requirement for a protein transporter on the membrane, the presence of sodium, and the requirement of energy in the form of ATP.

nomenclature has, therefore, been further developed. Amino acid transport systems use a lettering system: uppercase letters mean that sodium is required, and lowercase letters mean that the process is sodium independent; however, this is not always the case. Leucine, L, is sodium independent. Transporters such as y^+, t, $b^{o,t}$, and asc have passive mechanisms and are sodium independent. For instance, X_{AG}^- indicates that the process is sodium dependent due to the capitalized "X"; the A stands for aspartate; and the G indicates glutamate as possible amino acids transported (e.g., the X_{AG}^- transporter). Another transporter system, N, has glutamine, histidine, or asparagine with sodium ions entering the mucosal cell in exchange for a hydrogen ion. **TABLE 6.4** summarizes some of the amino acid transporting systems in the small intestine. However, the traditional system applies for most of the amino acid transports that occur.

Dipeptides, tripeptides, and tetrapeptides may be absorbed by humans, and this route of uptake may be more significant than once thought. In fact, the uptake of amino acids via this route may be faster than from

equivalent mixtures of free amino acids. Dipeptidases and aminopeptidases have been isolated from the cytosolic fractions of intestinal mucosal cells. This suggests that some of the final steps in peptide hydrolysis occur inside the cell.

Only amino acids leave the mucosal cell for entry into the portal blood. Evidence of this occurring comes from two human genetic diseases: Hartnup disease and cystinuria. In Hartnup disease, there is a defect in the ability to transport free neutral amino acids. In cystinuria, there is a reduced ability to absorb dibasic amino acids and cysteine. Despite their inability to transport certain essential amino acids, patients afflicted with those diseases show no evidence of protein malnutrition. Dipeptides given to those patients show a disappearance from the lumen, indicating uptake. The uptake of dipeptides occurs mostly in the jejunum and, for free amino acids, in the ileum. The available data suggest that neutral, basic, or acidic dipeptides all share the same carrier. The system appears to be sodium dependent, but evidence also suggests the coexistence of a sodium-independent mechanism. More recent data suggest a system for tripeptides as well as dipeptides. The transport system called PEPT1 appears to be able to transport dipeptides and tripeptides across the brush border of mucosal cells along with H^+ co-transport into the cell. The H^+ is pumped back out of the cell using sodium.

Tetrapeptidases in the brush border of the microvilli membrane hydrolyze tetrapeptides into tripeptides and free amino acids. Tripeptidases are present in both membrane and cytoplasm in equal amounts. Dipeptidases are found commonly in the mucosal cell cytoplasm. However, there is evidence that some peptides can be absorbed through a paracellular process, meaning that they are able to enter between adjacent enterocytes. Next, they can be hydrolyzed by proteases in the blood. In cases where the small intestine is compromised, such as in the case of celiac disease or inflammation, the uptake by this route may be more significant.

TABLE 6.4 Intestinal Cell Brush Border and Basolateral Membrane Amino Acid Transport Systems		
Transport System	**Substrate Transported**	**Sodium Required?**
B	Phenylalanine, tyrosine, tryptophan, isoleucine	Yes
$B^{o,+}$	Basic amino acids and most neutral amino acids	Yes
$b^{o,+}$	Basic amino acids and most neutral amino acids	No
L	Leucine, other neutral amino acids	No
Ag	Glutamate, aspartate	No
N	Asparagine, histidine, glutamine	Yes
Asc	Alanine, serine, cysteine	No
ASC	Alanine, serine, cysteine	Yes
T	Tyrosine, phenylalanine, tryptophan	No
y^+	Basic amino acids	No
IMINO	Glycine, proline	Yes

⬡ BEFORE YOU GO ON ...

1. The grams of protein in a food is determined by multiplying the grams of nitrogen by 6.25. Why?

2. What is the fundamental difference between carboxypeptidase A and carboxypeptidase B? How are they similar?

3. How is pepsin produced in the stomach mucosa?

4. What are five characteristics that all amino acid carriers have in the small intestine?

5. How can dipeptides and tripeptides be absorbed?

6. What are Hartnup disease and cystinuria?

▸ Dietary Protein Quality

Protein quality is different from quantity. *Quantity* refers to the amount of nitrogen in the food as discussed above. *Quality,* on the other hand, refers to the essential amino acid content in a protein compared with the needs of human cells, collectively. If the availability of essential amino acids is not adequate to meet the needs of cells to synthesize proteins, protein synthesis will be limited. The availability of essential amino acids in cellular pools largely reflects the composition and quantity of dietary protein. If the amount of an essential amino acid in a food protein is relatively low in comparison with human protein as a whole, that amino acid is referred to as limiting. Food proteins that are able to provide all essential amino acids in proportions meeting human proteins are called **complete proteins** or **high biological value proteins**. The following definition of terms may help:

- *High-quality protein (complete protein):* The protein has all nine essential amino acids in proportion to human protein and will support growth and maintenance. This is normally protein of animal origin.

- *Low-quality protein (incomplete protein):* The protein contains all nine essential amino acids but not in the proportional amounts to meet the body's need. Plant proteins often fall into this category. Corn is an example because it is low in the amino acid lysine.

Several methods are used to assess the relative quality of a protein. Some have advantages over others, and many of those methods are used in the food industry. The measures used to assess protein quality always compare the quality of a particular protein to a **reference protein** that is a high-quality protein. One such protein that is highly digestible and has an essential amino acid content similar to human protein is egg protein. Egg protein has long been considered the most "perfect" protein source for humans in that the correct balance of amino acids appears to be present and available. Another commonly used reference protein is the milk-based protein casein.

Biological value (BV) is the amount of nitrogen digested, absorbed, and used by the body but not excreted. Egg protein has a BV of 100 (i.e., is 100% efficient). The assessment of BV begins with an analysis of the nitrogen content of food, urine, and feces. A test diet that is protein free needs to be included in this method. Urinary nitrogen represents absorbed amino acids that have been deaminated. Fecal nitrogen represents unabsorbed amino acids and nitrogen from sloughed-off intestinal cells and the nitrogen composing the enzymes. To determine the endogenous protein excretion and the nitrogen from sloughed-off cells and digestive enzymes, a protein-free diet is needed to subtract the difference. The following formula best illustrates this concept:

$$BV = \frac{Dietary\,N - (Urinary\,N - U_o) - (Fecal\,N - F_o)}{Dietary\,N - (Fecal\,N - F_o)} \times 100$$

where

$$\begin{aligned}
Dietary\,N &= \text{Nitrogen content of the food consumed}\\
Urinary\,N &= \text{Nitrogen in the urine while consuming}\\
&\quad\text{the test protein}\\
U_o &= \text{Nitrogen content of the urine while}\\
&\quad\text{consuming the protein-free diet}\\
Fecal\,N &= \text{Nitrogen in the feces while consuming the test protein}\\
F_o &= \text{Nitrogen content of the feces while consuming the protein-free diet}
\end{aligned}$$

A protein with a BV of 70 or more is considered capable of supporting growth, assuming the caloric value of the diet is adequate. This value means that 70% of the nitrogen absorbed is retained.

One problem with BV is that this measure does not take into account differences in digestibility between various proteins. For instance, it is generally known that plant protein sources are less digestible than animal sources because the cell walls of the former may interfere with digestive enzymes binding to the substrates. To correct this problem, another measure can be applied—**net protein utilization (NPU)**. This measure expresses how efficiently protein is used by an organism such as a human. It accounts for both the digestibility of the protein and the BV. The NPU is, therefore, the BV multiplied by the digestibility:

$$Digestibility = \frac{Diet\,N - (F - F_o)}{Diet\,N} \times 100$$

The NPU represents the percentage of the dietary nitrogen retained; BV represents the percentage of the absorbed nitrogen retained. The NPU is almost always lower than the BV. For instance, the BV of an egg is 100%, and its NPU is 94%. However, for peanuts, both the BV and NPU are 55%.

Another commonly used measure of protein quality is the **protein efficiency ratio (PER)**. This is perhaps the simplest method of determining protein quality; however, it does require some chemical analysis. The basic idea is to calculate the weight gain of a growing animal in relation to its protein intake when energy is ample and the protein source is fed at an adequate level. The adequate level for protein when using a laboratory rat, which is the common approach, is 9% protein expressed on an energy basis. Growing rats are usually given the test protein at weaning (21 days of age) and allowed free access to the test diet for a 28-day period. A control group of rats is used that has casein as a control protein source. The expression for PER is as follows:

$$PER = \frac{\text{Weight gain (g)}}{\text{Protein intake (g)}}$$

Casein usually will yield a PER value of 2.5. This means that for every gram of protein consumed by the growing rat, a body weight gain of 2.5 grams was obtained. Egg protein usually has a PER value of 3.9, whereas soybeans have a value of 2.3 and peanuts a value of 1.7. Thus, the higher the PER number, the better the protein quality.

Another commonly used method for assessing protein quality is the **chemical score**, sometimes referred to as the **amino acid score**. This method requires that a particular test and reference protein be analyzed for specific amino acid content. The expression is as follows:

$$\text{Score} = \frac{\text{Amino acid (in mg) in 1g test protein}}{\text{Amino acid (in mg) in reference protein}} \times 100$$

The amino acids in the test and reference proteins are determined, and the smallest score is, by definition, the score applied to that particular protein because the amino acid found in the smallest amount is the **limiting amino acid**. Either egg or milk protein is typically used as the reference protein. Egg has a score of 100. When cow's milk is compared with egg, the former has a score of 95. Beef has a score of 69, soybeans 47, and corn 49.

A related protein quality assessment takes into account the percent protein digestibility. Plant proteins have lower protein digestibility compared with animal protein. Correcting the amino acid score for protein digestibility involves multiplying the amino acid score by the percent true digestibility. This term is called the **protein digestibility corrected amino acid score (PDCAAS)** and this system of assessing protein quality is considered the best standard to date, at least in the United States. The equation for calculating PDCAAS is:

$$\frac{\text{Limiting amino acid (in mg) in 1g test protein}}{\text{Same amino acid (in mg) in 1g of reference protein}} \times \text{Fecal true digestibility percentage}$$

The PDCAAS method is based on comparison of the concentration of the first limiting essential amino acid in the test protein with the concentration of that amino acid in a reference (scoring) pattern, which is the essential amino acid requirements of the preschool-age child. The chemical score obtained in this way is corrected for true fecal digestibility of the test protein. PDCAAS is corrected for digestibility by factoring in fecal protein estimates. PDCAAS values for foods or isolated proteins higher than 100% are not accepted as such but are truncated to 100%. For instance, the value for eggs and milk proteins is approximately 120% and they are truncated to a value of 100 while soy is 91. The methods used for PDCAAS has led to many debates, including the applicability of the school-age child and the truncating of certain proteins.

A newer method for determining protein quality advocated to replace the PDCAAS is the **Digestible Indispensable Amino Acid Score (DIAAS)** recommended by the Food and Agriculture Organization (FAO) of the United Nations. An indispensable amino acid is an essential amino acid. As noted above, the PDCAAS is truncated to be no greater than 100. This does not allow for a ranking of overall quality of various sources of protein. Using the DIAAS approach requires that the digestibility of amino acids be determined by the absorption of each indispensable amino acid at the terminal end of the ileum. That provides a more reliable measure of a protein contribution to human amino acid and protein requirements. If one protein has a score of 130 and another 110, the first protein is a higher quality than the second protein. The PDCAAS does not allow for this relative comparison for those higher quality proteins since the scores did not exceed 100 using this method.

● BEFORE YOU GO ON . . .

1. Distinguish between a high-quality protein and a low-quality protein.
2. What does a protein efficiency ratio of 3.3 mean, in your own words?
3. Distinguish between biological value and net protein utilization.
4. How is an amino acid score determined, and what does it mean?
5. What does the Protein Digestibility Corrected Amino Acid Score refer to and how does it compare with the Digestible Indispensable Amino Acid Score?

SPECIAL FEATURE 6.1

Do High-Protein Diets Lead to Weight Loss?

Most students of nutrition are well aware of the many diets promising quick weight loss. Several diets, such as the Atkins diet and the South Beach diet, feature low-carbohydrate diets. One problem with most low-carbohydrate diets is that they are relatively higher in fat and, in the case of the Atkins diet, may restrict fruits and vegetables too severely. Another type of diet where the macronutrient content of the diet is manipulated is high-protein diets. Like many other fad diets, that diet promises greater weight loss as well as sustained weight loss or weight maintenance. Is there evidence to support that this type of diet is effective?

The results of several studies have indicated that a high-protein diet may be effective at reducing body weight. Some of the weight loss is thought to be due to decreased energy intake because high-protein diets afford greater satiety compared with those that incorporate carbohydrates and fats. Many studies have, in fact, found that higher-protein diets do lead to better weight loss than those containing increased levels of other macronutrients. However, a complicating factor is that many high-protein diets are also low in carbohydrates, begging the question, which factor is at play here, the higher-protein or the lower-carbohydrate part of the diet? A study conducted in the Netherlands on 132 obese subjects compared high- with normal-protein diets, as well as low- and normal-carbohydrate diets in combination with different levels of protein. Those on the higher-protein/low-carbohydrate diet vs those on the high-protein/normal-carbohydrate diet did not differ in body weight or fat mass. The higher-protein/normal-carbohydrate diet resulted in greater loss of body weight and a greater reduction in fat mass compared with those fed the normal-protein/normal-carbohydrate diet. Furthermore, those on the higher-protein/low-carbohydrate diet lost more body weight and fat mass than those consuming a normal-protein/low-carbohydrate diet. Those data suggest that higher-protein diets, regardless of carbohydrate level, can promote greater loss of body weight and fat mass. That means that the body weight and fat mass losses were due to the higher-protein component, not the low-carbohydrate component, of the diets. However, in all of those cases, overall energy or calories was markedly reduced.

What about keeping the weight off? Researchers in Denmark conducted a study that looked at normal weight individuals on a diet where 25% of the calories were derived from protein compared with another group where 12% of the calories came from protein. After 6 months, the subjects on the high-protein diet had greater body weight and fat losses. Those findings were rechecked 1 and 2 years later, and greater weight loss was reported among those on the high-protein diets, indicating success at keeping the weight that was lost from being regained. Unlike the study discussed above, this diet did not have any energy restrictions. Some studies on the long-term effects of high-protein diets have also indicated that such diets result in greater weight maintenance after the initial weight loss. However, others have failed to show the ability of higher-protein diets to maintain the weight loss. In an attempt to resolve those conflicting findings, Lepe and colleagues performed a meta-analysis of 450 studies and found that the longer the subjects were on a higher-protein diet, the lesser the chance of maintaining the weight reduction.

Key aspects in the impact of a higher protein diet upon weight loss may be related to the protein level at meals as well as the amino acid composition of the diet as discussed later in this chapter. For instance, a higher percentage of calories from protein of a dramatic caloric restriction might not deliver enough protein at meals and total day to elicit benefit. Also, branched chain amino acid (BCAA) intake in combination with a complete protein can support weight loss as well as an increase in fat free mass when resistance exercise is included. The BCAAs are leucine, isoleucine and valine and of which, leucine appears to be the most efficacious.

The overwhelming majority of studies have shown that in the short term, high-protein diets are effective at promoting weight loss compared with normal protein-level diets and/or low-carbohydrate diets. Although the final verdict as to whether they are successful for long-term weight maintenance remains open for debate, the evidence that they are successful is promising.

▶ Roles of Amino Acids and Proteins in Metabolism

Proteins and amino acids have diverse roles in promoting optimal health (**TABLE 6.5**). Below is a discussion of each role.

Enzymes

All enzymes are proteins and function to catalyze biochemical reactions by lessening the energy requirements for a particular chemical reaction. In general, enzyme names end in -*ase* following the type of reaction they catalyze. For instance, a hydrogenase, such as pyruvate dehydrogenase, removes hydrogen from a reactant; transferases (e.g., alanine transferase) facilitate group transfers from one molecule to another. Chemical reactions, and the enzymes that facilitate their action, have been placed into six classes, each having numerous subclasses. The six classes of enzymes are oxidoreductases, transferases, hydrolases, isomerases, lyases, and ligases

TABLE 6.5 Biochemical, Structural, and Physiologic Roles of Proteins and Amino Acids

Enzymes
Blood components
Blood clotting
Muscle function and structure
Endocrine functions
Connective tissue structure
Fluid balance
Acid-base of pH balance
Immune function
Component of membrane receptors
Energy utilization
Precursor to other compounds
Source of methyl and carbon as donors

(**TABLE 6.6**). The following discussion describes the major functions of proteins.

Blood Components

Proteins are important transportation components of the blood. For example, hemoglobin in red blood cells endeavors to transport oxygen. An adult man contains about 3×10^{13} red blood cells and

TABLE 6.6 Classifications of Enzymes and Their General Functions

Enzyme Class	General Function
Oxidoreductase	In those reactions, one substrate is oxidized while another is reduced.
Transferases	In those reactions, a functional group is transferred between substrates.
Hydrolases	In those reactions, water splits an ester, ether, peptide, glycyl linkage, acid anhydride, carbon-carbon bond, carbon-halide bond, or phosphorus-nitrogen bond.
Lyases	In those reactions, two groups are removed from a substrate, leaving a double bond.
Isomerases	In those reactions, there is an interconversion of isomers—optical, geometric, and positional.
Ligases	In those reactions, a covalent bond is formed, utilizing the hydrolysis of ATP or some other high-energy compound.

about 900 grams of hemoglobin. Each subunit of hemoglobin contains one heme group with a centralized iron atom that can bind oxygen. Hemoglobin has a molecular weight of approximately 67,000 daltons and has four subunits: two α-chains of 141 amino acids each and two β-chains of 146 amino acids each. Hemoglobin in the form of 2α2β is often referred to as hemoglobin A. Approximately 2.5% of hemoglobin is in the form of hemoglobin A_2, in which the two β subunits are replaced by two δ subunits (2α2δ), also containing 146 amino acids each. Ten amino acid residues differ in the δ-chains compared with those in the β-chain. Fetal hemoglobin (hemoglobin F) is similar to hemoglobin A except that its two β subunits are replaced by two γ subunits (2α2γ). Here again, the β subunits and the γ subunits contain 146 amino acids each; however, this time, there is a difference in 37 amino acid residues.

Other important transport proteins include plasma proteins. With the exception of antibodies, gamma globulin, and some endothelially secreted proteins, plasma proteins are largely synthesized and secreted by the liver. The total protein content of plasma for an adult is 7.0 to 7.5 grams per 100 milliliters. Plasma proteins contain simpler molecules as well as conjugated proteins, such as glycoproteins and lipoproteins. **Albumin**, a 610-amino acid single-chain protein with a molecular weight of 69,000, is the principal plasma protein. Its concentration is usually between 3.5 and 5.0 grams per 100 milliliters. Albumin is a principal transporter for substances, such as fatty acids, bile acids in the portal circulation, and many other substances, including several minerals. Other transport proteins found in the blood include transferrin, ceruloplasmin, and vitamin D-binding protein (DBP). Protein-containing lipoproteins are major transporters of lipids and lipid-soluble substances (e.g., fat-soluble vitamins).

Blood Clotting

Clotting factors are synthesized in the liver and released in a zymogen form. Those include factors V, VII (proconvertin), VIII (antihemolytic factor), IX (Christmas factor), X (Stuart factor), XI (plasma thromboplastin), XII (Hageman factor), and XIII (**transaminase**); fibrinogen; and prothrombin. The mechanism of clotting incorporates a cascade of events or stages, each serving to amplify the process. The final reaction in the cascade results in the activation of **fibrinogen** to **fibrin**, which forms a cross-linking structure, the structural basis of the clot. The liver also secretes **plasminogen**, which, when activated to **plasmin**, serves to dissolve clots.

Muscle Structure and Function

Muscle contraction is based on contractile proteins such as myosin, actin, troponin, and tropomyosin. Myosin is a major body protein as well as a major muscle protein, accounting for 55% of muscle mass. It contains three pairs of proteins—one pair of heavy chains and two different pairs of light chains—and is approximately 460,000 daltons. The heavy chains alone are about 1,800 amino acids long, which are among the longest in the human body. Actin is a smaller protein with a molecular weight of about 45,000. As initially synthesized, actin is a globular protein (G-actin), which can then polymerize with other actin molecules to form a fibrous structure called F-actin.

Tropomyosin is also a fibrous protein that binds to F-actin and serves to cover myosin-binding sites on actin monomers when a muscle is not being stimulated to contract. There are three principal troponin molecules, all of which are in some manner associated with one another, as well as with tropomyosin. The C subunit binds calcium when intracellular calcium levels increase during stimulation. This results in a conformational change in the troponin complex that ultimately results in the uncovering of myosin binding sites on actin by physically moving tropomyosin structures.

Endocrine Functions

Several hormones are protein structures or modified amino acids. Insulin and glucagon, which are pivotal hormones involved in energy nutrient metabolism, are examples. The hypothalamus alone produces nine hormones of a protein or modified amino acid nature. Those are thyrotropin-releasing hormone (TRH), somatostatin, growth hormone-releasing hormone (GHRH), prolactin-inhibiting hormone (PIH), prolactin-releasing hormone (PRH), melanocyte-stimulating hormone (MSH)-inhibiting hormone, MSH-releasing hormone, gonadotropin-releasing hormone, and corticotropin-releasing hormone. The anterior pituitary gland produces eight protein-based hormones, including thyroid-stimulating hormone (TSH), growth hormone (GH), prolactin, MSH, luteinizing hormone (LH), follicle-stimulating hormone (FSH), and adrenocorticotropic hormone (ACTH). FSH, LH, and TSH are glycoproteins composed of two subunits: an α subunit, which is identical in both hormones and a β subunit, which differs between the hormones.

Connective Tissue

Connective tissue protein structures, such as collagen and elastin, provide strength and elastic properties to human tissue. As mentioned earlier, collagen is the most abundant protein in the human body. It is generally an insoluble fibrous protein found in tendons, bones, cartilage, skin, the cornea, and in interstitial spaces. Approximately 30% of its amino acids are glycine. Proline, hydroxyproline, and hydroxyserine contribute approximately 20%. Collagen as synthesized by fibroblasts is helical in structure, and three collagen helices are twisted together to form a larger left-handed helix called tropocollagen. Multiple tropocollagen helices are cross-linked together to form a strong collagen fiber. Copper, iron, and vitamin C are all vital in the production of collagen fibers. Elastin is a protein also found in connective tissue and is an especially important component to vascular tissue, such as the aorta and other arteries and arterioles. It allows for expansion of a vessel under pressure and for recoil as pressure subsides. Elastin is especially rich in lysine and glycine.

A major protein of hair, skin, and nails is α-keratin, which has a secondary protein structure in the form of an α-helix. Like collagen, several keratin helices are twisted together and stabilized by disulfide bonds to form thicker fibers. Commercially available permanent waves disrupt the disulfide bonds.

Fluid Balance

Protein is also an important factor in water balance. Because proteins cannot diffuse through a semipermeable membrane, they exert osmotic pressure in either the intracellular or extracellular fluid or across organelle membranes. A normal concentration of protein in the plasma, especially albumin, is fundamental in balancing water between tissue and the blood. If protein intake is insufficient, a decreased concentration of protein in the plasma results and water deposits into tissues, resulting in edema.

Acid–Base Balance

Acid–base balance is another function, because proteins act as natural buffers and amino acids can ionize and provide both acidic and basic groups. The carboxyl group helps neutralize excess base, and the amine group neutralizes excess acid. The natural buffering capacity of amino acids and some proteins (e.g., carbonic anhydrase) is critical for cellular and extracellular environments and for metabolic functions and biochemical reactions.

Immunity, Transport Carriers, and Membrane Receptors

Additionally, antibodies are composed of protein. It is not unusual to find decreased resistance to infections in areas of the world where protein intake is low or insufficient. Membrane transport carriers (e.g., GLUT4, Na^+–K^+ ATPase) and receptors are also proteins, as are many intra-cellular binding entities, such as metallothionein and ferritin. The visual pigment opsin is a protein found in the retina of the eye.

Energy Supply

In addition to being building blocks for proteins, amino acids may be used to construct other molecules or their carbon skeleton can be used in energy metabolic pathways. From an energy perspective, amino acids may be classified either as **ketogenic** or **glucogenic**. Phenylalanine, tyrosine, leucine, and isoleucine are degraded to acetoacetate and are ketogenic. Other amino acids are degraded to pyruvate, oxaloacetate, α-ketoglutarate, succinate, and fumarate, which can be used in gluconeogenesis to produce glucose, and thus are glucogenic.

Precursors to Other Biochemical Compounds

Beyond serving as intermediates of energy pathways, certain amino acids are also precursors of critical biochemical compounds. As alluded to already, some amino acids give rise to other amino acids, as in the conversion of phenylalanine to tyrosine. Tyrosine itself is a precursor of thyroid hormone (T_3/T_4), dopamine, epinephrine, and norepinephrine. Sulfur-containing amino acids give rise to bile compounds such as taurine. Tryptophan is metabolized to serotonin, a critical neurotransmitter. The simplest amino acid, glycine, is involved in the formation of the porphyrin ring of hemoglobin as well as creatine. Hydroxyproline and hydroxylysine are important components of collagen. **TABLE 6.7** summarizes some of the substances derived from amino acids.

Role as Carbon and Methyl Donors

The amino acid methionine is an important molecule involved in single-carbon-unit transfer mechanisms used in molecular synthesis operations. The enzyme methionine adenosyl transferase catalyzes the ATP-requiring conversion of methionine to S-adenosyl methionine (SAM). This enzyme is abundant in the liver, which is the primary site of methionine metabolism. SAM is the principal methyl donor in the human cells and is used to create molecules such as carnitine, creatine, epinephrine, purines, and nicotinamide. Removal of the methyl group from SAM creates the compound S-adenosyl homocysteine (SAH), which can be converted to homocysteine. For methionine to be regenerated from homocysteine, vitamin B_{12}, 5-methyl-tetrahydrofolate (a folate form), and betaine

TABLE 6.7 Amino Acid–Derived Substances

Substance	Amino Acids Utilized in the Synthesis
Choline	Serine
Niacin	Tryptophan
Glutathione	Cysteine, glycine, glutamic acid
Serotonin	Tryptophan
Carnitine	Lysine, methionine
Carnosine	Histidine, β-alanine
Creatine	Arginine, glycine, methionine
Pyrimidines	Aspartate, glutamine
Purines	Aspartate, glutamine, glycine
Epinephrine, norepinephrine, dopamine, thyroid hormone	Tyrosine or phenylalanine

must be present, with the latter compound donating a single carbon unit. Homocysteine can also be converted to the nonessential amino acids serine and cysteine. Recently, attention has been focused on the relationship between homocysteinemia and the risk of heart disease (see Special Feature 6.2).

Other Functions

Taurine and ornithine are two amino acids that have fundamental roles in the human body but are not incorporated into protein. Taurine has a fundamental role in retinal operations related to vision, in membrane stability, as a component of bile acids, and possibly as a neurotransmitter. Ornithine is vital in the disposal of nitrogenous waste molecules (ammonia) via the **urea cycle**, which is discussed later in this chapter.

⬢ BEFORE YOU GO ON . . .

1. What are the major muscle proteins?
2. With what are the proteins fibrinogen and prothrombin involved?
3. What are the protein hormones produced by the hypothalamus of the brain?
4. How do proteins moderate acid–base balance?

SPECIAL FEATURE 6.2

Homocysteine and the Risk of Coronary Heart Disease

Elevated homocysteine levels have recently been implicated as a risk factor for heart disease. A deficiency of folate, vitamin B_6, or vitamin B_{12} can interfere with the enzymatic conversion of homocysteine to methionine. Even moderate elevations in blood homocysteine levels are associated with an increased risk of heart disease. For example, an increase of 5 micromoles per liter in plasma homocysteine levels is estimated to increase heart disease risk by 70%. This is equivalent to an increase in risk when serum cholesterol levels increase by 0.5 micromoles per liter. An increased intake of folic acid by 200 micrograms per day reduces homocysteine levels by about 4 micromoles per liter.

Homocysteine levels can be regulated by both genetic and environmental (nutritional) factors. Genetic defects in the enzymes cystathione β-synthase, methionine synthase, and methylenetetrahydrofolate reductase can all lead to an augmentation of homocysteine levels. However, folic acid, riboflavin, methionine, choline, and vitamins B_6 and B_{12} may all affect homocysteine metabolism.

Elevated serum homocysteine has been suggested to cause oxidative damage, in particular that of LDL. However, it may also interfere with the blood coagulation process, in particular, those events associated with dissolution of the fibrin clot. In general, it is thought that elevated homocysteine injures blood vessels and accelerates the deposition of fat on the lining of blood vessels. As a result of this link, some scientists have suggested that folic acid supplements be used to control blood homocysteine levels. One study suggested that 400 micrograms of folic acid per day reduces blood homocysteine levels. The American Heart Association (AHA) does not believe that there is sufficient evidence to warrant consumption of folic acid supplements to prevent heart disease. However, the AHA does recommend that those at risk for heart disease consume the DRI for both folate and vitamin B_{12} through food consumption.

▶ Metabolism of Amino Acids

Transamination and Deamination

Amino acids are different from other energy nutrients in that they contain the element nitrogen. The removal or transfer of nitrogen is necessary for the utilization of amino acids as an energy source as well as the creation of nonessential amino acids and other molecules. **Transamination** reactions, involving an amino transferase enzyme, transfer the amino group to an α-keto acid, whereas **deamination** reactions, catalyzed by deaminases, remove amine groups to form ammonia (**FIGURE 6.7**).

Amino transferases bind to the substrate amino acid and pass the amine group to pyridoxal phosphate (PLP), which is a form of vitamin B_6. Pyridoxal phosphate is also bound to the amino transferase. The amine group is then passed to an acceptor α-keto acid that binds with PLP and the enzyme. Amino transferase enzymes are specific to an α-keto acid and an amino acid. Pyruvate and α-ketoglutarate are the two α-keto acids used most in transamination reactions. Alanine-pyruvate transaminase and glutamate-α-ketoglutarate transaminase are present in most human cells, and an increase in their cardiac and hepatic isomeric forms present in

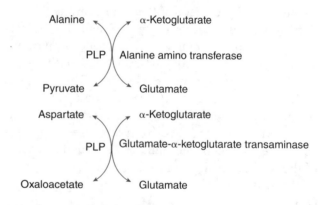

(a) Transamination

$$\text{Glutamate} + NAD^+ + H_2O \xrightarrow{\text{Glutamate dehydrogenase}} \alpha\text{-Ketoglutarate} + NADH + H^+ + NH_3$$

(b) Oxidative deamination

$$\text{Amino acid} + H_2O \xrightarrow[\text{Reduced flavin-bound enzyme}]{\text{Flavin-bound enzyme}} \text{Ketoacid} + NH_3$$

(c) Amino acid oxidases

FIGURE 6.7. General Reactions Involving the Transfer or Removal of Amino Groups. (a) Transamination, (b) Oxidative deamination (c) Amino acid oxidation

the plasma is a diagnostic tool for cardiac and hepatic pathology.

Nitrogen can also be removed from amino acids by deamination. For instance, oxidative deamination of glutamate yields α-ketoglutarate and free ammonia (see Figure 6.7). This deamination is catalyzed by glutamate dehydrogenase, an enzyme that uses nicotinamide adenine dinucleotide (NAD) or nicotinamide adenine dinucleotide phosphate (NADP) as electron acceptors. In peroxisomes, d-amino acids undergo oxidative deamination by amino acid oxidases that use flavin adenine dinucleotide (FAD) and flavin mononucleotide (FMN) as electron acceptors.

As discussed in more detail later in this chapter, amino groups can be removed from amino acids to create free ammonia (see Figure 6.7). Glutaminase, asparaginase, and the amino acid oxidases all produce ammonia; however, glutamate dehydrogenase generates the most ammonia. This hepatic enzyme is pivotal in amino acid disposal via urea synthesis.

Synthesis of Amino Acids

Discussion of the **synthesis of amino acids** is limited to nonessential amino acids and post-translational derivatives of nonessential amino acids (e.g., hydroxyproline). Glutamate provides most of the nitrogen used in the synthesis of nonessential amino acids. As mentioned previously, two nonessential amino acids rely on the presence or appropriate metabolism of essential amino acids for their creation. Tyrosine is synthesized by hydroxylation of phenylalanine, and cysteine is formed with the help of methionine. Many amino acids are derived from intermediates of glycolysis and the Krebs cycle. Serine can be synthesized from the glycolytic intermediate 3-phosphoglycerate. Serine can then serve as a precursor for glycine and cysteine. Although the carbon skeleton and nitrogen of cysteine are derived from serine, methionine is needed to supply sulfur. Alanine is produced via the transamination of pyruvate.

The nonessential amino acids derived from Krebs cycle intermediates include aspartate, asparagine, glutamate, glutamine, proline, and arginine. Aspartate is derived from oxaloacetate via transamination, and asparagine can then be synthesized from aspartate by amidation. Glutamate is derived from α-ketoglutarate either by transamination or by the addition of ammonia via glutamate dehydrogenase. Glutamine, proline, and arginine are also produced from glutamate. Glutamine is generated via amidation, whereas proline and arginine are derived from glutamate semialdehyde, which is the result of the reduction of glutamate. Proline requires the cyclization of glutamate semialdehyde,

whereas the creation of arginine requires glutamate semialdehyde to first be converted to ornithine, which is eventually converted to arginine by way of urea cycle reactions.

Several proteins contain modifications of nonessential amino acids, such as hydroxyproline, hydroxylysine, and homocysteine. The modifications occur after the initial protein chain has been synthesized on ribosomes; thus, the modifications are called post-translational events. Hydroxylysine and hydroxyproline occur almost exclusively in collagen. Those amino acids are formed by dioxidation reactions, and iron, vitamin C, and α-ketoglutarate are required. 3-Methyl histidine is formed posttranslationally from the amino acid histidine. This amino acid is found almost exclusively in actin protein. Although quantitatively, most actin is found in muscle, some actin is found in other tissues, such as the intestines, where actin shafts provide support to microvilli. Some actin is also found in platelets as well. Upon proteolysis, 3-methyl histidine is released from those cells; it is not reincorporated into new proteins. It diffuses out of cells and is excreted in the urine. Because of the greater relative mass of muscle compared with other actin-containing tissue, most of the 3-methyl histidine in the urine is attributable to muscle catabolism during fasting, starvation, or prolonged activity.

Degradation of Amino Acids

Once nitrogen is removed from amino acids, the remaining molecule is referred to as the carbon skeleton. When carbon skeletons of amino acids are degraded, the major products are pyruvate, acetyl CoA, intermediates of the Krebs cycle, and the ketone body acetoacetate (**FIGURE 6.8**). As alluded to earlier, amino acids whose carbon skeletons form pyruvate or intermediates of the Krebs cycle are deemed glucogenic because they can be used to form glucose in the liver via gluconeogenesis. Those amino acids whose skeletons become acetyl CoA and acetoacetate are deemed ketogenic because they can form ketone bodies. Although most amino acids are either glucogenic or ketogenic, a few amino acids—namely, tryptophan, phenylalanine, threonine, tryosine, and isoleucine—are both.

Those amino acids whose carbon skeletons are used to form pyruvate include serine, glycine, cysteine, hydroxyproline, threonine, tryptophan, and alanine, with the latter forming pyruvate directly via a transamination reaction. Serine dehydratase converts serine to pyruvate by first removing water; a hydrolysis reaction then removes ammonia. Glycine, in contrast, is first

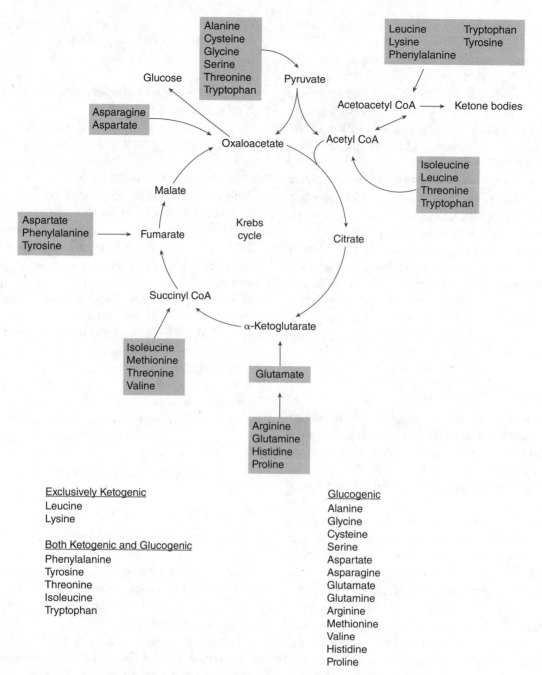

FIGURE 6.8. **Catabolism of Amino Acids and Their Fate in Terms of Ketone Body.** Different amino acids may enter the Krebs cycle at different points in the pathway. Also, note in the bottom of the figure that some amino acids are exclusively ketogenic, some glucogenic, and some both ketogenic and glucogenic.

converted to serine and then to pyruvate. In the first reaction, a single carbon unit is donated to glycine by N^5,N^{10}-methylenetetrahydrofolate, a folic acid form.

Hydroxyproline, which is prominent in collagen yet is not found in most other proteins, undergoes a series of reactions that ultimately produces pyruvate and glyoxylate. The nitrogen of hydroxyproline is removed by transamination. Cysteine's carbon skeleton forms pyruvate by one of two mechanisms. In the first, cysteine must first be transaminated to form thiopyruvate, after which sulfur is removed to form

pyruvate; in the second, sulfur is first removed and then cysteine dehydratase removes ammonia in a hydrolytic reaction. In either case, the removal of sulfur creates sulfuric acid (H_2SO_4).

The initial reaction in the catabolism of threonine creates glycine and acetaldehyde. Glycine can be converted to pyruvate, as mentioned previously, whereas acetaldehyde is oxidized by FAD to create acetate, which itself is condensed with coenzyme A to yield acetyl CoA (see Figure 6.8). Thus, threonine is both glucogenic and ketogenic, as is tryptophan.

Tryptophan catabolism results in the formation of pyruvate and acetoacetate.

Those amino acids whose carbon skeletons form Krebs cycle intermediates are glutamate, glutamine, proline, arginine, histidine, asparagine, aspartate, threonine, methionine, homocysteine, valine, and isoleucine. Aspartate is converted into oxaloacetate via a transamination reaction involving α-ketoglutarate and forming glutamate in the process. Asparagine's carbon skeleton is also converted to oxaloacetate; however, asparagine must first be deaminated by asparaginase to aspartate.

The carbon skeletons of arginine, histidine, proline, and glutamine can all be converted to α-ketoglutarate. However, they are first converted to glutamate, which, via oxidative deamination, is converted to α-ketoglutarate. Glutamate can also be used in a transamination reaction that forms alanine and α-ketoglutarate.

Parts of methionine, isoleucine, and valine are used to form succinyl CoA. The catabolism of those amino acids allows for the formation of either propionyl CoA or methylmalonyl CoA, which are oxidized to succinyl CoA in the same reactions that oxidize odd-chain-length fatty acids. The catabolism of methionine first involves the production of SAM, which subsequently loses its methyl group, producing S-adenosyl homocyteine (SAH). Further enzymatic processing results in the cleavage of adenosine and the addition of serine to yield cystathionine. Cystathionine is subsequently cleaved to form cysteine and homoserine. Cysteine is converted to pyruvate, as discussed previously. Meanwhile, oxidative deamination of homoserine yields α-ketoglutarate, which is then decarboxylated and activated by the attachment of coenzyme A to form propionyl CoA. Further carboxylation to methylmalonyl CoA and subsequent molecular rearrangement produces succinyl CoA.

Phenylalanine and tyrosine are converted to fumarate. The first step in phenylalanine breakdown is the formation of tyrosine (**FIGURE 6.9**). The first reaction is catalyzed by phenylalanine hydroxylase. A genetic predisposition resulting in diminished activity of this enzyme results in the increased formation

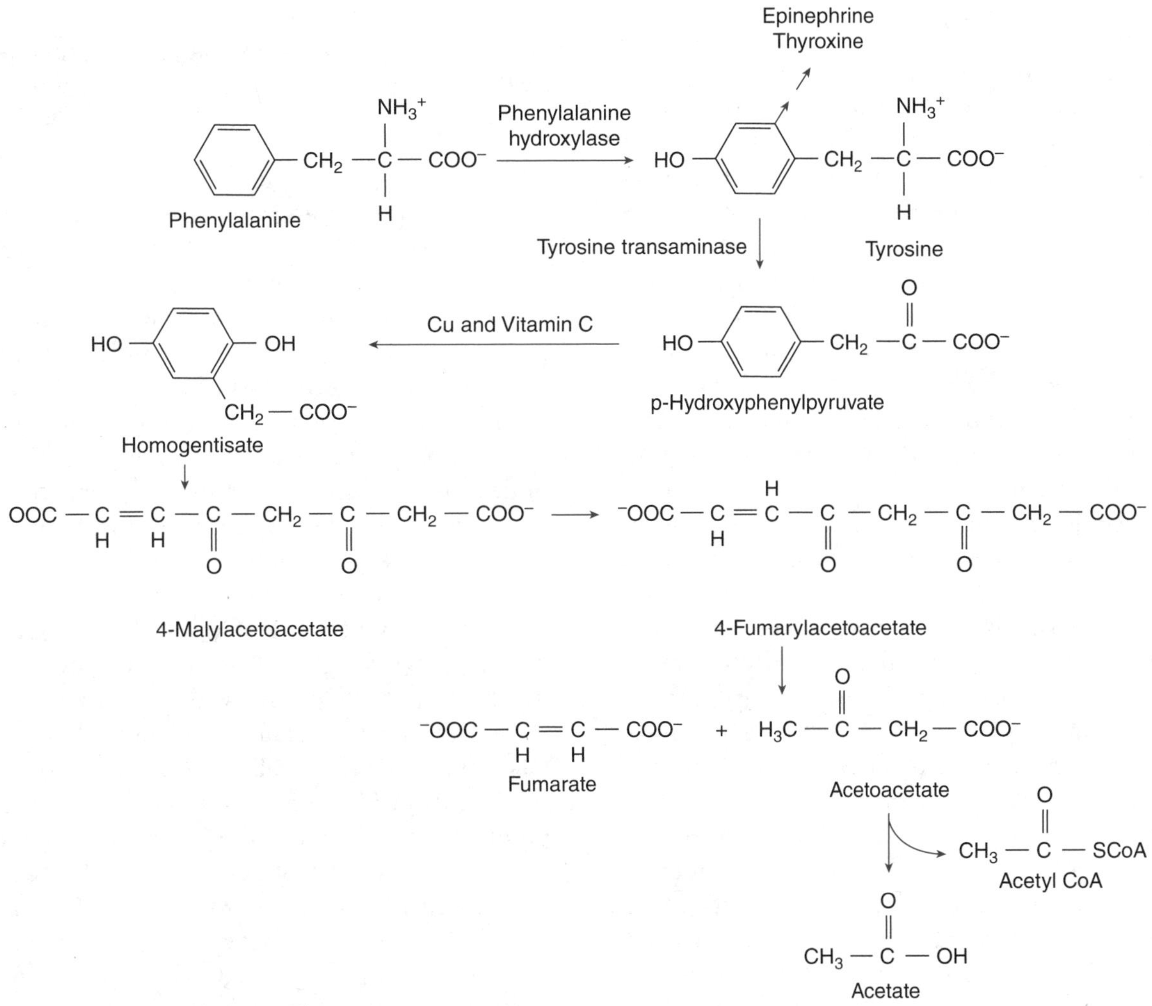

FIGURE 6.9. Catabolism of Phenylalanine. Phenylalanine and tyrosine, through a series of reactions can be converted to fumarate and acetoacetate. Acetoacetate can be converted to Acetate and Acetyl CoA.

of alternative phenylalanine metabolites (phenyletha-nolamine, phenylpyruvate, phenylacetate), which can result in poor growth and development, especially of the brain. This disease is called phenylketonuria (PKU) and is discussed later in this chapter. Tyrosine is transaminated by tyrosine transaminase to form p-hydroxyphenylpyruvate. The acceptor of the transferred amino group is α-ketoglutarate. A copper-containing enzyme that also requires ascorbate yields homogentisate, which is then ultimately metabolized to fumarylacetoacetate, which is split to yield fumarate and acetoacetate.

Five amino acids are converted to acetoacetate: lysine, leucine, phenylalanine, tyrosine, and tryptophan. The latter three have been discussed previously. Leucine and lysine are the only amino acids that are only ketogenic; that is, they do not produce glucogenic intermediates. The product of leucine metabolism is similar to isoleucine and valine, except that leucine yields acetoacetate and acetyl CoA. The breakdown of lysine yields acetoacetate.

Glutamine Metabolism

Glutamine is a nonessential amino acid that plays a critical role in interorgan transport of nitrogen and carbon. It is found in almost all organ tissues, including the small intestine, skeletal muscle, liver, kidneys, lungs, and, of course, blood. The primary sites of synthesis are skeletal muscle, lungs, and adipose tissue, but all tissues can synthesize glutamine. Whereas ammonia from the liver can be shuttled into the urea cycle, other tissues need another mechanism to get rid of ammonia because elevated levels are toxic. One such method to dispose of ammonia is through the production of glutamine. This reaction requires the amino acid glutamate and the enzyme glutamine synthetase, along with ATP, magnesium, or manganese (**FIGURE 6.10**). Cells and tissues are permeable to glutamine; thus, it can find its way to other parts of the body. In terms of catabolism, the enzyme glutaminase removes the amide group. The glutamate can be further metabolized by glutamate dehydrogenase to α-ketoglutarate plus ammonia. The ammonia may enter the urea cycle, explained later in this chapter.

Glutamine is used extensively by the mucosal cells of the intestine. It can stimulate cell proliferation or it can be degraded and used as a source of energy by the small intestine. The integrity of the small intestine is thought to be maintained by glutamine, preventing bacterial invasion into the mucosal cells. As already described, glutamine in the small intestine can be converted to glutamate with the liberation of ammonia; glutamate can then give up

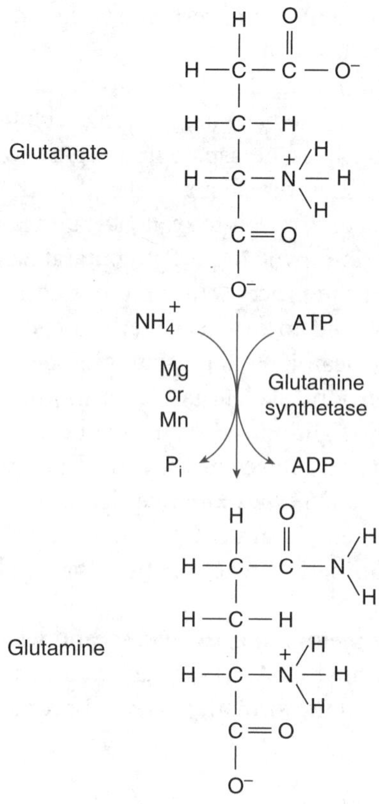

FIGURE 6.10. Synthesis of Glutamine from Glutamate. Production of glutamine is one method to dispose of ammonia.

its remaining amide group to pyruvate to produce alanine and α-ketoglutarate. The latter can then enter the Krebs cycle for energy production.

A significant function of glutamine is that it is the precursor to the purine and pyrimidine nucleotide bases used in the synthesis of RNA and DNA. It also is the precursor for glucosamines, asparagines, and nicotinamide adenine dinucleotide. For the nucleotides, the reactions occur in the liver. For pyrimidines, the initial step in this synthesis is the creation of carbamoyl phosphate from glutamine, carbon dioxide, and ATP in the presence of the enzyme carbamoyl PO_4 synthetase II (**FIGURE 6.11**). Glutamate is liberated through the process. The next reaction involves aspartate reacting with the carbamoyl PO_4 to form carbamoylaspartate. The enzyme here is aspartate transcarbamoylase. Several other reactions occur to produce uridine monophosphate (UMP). At this point, UMP can serve as the precursor to the remaining pyrimidine nucleotides. Through the action of a kinase and ATP, uridine diphosphate (UDP) is produced. Another phosphorylation reaction results in uridine triphosphate (UTP), which is used for RNA synthesis. UTP can react with glutamine, ATP, and water in the presence of cytosine triphosphate (CTP) synthase to produce cytosine triphosphate, which can

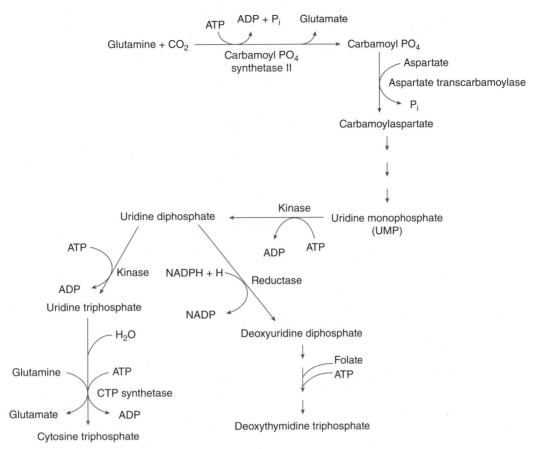

FIGURE 6.11. Synthesis of Pyrimidine Nucleotide Bases. Glutamine is also a precursor to pyrimidine nucleotide bases for DNA and RNA production.

be used in both DNA and RNA synthesis. UDP can take another path in the presence of a reductase and NADPH to yield deoxyuridine diphosphate. Through a series of reactions that involve folate, deoxyuridine diphosphate can yield deoxythymidine triphosphate, which is needed for DNA synthesis.

The production of purines is dependent on glutamine and involves the hexose monophosphate (HMP) shunt. Ribose-5-phosphate is produced by the HMP shunt and enters the pathway for purine synthesis to synthesize inosine monophosphate (IMP) **(FIGURE 6.12)**. Glutamine is required for two reactions in this pathway. After IMP is produced, two diverging pathways are possible. IMP can react with aspartate and eventually produce deoxy-ATP for DNA synthesis of ATP for RNA synthesis. Alternatively, the purine guanosine triphosphate (GTP) can be synthesized (through a series of reactions that involve glutamine) for RNA synthesis, or deoxy-GTP can by synthesized for DNA synthesis.

The Alanine–Glucose Cycle

We have already discussed how important glutamine is in the intertissue transfer of amino groups that result from amino acid degradation. Alanine is another important amino acid used for this function. The alanine–glucose cycle allows for the interchange of alanine between skeletal muscle and the liver **(FIGURE 6.13)**. Alanine comes from the muscle via the transamination of pyruvate. Alanine leaves the muscle and can be taken up by liver cells. When in the liver, alanine is transaminated with α-ketoglutarate; the resulting pyruvate enters gluconeogenesis, and the resulting glutamate may enter the urea cycle. When the glucose is produced by the liver, it is released to the bloodstream and can go back to the muscle to be used for energy. Alanine amino transferase is used in both the liver and muscle to facilitate those reactions.

Amino Acids and Neurotransmitters

A discussion of amino acids would not be complete without acknowledging the role they play in neurotransmission. One amino acid that is a well-known neurotransmitter is glutamate, which we have already mentioned in other contexts. It is excitatory in terms of its physiologic action and is well distributed among various brain regions. Another such amino acid is aspartate. Both glutamate and aspartate are found in axon terminals. The brain synthesizes those two

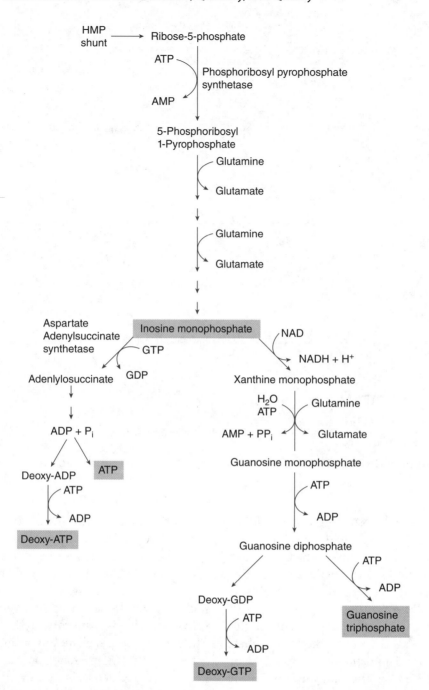

FIGURE 6.12. Synthesis of Purine Nucleotide Bases. Glutamine is also a precursor to purine nucleotide bases for DNA and RNA production. The hexose monophosphate (HMP) shunt is required for the reaction involving glutamine.

amino acids, and their levels do not appear to be related to dietary levels. Specific receptors have been identified for those two amino acids in the brain. Glutamate can be converted to another neurotransmitter, γ-aminobutyric acid (GABA), which has inhibitory effects on neurons. The conversion of glutamate to GABA depends on the enzyme glutamate decarboxylase and vitamin B_6 and liberates carbon dioxide from the α-carbon (**FIGURE 6.14**).

Glycine, the simplest of amino acids, is an inhibitory neurotransmitter. It is found primarily in the brain stem and spinal cord. Taurine is another amino acid that is an inhibitory neurotransmitter. Taurine has sometimes been used to treat epilepsy because it lessens neuroactivity and can function as a mild sedative.

The most significant amino acids involved with neurotransmission are tyrosine and tryptophan. As shown in Figure 6.9, tyrosine is synthesized from phenylalanine. **FIGURE 6.15** shows how tyrosine may be metabolized into a group of neurotransmitters known as catecholamines. Tyrosine is first converted to DOPA (3-4,dihydroxyphe-nylalanine) via tyrosine hydroxylase. The reaction converting DOPA

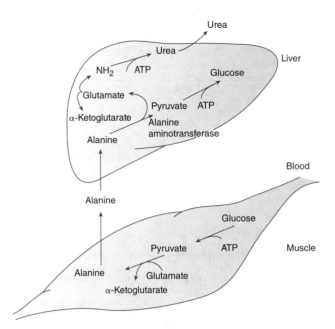

FIGURE 6.13. The Alanine–Glucose Cycle. This cycle allows for the interchange of alanine between the liver and skeletal muscle.

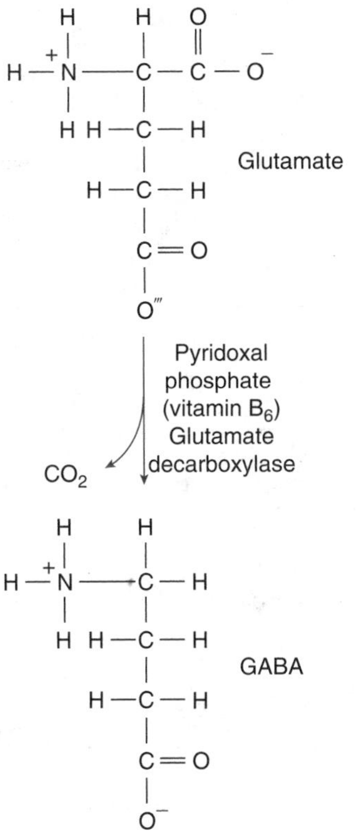

FIGURE 6.14. Synthesis of GABA from Glutamate. GABA has an inhibitory effect on neurons. Note the requirement for vitamin B_6.

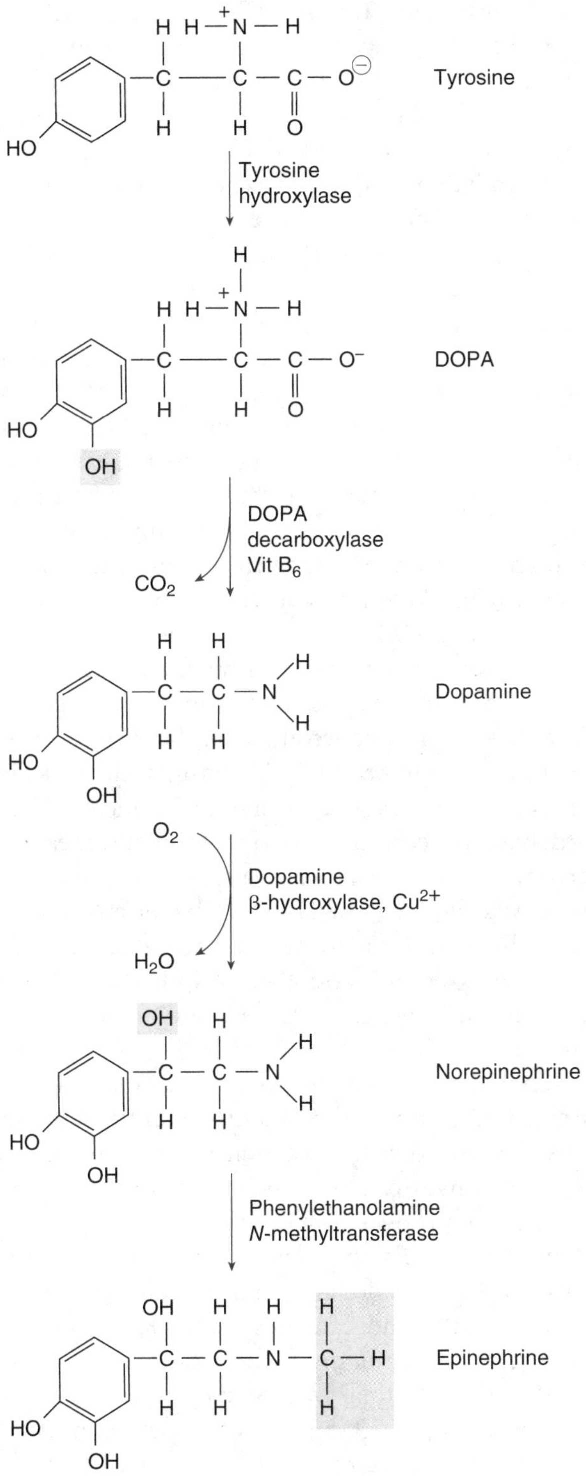

FIGURE 6.15. Catecholamine Neurotransmitter Synthesis from Tyrosine. Tyrosine is a precursor to a rather large number of neurotransmitters as revealed by these reactions.

to dopamine requires vitamin B_6, and the enzyme that converts dopamine to norepinephrine (namely, dopamine β-hydroxylase) is a copper-dependent enzyme. Those catecholamines have profound effects on metabolism, including stimulating glycogenolysis and lipolysis and increasing metabolic rate. After those catecholamines have exerted their effects on target cells, they must be inactivated by a mitochondrial enzyme called monoamine oxidase (MAO). This enzyme removes the amine group from those neurotransmitters. That reaction occurs in the brain tissue. The liver may also degrade catecholamines via the enzyme catechol-O-methyltransferase.

MAO metabolism may be affected by drugs. A group of drugs known as MAO inhibitors decreases the degradation of those catecholamines to increase their levels in the brain. Those drugs historically have been very effective in treating depression and various anxiety disorders. However, they also inhibit the breakdown of other biogenic amines, such as tyramine, which can be found in foods. Normally, tyramine, absorbed by enterocytes, is degraded by MAO. Drugs, such as Nardil and Parnate, inhibit MAO and allow tyramine to be absorbed, which can increase blood pressure to life-threatening levels. Patients on those drugs must follow a diet low in tyramine. Foods that are high in tyramine include aged foods, such as aged cheeses (e.g., American, processed, blue, Boursault, brick [natural], brie, camembert, cheddar, Emmentaler, gruyere, mozzarella, Parmesan, Romano, sour cream, Roquefort, Stilton, and Swiss); meats, such as sausage, bologna, pepperoni, and salami; aged meats; fava beans; fermented or pickled fish, such as pickled herring; red wines and vermouth; fermented bean curd; banana peels; and sauerkraut. Finally, meat tenderizer, meat extracts, caviar, salted herring, and other dried fish should be avoided. A hypertensive crisis caused by consuming those foods while taking MAO inhibitors is serious, and affected individuals should be taken to an emergency room as soon as possible for treatment.

Tryptophan is converted to a hormone known as melatonin and to the neurotransmitter serotonin (**FIGURE 6.16**). The first reaction is with the enzyme tryptophan hydroxylase, which is an iron-dependent enzyme, to produce 5-hydroxytryptophan. This is followed by a decarboxylation reaction to produce 5-hydroxytryptamine (serotonin). Serotonin elicits neuroexcitation and can cause vasoconstriction and contraction of smooth muscle. Serotonin is also found in the intestinal wall. Serotonin has numerous functions, including control of appetite, memory, sleep, mood, behavior, body temperature, sexual and hallucinogenic behavior, cardiovascular and endocrine function, muscle contraction, and depression. Depression has been linked to decreased brain levels of serotonin. More important has been the identification of several types of serotonin receptors in the brain that, when stimulated, have an excitatory effect. When serotonin is released at the synapse, it can either be degraded or taken back up by the axon and reused. To keep the concentration of serotonin elevated at the synapse, a class of drugs known as selective serotonin

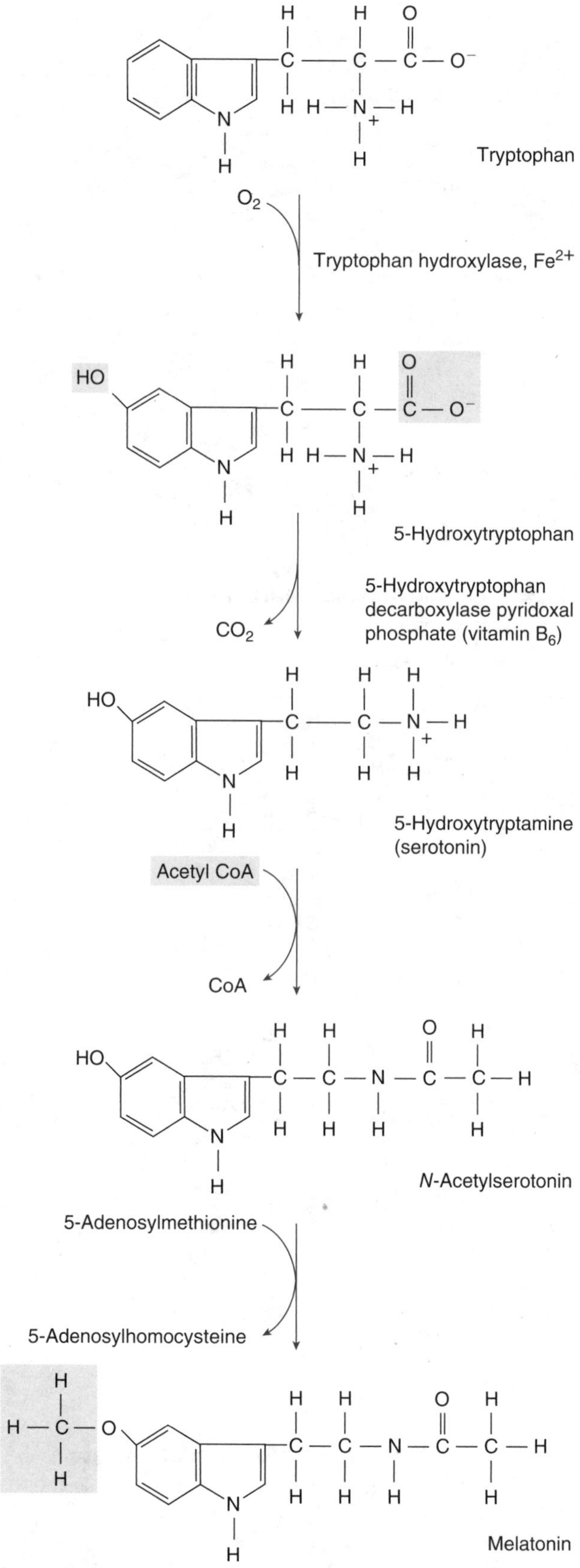

FIGURE 6.16. Synthesis of Serotonin (5-hydroxytryptamine) and Melatonin. Note that for both neurotransmitters, the amino acid tryptophan is the precursor.

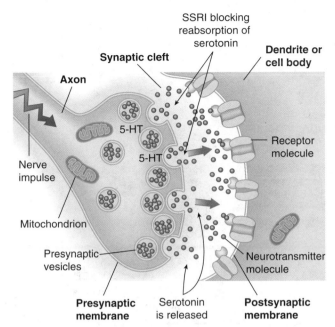

FIGURE 6.17. Serotonin Release at the Synapse and the Function of Selective Serotonin Reuptake Inhibitors (SSRIs). The presence of SSRI drugs maintains the serotonin levels to allow greater uptake by adjoining neurons to continue neurotransmission. SSRIs are used in the treatment of various psychiatric disorders, including depression.

reuptake inhibitors (SSRIs) block the reuptake of serotonin (**FIGURE 6.17**), making more serotonin available to be taken up by the adjoining neuron to continue neurotransmission. Like the catecholamines, serotonin is degraded by MAO.

If serotonin is not degraded, it is converted to *N*-acetylserotonin with acetyl CoA. Finally, the methyl donor S-adenosyl methionine methylates *N*-acetylserotonin to produce melatonin. Melatonin is synthesized mostly in the pineal gland of the brain during the dark phase of a daily cycle. Melatonin is involved with the regulation of sleep patterns and circadian rhythms.

Disposal of Amino Acid Nitrogen

Disposal of amino acid-derived nitrogen in the form of ammonia is crucial for the survival of humans. Increased serum levels of ammonia result in a toxicity syndrome, with the brain being a major site of impact. Ammonia is produced either by cellular degradation of amino acids and nucleic acids or by the metabolism of intestinal bacteria. Glutaminase, asparaginase, histidases, serine dehydratase, cysteine dehydratase, and amino acid oxidases all produce ammonia; the major source of cellular ammonia, however, is glutamate dehydrogenase. This mitochondrial enzyme catalyzes the removal of glutamate nitrogen collected from

amino acid transaminase reactions. Because urea synthesis occurs within the mitochondria primarily in the liver and secondarily in the kidneys, the liberated ammonia can be immediately used.

Tissues other than the liver and kidneys do not synthesize urea. Therefore, ammonia liberated in cellular reactions can be used to convert glutamate to glutamine. In fact, if a cell starts with α-ketoglutarate, two ammonia molecules can be transported as glutamine. Glutamine can then recirculate to the liver. Muscle tissue forms alanine and glutamine in an effort to transport excess nitrogen generated by the degradation of amino acids. Alanine is produced in muscle by the transamination of pyruvate via alanine transaminase. During a fasting state, alanine and glutamine account for as much as 50% of the amino acids released from skeletal muscle into circulation. During fasting and protracted aerobic exercise, branched-chain amino acids are oxidized in muscle and some of their carbon skeletons are converted to alanine and glutamine. Alanine circulates to the liver and is transaminated to pyruvate, which serves as a gluconeogenic precursor, whereas glutamine serves as an energy source for the intestines and a gluconeogenic precursor for the kidneys.

Urea Cycle

The urea cycle consists of five reactions that convert ammonia, carbon dioxide, and the α-amino nitrogen of aspartate into urea. Two of the reactions occur within the mitochondria, and the remaining reactions occur in the cytoplasm (**FIGURE 6.18**). In the preliminary reaction, carbon dioxide in the mitochondria is phosphorylated via ATP and subsequently condensed to ammonia using the energy released by the hydrolysis of another ATP molecule. The enzyme catalyzing the reaction is carbamoyl phosphate synthase, and the product is **carbamoyl phosphate**. While still in the mitochondria, carbamoyl phosphate is condensed with ornithine, via ornithine transcarbamoylase, to form citrulline. Phosphate is released in the reaction, and citrulline enters the cytosol. Next, citrulline condenses with aspartate via arginosuccinate synthase to form arginosuccinate, which is subsequently split by argininosuccinase into fumarate and arginine. The arginase enzyme then hydrolyzes arginine to form ornithine and urea.

There is some disagreement as to the fate of the fumarate formed by the splitting of arginosuccinate. It is most probable that fumarate is hydrated in the cytosol to form malate, which is then oxidized to oxaloacetate by cytosolic malate dehydrogenase. Finally, oxaloacetate accepts an amino group from glutamate to reform aspartate.

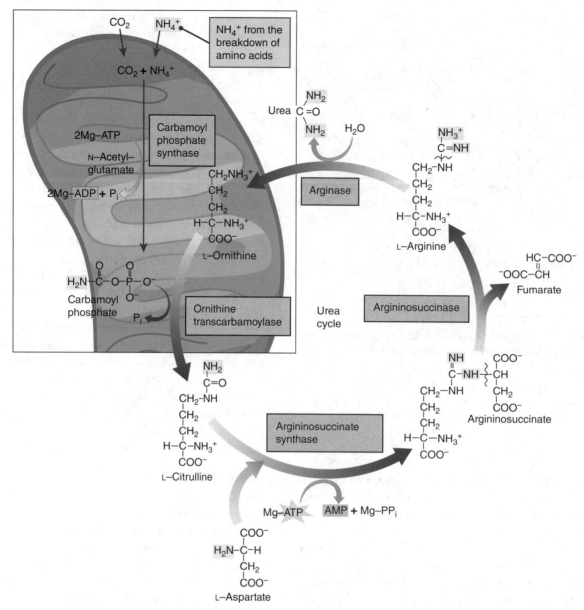

FIGURE 6.18. The Urea Cycle. The pathway responsible for the production of urea to eliminate ammonia generated from the breakdown of amino acids.

● BEFORE YOU GO ON . . .

1. What is meant when an amino acid is referred to as ketogenic? Glucogenic? Can an amino acid be both ketogenic and glucogenic?

2. How are purine and pyrimidine nucleotide bases produced?

3. What are the advantages of the alanine–glucose cycle and of the amino acid glutamine?

4. Describe the importance of tyrosine and tryptophan in terms of neurotransmission.

5. Outline the first key step of the urea cycle in which carbon dioxide is used.

▶ Protein and Amino Acid Requirements

Protein

The measures discussed in the section "Dietary Protein Quality" are methods of determining the quality of proteins. The *amount* of protein, or nitrogen, required by a human is another matter, a concept known as **nitrogen balance**. If the amount of nitrogen from protein consumed per day (N_{in}) is equal to the amount of protein nitrogen lost per day (N_{out}), the individual is said to be in nitrogen equilibrium ($N_{in} = N_{out}$). To measure nitrogen balance, the amounts of nitrogen lost in urine, feces, and sweat are determined, and the sum of those is subtracted from the amount ingested. A positive nitrogen balance occurs when the body is building up tissues so that more nitrogen is retained than is excreted by the body ($N_{in} > N_{out}$). A negative nitrogen balance occurs when the amount of nitrogen lost is greater than the amount of nitrogen retained ($N_{in} < N_{out}$). In such a case, tissue proteins are being catabolized in excess of synthesis. However, there is a growing consensus that measuring nitrogen balance may not be the best method to determine protein requirement. Instead, the oxidation of amino acids has recently gained a great deal of attention as a preferred method. Using this method reveals that the requirement for dietary protein may be much higher than those studies using nitrogen balance. We will first discuss two balance methods followed by oxidation of amino acids as a method of determining protein requirements.

The **factorial method** is used to determine obligatory nitrogen losses, that is, nitrogen loss through urine, feces, sweat, nails, and dermal sources when a protein-free diet is given to test subjects. Adequate energy is given in the diet to prevent endogenous muscle being used for energy. The grams of nitrogen lost through each of the routes is assessed daily until the loss levels out. The point of leveling is referred to as the endogenous loss. Fecal nitrogen will be present, even in a protein-free diet, because enzymes and sloughed-off cells will be present. All of the nitrogen loss sources are then added up for a given individual. **TABLE 6.8** presents the estimated daily nitrogen loss for a 70-kilogram adult male.

A 70-kilogram male loses about 54 milligrams of nitrogen per kilogram body weight per day (±2 SD). This loss increases the estimated nitrogen requirement to 70 milligrams nitrogen per kilogram body weight per day. To convert this figure to the amount of protein, the factor 6.25 is used, because 16% of the protein by weight is nitrogen (100/16 = 6.25); thus, the example value converts to 0.44 gram of protein per kilogram of body weight per day.

However, the conceptual nitrogen requirement assumes a linear response, which does not exist in reality. As the level of nitrogen in the diet increases toward the balance figure, efficiency declines. Said another way, the relationship is curvilinear as the nitrogen in the diet approaches the requirement level. The efficiency of protein utilization, therefore, declines. The reduction in efficiency is estimated to be 30%. Therefore, the requirement for dietary protein is increased by that percentage, or from 0.44 to 0.57 gram protein per kilogram body weight per day. In this example, egg protein is the sole source of nitrogen considered. If other proteins are used, the protein requirement must be adjusted upward accordingly. In American and other Western diets, the dietary protein quality is about 75% of the quality of egg protein. The requirement for protein when this fact is taken into account is as follows:

$$0.57 \text{ g protein/kg body weight/day} \times \frac{100}{75}$$
$$= 0.8 \text{ g protein/kg body weight/day}$$

Thus, for a 70-kilogram male, 56 grams of protein per day is needed to meet the nitrogen requirement. This is essentially the Dietary Reference Intake (DRI) for males.

This calculation assumes that the energy levels are adequate because energy levels may influence protein requirements. When calories are supplied at a level of 45 kilocalories per kilogram body weight per day, egg protein has a nitrogen requirement of 0.65 gram per kilogram body weight per day. At higher energy levels of 57 kilocalories per kilogram body weight per day, the protein requirement declines to 0.45 gram protein per kilogram body weight per day. Also, the 30% decline in efficiency in egg protein as the nitrogen level approaches balance levels may not apply to other protein sources.

An alternate method for calculating protein requirements is the **nitrogen balance method**. For adults, the minimum amount of dietary protein needed to keep the subject in nitrogen equilibrium is the objective. For infants and children, optimal

TABLE 6.8 Estimated Daily Loss of Nitrogen via Various Routes	
Route	**Daily Loss (mg N/kg body weight/day)**
Urine	37
Feces	12
Cutaneous	3
Minor routes (nasal secretions, expired breath, seminal fluid)	2
Total	**54**

growth, not zero nitrogen balance, is the criterion used. The expression for this approach is simple:

$$\text{Balance} = \frac{\text{Diet}}{\text{intake}} - (\text{Urinary N} + \text{Fecal N} + \text{Skin N}) \times 6.2$$

A positive nitrogen balance is considered anabolic as it suggests net deposition, whereas a negative balance is considered catabolic and suggests a net loss of nitrogen. A limitation of this method is that at zero balance, it does not reveal whether there have been shifts within organs or body compartments. The loss of nitrogen by one route may be compensated by decreased loss from another route.

A newer method used to determine dietary protein requirements is referred to as the **indicator amino acid oxidation (IAAO) method**. The rationale for using this method over balance approaches is that, as stated above, the efficiency of protein utilization as it reaches zero balance, is curvilinear and results in a decrease in protein efficiency. This limitation resulted in the research and development of an alternate method of estimating protein requirements.

How does this method work? The principle is that when there are limiting amino acids in the diet that are of insufficient quantities, protein synthesis ceases and the amino acids are oxidized. The method requires an "indicator amino acid". This is an amino acid that is labelled and in excess. A commonly used amino acid is L-1-^{13}C-phenylalanine. At low levels of protein, the oxidation of this amino acid is greater. As the dietary protein levels increase, the oxidation of phenylalanine decreases. When the point is reached that all of the essential amino acids are present in the amounts required for protein synthesis, the oxidation of the phenylalanine plateaus. The point at which the plateau occurs is the Estimated Average Requirement (EAR). Two standard deviations above the EAR is the RDA (**FIGURE 6.19**).

In comparing the balance method to the IAAO method, we can compare the EAR and RDA for each method. For an adult, using the balance method, the EAR and RDA are 0.66 and 0.80 g/kg body weight/day, respectively. Using the IAAO method would result in an EAR and RDA of 0.93 and 1.2 g/kg body weight/day, respectively. Estimates of an EAR and RDA for other age groups (e.g., children, pregnant women, and elderly women) have been determined. In each case, the EAR and RDA using the IAAO methods are much higher than previous values using the balance study. However, those values have not yet been officially adopted by the Food and Nutrition Council as official EAR and RDAs as of this writing. However, later in this chapter (see clinical insight), those values have a significant impact on muscle mass, particularly in older adults.

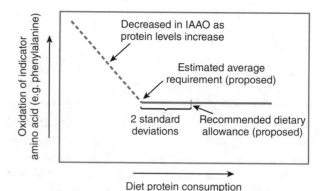

FIGURE 6.19. Theoretical Determination of Protein Requirements and RDA using the Indicator Amino Acid Oxidation Method. Using this technique, the requirement and, therefore, the current RDA, may be underestimated compared with traditional methods to estimate nitrogen requirements.

Modified from Arentson-Lenz et al. *Appl. Physiol. Nutr. Metab.* 2015;40:755-761.

Amino Acids

Determining how much of an essential amino acid should be consumed is not a simple process. Minimum levels of the nonessential amino acid nitrogen may be required when determining the minimal intake needed for an essential amino acid. To study amino acid requirements, a partially purified diet in which synthetic amino acids are incorporated must be used. When any one of the essential amino acids is excluded from the diet, subjects will immediately fall into negative nitrogen balance. The missing amino acid is then fed at graded levels until the criteria for adequacy is met. **TABLE 6.9** lists the requirements for the essential amino acids.

TABLE 6.9 Essential Amino Acid (EAA) Requirements (mg/kg/day) by Age Category			
Amino Acid	**Adults**	**10–12 Years**	**2 Years**
Tryptophan	3.5	4	12.5
Threonine	7	35	37
Isoleucine	10	30	37
Leucine	14	45	73
Lysine	12	60	64
Methionine + cysteine (S-containing)	13	27	27
Phenylalanine + tyrosine (aromatic)	14	27	69
Valine	10	33	38

When an essential amino acid is present in an inadequate amount, protein synthesis ceases. This process is believed to have a molecular basis or control point. More specifically, the initiation complex is most likely affected by the lack of an essential amino acid. A **eukaryotic initiation factor (eIF)** is thought to play a pivotal role. eIF-2 is phosphorylated with GTP to produce an eIF-2-GTP complex. The tRNA for methionine normally forms a complex with eIF-2-GTP. However, when one essential amino acid is missing, the enzyme eIF-2 α-kinase is activated and will phosphorylate the eIF-2-GTP, which blocks the formation of the 43S initiation complex required to initiate protein synthesis (**FIGURE 6.20**).

Organisms have adaptation mechanisms to deal with low protein intakes and, in particular, low intakes of the essential amino acids. In rats and humans fed a

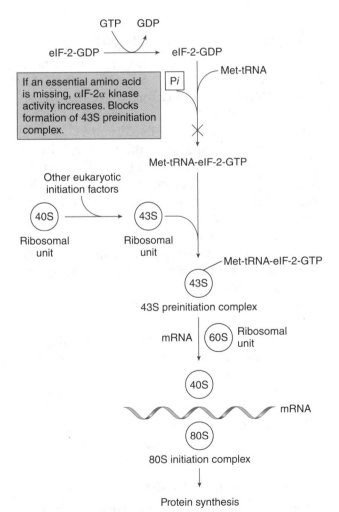

FIGURE 6.20. Initiation of Protein Synthesis Through the Formation of the 43S Preinitiation Complex. When an essential amino acid is depleted, the formation of the 43S preinitiation complex is blocked by phosphorylation via increased αIF2-2α kinase activity. This results in decreased protein synthesis

low-protein diet, amino acid oxidation is minimized. When the dietary protein levels of specific essential amino acids are increased, oxidation will increase only after a level is reached that will meet the needs of optimal growth.

The K_m, or Michaelis-Menton constant, of the enzymes responsible for both amino acid oxidation and mRNA synthesis is critical. The K_m value for an enzyme is an index of the affinity of that enzyme for a particular substrate. Basically, the lower the value, the greater the affinity, and vice versa. Thus, if the K_m is high for a particular enzyme, a relatively higher concentration of a substrate is needed to have an appreciable effect on the enzyme activity because a high K_m means lower enzyme affinity for the substrate. K_m values for amino acid oxidative enzymes are high, and for mRNA, they are low. A low-protein diet provides a reduced amino acid substrate for the enzymes. Because the oxidative enzymes require a higher concentration of amino acids to increase the reaction rate, a low-protein diet decreases the activity of those enzymes, and thus, amino acid catabolism is kept to a minimum. However, mRNA synthesis will still proceed because the K_m values are low. Therefore, for a human consuming a low-protein diet, protein synthesis will continue; that is, humans will direct more of the limited amino acids into protein synthesis.

Some mention of the urea acid cycle enzymes is appropriate with regard to conditions in which protein intake is limited. The liver is the site for excretion of the nitrogenous waste and toxic ammonia compounds of the urea cycle. Altering dietary protein intake alters the activity of urea cycle enzymes. For instance, when protein synthesis decreases, so does the activity of the urea cycle enzymes. Liver arginosuccinate synthetase, for example, declines in activity when rats are fed a low-protein diet. Furthermore, the mRNAs responsible for the coding of urea cycle enzymes also decline in a parallel fashion.

The enzymes responsible for nitrogen removal through the urea cycle and those enzymes used by tissue amino acid metabolism respond to a low-protein diet in different ways with respect to their actions on essential vs nonessential amino acids. As protein intake increases, the activity of enzymes responsible for the catabolism of nonessential amino acids varies in direct response to the dietary protein intake in a linear fashion. For essential amino acids, however, such as branched-chain ketoacid dehydrogenase, activity is relatively low when protein intake is low or below the requirement. Once the protein level has increased to the requirement level or above, enzyme activity increases in a linear fashion. Thus, organisms must have at their disposal unique mechanisms to derive as much gain from the essential amino acids as possible when protein intake is low.

▶ Amino Acid Inborn Errors of Metabolism

A number of inherited diseases pertain to the inability to properly metabolize certain amino acids. We have already discussed issues with homocysteine metabolism as it relates to risk of cardiovascular disease in Special Feature 6.2. This inability to metabolize amino acids is often due to a defect in a rate-limiting enzyme that is critical for the disposal of the amino acid or its role as a precursor to other significant compounds to maintain optimal health. The defects in those enzymes are at the gene level, but there may be several points of gene mutation that differ among individuals but have the same result. At the same time, there may be mutations in the gene that encode for a specific enzyme that have no effect on enzyme activity or result in any significant issue with health. Here, we focus on those genetic defects in enzyme function that result in abnormal amino acid metabolism that compromises health.

Issues with Phenylalanine Metabolism: Phenylketonuria

Phenylketonuria, or **PKU**, is perhaps the best known of the amino acid inborn errors of metabolism. The disease has many genetic variants and is the most common inborn error of amino acid metabolism in Caucasians. Both parents must have the defective gene for this disease to become apparent. PKU is present in 1 out of every 20,000 births.

With PKU, the essential amino acid phenylalanine is unable to be metabolized to the nonessential amino acid tyrosine. The enzyme phenylalanine hydroxylase is defective, thereby blocking the conversion of phenylalanine to tyrosine (see Figure 6.9). As phenylalanine accumulates, it takes a different pathway through a transamination reaction and is converted to phenylpyruvic acid (see Figure 6.9). Urine tests of patients with PKU show a buildup of phenylpyruvic acid. If the disease is not diagnosed in the newborn, high levels of phenylpyruvic acid can build up, leading to mental retardation, unusual irritability, epileptic seizures, and skin lesions. Furthermore, unless there is ample dietary tyrosine, metabolites of tyrosine metabolism, such as DOPA, dopamine, norepinephrine, and epinephrine, are likely to be decreased (see Figure 6.15). The standard treatment for this disease has been restricted dietary phenylalanine, with most of the protein requirement being met by use of phenylalanine-free medical food containing free amino acids. This diet must be continued over a lifetime.

Issues with Tyrosine Metabolism

As mentioned above, tyrosine is important in the synthesis of some key neurotransmitters (see Figure 6.15). However, tyrosine may take another metabolic pathway where it can eventually be metabolized to acetyl CoA (**FIGURE 6.21**). Two disorders can result from defects in enzymes along this pathway. Tyrosine can be converted to a metabolite, p-hydroxyphenylpyruvate, which requires the vitamin B_6-dependent enzyme tyrosine aminotransferase. A defect in this enzyme can result in an accumulation of tyrosine, resulting in a disorder called **tyrosinemia type II**. People afflicted with this disorder require treatment with both a phenylalanine- and tyrosine-restricted diet. If left untreated, mental retardation and skin and eye lesions can develop.

In this same pathway, a disease called **alkaptonuria** can result if there is a defect in the enzyme homogentisate dioxygenase. This enzyme is involved in converting homogentisate, a metabolite generated during the breakdown of tyrosine, to maleylacetoacetate. The defective enzyme results in increased levels of homogentisate in the blood, which can lead to problems with joints and connective tissues.

Issues with Valine, Leucine, and Isoleucine Metabolism: Maple Syrup Urine Disease

Maple syrup urine disease (MSUD) is so named because the urine and feces (cerumen) of untreated neonates have a maple syrup smell. Affected infants have elevated plasma branched-chain amino acids and disturbed plasma amino acid concentration ratios in

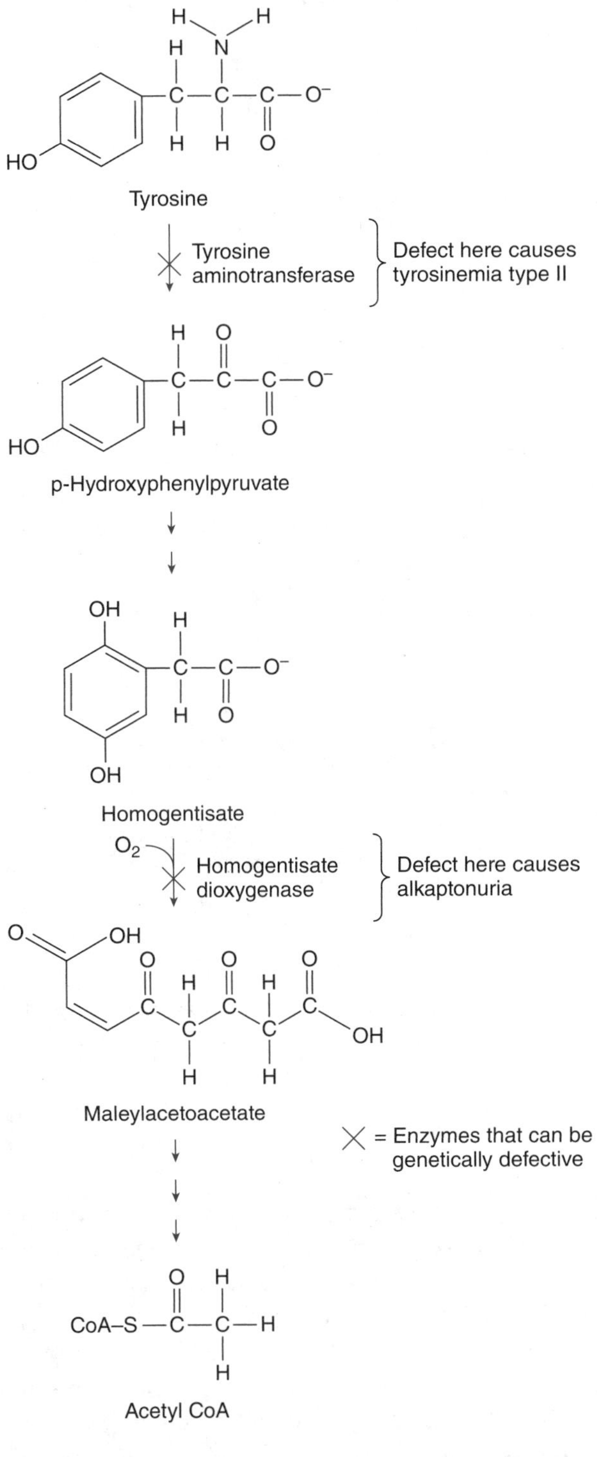

FIGURE 6.21. Metabolism of Tyrosine to Acetyl CoA.
Note that genetic defects in the enzymes tyrosine aminotransferase or homogentisate dioxygenase can lead to the diseases tyrosinemia type II or alkaptonuria, respectively.

the first day of life. They demonstrate ketonuria, irritability, lethargy, and poor feeding. The condition may lead to respiratory difficulties, coma, and death within 1 week.

MSUD can be diagnosed not only by clinical symptoms but also by the decreased activity of the branched-chain α-ketoacid dehydrogenase (BCKAD) complex, the second enzymatic step in the degradative pathway of the branched-chain amino acids. BCKAD has four components (E1a, E1b, E2, and E3), and mutations in both alleles of any subunit can result in decreased activity of the enzyme complex, which, in turn, results in the accumulation of branched-chain amino acids and corresponding branched-chain ketoacids in tissues and plasma (**FIGURE 6.22**).

The most problematic amino acid in this disease is leucine. Neurologic signs of leucine intolerance and intoxication in older individuals vary and can include cognitive impairment, hyperactivity, anorexia, sleep disturbances, hallucinations, mood swings, focal dystonia, choreoathetosis, and ataxia. Treatment requires limiting the intake of branched-chain amino acids, especially leucine. During acute flare-ups, protein restriction or protein-free diets may be used. Intravenous nutrients may be administered, and hemodialysis or peritoneal dialysis may be used until amino acid levels normalize in blood. Special foods that are limited in those branched-chain amino acids are available.

Issues with Methionine Metabolism

An earlier discussion in the chapter noted the role that a derivative of methionine, homocysteine, has on increasing the risk of cardiovascular disease. A defect in cystathionine β synthase can lead to increased levels of homocysteine, which is thought to be a risk factor for heart disease (**FIGURE 6.23**).

Methionine is a critical amino acid because it contains sulfur and is a precursor to cysteine, another critical sulfur-containing amino acid. However, another major role of methionine is as a methyl donor in biochemical reactions. The form of this methyl donor is referred to as **S-adenosyl methionine (SAM)**. SAM is needed for the synthesis of carnitine, creatine, melatonin, and epinephrine. The enzyme that converts methionine to SAM is methionine adenosyl transferase. In some instances, this enzyme may be genetically defective, resulting in increased blood methionine levels. People with this condition (**hypermethioninemia**) require a methionine-restricted diet and supplementation with extra cysteine.

In the catabolism of methionine to succinyl CoA, two enzymes may be defective: propionyl CoA carboxylase and methylmalonyl CoA mutase. Those two defects results in **propionic acidemia** and

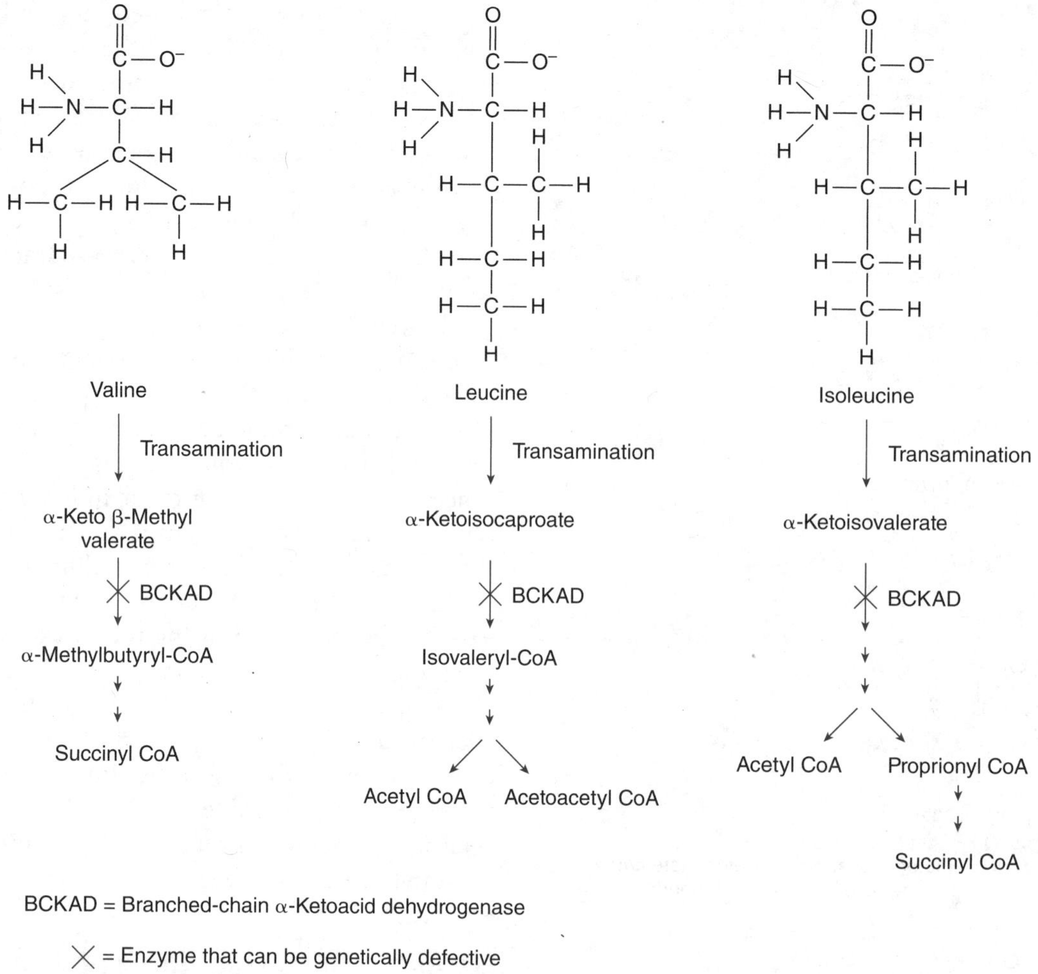

FIGURE 6.22. Metabolism of Branched-Chain Amino Acids: Valine, Leucine, and Isoleucine. These branched chain amino acids may have a defective gene encoding for branched-chain α-ketoacid dehydrogenase. This results in an accumulation of branched-chain amino acids known as Maple Syrup Urine Disease.

methylmalonic acidemia, respectively. Defects in those enzymes can result in a number of clinical defects in newborns, such as failure to thrive, ketosis, and respiratory difficulties. Methionine levels need to be restricted for infants with either enzyme defect.

Issues with Tryptophan Metabolism

A major function of tryptophan in human nutrition is that one of its breakdown products is niacin, or vitamin B_3. The ratio of the conversion of tryptophan to niacin is about 60 to 1. Another pathway leads to the production of acetyl CoA (**FIGURE 6.24**). It is in this latter pathway where two genetic defects have been identified. One disorder occurs due to a defect in the gene that encodes for the enzyme α-ketoadipic dehydrogenase (**α-ketoadipic aciduria**). That enzyme converts an intermediate, α-ketoadipic acid, to glutaryl CoA.

When the enzyme is defective, a number of metabolites, including tryptophan, lysine, and metabolic acids, build up. Infants born with this disorder have difficulty with motor skills and may have seizures. A tryptophan- and lysine-restricted diet is essential for those individuals. Lysine is implicated here because when lysine is degraded it is also converted into α-ketoadipic acid.

Glutaric aciduria type 1 is the second disorder of tryptophan metabolism. It is the result of a defect in the enzyme glutaryl CoA dehydrogenase. This enzyme converts glutaryl CoA to glutaconyl CoA. As stated above, this enzyme is also critical to the breakdown of lysine. The glutaryl CoA is converted to glutaric acid and accumulates in fluids. This accumulation can lead to seizures, acidosis, and an enlarged head. As stated above, the treatment is a tryptophan- and lysine-restricted diet. Sometimes, vitamin B_2 may be given because it is a cofactor for glutaryl CoA dehydrogenase.

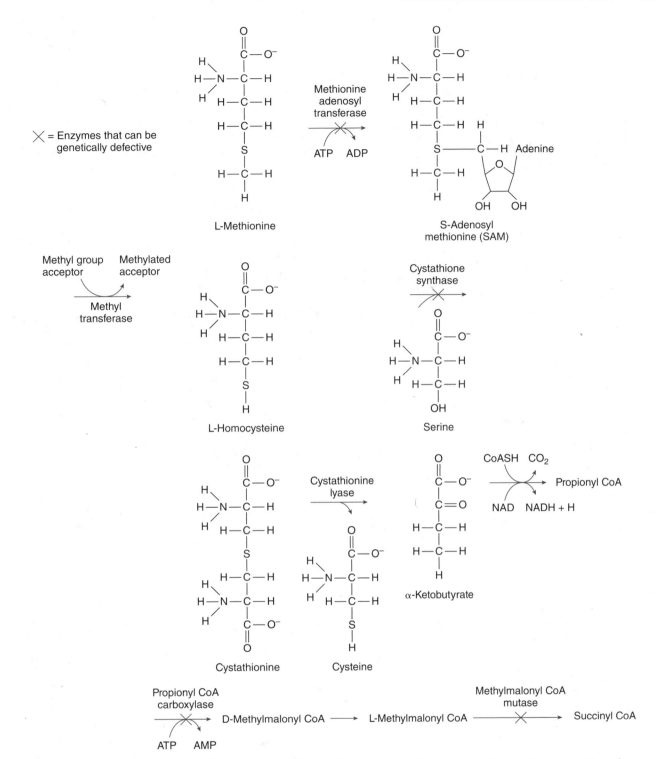

FIGURE 6.23. Metabolism of Methionine to Succinyl CoA. There are multiple genetic defects in the conversion of methionine to succinyl CoA. Often, methionine restricted diets are given to infants with those defects.

Issues with Lysine, Glycine, and Threonine Metabolism

As has been discussed previously, with disorders of tryptophan metabolism, lysine needs to be restricted due to the degradation of lysine sharing a common pathway when lysine is broken down to glutaryl CoA.

Threonine is a precursor to glycine, and glycine is a precursor to serine. However, threonine can be converted to either succinyl CoA or pyruvate, making them glucogenic and ketogenic. When it is converted to succinyl CoA, two enzymes are defective in the process: propionyl CoA carboxylase and methylmalonyl CoA mutase

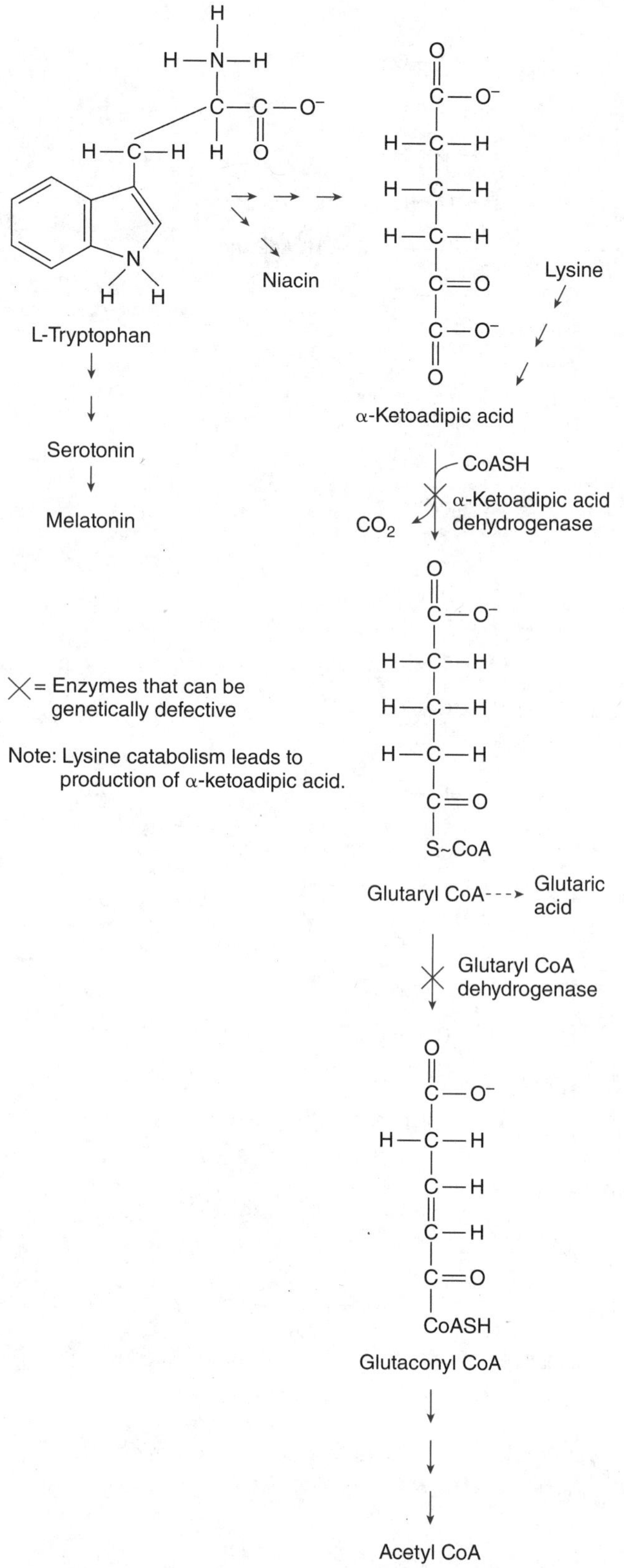

= Enzymes that can be genetically defective

Note: Lysine catabolism leads to production of α-ketoadipic acid.

FIGURE 6.24. Metabolism of L-Tryptophan to Niacin and Acetyl CoA. Genetic defects in the enzymes α-ketoadipic acid or glutaryl CoA dehydrogenases may occur and various metabolites accumulate that have serious health consequences. Treatment often requires a tryptophan- and lysine-restricted diet.

(FIGURE 6.25). The blockage in those two enzymes leads to propionic acidemia and methylmalonic acidemia, respectively.

Finally, the simplest of all of the amino acids, glycine, may also have impaired catabolism due to genetic defects in not one enzyme, but rather an enzyme complex. This complex will convert glycine in some cases to carbon dioxide and ammonia. However, when there are defects in the genes that encode the enzymes in the complex, increased blood glycine levels (**hyperglycinemia**) can result. Elevated blood glycine levels in infants may lead to neurologic impairment and seizures. A low-protein diet is used to treat those with this disorder because glycine is found in almost all proteins.

⬡ BEFORE YOU GO ON . . .

1. In PKU, which metabolite accumulates in the blood, and which health issues affect infants?

2. List two genetic disorders of tyrosine metabolism. Which type of diet is needed to control those disorders?

3. What is the basic cause of maple syrup urine disease, and how is it treated?

4. What is glutaric aciduria type 1?

5. Defects in which two enzymes result in the conversion of the amino acid threonine to succinyl CoA?

▸ Leucine and other Branched Chain Amino Acids as Related to Body Composition and Obesity

Recent studies have reported that increased intake of branched chain amino acids, in particular, leucine, can increase lean body (muscle) mass as well as decreasing body weight and adiposity, particularly in energy-controlled studies and more so in combination with exercise. Studies in both rodents and humans have yielded some consistent findings on this issue, but studies have not been 100% in agreement. Nonetheless, it would appear that the overall evidence supports some role of those amino acids and, in particular, leucine, in activating a key signaling pathway (mTOR-discussed below) that leads to protein production in muscle and other body tissue. With respect to the enhancement of lean body mass, leucine and other branched chain amino acids appear to

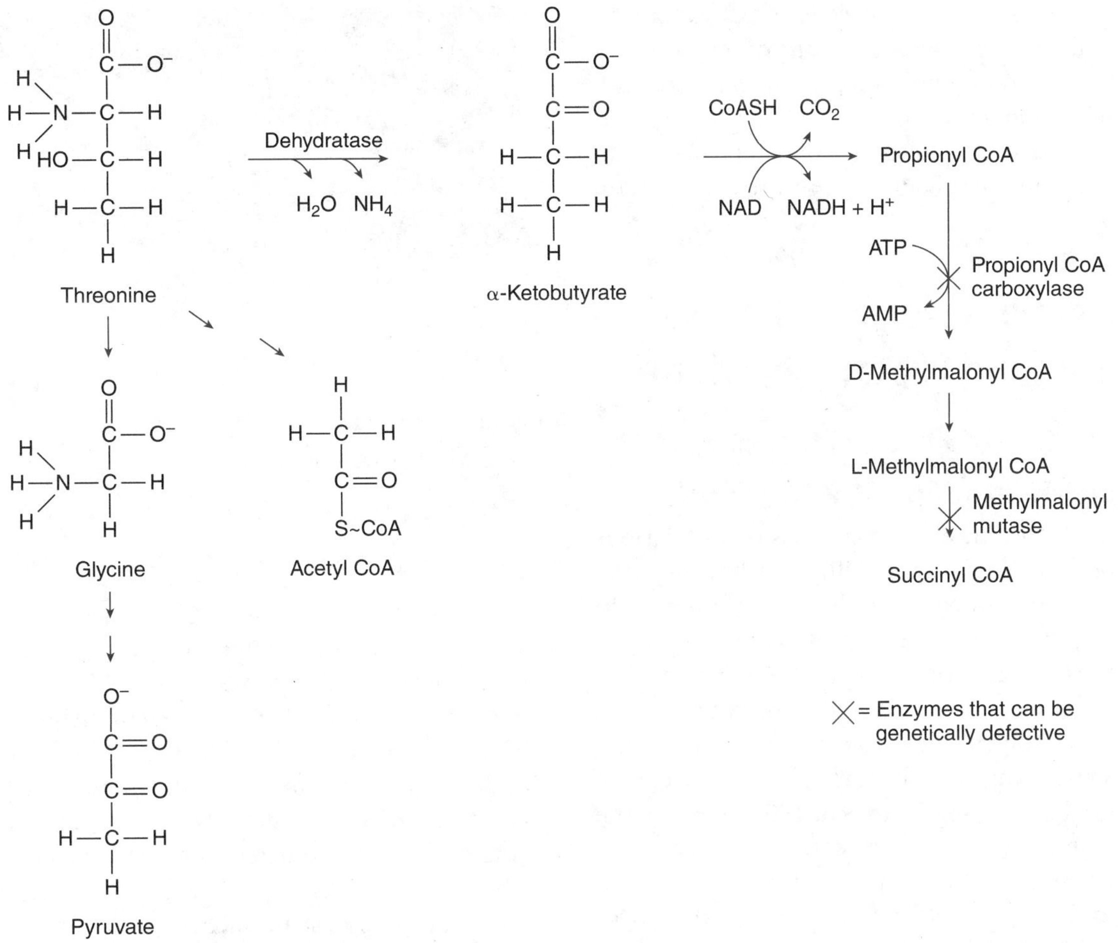

FIGURE 6.25. Metabolism of Threonine. Threonine can be metabolized via two pathways. One pathway can lead to the conversion of threonine to acetyl CoA and the other to succinyl CoA. Note that two enzymes in the synthesis of succinyl CoA from threonine may be defective.

increase or at least prevent the loss of lean body mass when consumed in combination with a complete protein. One study suggested that slightly more than 7 g of leucine per day resulted in lean body mass in older adults. Furthermore, this would amount to 2.3 to 2.8 grams of leucine at each meal for those over 65 years of age. This level of leucine appears to stimulate muscle protein synthesis and this threshold level appears to be relatively higher in older individuals than their younger counterparts.

In addition to leucine's potential role in preventing the loss of lean body mass, it would appear that obesity development could be lessened and/or reversed by increased intake. Studies in both humans and rodents suggest that branched-chain amino acids and leucine, in particular, can reduce the potential for obesity resulting from a high-fat diet in addition to reducing high blood glucose levels and abnormal blood lipid levels. It would appear that not only obesity per se is modulated but metabolic syndrome may

also be attenuated. One potential mechanism is a pathway, mTOR, that is a cell signaling and transduction pathway. It is involved via a group of kinases in cell growth, survival and proliferation, and protein transcription and translation. **mTOR** appears to increase protein synthesis that enhanced lean body mass while blocking proinflammatory cytokines. Another mechanism implicated in the reduction of obesity with increased leucine involves the **SIRT1-AMPK-PGC-1α complex**. SIRT1 is also known as sirtuin and NAD-dependent deacetylase sirtuin-1. Its function is to deacetylate regulatory transcription factors, thereby activating them. One such regulatory factor is PGC-1α, which is the master regulator of mitochondrial biogenesis. Increased SIRT1 activity improves insulin sensitivity. 5' adenosine monophosphate-activated kinase (AMPK) is an enzyme that enhances fatty acid oxidation in the liver, blocks cholesterol and triglyceride biosynthesis, decreases lipogenesis, and helps to maintain normal insulin secretions in pancreatic beta cells. Taken together, the results of related studies suggest that a diet with a higher leucine content, particularly where protein makes a higher contribution to an appropriate total energy intake could be incrementally beneficial in improving certain metabolic aberrations.

▶ Protein Quality, Protein Excess, and Protein Deficiency

Determination of Protein Intakes by Food Source Based on Limiting Amino Acids

Knowledge of the amino acid composition of various protein sources facilitates the ability to determine what levels of protein are needed in the diets of humans to meet minimum needs. Protein quality differs substantially in different areas of the world. Protein digestibility and the amino acid score, as discussed previously, are critical in determining protein requirements. The U.S. Food and Drug Administration (FDA), as part of its nutrition labeling regulations of 1993, required the use of the protein digestibility-corrected amino acid scoring method of protein quality evaluation for the labeling of food products intended for children over 1 year of age and adults.

To calculate the protein intake for a person of a particular age, the Food and Agriculture Organization (FAO) of the World Health Organization (WHO) developed guidelines, including publishing safe levels of protein intake. Those are levels of protein that, when consumed on a daily per kilogram body weight basis, will meet the amino acid requirements for an individual of a certain age. Safe levels have been established for the reference proteins milk, eggs, meat, and fish in three different age ranges (**TABLE 6.10**). The age groups are adults, children aged 1 to 6 years and children aged 6 to 12 years. After age 12 years, adult values are used. To apply this information, the protein digestibility needs to be known. However, rather than analyzing a meal for each protein fraction and determining separate digestibility, the WHO has simplified the process by using one of two values. If a diet is composed of coarse food items, whole grain cereals, and vegetables, a digestibility of 85% may be a close approximation. If refined cereals are more likely to be found in the diet, a digestibility of 95% is suggested.

Critical pieces of information that are needed are the amino acid scores for the essential amino acids of the diet consumed. This information allows for the determination of one or more limiting amino acids. Lysine,

TABLE 6.10 Safe Levels of Reference Protein (Milk, Eggs, Meat, and Fish) for Different Age Groups	
Age	**Safe Level of Reference Protein (g/kg/day)**
Adults	0.75
Children (preschool; ages 1–6 years)	1.10
Children (school aged; 6–12 years)	0.99

methionine (plus cysteine), threonine, and tryptophan are the amino acids that are most limiting in the world's diets. The minimum levels of each of these amino acids have been determined for the three age ranges, as well as the levels of the amino acids present in a typical diet. From such data, the amino acid scores for those four amino acids can be determined and thus the limiting amino acid(s) determined in each diet. With this information, it is possible to calculate the amount of dietary protein required for either maintenance or growth.

For example, a preschool-aged child has a reference requirement for lysine of 58 milligrams per gram of protein. A rural Tunisian diet provides 33 milligrams per gram of protein with respect to lysine. The amino acid score is $(33/58) \times 100\%$, or 57%. The safe level of protein intake for a preschool-aged child is 1.10 grams per kilogram body weight per day. The diet is likely to be coarse, and thus a digestibility of 85% may be assumed. From this information, one can calculate the amount of protein that this child should consume from the available diet to meet the minimum amino acid requirement:

1.10 grams of protein/kilogram body weight/day × (100%/85%) × (100%/57%) = 2.27 grams of protein/kilogram body weight/day

Thus, 2.27 grams of protein per kilogram body weight per day from a rural Tunisian diet needs to be consumed for this child to stay in positive nitrogen balance.

If one knows the protein content of various foods, the amount or total quantity of food needed can be determined. Although this approach is not likely to be practical on an individual basis, it does give relief agencies, government agencies, and related institutions some guidelines to use in estimating food production needs, import requirements, and emergency food aid.

Excess Dietary Protein

Is it possible to eat too much protein? In the United States, a lack of protein is seldom a problem, unlike in other parts of the world. However, there is some concern that Americans may be consuming too much protein. Most studies suggest that America as a nation consumes twice the required levels needed. The question must then be posed: Can this have a detrimental influence on human health? Although the subject is still being debated, some causes for concern have been suggested, including increased renal stress leading to impaired function; bone demineralization; an increased incidence of colon cancer due to the type of bacteria present in a high-nitrogen environment; and obesity, particularly in America, where high-protein foods are often high in fat.

The consumption of individual amino acid supplements has also been suggested to have detrimental possibilities. Because amino acid absorption transport systems are shared, increased consumption of a particular amino acid may reduce the absorption of other amino acids, potentially leading to imbalance. Supplements of individual amino acids should not be taken in conjunction with protein-rich meals unless these amino acids are deficient in the meal.

Protein Undernutrition

Protein-energy malnutrition (PEM) [also known as protein-calorie malnutrition (PCM)] is the most prevalent form of undernutrition in the world. Whether the problem is lack of total protein or poor protein quality, **kwashiorkor** is often the result. **Marasmus** may also occur, or a combination of both diseases. Kwashiorkor is a disease resulting from a lack of dietary protein. Marasmus results from a lack of energy or calories (lack of food) and protein. In kwashiorkor, one may consume seemingly adequate energy, but not enough protein. In this disease, the subject appears pot-bellied due to edema, has depigmented (red and white) and easily pluckable hair, a moon-faced appearance, facial expressions that resemble agony, skin lesions, a fatty liver, and decreased antibodies and is more susceptible to disease. The victim does have some body fat.

Individuals suffering from marasmus, in contrast, are emaciated from excessive muscle wasting and have minimal body fat. Clinically, marasmus is most commonly observed in 6- to 18-month-old children who were not breast-fed or who were weaned to poor diets. Even when adequate protein is present, the body will use it for energy, and thus symptoms similar to kwashiorkor may appear in the individual suffering from marasmus. Marasmus victims display excessive crying, mostly due to hunger. In contrast, individuals with kwashiorkor experience increased pain and possess a decreased ability to cry due to impaired brain functions.

Protein-malnourished females will often give birth to small or premature infants who are underdeveloped neurologically as well as physically. Brain damage can result in the toddler stage even if the undernutrition does not occur until after birth. Undernutrition at practically any point in the life cycle

---

SPECIAL FEATURE 6.3

Causes of Global Protein Undernutrition

The causes of protein undernutrition may be debatable, but certain elements are common in areas where protein undernutrition and simple undernutrition are prevalent. It was once dogma that overpopulation and inadequate food production were the primary causes of undernutrition. Although those aspects contribute, there are other factors, such as the greed of those in power or in control; unemployment; lack of productive resources, including natural resources; lack of available land, credit, and proper tools; and lack of technology in many areas. Also, there is a problem with developed nations not transferring their technology to those who could benefit from it. Debt and trade imbalances play a role: the high cost of oil means that more is spent to buy that commodity than what a nation may get for a crop. Cultural traditions may also make things worse. Women often will perform heavy physical labor, even when pregnant, to help support the family and will often feed their husbands and older children first. Often, the mother will eat last or an infant who is already weaned will get what is left over.

Catastrophes and weather-related issues, such as droughts, may influence food supply. War and civil unrest are man's own creation of misery on earth. The sub-Saharan region is an example of an area in which the ecology for agriculture

(continues)

SPECIAL FEATURE 6.3 *(continued)*

production is deteriorating. Many nations do not have adequate food reserves to get by in case of an emergency. Lack of economic incentives may exist, and farmers may not own their land. Disease and parasites play a large role and one that often is ignored. When considering undernutrition, one must also look at the disease states of those afflicted. Many have parasites and infections (malaria, cholera, dysentery, etc.) that will increase their nutritional requirements even more.

The United States is not without its own undernutrition problems. However, those problems are not likely to be related to protein issues. Undernutrition in the United States traditionally has been restricted to economically poor African Americans, southern Americans, immigrant workers, unemployed minorities, and some of the elderly; however, it is now extending into other parts of the population. Those include such diverse groups as youngsters (500,000 of whom are believed to be malnourished); the "new poor," namely, displaced farm families and laid-off blue-collar workers; the elderly; and the homeless. Problems with lack of health insurance, the rising costs of living, and inflation contribute to undernutrition. The homeless are often malnourished. Estimates of the homeless in the United States range from 3 to 5 million, which are staggering figures. More than half of the homeless are single mothers. Many were once in mental institutions. Low-income women, especially single mothers with children, often have undernutrition problems. Ethnic minorities, such as African Americans and Hispanics, experience a greater prevalence of malnutrition. The unifying factor in this list of affected groups is a lack of income with which to buy nutrient-dense foods.

lessens resistance to illness and infection. Height and head size may be relatively low in a child or infant. Malnourished children show little curiosity or eagerness to learn. They often have difficulty learning in school because they may have shorter attention spans and are unable to concentrate. Malnourished adults are usually less physically active, may work at a slower pace, and often have poor general health. Also, malnourished individuals may suffer nutritionally from more than just a lack of protein and energy. They may have vitamin and mineral deficiencies superimposed on the lack of the macronutrients. Around half of the 5 billion people in the world suffer from undernutrition of some type.

⬡ BEFORE YOU GO ON . . .

1. Explain from a mechanism perspective how dietary leucine may reduce obesity and metabolic syndrome?

2. What two pieces of information do you need to determine the safe and adequate intake of a protein source for a child?

3. What would be the safe protein intake for a 10-year-old boy consuming a coarse diet with an amino acid score of 65%?

4. What are some potential problems of consuming a high-protein diet?

5. What are the major differences between marasmus and kwashiorkor?

🩺 CLINICAL INSIGHT

Debate on the Levels of Protein Intake, Exercise, and Sarcopenia

While the adult RDA for protein is currently 0.8 g/kg body weight per day, recently, there has been a debate on this figure. A higher protein intake has been debated in the last several years. This increase has focused on the elderly; more specifically, on approaches to prevent sarcopenia. Sarcopenia is a decrease in muscle mass and strength, and this is a frequent condition in the older adult. This results in an increase frailty and the likelihood of falls among older adults. While many Americans do consume more than the RDA for protein, there are a number who fail to consume even this level of 0.8 g/kg/day. The older adult may be more challenged in consuming adequate levels of food and, consequently, less protein. Adequate dietary protein intake is essential for muscle protein synthesis. In addition to the older adult, there is a growing concern over protein malnutrition in the hospitalized patients at various parts of the life cycle.

As indicated above, the RDA was developed using balance studies. This may best reflect a minimal level of protein rather than an optimal protein level as it relates to overall health. While more recent research suggests that higher protein recommendations are appropriate for athletes as well as during aging and weight loss, this has led to some debate as to whether a higher protein intake is potentially problematic in the long run. The conventional dogma from a clinical perspective is that increased protein intake may present issues with kidney integrity. However, the issue with protein and renal function may be more linked to those who have developed kidney disease and require significant dietary modifications to maintain renal function. Said differently, this does not mean that increased dietary protein intake leads to negative issues in renal function. In fact, when one reviews available research addressing protein intake and renal health, it is indeed difficult to determine that a link between elevated protein intake and kidney disease exists.

Muscle loss is lowest in subjects consuming 1.2 g/kg/day of protein than those consuming 0.8g/kg/day. The increase in protein intake goes beyond minimizing muscle loss but, in fact, it leads to increased muscle mass, especially when combined with weight bearing exercises. Intake above the 0.8 g/kg/day figure, especially when skewed toward one meal, was discouraged because the amino acids needed to be present for protein synthesis to occur. Those amino acids that were in excess are thought to be lost or catabolized and thus wasted. This may not be the case in older adults who appear to require relatively higher intake to achieve a similar response.

The distribution of protein intake throughout the day has received attention. Having most protein at one meal (e.g. dinner) rather than evenly spread throughout the day has been the norm for protein intake. The minimum amount of protein is consumed at breakfast and evidence suggests that this should be increased. Some studies suggest that a more even intake of protein throughout the day supports more desirable body composition changes, especially when paired with exercise. Furthermore, the most effective level of protein to maximize muscle protein response immediately after exercise can be influenced by the type of exercise and how muscle body musculature is involved. Said differently, more protein would be needed after a whole body workout versus a workout that involved limited muscle groups. Moreover, the quality of protein must be considered. For instance, the amino acid leucine has been shown to increase muscle protein synthesis, as discussed previously.

In addition to the role of an increased diet protein intake as it relates to preventing or slowing down sarcopenia progression, a higher level of protein is likely to lead to better weight maintenance. Controlled studies have demonstrated greater weight loss on high protein diets, as well as appetite control. Taken together, an intake of 1.2 to 1.6 g protein/kg/day may provide better health benefits than the current RDA or the proposed one of 1.2 g/kg/day; and some recommend even a greater intake of 1.5 to 2.0 g/kg/day to account for higher energy expenditure than assumed for the RDAs, such as for performance athletes.

Dealing with minimizing the impact of sarcopenia is more than simply increasing dietary protein. Lifestyle activities play a role. One lifestyle factor that has to be considered is the issue of exercise, particularly, resistant exercise, singly or in combination with increased protein intake. Resistance training attenuates muscle loss in older adults and with increased protein levels combined with resistance exercise, the attenuation is even greater. There have been a number of studies that have reported consistent results on the slowing of muscle loss with resistance exercise; and many report that having increased dietary protein levels with resistance exercise results in increased muscle mass. From a clinical perspective, it is likely that both increased protein intake and exercise are likely to minimize muscle frailty in the older adult and reduce the incidence of sarcopenia.

▶ **Here's What You Have Learned**

1. Although approximately 140 amino acids are found in nature, only 20 are genetically encoded. A common characteristic of amino acids is that they have an asymmetric, or α-carbon, which has attached to it an amino group, a carboxyl group, and a hydrogen atom. The fourth entity attached to the asymmetric carbon is unique from one amino acid to the next.

2. Human cells are unable to synthesize eight to nine amino acids, either at all or in adequate amounts to meet the needs for growth and maintenance. Those amino acids, termed dietary essential amino acids, are lysine, tryptophan, methionine, valine, phenylalanine, leucine, isoleucine, threonine, and, for infants, histidine. A limiting amino acid is an essential amino acid present in a food that is found in an amount that would be insufficient to support growth or maintenance if it were the sole source of protein.

3. Proteins take on varying degrees of complexity. The primary structure is that determined by the genetic code and is simply a polymer of amino acids. The secondary structure refers to chemical interactions among the amino acids forming the primary structure via hydrogen bonds and disulfide linkages. Spiral (e.g., α-helix), globular, or flat sheet (e.g., β-pleated sheet) arrangements

are common. The tertiary structures of proteins are produced by the coiling of molecules and bonding within molecules that determine the general shape of proteins.

4. Protein digestion begins in the stomach, where HCl is secreted. This HCl causes pepsinogen to be activated to pepsin, an enzyme capable of hydrolyzing proteins. HCl also causes proteins to be denatured and linearized so that pepsin may better hydrolyze proteins. Further protein digestion occurs in the small intestine, where the pancreatic enzymes trypsin, chymotrypsin, and carboxypeptidases A and B hydrolyze the proteins into smaller polypeptide units. The final hydrolysis of the peptides produced by those series of reactions via pancreatic enzymes occurs at the surface of the microvilli membranes of the intestinal mucosal cells. The aminopeptidases take the peptides and yield individual amino acids and oligopeptides (three or four amino acid fragments). Thus, the net result of luminal digestion in the small intestine is short oligopeptide fragments, dipeptides, and amino acids.

5. Free amino acid absorption is an energy-dependent, carrier-mediated mechanism. There are several transport carriers for amino acids. All of those carriers have the following elements in common: (1) transport is against a concentration gradient; (2) the carrier is specific for L-isomers and will not absorb D-isomers; (3) energy in the form of ATP is required; (4) sodium and vitamin B_6 are required; and (5) carboxyl, amino, and α-H groups are required. There are also four separate types of amino acid carriers: neutral amino acids, imino amino acids, basic amino acids, and dicarboxylic acid amino acids. Tetrapeptidases in the brush border of the microvilli membrane hydrolyze tetrapeptides into tripeptides and free amino acids. Tripeptidases are present in both membrane and cytoplasm in equal amounts. Dipeptidases are found commonly in the mucosal cell cytoplasm.

6. The quality of a protein depends on the amount of essential amino acids and, most important, the concentration of the limiting amino acid in a food. Many measures of protein quality have been developed, including biological value, net protein utilization, protein efficiency ratio, and amino acid score.

7. Proteins have many functions and roles: enzymes; blood transporters; plasma proteins that not only transport other constituents but also control water balance; clotting factors; muscle proteins for contraction; hormones, such as glucagons and insulin, as well as hypothalamic hormones; connective tissue proteins (elastin, collagen); acid–base balance; immune function; the use of amino acids for energy; and the use of amino acids as precursors for other compounds, such as biogenic amines.

8. Amino acids are different from other energy nutrients in that they contain the element nitrogen, which can be removed or transferred to another carbon skeleton to create a different amino acid. Transamination reactions involve an amino transferase enzyme that transfers the amino group to an α-keto acid, whereas deamination reactions, catalyzed by deaminases, remove amine groups to form ammonia. Vitamin B_6 is needed for transamination reactions to occur.

9. Synthesis of amino acids is limited to nonessential amino acids and post-translational derivatives of nonessential amino acids (e.g., hydroxyproline). Many amino acids are derived from intermediates of glycolysis and the Krebs cycle. Serine can be synthesized from the glycolytic intermediate 3-phosphoglycerate and can then serve as a precursor for glycine and cysteine. Whereas the carbon skeleton and nitrogen of cysteine are derived from serine, methionine is needed to supply sulfur. Alanine is produced via the transamination of pyruvate.

10. The nonessential amino acids derived from Krebs cycle intermediates include aspartate, asparagine, glutamate, glutamine, proline, and arginine. Aspartate is derived from oxaloacetate via transamination, and asparagine can then be synthesized from aspartate by amidation. Glutamate is derived from α-ketoglutarate either by transamination or by the addition of ammonia via glutamate dehydrogenase. Glutamine, proline, and arginine are also produced from glutamate. Glutamine is generated via amidation, whereas proline and arginine are derived from glutamate semialdehyde, which is the result of the reduction of glutamate. Proline requires the cyclization of glutamate semialdehyde, whereas the creation of arginine requires glutamate semialdehyde to first be converted to ornithine, which is eventually converted to arginine by way of urea cycle reactions.

11. When the carbon skeletons of amino acids are degraded, the major products are pyruvate, acetyl CoA, intermediates of the Krebs cycle,

and the ketone body acetoacetate. Amino acids whose carbon skeletons form pyruvate or intermediates of the Krebs cycle are deemed glucogenic. Those whose amino acid skeletons become acetyl CoA and acetoacetate are deemed ketogenic because they can form ketone bodies. Although most amino acids are either glucogenic or ketogenic, a few amino acids—namely, tryptophan, phenylalanine, tyrosine, and isoleucine—are both. Leucine is the only amino acid that is only ketogenic. That is, it does not produce glucogenic intermediates.

12. Glutamine is a nonessential amino acid that plays a critical role in the interorgan transport of nitrogen and carbon. Glutamine can be used to rid cells and tissues of excess ammonia if the latter does not enter the urea cycle. Other significant functions of glutamine include its precursor role in the creation of the purine and pyrimidine nucleotide bases used in the synthesis of RNA and DNA and its role in the production of glucosamines, asparagines, and nicotinamide adenine dinucleotide.

13. The alanine–glucose cycle is a key method of supplying energy to muscle. Alanine comes from the muscle via the transamination of pyruvate. Alanine leaves the muscle and can be taken up by liver cells. When in the liver, alanine is transaminated with α-ketoglutarate; the resulting pyruvate enters gluconeogenesis, and the resulting glutamate may enter the urea cycle.

14. A number of amino acids are involved in neurotransmission and brain function. Among those are glutamate, aspartate, GABA, glycine, taurine, tyrosine, and tryptophan. Tyrosine is a precursor to serotonin and melatonin, whereas tryptophan is a precursor to the catecholamine class of neurotransmitters. Drugs have been developed to augment those amino acid derivatives that stimulate the nervous system in order to help combat depression and anxiety disorders.

15. The buildup of ammonia from deamination reactions is toxic to human cells and organs and needs to be dealt with. Ammonia is, therefore, converted to urea through a metabolic pathway known as the urea cycle. The urea cycle consists of five reactions that convert ammonia, carbon dioxide, and the α-amino nitrogen of aspartate into urea. Two of the reactions occur within the mitochondria, and the remaining reactions occur in the cytoplasm.

16. Protein requirements can be determined by the factorial method or the nitrogen balance method. The factorial method relies on feeding a human subject an energy-sufficient but nitrogen-free diet and measuring the nitrogen losses in the feces, urine, skin, and so on to determine how much protein needs to be replaced. Factors, such as protein quality and digestibility, are considered to arrive at an estimate. The nitrogen balance method measures diet nitrogen intake and subtracts the level of nitrogen appearing in the urine, feces, and skin. A newer method suggests that protein requirements may be greater. The indicator amino acid oxidation method may be superior to other older methods in overcoming some of their limitations.

17. If a limiting amino acid is not present in sufficient amounts, protein synthesis ceases. A particularly important molecular mechanism is the eukaryotic initiation factor (eIF). eIF-2 is phosphorylated with GTP to produce an eIF-2-GTP complex. The tRNA for methionine normally forms a complex with eIF-2-GTP. However, when one essential amino acid is missing, the enzyme eIF-2 α-kinase is activated and phosphorylates the eIF-2-GTP, which blocks the formation of the 43S initiation complex required to initiate protein synthesis.

18. When protein intake is low, human enzymes can adapt. For instance, with limited protein intake, catabolic enzymes directed at amino acids have lower activity. Liver arginosuccinate synthetase, for example, declines in activity when rats are fed a low-protein diet. Furthermore, the mRNAs responsible for the coding of urea cycle enzymes also decline in a parallel fashion.

19. Branched chain amino acids and leucine, in particular, may prevent weight gain and/or even reverse obesity.

20. A number of inborn errors of metabolism impair the metabolism of amino acids. Phenylketonuria (PKU) and maple syrup urine disease (MSUD) are two of the most well-known of those disorders, affecting the catabolism of phenylalanine and branched-chain amino acids, respectively. Other amino acids in which metabolism may be impaired include methionine, L-tryptophan, threonine, lysine, and glycine.

21. Because protein quality may vary worldwide, the World Health Organization has determined guidelines as to what constitutes safe levels of protein intake by age in terms of grams per kilogram body weight per day for a reference protein (usually meat, milk, egg, or fish). From those values and knowing the limiting amino

acid in the food supply and whether the diet is coarse or refined (to estimate percent digestibility), one can calculate how many grams per day a person needs to achieve adequate amino acid intake.

22. Consuming more protein than that needed for energy balance does not result in more muscle mass, but more likely in more body fat. In contrast, protein deficiency is a much more serious and worldwide problem. A lack of protein with adequate calories in young children leads to kwashiorkor, in which the classic pot-belly appearance is common. A lack of overall calories leads to emaciation and is called marasmus.

▶ Suggested Reading

Antonio J, Ellerbroek A, Silver T, et al. A high protein diet has no harmful effects: a one-year crossover study in resistance-trained males. *J Nutr Metab.* 2016;2016:9104792. Epub 2016 Oct 11.

Arentson-Lantz E, Clairmont S, Paddon-Jones D, Tremblay A, Elango R. Protein: a nutrient in focus. *Appl Physiol Nutr Metab.* 2015;40(8):755–761.

Brosnan JT. Glutamate, at the interface of amino acid and carbohydrate metabolism. *J Nutr.* 2000;130(4S suppl):988S–990S.

Creighton TE. *Protein Structure: A Practical Approach.* Washington, DC: IRL Press; 1997.

Curthoys NP, Watford M. Regulation of glutaminase activity and glutamine metabolism. *Ann Rev Nutr.* 1995;15:133–159.

Layman DK, Boileau RA, Erickson DJ, et al. A reduced ratio of dietary carbohydrate to protein improves body composition and blood lipid profiles during weight loss in adult women. *J Nutr.* 2003;133(2):411–417.

Layman DK, Evans E, Baum JI, Seyler J, Erickson DJ, Boileau RA. Dietary protein and exercise have additive effects on body composition during weight loss in adult women. *J Nutr.* 2005;135(8):1903–1910.

Lepe M, Gascón B, Cruz J. Long-term efficacy of high-protein diets: a systematic review. *Nutr Hosp.* 2011;26(6):1256–1259.

Liepa GU, ed. *Dietary Proteins: How They Alleviate Disease and Promote Better Health.* Champaign, IL: American Oil Chemists Society; 1992.

McDonald CK, Ankarfeldt MZ, Capra S, Bauer J, Raymond K, Heitmann BL. Lean body mass change over 6 years is associated with dietary leucine intake in an older Danish population. *Br J Nutr.* 2016;115(9):1556–1562.

Millward DJ, Layman DK, Tomé D, Schaafsma G. Protein quality assessment: impact of expanding understanding of protein and amino acid needs for optimal health. *Am J Clin Nutr.* 2008;87(5):1576S–1581S.

Moughan PJ. Dietary protein quality in humans—an overview. *J AOAC Int.* 2005;88(3):874–876.

Pencharz PB, Elango R, Wolfe RR. Recent developments in understanding protein needs-how much and what kind should we eat? *Appl Physiol Nutr Metab.* 2016;41(5): 577–580.

Petsko GA, Ringe D. *Protein Structure and Function.* London: New Science Press; 2005.

Rand WM, Scrimshaw NS, Young VR. Determination of protein allowances in human adults from nitrogen balance data. *Am J Clin Nutr.* 1977;30(7):1129–1134.

Phillips SM, Chevalier S, Leidy HJ. Protein "requirements" beyond the RDA: implications for optimizing health. *Appl Physiol Nutr Metab.* 2016;41(5):565–572.

Sarwar G. The protein digestibility-corrected amino acid score method overestimates quality of proteins containing antinutritional factors and of poorly digestible proteins supplemented with limiting amino acids in rats. *J Nutr.* 1997;127(5):758–764.

Schaafsma G. The protein digestibility-corrected amino acid score (PDCAAS)—a concept for describing protein quality in foods and food ingredients: a critical review. *J AOAC Int.* 2005;88(3):988–994.

Soenen S, Bonomi AG, Lemmens SG, et al. Relatively high-protein or 'low-carb' energy-restricted diets for body weight loss and body maintenance? *Physiol Behav.* 2012;107(3):374–380.

Strauss KA, Puffenberger EG, Morton DH. Maple syrup urine disease. Gene Reviews. Updated May 9, 2013. Available at: http://www.ncbi.nlm.nih.gov/bookshelf/br.fcgi?book=gene&part=msud

Uauy R, Scrimshaw NS, Rand WM, Young VR. Human protein requirements: obligatory urinary and fecal nitrogen losses and the factorial estimation of protein needs in elderly males. *J Nutr.* 1978;108(1):97–103.

Wolfe RR, Rutherfurd SM, Kim IY, Moughan PJ. Protein quality as determined by the Digestible Indispensable Amino Acid Score: evaluation of factors underlying the calculation. *Nutr Rev.* 2016; 74(9):584–599.

Yao K, Duan Y, Li F, et al. Leucine in obesity: therapeutic prospects. *Trends Pharmacol Sci.* 2016;37(8):714–727.

Young VR, Marchini JS. Mechanisms and nutritional significance of metabolic responses to altered intakes of protein and amino acids, with reference to nutritional adaptation in humans. *Am J Clin Nutr.* 1990;51(2):270–289.

Young VR, Pellett PL. Plant proteins in relation to human protein and amino acid nutrition. *Am J Clin Nutr.* 1994;59 (5 suppl):1203S–1212S.

Zello GA, Wykes LJ, Ball RO, Pencharz PB. Recent advances in methods in assessing dietary amino acid requirements for adult humans. *J Nutr.* 1995;125(12):2907–2915.

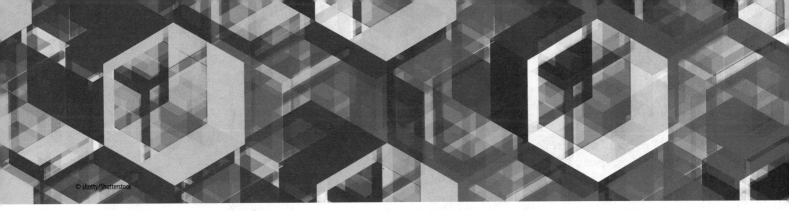

CHAPTER 7

Water

← HERE'S WHERE YOU HAVE BEEN

1. You have covered all of the nutrients that are capable of harnessing energy for the tissues and cells of our bodies.
2. Protein is critical for growth and maintenance, and carbohydrates and fats are critical for energy demands in addition to their own unique functions.
3. Digestion of the macronutrients is dependent on specific enzymes for each macronutrient class, and the absorption of each end product is unique.
4. The key metabolic pathways, such as glycolysis, the Krebs cycle, the HMP shunt, and the urea cycle, among others, have been detailed.
5. The form and composition of each class of macronutrients can affect human health either positively or negatively.

HERE'S WHERE YOU ARE GOING →

1. Water is considered a macronutrient but is the only macronutrient that does not provide the body with energy.
2. Besides consuming water through beverages and food, the human body produces water as a part of energy metabolism.
3. Water balance is extremely important in maintaining health and life. The amount of water lost through various routes may differ based on an individual's health status and physical activity.
4. The body has unique biochemical mechanisms in place to ensure that water and electrolyte balances are held in check. Central to this task are endocrine compounds and the kidney.
5. Retention of water in interstitial spaces is known as edema. It occurs through several physiologic mechanisms and is associated with multiple disease states.

▶ Introduction

An argument can be made that water is the most essential nutrient to humans. First, adults need approximately 2 to 3 kilograms of water daily to balance losses. This amount is substantially greater than the requirements for all other essential nutrients. For example, the average daily need for water for an adult is approximately 40 to 50 times greater than an adult's protein needs and about 5,000 times greater than his or her vitamin C requirement. Second, signs and/or symptoms of water deficiency, or **dehydration**, are apparent within the first day without water, and a complete lack of water influx may result in death in as few as 3 to 4 days. Therefore, a deficiency of water leads to the development of signs at a rate greater than a deficiency of other nutrients. Finally, because water is the medium of intracellular and extra-cellular fluids, dehydration (or its opposite, overhydration) cannot occur without affecting the metabolism of all other nutrients.

▶ Properties and Body Distribution of Water

Properties

The chemical and physical properties of water, such as its ability to function as a general solvent and its high specific heat, make it a well-suited medium for the human body. Water differs from the other macronutrients in that it is an inorganic molecule, consisting of two atoms of hydrogen bonded to one atom of oxygen. The bonding is covalent; however, the sharing of electrons is far from equal. Oxygen, with eight protons within its nucleus vs hydrogen's lone proton, is able to generate a greater electric pulling force on the shared electrons (**FIGURE 7.1**). This results in a partially positive charge associated with the hydrogen atoms and a partially negative charge associated with the oxygen atom. It is this arrangement that allows

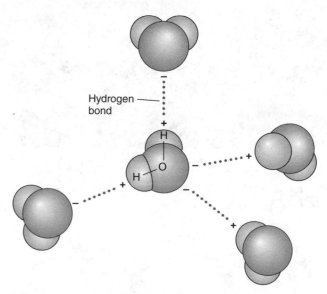

FIGURE 7.2 Water Molecules Held Together by Hydrogen Bonds. Gray denotes hydrogen; color denotes oxygen.

for the cohesiveness between water molecules. The hydrogen atoms of one water molecule are electrically attracted to the oxygen atoms of nearby molecules (**FIGURE 7.2**). In fact, in a solution containing pure water, individual water molecules can interact with up to four other water molecules in somewhat of a tetrahedral arrangement, which results in the formation of a water lattice. The association between water molecules decreases as temperature increases, or as its phase goes from solid to vapor. Water is solid below 0°C and vaporizes above 100°C. Water also has a relatively low thermal conductivity and, as mentioned earlier, a relatively high specific heat.

The dipolar nature of water molecules allows for the solubility of many substances. In general, substances having ionic character, such as sodium chloride (**FIGURE 7.3**), and polar molecules possessing the ability to hydrogen-bond (i.e., alcohols, ketones, and sugars) demonstrate water solubility. Larger molecules, such as proteins, form colloidal suspension solutions consisting of particles measuring between 1 and 100 nanometers. Furthermore, water provides a medium for the formation of emulsions. For example, homogenized milk contains emulsions of fat globules, protein, and other solutes in aggregates with diameters ranging between 1 and 100 micrometers.

Distribution of Water in the Human Body

The human body is about 60% water by mass. Because adipose tissue is relatively void of water, whereas skeletal muscle is approximately 73% water, it is the ratio of skeletal muscle to body fat that is

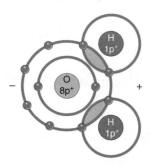

FIGURE 7.1 Water Molecule. A partial negative charge is associated with the oxygen atom, and a partial positive charge with the hydrogen atoms.

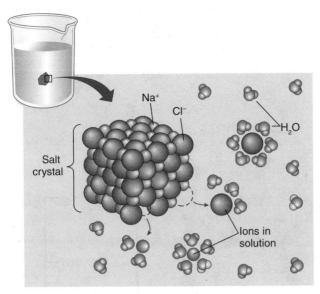

FIGURE 7.3 Ionization of Sodium Chloride into Water.
Due to the dipole nature of water, other substances that are ionized, such as sodium chloride, are soluble in water. Other polar molecules such as alcohols and sugars are soluble due to the dipole nature of water. Larger molecules such as proteins can form emulsions.

TABLE 7.1 Distribution of Water	
Compartment	**Approximate Percentage of Total Body Water**[a]
Plasma	7
Interstitial fluid (including lymph)	20
Cartilage and connective tissue	8
Contents of lumen of gastrointestinal tract	1
Cerebral spinal fluid	1
Bile	1
Intracellular Fluid	60

[a]Values are for a 70-kilogram man (42 liters total).

the primary factor in determining body water mass. Because men typically have a greater skeletal muscle-to-body fat ratio, they tend to have higher percentages of body water.

Water is compartmentalized into extracellular and intracellular fluids. About 55% to 60% of total body water in an adult is intracellular, with the remainder being extracellular. The extracellular compartment is composed of interstitial (between cell) fluid, including lymph and the fluid within connective tissue, plasma, fluids within the intestinal tract lumen and joints, and cerebrospinal fluid (**TABLE 7.1**). Collectively, plasma and the interstitial fluid account for about 27% of the total body water mass. Blood plasma is about 90% water and 10% dissolved and suspended substances such as proteins, electrolytes, urea, and lipoproteins. The daily secretion of water-based intestinal juices is approximately 6 to 7 liters for a typical adult, which includes saliva (1,000 milliliters), gastric secretions (1,500 milliliters), pancreatic secretions (1,000 milliliters), and bile (1,000 milliliters), along with secretions from the small intestine (2,000 milliliters) and large intestine (200 milliliters).

Sweat Water

Water provides the basis for **sweat**, which is a primary mechanism for removing excessive body heat. The core

temperature of the human body on average is 37°C (98.6°F). For this temperature to remain constant, excessive heat generated through the metabolic operations of deep organs or exercising muscle must be dissipated by conduction, radiation, convection, or evaporation. Evaporation of sweat occurs continually throughout the day and is particularly augmented during exercise. The evaporation of 1 gram of water from the skin surface dissipates 0.58 kilocalorie. Thus, 1 liter of water evaporation can remove about 580 kilocalories of heat.

Sweating is largely controlled autonomically and is initiated by stimulating the preoptic-anterior hypothalamus area of the brain. Sweat glands are located in skin tissue throughout the body and are innervated by sympathetic cholinergic fibers. Sweat gland activity may also be stimulated by circulating epinephrine and norepinephrine. This becomes particularly important during exercise bouts, when the circulating level of those chemicals increases.

Sweat glands, as depicted in **FIGURE 7.4**, are long tubular structures consisting of a deep subdermal coiled portion and a duct that reaches to the skin's surface. The deep coiled portion consists of epithelial cells, which, when stimulated, secrete a primary sweat solution that is very similar to plasma in its sodium (142 mEq/l) and chloride (104 mEq/l) content. However, the primary secretion contains relatively little of the other plasma solutes, including proteins.

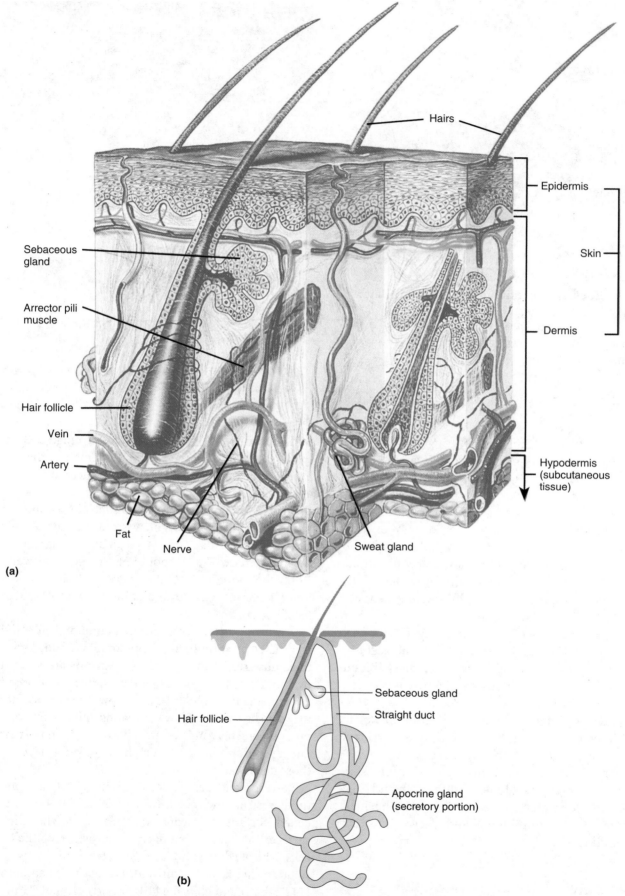

FIGURE 7.4 Sweat Glands. (a) The skin is composed of an epidermis from which hair follicles, sweat glands, and sebaceous glands descend into the underlying dermis. (b) A sweat gland showing the sebaceous gland and the secretory (apocrine) gland. The secretory gland also has sympathetic nerve fibers (not shown) associated with it.

As the primary solution flows through the duct, it is modified in solute concentration. If the rate of sweating is slow, resulting in a slow rate of flow through the tubule, almost all of the sodium and chloride will be reabsorbed, as well as a large portion of the water. Reabsorption of sodium by the sweat glands is under the influence of the hormone aldosterone (discussed later in this chapter). Water reabsorption is primarily attributed to the osmotic gradient developed by the reabsorption of sodium and chloride. The reabsorption of water leads to the concentration of the other components of sweat, such as lactic acid, urea, and potassium.

As the rate of sweating increases, the transit time through the duct decreases. This results in decreased reabsorption of sodium, chloride, and water. When sweat release is strongly stimulated and copious amounts of primary secretion flow through the duct, only about half of the sodium and chloride, along with a minimal amount of water, is reabsorbed. This results in a final concentration of sodium and chloride that is about half that of plasma levels.

Urinary Water

Water also provides the basis of urine, which serves as the primary route of excretion of metabolic waste and regulates the composition of the extracellular fluid. Each human kidney contains about 1,000,000 nephrons. Collectively, they typically generate approximately 1 to 2 liters of urine daily for adults and relative to fluid intake. Urine is a composite of water, electrolytes, urea, creatinine, and trace amounts of glucose, amino acids, and proteins. **FIGURE 7.5** displays a nephron unit.

At rest the kidneys receive approximately 20% of the left ventricular cardiac output, or about 1 liter per minute. In nephrons, water and plasma solutes having a size smaller than about 3 to 7 nanometers in diameter are filtered into the Bowman, or glomerular, capsule under a glomerular capillary pressure that is about three times greater than in capillaries of other tissue. On a daily basis, about 180 liters of renal filtrate, or ultrafiltrate, is produced. At this point, ultrafiltrate has many compositional similarities to plasma.

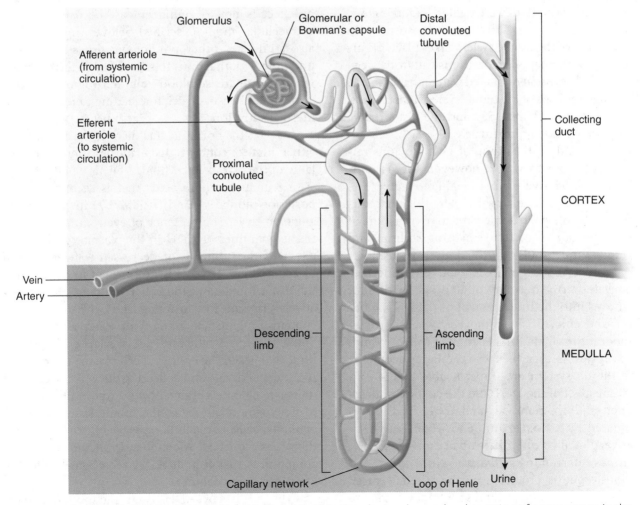

FIGURE 7.5 The Kidney Nephron Unit. Blood is filtered within the glomerulus, and reabsorption of water occurs in the various tubules, but mostly in the distal convoluted tubule and the collecting duct.

However, it lacks plasma proteins and lipoproteins as well as platelets and blood cells. As ultrafiltrate flows through the tubule system, its composition changes and its volume greatly decreases. In fact, reabsorptive operations reduce the filtered fluid volume by about 99%, or from 180 liters to about 1 to 2 liters.

The first part of the renal tubule system, the **proximal convoluted tubule (PCT)**, is designed for massive reabsorptive operations. The epithelial cells lining the tubule are endowed with microvilli that are heavily studded with transport proteins and channels. PCT epithelial cells also have a rich complement of mitochondria, which provide ATP for the extensive active transport operations associated with reabsorption. Glucose and amino acids are completely reabsorbed in the PCT, along with much of the electrolytes and water.

Water reabsorption along the length of the nephron tubule system occurs entirely by osmotic diffusion. Water moves largely through relatively loose junctions between PCT epithelial cells to reenter the extracellular fluid. This allows significant amounts of osmotic water reabsorption to occur, concomitant with the large reabsorption of ultrafiltrate solutes in the PCT. However, the junctions in the **loop of Henle** and **distal convoluted tubule (DCT)** are tighter, and, therefore, less permeable to water. Thus, water reabsorption in the latter parts of the tubule system takes place mostly by moving through epithelial cells instead of between them. The reabsorption of filtered water attributable to the varying segments of the tubule system is as follows: PCT, 65%; loop of Henle, 15%; and the distal tubule and collecting ducts, approximately 10% each.

The descending thin loop of Henle begins relatively permeable to water; however, the ascending portion is relatively impermeable to water. The DCT is also water impermeable. The thick ascending loop of Henle participates in active transport of about three-fourths of the remaining sodium and chloride in the tubular fluid to the extracellular fluid. Because this segment is relatively impermeable to water, urine becomes diluted. As the tubular fluid moves into the first segment of the DCT, more sodium and chloride are removed by active transport operations. This further dilutes urinary fluid. The exception is urea, because the latter segments of the tubule system are impermeable to urea. In the latter aspect of the DCT and the cortical collecting duct, sodium removal (and water, indirectly) is regulated by **aldosterone**, and water reabsorption is regulated by **antidiuretic hormone (ADH)**, sometimes referred to as **vasopressin**.

Aldosterone is produced by the adrenal cortex in response to low tubular fluid sodium levels via the renin-angiotensin system. Aldosterone stimulates sodium reabsorption by the DCT and the cortical collecting duct. This sodium reabsorption results in increased water reabsorption, leading to increased plasma volume in addition to the independent effects of ADH. Potassium is simultaneously secreted into the tubules. How does this work? The renin-angiotensin-aldosterone system is pivotal in maintaining the correct balance of water and electrolytes (**FIGURE 7.6**). In this system, a protein called **renin** is produced by afferent arteriole cells in the kidney glomerulus. Those cells are part of the **juxtaglomerular apparatus**. Renin is produced in response to either low blood volume, decreased blood pressure, or low plasma sodium levels. Renin is released into the blood and then travels to the liver, where it converts the liver protein **angiotensinogen** to **angiotensin I**, which is an inactive peptide consisting of 10 amino acids. Angiotensin I is released into the blood and flows to the lung, where an **angiotensin-converting enzyme (ACE)**, converts angiotensin I into **angiotensin II**, which has eight amino acids. Angiotensin II stimulates the synthesis and release of aldosterone from the adrenal cortex and the release of ADH by the pituitary gland. Although angiotensin II can stimulate ADH release, its effect is not as significant as the osmolarity of extracellular fluids described below. Angiotensin II also stimulates other physiologic processes. It acts upon the hypothalamus to stimulate the thirst center, which will increase blood volume. Angiotensin II is also a potent vasoconstrictor, leading to reduced glomerular filtration.

ADH is the hormone that dictates the excretion of either dilute or concentrated urine based on the osmolality of the extracellular fluid. ADH is a peptide consisting of nine amino acids that is secreted by the posterior pituitary gland (**FIGURE 7.7**) in response to angiotensin II. The presence of even minute changes in the quantities of ADH in the plasma can result in either marked diuresis or decreased water excretion by the kidneys. If ADH is not present in the plasma, the distal tubule and the collecting duct remain relatively impermeable to water. Thus, the urine would contain a significant amount of water and be very dilute. In contrast, the presence of ADH evokes structural changes in the epithelial cell plasma membranes in the distal tubule and collecting duct. Those changes increase channels (aquaporins) that allow water to flow osmotically from the tubule lumen into the epithelial cells. Large fluid or water intake can inhibit the release of ADH. Alcohol and caffeine are known compounds that inhibit ADH secretion, leading to expanded urine volume.

The release of ADH from the posterior pituitary gland is regulated by specialized neurons called

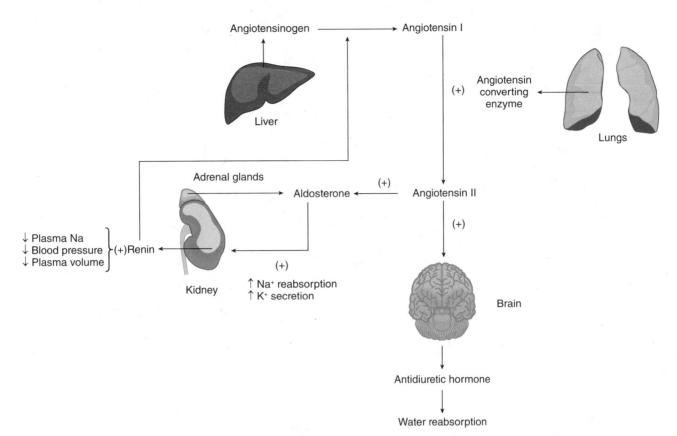

FIGURE 7.6 Regulation of Electrolytes (Na⁺, K⁺) and Water by the Renin-Angiotensin-Aldosterone System.
Electrolyte and water balance depend on several compounds produced by a variety of organs or tissues such as the kidneys, adrenal glands, liver, lungs and brain. A decrease in plasma sodium, blood pressure, and or plasma volume can cause the release of renin by the kidneys which initiates a sequence of events among the various organs to normalize electrolyte and water balance.

osmoreceptors in the hypothalamus (**FIGURE 7.8**). For example, if a concentrated electrolyte solution is injected into the hypothalamic vasculature, ADH neurons in the supra-optic and paraventricular nuclei carry impulses to the posterior pituitary, evoking the release of ADH. In contrast, injection of a dilute electrolyte solution into an artery serving the hypothalamus ultimately results in an inhibition of ADH release. Normally functioning kidneys can adjust the concentration of urine osmolality from 40 to 1,400 milliosmol per kilogram (mOsm/kg), depending on the water status of the human body. The highest solute concentration of urine is limited by the minimum **urinary water** necessary to excrete nitrogenous waste (principally urea), sulfates, phosphates, and other electrolytes. The maximal concentration is about 1,400 mOsm/kg for adults and 700 mOsm/kg for infants.

The urine solute concentration, or osmolality, can have clinical significance. A urine osmolality above 1,400 mOsm/kg suggests a fluid volume deficit. Renal disease, congestive heart failure, Addison disease, dehydration, diabetes, and excess alcohol ingestion are some of the diseases and health conditions that may lead to a fluid volume deficit. In contrast, lower urine osmolality

indicates that there is a fluid volume excess (i.e., water intoxication), or it may reflect increased fluid intake or the use of diuretics. It could also reflect an inability of the kidneys to concentrate urine, which, in turn, could be the result of inadequate production of ADH or reduced ability to augment aquaporin activity. This latter condition is termed **diabetes insipidus**, in which there is an increased output of urine that is dilute in solutes.

⬢ BEFORE YOU GO ON . . .

1. What percentage of body water is in the extracellular compartment, and where is the extracellular water distributed within the body?

2. What is the juxtaglomerular apparatus?

3. How is the amount of sweat controlled, as well as the concentration of sodium and chloride?

4. How do renin, angiotensin, and aldosterone affect one another? Collectively, what roles do they have in maintaining electrolyte and water balance?

5. What is diabetes insipidus, and what is the underlying cause?

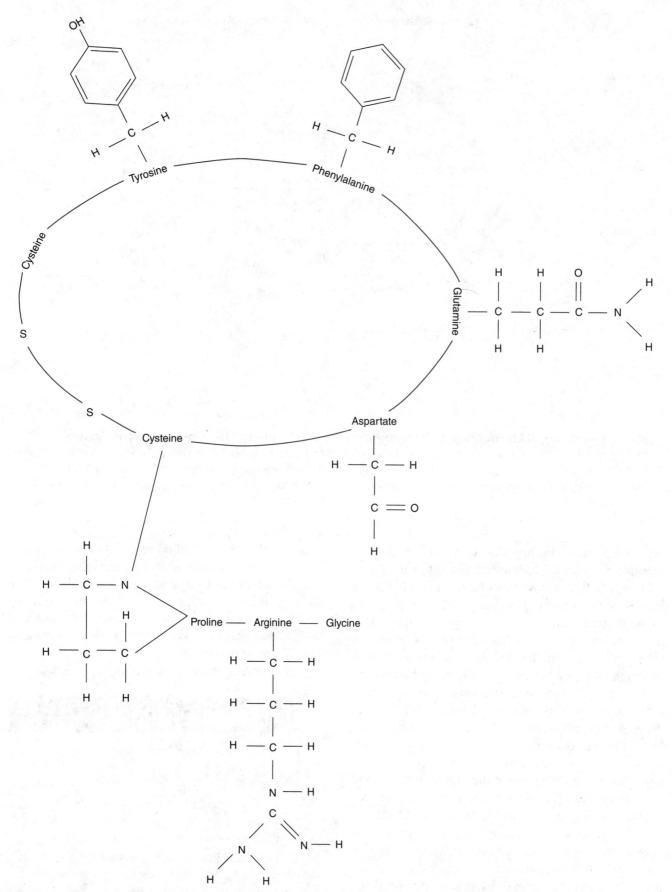

FIGURE 7.7 Antidiuretic Hormone (Vasopressin) Structure and Amino Acid Composition. The hormone is composed of these nine amino acids that are produced by the pituitary gland.

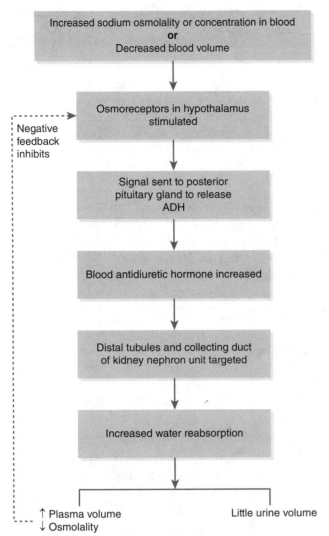

FIGURE 7.8 Regulation of Urine Volume and Plasma Osmolality by Control of Antidiuretic Hormone (ADH) Release by the Hypothalamus. An increase in sodium osmolarity (increased sodium concentration) in the blood or decreased blood volume results in ADH output, which increases plasma volume and decreases plasma osmolarity.

▶ Water Balance

No other nutrient experiences as much flux (in/out) on a daily basis as water. Daily water loss from the human body is about 4% of body mass for a nonexercising adult. For infants, the percentage of body water lost daily is approximately 15% of total body weight. This loss must be balanced by water ingestion or infusion to avoid the development of deficiency. Furthermore, unlike all other essential nutrients, water does not have an appreciable storage reservoir in the human body. For instance, a reduction in extracellular water content is not buffered by a mobilization of water from some inert storage site. In reality, the increased osmolality of the extracellular fluid evokes an osmotic pull on intracellular water. Continuation of extracellular water loss will dehydrate cells. Thus, even a slight inadequacy of water supply can result in alterations of physiologic function.

Water loss from the human body occurs primarily by the following routes: sweat, excretion of urine and feces, and exhalation of air humidified by the lungs. Generally, about 900 to 1,200 milliliters of water are lost daily as urine (**TABLE 7.2**). This quantity increases relative to water ingestion and decreases relative to increased losses by other means. Urinary water loss is strongly influenced by ADH, as discussed earlier, allowing for urine to be very concentrated or very dilute. However, to remove potentially deleterious nitrogenous waste molecules, such as urea, obligatory water loss must be about 400 to 600 milliliters per day.

About 200 milliliters of water are lost daily within feces, about 400 milliliters are lost in mild sweating, and 300 milliliters are lost through exhalation of humidified air. Thus, the daily loss is roughly 1,800 to 2,100 milliliters. Because mild daily sweating and the exhalation of air

TABLE 7.2 Water Balance from Intake and Output			
Source	**Water Intake (ml)**	**Source**	**Water Loss (ml)**
Drinking water, including beverages	1,000	Urine	900–1,200
Water from food	600–800	Mild sweating	400
Metabolic water	200–300	Lungs	300
		Feces	200
Total	1,800–2,100	Total	1,800–2,100

SPECIAL FEATURE 7.1

Hydration While Exercising

It is important to remain hydrated during exercise, particularly in events of longer duration in which sweating is moderate to heavy. The American College of Sports Medicine has developed guidelines on fluid intake before, during, and after exercise and their recommendations are included in the guidelines below. In addition, they recommend that individuals weigh themselves before and after exercise and to convert the change in body weight to ml (or ounces) of water loss to help gauge fluid needs to stay hydrated during exercise. Another gauge for potential water loss is based on calories burned during exercise as each liter of sweat dissipates about 580 kcals.

Before Exercise

Proper hydration status should exist before exercise begins. Whether an athlete has proper hydration may depend on how long ago the person last exercised and whether he or she rehydrated. If there was a recovery period of 8 to 12 hours and sufficient meals and beverages were consumed after the most recent period of exercise, the person should be hydrated. As a rule of thumb, a person should drink beverages at least 4 hours before an event totaling 500–600 ml (16–20 oz) of water or sports beverage. The person should then drink 250–350 ml (8–12 oz) 10–15 minutes prior to starting.

During Exercise

Making recommendations for fluid intake during exercise is much more difficult because of differences in the duration and intensity of the exercise, weather, clothing worn, and other variables. The goal is to prevent excessive dehydration, or fluid loss of greater than 2% body weight, and to minimize electrolyte loss. Again, athletes are encouraged to weigh themselves before and after events during training to get an idea of how much weight they lose in a defined time so that they can customize their fluid intake. Athletes should strive for 100–250 ml (3–8 oz) of water every 15–20 minutes of exercise when exercising for less than 60 minutes. If they are training or competing longer, a sport beverage is recommended containing 5–8% carbohydrate.

After Exercise

The goal after exercise is to replace the water and electrolytes lost. In most instances, intake of normal meals with sufficient plain water will rehydrate the body. The food should contain sufficient sodium to replace the losses. In most instances, our diets have ample salt for this purpose. However, a little extra salt added to meals may be useful, especially if the athlete experienced excessive sweating. The athlete should drink 20–24 oz for every pound of weight loss or roughly 45–50 ml for every kilogram lost.

humidified by the lungs generally go unnoticed, they, and other minor water-loss mechanisms, such as lacrimal secretions from the eyes, are often referred to as **insensible water losses**. Mild sweating is often separated from activity-induced sweat; the latter has a higher mineral content and is visually obvious. The amount of water loss by mild sweating is related to body surface area. On average, this process allows a continual removal of excessive body heat, totaling about 250 to 400 kilocalories per day.

Sweating becomes a significant route of water loss during athletic training or competition and for individuals in warmer climates. Over a span of a few weeks, a person can acclimate to increase his or her sweat rate from about 700 to 2,000 milliliters per hour. The increased production of sweat is attributable to increased capabilities of the sweat glands. In addition, the sweat produced will be much more dilute than that of a nonacclimated individual.

To prevent dehydration, cumulative water output must be balanced by water made available to the body. Water is made available primarily by oral ingestion. Approximately two-thirds enters as pure water or other water-based fluids, and the remaining third is consumed as part of food or produced metabolically. Several foods are excellent sources of water because of their high water content. For instance, many fruits and vegetables are 85 to 95% water by mass (**TABLE 7.3**). Drinking water and other beverages contribute around 1,000 milliliters per day, and water in food contributes 600 to 800 milliliters per day.

The metabolic generation of water accounts for about 200 to 300 milliliters of water daily (see Table 7.2). The complete oxidation of fuel substrates results in the production of water. For instance, the oxidation of 1 mole of glucose generates 6 moles of water:

$$C_6H_{12}O_6 + 6\,O_2 \rightarrow 6\,CO_2 + \mathbf{6\,H_2O}$$

Water requirements are based on replenishing water lost by the processes just discussed. It is often difficult to accurately estimate water losses because

TABLE 7.3 Water Content of Various Foods

Food	Approximate Percentage of Water in Total Weight
Tomato	95
Lettuce	95
Cabbage	92
Beer	90
Orange	87
Apple juice	87
Milk	87
Potato	78
Banana	75
Chicken	70
Bread, white	35
Jam	28
Honey	20
Butter	16
Rice	12
Shortening	0

approximately half is lost by insensible routes (mild sweating and humidification of breath). For an average adult, intake of water should total 1,800 to 2,100 milliliters per day to equal loss. However, the Adequate Intake (AI) for water is set much higher because the Food and Nutrition Board recognizes that environmental and physical activity factors may cause wide variability in addition to the existence of wide variability among individuals. An Estimated Average Requirement (EAR) was rejected by the Food and Nutrition Board because, by definition, half of the individuals in a particular life-stage group would have inadequate intakes. An AI allows for a large safety margin. One to 3.1 liters per day is the range estimated to replace urinary, fecal, and insensible water losses (respiratory and skin), which is a wide range.

Data from the Third National Health and Nutrition Examination Survey (NHANES III) were used to determine the AI for water. The median intakes of total water from beverages, drinking water, and food rounded to the nearest 0.1 liter were used in setting the values. That method assumed that this amount would cover the minimal losses that occur on a routine basis in temperate climates for people who are somewhat sedentary. Those recommendations translate into an AI of 3.7 liters per day of total water for adult men and 2.7 liters per day for adult women (ages 19 to more than 70 years). Those values include total beverages and water in food.

Water requirements are augmented during pregnancy and lactation. The expanded extracellular fluid space and the needs of both the fetus and the amniotic fluid increase water requirements by approximately 30 milliliters per day. This shows an increase from 2.7 to 3.0 liters per day. Human breast milk is approximately 87% water. Because the average milk secretion is 750 milliliters per day for the first 6 months, the increased water need approximates 600 to 700 milliliters per day. The AI during lactation is 3.8 liters per day.

The perceived need for water is commonly called **thirst** and is controlled by the hypothalamus. There is a direct correlation between plasma osmolality and the intensity of thirst. This also means that an individual must be slightly dehydrated prior to the initiation of thirst. Reductions in extracellular fluid volume also evoke thirst, independent of plasma osmolality. For example, a hemorrhage and subsequent reduction in extracellular fluid volume will result in thirst without changes in plasma osmolality. The effect of a reduced extracellular fluid volume on thirst is mediated in part by the renin-angiotensin mechanism. Renin secretion is increased by hypovolemia and subsequently results in an increase in angiotensin II. Angiotensin II acts on a specialized region in the diencephalon to stimulate neural activity associated with thirst.

● BEFORE YOU GO ON . . .

1. What is the percentage of body water loss of a nonexercising adult compared with that of an infant?
2. List the sources of water loss in humans.
3. How much water comes from metabolic water on a daily basis for the average adult, and how does this come about?
4. How much additional water should a lactating woman consume per day?
5. What are the physiologic factors associated with thirst?

▶ Edema

Thus far, we have discussed the physiologic basis of water balance and dehydration. However, attention to the distribution of water is critical in optimizing health. Excess accumulation of water can lead to **edema**, or swelling. In most cases, edema is the accumulation of water in interstitial spaces. In some instances, the water accumulation may be intracellular, in which case it is still considered edema. In almost all cases, edema is not normal, but a sign of illness, such as renal disease, cardiac failure, or cirrhosis of the liver. It can also result from nondisease factors, such as excess dietary salt, dietary protein deficiency, or pregnancy. Edema is also correlated with obesity and can be caused by non-life-threatening injury, such as a sprained joint or localized inflammation. Some medications may also cause edema, including ibuprofen; some antihypertensive or steroid medications; calcium channel blockers; and cholesterol-lowering drugs, such as Lipitor and Crestor, to name a few.

Mechanisms for Edema Formation

Most edema is due to the accumulation of water in interstitial spaces. Three physiologic forces within the capillary beds need to be considered with regard to the etiology of edema (**TABLE 7.4**). The first force is hydrostatic pressure. Hydrostatic pressure is simply the pressure exerted by the weight of the water in the capillaries or, more specifically, the pressure exerted against the capillary walls. The second force is osmotic pressure (sometimes called oncotic pressure). Although a bit more complicated than hydrostatic pressure, it is equally as important. This is the pressure that is needed to prevent the flow of water, either into the capillary or out of the capillary, depending on the circumstances. The flow of water across a semipermeable membrane to equal concentration gradients of materials that cannot cross the membrane is the essence of osmosis. With regard to edema, protein levels may change in disease conditions. In many disease states, protein levels decrease in the blood but are higher in the interstitial tissues. This will result in water leaking into the interstitial tissues to equalize the concentration of protein. The osmotic pressure is simply the pressure needed to stop the flow of water. The third force is the development of leaky capillaries. The loss of protein through the capillaries will also cause water to leak into the interstitial fluid. A fourth force that is independent of

TABLE 7.4 Edema: Mechanisms and Pathological States
Mechanisms

1. Accumulation of water in interstitial spaces
  a. Increased hydrostatic pressure increases in capillaries
  b. Increased osmotic (oncotic) pressure in the interstitial spaces
  c. Leaky capillaries
  d. Inability of lymphatic system to drain interstitial fluid accumulation

2. Accumulation of water intracellularly   a. Hyponatremia or low plasma sodium
Pathologic states associated with edema

1. Decreased blood protein concentration leads to edema in:
  a. Kwashiorkor
  b. Nephrotic syndrome
  c. Cirrhosis of the liver

2. Inflammation
3. Parasites that block lymph drainage
4. Heart failure

the three physiologic forces dealing with capillaries involves the lymphatic system's ability to drain the interstitial tissue of fluid buildup.

Intracellular edema occurs when there is a redistribution of sodium and water. In hyponatremia, plasma sodium is low. Consequently, extracellular sodium levels are low and the water level is high. This leads to a greater intracellular concentration of solutes compared with the extracellular compartment. Water will move from the extracellular compartment to the intracellular compartment in order to normalize solute concentration. This leads to swelling of the cells. This condition is the most likely cause of brain edema.

Edema in Pathologic States

Let's consider the link between the mechanisms of edema with actual edemas that accompany diseases. A decrease in protein concentration can lead to a change in the osmotic force across capillaries. For instance, if there is a decrease in plasma proteins, such as occurs with Kwashiorkor, nephrotic syndrome, and cirrhosis of the liver, water will redistribute from the plasma compartment to the interstitial compartment of tissues. Increased permeability of capillary endothelium and cell membranes is also a force behind edema formation. Inflammation may lead to increased permeability of capillaries to plasma proteins. This will result in water moving into the interstitial compartment due to osmotic forces. However, inflammation can also lead to an increase in hydrostatic pressure by causing the capillaries to contract, further pushing water from the plasma to the interstitial compartment. The latter mechanism may lead to edema, which is caused by allergic reactions. Edema may also occur when there is a decrease in fluid drainage via the lymphatic system. Under normal conditions, the lymphatic system drains excess fluid from the interstitial compartment. Any time the accumulation of water in the interstitial compartment is greater than lymphatic drainage, edema will occur. Edema may also result from parasites blocking lymphatic drainage or surgeries that affect the lymph nodes (e.g., breast cancer surgery or mastectomy).

Edema may also result from heart failure (**FIGURE 7.9**). In heart failure, the hydrostatic pressure in the vasculature increases. How does this happen? Normally, this disease starts in the left ventricle. In heart failure, the blood in the heart fails to empty completely, primarily because ventricular contraction is less forceful. That causes a decrease in stroke volume as well as cardiac output. This also means that there is more blood in the left ventricle during relaxation (or increased end-diastolic volume), increasing left ventricular end-diastolic pressure. If the pressure rises sufficiently, the pressure will also increase in the left atria, which will also cause pressure to rise in the lungs. When the hydrostatic pressure increases in the lungs sufficiently, water will move into the interstitial compartment, leading to pulmonary congestion. However, there is also another issue. With reduced stroke volume or cardiac output, the cardiovascular system responds with not only an increased ventricular end-diastolic pressure but also an increase in heart rate and vasoconstriction to maintain cardiac output. Next, peripheral vasoconstriction will occur to redirect blood flow from the kidney to other, more vital organs. This results in increased pressure for the venous return of blood to the heart, which increases the overall hydrostatic pressure, leading to edema. Furthermore, due to the redistribution of blood away from the kidney,

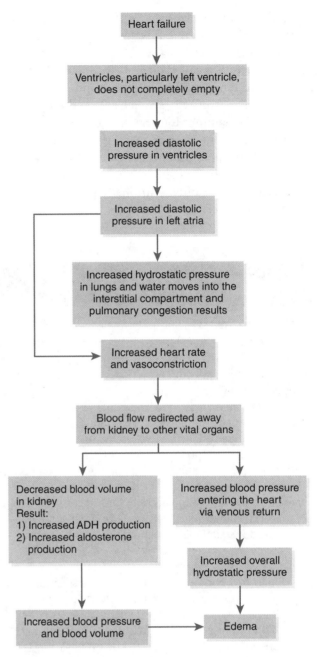

FIGURE 7.9 Sequence of Events That Lead to Edema as a Result of Heart Failure. Edema that results from heart failure involves both numerous and complex series of events. The underlying pathology in heart failure is an increase in hydrostatic pressure that results in edema.

the kidney senses less blood volume and consequently releases more ADH and aldosterone. This will increase the amounts of sodium and water reabsorbed, leading to increased blood volume and hydrostatic pressure. This turns into a vicious cycle that leads to a systemic edema. Often, this edema is more apparent in the lower extremities upon standing for a period of time.

When edema is observed in the extremities, it is termed peripheral edema. If water accumulates in the abdomen, it is referred to as ascites. If the edema is in the chest cavity, it is called pleural effusion. In general, there are two types of edemas: pitting and nonpitting. If one applies pressure to a swollen area and there is an indentation remaining after release of the pressure, it is pitting edema. Nonpitting edema is the opposite, with no indentation apparent upon release of the pressure. Pitting edema is the most common type. Nonpitting edema occurs most often with inadequate lymphatic drainage and hyperthyroidism.

● BEFORE YOU GO ON . . .

1. What three physiologic forces contribute to edema?
2. What conditions can lead to edema?
3. What is intracellular edema, and what may cause it to occur?
4. What processes lead to edema as a result of heart failure?
5. Explain the difference between pitting and nonpitting edema.

CLINICAL INSIGHT

Dehydration

In extreme situations, failure to ingest or infuse water can result in death within several days. Mild or early dehydration can result in significant alterations in physiologic operation. Perhaps, those most affected by early dehydration are training or competing athletes. A loss of water approximating 2% of body weight can result in significant reduction in athletic ability. If dehydration continues, allowing a loss of approximately 5% in body weight as water, cramping and heat exhaustion can result. A reduction in body water approximating 7 to 10% of body weight can result in hallucinations and the development of heat stroke. Coma, shock, and death may soon follow.

One of the most vulnerable groups susceptible to dehydration are infants and children when compared with adults. Part of this is due to the fact that the surface area per unit volume is greater in a smaller person, such as an infant. That allows for greater relative evaporation of water from the skin's surface in particular. The water requirement is more critical for premature infants as the surface per unit volume is even greater. Insensible water losses from the surface of the skin and respiration account for the most significant loss of water. Additionally, the metabolic rate is greatest in infants and gradually declines through the lifespan. Water is able to regulate heat effectively, and heat stress can occur in infants due to dehydration at a much easier rate than adults or even older children. In infants, the ability of the kidney to regulate the concentration of urine produced is less developed than adults. Loss of fluids can lead to increase plasma sodium levels of hypernatremia.

Breast milk and bottle feeding, in most cases, do provide sufficient water. There are times when some formula mixtures may be more concentrated due to a relative lack of water and this can lead to dehydration.

Often ignored are other issues that can lead to dehydration. Clinical nutritionists often recognize that vomiting and diarrhea that can occur in children and infants is likely the chief cause of dehydration. If a fever is present, the loss is even greater. Dehydration is a very serious health issue in infants and children and requires instant medical intervention. Remember that water is the chief manner in which humans regulate body temperature. A loss of water will compromise temperature regulation.

Factors that can expedite the development of critical dehydration include severe protracted diarrhea and sodium deficiency. Severe dehydration causes a shift in fluid from intracellular and interstitial fluids to the vascular compartment. Eventually, the vascular volume is reduced to a critical level and results in reduction in venous return to the heart and ultimately in a diminished cardiac output and reduced blood pressure. Tissue perfusion is reduced, and organs, such as the brain, are starved of oxygen and nutrients. Furthermore, dehydration reduces the ability to remove excessive heat in sweat, leaving an individual prone to hyperthermia and heat stroke. **TABLE 1** details some clinical signs of mild dehydration and moderate to severe dehydration.

A simple method to determine hydration status is urine color. Normal urine color is a pale yellow. Dark yellow signals dehydration. However, if taking a riboflavin supplement, this can result in a false reading of dehydration as this vitamin is excreted in the urine and can turn urine a bright yellow. Color charts are available that correlate color with hydration status.

In infants, diarrhea that leads to dehydration is among the leading causes of death in some underdeveloped portions of the world. In such diseases, it is important to replace the loss of essential electrolytes that accompanies diarrhea. A sodium deficit can easily occur. The first line of rehydration is giving extra fluids initially in mild dehydration cases. In more severe cases, it can be treated with a glucose plus electrolyte solution, often referred to as Oral

TABLE 1 Signs of Dehydration

Mild Dehydration	Moderate to Severe Dehydration
Dry and sticky mouth	Extreme thirst
Feeling of tiredness and sleepiness	Lack of sweating
Thirst	Very dry mouth and skin
Decreased urine output	Little or no urine output; dark-colored urine
Lack of tears when crying	Sunken eyes
Muscle weakness	Shriveled skin and lack of elasticity
Headache	Low blood pressure
Dizziness	Rapid heartbeat
Cramping in arms and legs	Rapid deep breathing
	Fever
	Unconsciousness and convulsions

Rehydration Salts (ORS). A rehydration solution that is recommended by the World Health Organization (WHO) is composed of the following on a per-liter basis:

- 2.6 g NaCl
- 13.5 g glucose
- 1.5 g KCl
- 2.9 g trisodium citrate, dehydrate

Children can also be affected by dehydration not only due to an increase surface area to body volume compared with adults but due to their activity level. In hot, humid areas, there may be a lack of hydration among children in which they also do not consume sufficient fluids. If they are involved in sports activities, fluids need to be administered to children to satisfy their thirst. They should do so every 20 to 30 minutes, regardless of thirst, if playing sports. To be on the safe side, it is often recommended that children less than 10 years old drink until there is no thirst and add another ⅓ to ½ cup of fluid on top of what has already been consumed.

Regardless of whether infants, children, or older age groups are involved, dehydration is too often ignored as an issue. Not only is water intake critical but the concentration of electrolytes is also a critical health issue that needs to be considered.

▶ Here's What You Have Learned

1. Water deficiency, or dehydration, occurs much more rapidly than for any other nutrient; death can result within 3 to 4 days.

2. Water atoms are covalently bonded to one another. Oxygen is able to generate a greater electric pulling force on the shared electrons with hydrogen that results in a partially positive charge associated with the hydrogen atoms and a partially negative charge associated with the oxygen atom. This allows for cohesiveness between water molecules.

3. The dipolar nature of water molecules allows for the solubility of many substances within water. In general, substances having an ionic character, such as sodium chloride, possess the ability to hydrogen-bond with water.

4. The human body is about 60% water by mass. Approximately 55 to 60% of total body water in an adult is intracellular, with the remainder being extracellular. The extracellular compartment is composed of interstitial fluid, including lymph and the fluid within connective tissue,

plasma, fluids within the intestinal tract lumen and joints, and cerebrospinal fluid.

5. Sweat is an important factor in body temperature regulation. One liter of water evaporation can remove approximately 580 kilocalories of heat. Sweat is produced by sweat glands in the skin, and the composition of sweat is highly regulated by autonomic nerve processes.

6. Urine production is the primary route of water loss, with an average of 1 to 2 liters of urine produced per day. The kidney nephron unit produces urine, and the water and salt concentration of urine is highly regulated by endocrine and blood pressure factors. Antidiuretic hormone is produced by the posterior pituitary gland and is secreted whenever water conservation is required.

7. Sodium reabsorption is closely linked to water reabsorption. Sodium levels are regulated by renin, angiotensin II, and aldosterone. When plasma sodium, blood pressure, or blood volume decrease, renin is released by the kidney to eventually produce angiotensin II. Angiotensin II will increase production and release of the hormone aldosterone from the adrenal glands, which stimulates sodium reabsorption by the kidney tubules.

8. The perceived need for water is thirst. Osmolality of plasma and blood volume are key determinants of thirst mechanisms within the hypothalamus. The effect of a reduced extracellular fluid volume on thirst is mediated in part by the renin-angiotensin mechanism. Renin secretion is increased by hypovolemia and subsequently results in an increase in angiotensin II. Angiotensin II acts on a specialized region in the diencephalon to stimulate neural activity associated with thirst. Additionally, angiotensin II will lead to the release of antidiuretic hormone of the pituitary, stimulating water reabsorption by the kidney tubules.

9. Water loss must be balanced by water intake. Water loss from the human body occurs by the following routes: sweat, excretion of urine and feces, and exhalation of air humidified by the lungs. Water is made available primarily by oral ingestion. Approximately two-thirds enters as pure water or other water-based fluids, and the remaining third is consumed as part of food or produced metabolically.

10. Edema is caused by a redistribution of water among body compartments, most notably water accumulation in the interstitial compartment. It can be caused by inflammation, renal disease, cardiac failure, blockage of the lymph nodes, and some medications. The most common type of edema is pitting edema.

▶ Suggested Reading

American College of Sports Medicine, Sawka MN, Burke LM, et al. American College of Sports Medicine position stand. Exercise and fluid replacement. Position stand of the American College of Sports Medicine. *Med Sci Sports Exerc.* 2007;39(2):377–390.

Ball SG. Vasopressin and disorders of water balance: the physiology and pathophysiology of vasopressin. *Ann Clin Biochem.* 2007;44(pt 5):417–431.

Burke L. *Practical Sports Nutrition.* Champaign, IL: Human Kinetics; 2007.

Coyle EF. Fluid and fuel intake during exercise. *J Sports Sci.* 2004;22(1):39–55.

Food and Nutrition Board, Institute of Medicine. *Dietary Reference Intakes for Water, Potassium, Sodium, Chloride, and Sulfate.* Washington, DC: The National Academies Press; 2005;1–638. http://doi.org/10.17226/10925

Jain V, Ravindranath A. Diabetes insipidus in children. *J Pediatr Endocrinol Metab.* 2016;29(1):39–45.

Rodriguez NR, DiMarco NM, Langley S, et al. Position of the American Dietetic Association, Dietitians of Canada, and the American College of Sports Medicine: nutrition and athletic performance. *J Am Diet Assoc.* 2009;109(3):509–527.

Shils ME, Shike M, Ross AC, Cabellero B, Cousins RJ. *Modern Nutrition in Health and Disease.* 10th ed. Philadelphia: Lippincott Williams & Wilkins; 2005.

Shirreffs SM, Armstrong LE, Cheuvront SN. Fluid and electrolyte needs for preparation and recovery from training and competition. *J Sports Sci.* 2004;22(1):57–63.

Shirreffs SM, Watson P, Maughan RJ. Milk as an effective post-exercise rehydration drink. *Br J Nutr.* 2007;98(1):173–180.

Stipanuk MH. *Biochemical, Physiological, and Molecular Aspects of Human Nutrition.* St. Louis, MO: Saunders; 2006.

Thomas DT, Erdman KA, Burke LM. Position of the Academy of Nutrition and Dietetics, Dietitians of Canada, and the American College of Sports Medicine: Nutrition and Athletic Performance. *J Acad Nutr Diet.* 2016;116(3):501–528.

Wildman REC, Miller BS, Wilborn C. *Sports and Fitness Nutrition* (2nd ed). Kendall Hunt Publishing, 2013.

Wilson JL, Miranda CA, Knepper MA. Vasopressin and the regulation of aquaporin-2. *Clin Exp Nephrol.* 2013;17(6):751–764.

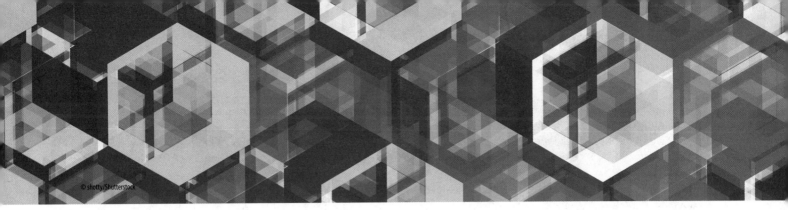

CHAPTER 8

Metabolism, Energy Balance, and Body Weight and Composition

← HERE'S WHERE YOU HAVE BEEN

1. The human body is composed of trillions of cells operating independently, which also combine in a synergistic fashion to create tissue.
2. Digestion is a complex synergy of the physical actions of chewing, mixing, and moving and the chemical actions of saliva, enzymes, and emulsifiers. Absorption refers to the movement of nutrients from the digestive tract into the blood or lymphatic circulation, whereas the concept of bioavailability also includes the uptake and utilization of nutrients by cells or tissue.
3. Carbohydrates are a class of nutrients that include sugars, starches, fibers, and related molecules, such as glycosaminoglycans, amino sugars, and more.
4. Proteins consist of amino acids and vary in size, shape, and function. Proteins serve as key structural molecules in cells and tissues and also function as enzymes and hormones. They are involved in blood clotting, transport, cell signaling, and more.
5. Fat is composed of glycerol and one to three fatty acids and serves as a key energy source for many cells in the body. Additionally, certain fatty acids can play a regulatory role in the body by serving as precursors for eicosanoids. Meanwhile, cholesterol is a lipid substance that plays a structural role in cell membranes and is a precursor to steroid hormones.

HERE'S WHERE YOU ARE GOING →

1. Metabolism refers to internal chemical reactions that occur in tissues throughout the body and is measured directly by heat release from the body or indirectly via respiratory gas exchange.
2. Cellular metabolism of the energy macronutrients is regulated by hormones, such as insulin, epinephrine, glucagon, and cortisol.

(continues)

(Continued)

3. Different metabolic states occur throughout the day and include fasting, fed, and exercising; those states are regulated by hormones.
4. Body weight control, including prevention of obesity, is primarily influenced by the level of kilocalories consumed chronically. The type of kilocalories consumed may also play a role in body weight control, although this is still being debated.
5. Body composition can be assessed at the levels of elements and molecules (e.g., water, protein, carbohydrate), specific tissue (e.g., muscle, adipose tissue, bone), or major tissue groups (e.g., fat mass, fat-free mass).

▶ Introduction

Every minute of every day, the human body is engaged in a myriad of metabolic reactions in an effort to maintain homeostatic operations and other human functions and activities. The daily metabolic cost, or energy expenditure, is very large, equaling 1,500 to 3,500 kilocalories for most adults. This number is the sum of the energy-releasing operations in tissue throughout the body. Human cells are tireless in their efforts to maintain ATP levels to support homeostasis and other functions. Furthermore, many cells are generally indiscriminate in their selection of energy substrates for ATP production. Cells tend to use energy substrates as dictated by their availability and hormonal and central influences upon metabolic pathways. Energy expenditure, or metabolism, can be assessed by directly measuring heat dissipation from the body or by oxygen utilization. Body composition, which influences metabolism, is most commonly assessed into two tissue groupings (e.g., fat mass and fat-free mass). This chapter presents an overview of total, tissue-level, and cellular-level energy metabolism and discusses metabolic states, **energy balance**, and body weight and composition. The obesity epidemic and impact upon health is highlighted here.

▶ Total Energy Expenditure and Components

Energy is constantly expended by the body. As trillions of cells engage in metabolic operations, energy molecules are used and byproducts are generated. Energy expenditure can be assessed for the entire body and can be divided into somewhat distinct, yet interrelated, components.

Measurement of Total Energy Expenditure

The amount of energy released from the body is directly or indirectly quantifiable. Adenosine triphosphate (ATP), along with other high-energy phosphate molecules, such as guanosine triphosphate (GTP), power those operations.

Those molecules, principally ATP, are derived from the catabolism of energy substrate molecules, such as carbohydrates, proteins (amino acids), fat, ethanol, and their metabolic intermediates; such as pyruvate and lactate. Those substrates are initially provided by the diet and can be used immediately or incorporated into storage forms, such as glycogen, triglyceride, and even protein. All energy-requiring operations in cells fall into three broad groups:

- Membrane transport
- Synthesis of molecules
- Mechanical work

With the exception of small amounts of energy transferred to objects and other entities during skeletal muscle efforts (mechanical work), energy released from the body ultimately becomes heat energy. Because body temperature is generally maintained within a narrow range, typically around 37°C (98.6°F), excessive heat must be dissipated. Measurement of that energy liberation within a given period of time, such as a minute, hour, or day, is called the **metabolic rate**. Metabolic rate becomes a more accurate reflection of human energy metabolism as the time period is extended. A 24-hour period, for example, takes into account periods in which the metabolic rate is both higher, such as during activity or exercise; and lower, such as during rest or sleep (**FIGURE 8.1**).

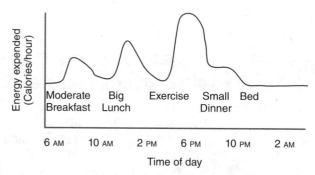

FIGURE 8.1 Example of Metabolic Fluctuations Throughout the Day. Note the periods of lower metabolism, such as sleep, versus periods of higher metabolism, such as during exercise.

Direct or Human Calorimetry

Metabolic rate can be measured directly using a human calorimeter, a method referred to as **direct calorimetry**. *Calorimetry* literally means the measurement of heat. Basically, direct calorimetry uses an insulated chamber in which heat dissipated from a person is measured by the warming of a layer of water associated with the wall of the chamber (**FIGURE 8.2**). Heat lost from the body in the form of water vapor is also measured as it interacts with sulfuric acid. All environmental factors are controlled. Facilities of this nature are expensive to maintain and are only available at a handful of universities and research institutions.

Indirect Calorimetry

Whereas direct calorimetry measures body heat production, an indirect method is more commonly used to estimate energy expenditure. Because ATP is generated from the combustion of energy molecules, and because combustion requires oxygen (O_2) and produces carbon dioxide (CO_2), it is possible to estimate energy expenditure based on the exchange of those gases with the environment (**FIGURE 8.3**). Because energy expenditure is estimated indirectly from gas exchange driven by metabolism, that method is called **indirect calorimetry**; it is typically assessed using a **metabolic cart**.

Representative chemical reactions for the combustion of carbohydrates, protein, and fat are shown below. Oxygen is used as a reactant for each reaction, and carbon dioxide is a product. By using mathematical equations generated from direct calorimetry, it is possible to estimate the amount of heat produced in a given period of time based on the amount of O_2 inhaled and used or the amount of CO_2 produced and expired. Indirect calorimetry is an accurate indicator of metabolism and can also be used to estimate the

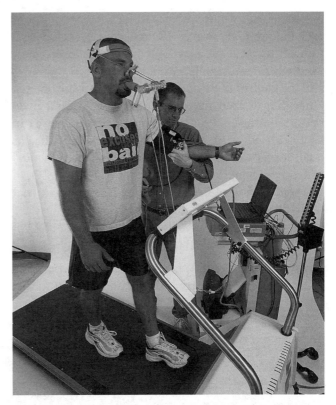

FIGURE 8.3 Indirect Calorimetry via Metabolic Cart. Oxygen consumption and carbon dioxide production is used to estimate caloric expenditure.

energy substances being combusted during the time of measurement.

$$\text{Carbohydrate:}$$
$$C_6H_{12}O_6 + 6\,O_2 \rightarrow 6\,CO_2 + 6\,H_2O$$

$$\text{Triglyceride (fat):}$$
$$2\,C_{57}H_{110}O_6 + 163\,O_2 \rightarrow 114\,CO_2 + 110\,H_2O$$

$$\text{Protein:}$$
$$C_{72}H_{112}N_2O_{22}S + 77\,O_2 \rightarrow 63\,CO_2 + 38\,H_2O + SO_3$$
$$+ 9\,CO\,(NH_2)_2$$

Balanced chemical equations, such as those can be used to calculate the **respiratory quotient (RQ)** for energy substrates. The RQ is equal to the amount of CO_2 exhaled divided by the amount of O_2 inhaled:

$$RQ = CO_2/O_2$$

For example:

RQ of glucose	$6\,CO_2/6\,O_2 = 1.0$
RQ for the example triglyceride	$114\,CO_2/163\,O_2 = 0.70$
RQ for the example protein	$63\,CO_2/77\,O_2 = 0.82$

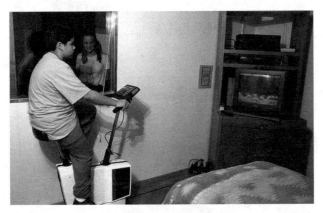

FIGURE 8.2 Direct Calorimetry Chamber. Heat dissipated from a person in a sealed water lined chamber is measured to obtain caloric expenditure.

RQ is used synonymously with RER, or respiratory exchange ratio. However, RQ reflects gas exchange at the cell/tissue level, and RER is more appropriately used when assessing gas exchange between the lungs and the environment and measured with a spirometer. Once the gas exchange quantities and RER for a given period of time are known, the energy expenditure can be calculated using the thermal equivalent of the gas quantities (**TABLE 8.1**). For instance, if an individual consumes 15 liters of O_2 and expires 12 liters of CO_2 in a 1-hour period of time, one could first calculate that individual's RER for that hour:

$$RER = 12/15 = 0.80$$

At an RER of 0.80, an individual would be using approximately 33% carbohydrates and 66% fat to fuel his or her metabolism (see Table 8.1). Under typical conditions, the contribution of amino acids to energy production is assumed to be minimal. Protein should be considered significant during extended fasting and/or prolonged exercise or during and after a high-protein meal. The metabolic rate is estimated by multiplying the amount of O_2 consumed (15 liters) by the caloric value for 1 liter of O_2 at an RER of 0.80:

$$15 \times 4.801 = 72 \text{ kilocalories/hour}$$

Doubly Labeled Water

Doubly labeled water (DLW) refers to water molecules containing the stable isotopes of hydrogen and oxygen: ^2H (deuterium) and ^{18}O. Estimating energy expenditure

TABLE 8.1 Thermal Equivalents of Oxygen and Carbon Dioxide for Nonprotein Respiratory Exchange Ratio (RER)

Nonprotein RER	Caloric Value, 1 L O_2	Caloric Value, 1 L CO_2	Carbohydrate (%)	Fat (%)
0.707	4.686	6.629	0	100.0
0.71	4.690	6.606	1.1	98.9
0.72	4.702	6.531	4.76	95.2
0.73	4.714	6.458	8.4	91.6
0.74	4.727	6.388	12.0	88.0
0.75	4.739	6.319	15.6	84.4
0.76	4.751	6.253	19.2	80.8
0.77	4.64	6.187	22.8	77.2
0.78	4.776	6.123	26.3	73.7
0.79	4.788	6.062	29.9	70.1
0.80	4.801	6.001	33.4	66.6
0.81	4.813	5.942	36.9	63.1
0.82	4.825	5.884	40.3	59.7
0.83	4.838	5.829	43.8	56.2
0.84	4.850	5.774	47.2	52.8
0.85	4.862	5.721	50.7	49.3

TABLE 8.1 *(continued)*

Nonprotein RER	Caloric Value, 1 L O$_2$	Caloric Value, 1 L CO$_2$	Carbohydrate (%)	Fat (%)
0.86	4.875	5.669	54.1	45.9
0.87	4.887	5.617	57.5	42.5
0.88	4.899	5.568	60.8	39.2
0.89	4.911	5.519	64.2	35.8
0.90	4.924	5.471	67.5	32.5
0.91	4.936	5.424	70.8	29.2
0.92	4.948	5.378	74.1	25.9
0.93	4.961	5.333	77.4	22.6
0.94	4.973	5.290	80.7	19.3
0.95	4.985	5.247	84.0	16.0
0.96	4.998	5.205	87.2	12.8
0.97	5.010	5.165	90.4	9.58
0.98	5.022	5.124	93.6	6.37
0.99	5.035	5.085	96.8	3.18
100	5.047	5.047	100	0

using DLW is based on the quantification of those two elements in body water to estimate the production of CO_2 during energy metabolism. To begin, ^2H_2O and $H_2^{18}O$ are ingested by an individual or infused into his or her circulation. After ^2H_2O and $H_2^{18}O$ equilibrate throughout body fluid, they are slowly lost from the body. ^2H remains as a component of body water and is excreted during normal water loss (e.g., urine, sweat, expiration). At the same time, some of the ^{18}O from $H_2^{18}O$ becomes part of the CO_2 produced by the carbonic anhydrase system in the blood. **FIGURE 8.4** provides an overview of this system, which serves as a means of circulating greater amounts of CO_2 from tissue to the lungs. ^2H_2O is lost only through the urine and evaporation. The ^{18}O from $H_2^{18}O$ can be lost via the lungs, urine, and evaporation. CO_2 production over time can be estimated by the difference in the levels of ^2H_2O and $H_2^{18}O$ in saliva and urine. Then the

volume of CO_2 (Vco_2) can be used to estimate energy expenditure by applying a specific factor.

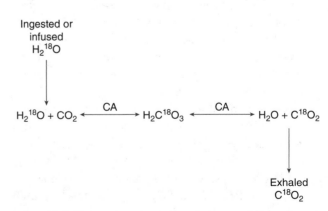

FIGURE 8.4 Carbonic Anhydrase System. Carbonic anhydrase (CA) catalyzes a reversible reaction that converts H_2O and CO_2 to carbonic acid and vice versa. (Shows labeled oxygen, ^{18}O, as a means of measuring activity).

Components of Energy Metabolism

Total energy metabolism is a reflection of all cellular activities in the body combined. However, human metabolism can fluctuate during a given period of measurement based on activity; environmental conditions; and the digestion, absorption, and processing of ingested substances. Therefore, **total energy expenditure (TEE)** can be subdivided into four principal components that are for the most part distinct: basal metabolism (BM), thermic effect of activity (TEA), the thermic effect of food (TEF), and adaptive thermogenesis (AT).

$$TEE = BM + TEA + TEF + AT$$

Basal Metabolism (Resting Metabolism)

Basal metabolism is the energy expended by internal processes during a period of complete rest (nonactive state) in a climate-controlled environment (not unusually cold or warm) at least 10 to 12 hours after the consumption of the most recent meal. **Basal metabolic rate (BMR)** is simply the basal metabolism within a specific time period, such as a minute, hour, or day. The processes that take place during basal metabolism include those that fundamentally support life and homeostasis—for example, the energy expended to support resting heart rate and basal respiration; the active processes of urine formation, cellular turnover, and the synthesis of proteins, nucleic acids, and other substances; as well as the tight regulation of ion concentrations across cellular membranes.

BMR is often used interchangeably with **resting metabolic rate (RMR)** and **resting energy expenditure (REE)**; however, the major difference is that an individual does not have to be in a fasting state to measure RMR. Consumption of a meal within a few hours prior to measurement of metabolic rate is typical, and thus, RMR is viewed as more representative of a real-world or daily base metabolism. Typically, 50 to 65% of TEE is attributable to BMR, and 65 to 75% to RMR.

Because the various tissues and organs in the human body have specific operations and masses, their contribution to basal metabolism differs. For instance, the most metabolically active tissues are organs, such as the heart, kidneys, lungs, brain, and liver. Collectively, those organs only contribute about 5% to adult body weight; however, the energy expended by those organs accounts for as much as 50 to 60% of REE (**TABLE 8.2**). Skeletal muscle, which makes up approximately 36 and 45% of a woman's and man's body weight, respectively, is not as metabolically active as the organs just mentioned when muscle is inactive. However, based on mass contribution to

TABLE 8.2 Estimated Metabolic Rates of Tissue and Percentage Contribution to Total Metabolism

	REE	MEN	WOMEN
	kcal/kg/day	% Total REE	% Total REE
Liver	200	17	18
Brain	240	19	21
Heart	440	9	8
Kidneys	440	8	8
Skeletal Muscle[a]	13	24	20
Adipose Tissue	4.5	4	7
Other[b]	12	19	18
		100	100

[a]Resting and nonexercise recovery state.
[b]Skeleton, blood, skin, GI tract, lungs, spleen, and other organs present in small amounts.
Data from Wang et al. Evaluation of specific metabolic rates of major organs tissues: Comparison between men and women. *Am J Hum Biol* 2011 23(3):333–338.

total body weight, resting skeletal muscle metabolism, which is mostly composed of protein turnover and tissue remodeling operations, contributes about 20 to 25% to REE for inactive people and 30 to 40% in athletes. Adipose tissue, in contrast, contributes relatively little unless its total mass is excessive.

Because most other aspects of RMR are generally static, increasing the ratio of skeletal muscle to fat is perhaps the most significant nonpharmacologic way of increasing RMR. For example, based on metabolic assumptions, a 90-kilogram (approximately 200-pound) man with 12% body fat would be expected to have a higher RMR than another man who weighed the same yet possessed 25% body fat. That's because skeletal muscle tends to be roughly 3X more metabolic (kcal/kg) than adipose tissue in a resting state (see Table 8.2). Furthermore, that differential will become higher in a postexercise resting state exponentially. Collectively, energy expenditure (at rest) of fat-free mass (FFM) approximates 13 to 28 kilocalories per kilogram per day (kcal/kg/day). In contrast, adipose tissue has a very low metabolic rate relative to its mass and normally contributes less than muscle to BMR or

RMR; estimations are approximately 4.5 kcal/kg/day. Variations in FFM have been shown to explain 65 to 90% of the variation in BMR or RMR energy expenditures between people of similar gender and weight.

Men tend to have a greater skeletal muscle-to-adipose tissue ratio than women; thus, the RMR for men is, on average, greater than the RMR for women on a per-weight basis. That concept is easily supported by the difference in O_2 consumption for women vs men. On average, women tend to consume only about 80% of the O_2 (milliliters per minute per kilogram) as men. RMR per kilogram body weight is highest during infancy and declines with age. Here again, RMR is mostly related to lean body mass (LBM), which tends to be higher during infancy (kcal/kg LBM) and lower in older individuals.

Several equations are available to quickly estimate BMR for a day without the assistance of a human calorimeter or a metabolic cart to measure gas exchange. A limitation of those calculations is that they tend to overestimate basal metabolism in heavier individuals with a higher percentage of body fat. The following are three commonly used equations for BMR. Note that in those equations, body weight (BW) is in kilograms (1 pound = 0.454 kilogram), and height (Ht) is in centimeters (1 inch = 2.54 centimeters).

Rule of Thumb

$$BMR = BW \times 24 \text{ hours}$$

Body Weight Raised to the Power of Three-Fourths

$$BMR = 70 \times BW^{0.75}$$

Harris and Benedict Equation

Men: BMR = 66.5 + (13.75 × BW) + (5.0 × Ht) – (6.78 × Age)
Women: BMR = 655.1 + (9.56 × BW) + (1.85 × Ht) – (4.68 × Age)

The following two equations are for RMR. Again, BW is in kilograms as is fat-free mass, and height (Ht) is in centimeters.

Mifflin–St. Jeor Equation

Men: (10 × BW) + (6.25 × Ht) – (5 × Age) + 5
Women: (10 × BW) + (6.25 × Ht) – (5 × Age) – 161

Cunningham Equation

$$RMR = 500 + (22 \times \text{fat-free mass})$$

The Cunningham equation uses FFM in kilograms to estimate RMR. Estimating FFM is simple once the percentage of fat mass (%FM) has been determined.

First, the fat mass (FM) is calculated, which is body weight multiplied by the percentage of body fat (%BF). Then FM is subtracted from body weight to determine the FFM.

The Mifflin–St. Jeor equation is adequate for the typical population of generally healthy, adults who do not engage in regular exercise training. For leaner, muscular people, such as athletes and fitness enthusiasts, estimating RMR based on body composition via the Cunningham equation is more appropriate. The following is a comparison of RMR estimates calculated via the Mifflin–St. Jeor and Cunningham equations for a 35-year-old man who weighs 180 pounds (82 kilograms) and is 5 feet, 11 inches tall (180 centimeters) with 15% FM. As shown, the estimated RMR is 13% higher using the Cunningham equation.

Mifflin–St. Jeor Equation

$$RMR = (10 \times 82) + (6.25 \times 180) - 5 \times 35) + 5$$
$$= 1{,}775 \text{ kilocalories}$$

Cunningham Equation

Step 1. Determine %FFM: 100% – 15% = 85% FFM
Step 2. Determine FFM: 82 kg × 0.85 = 70 kg FFM
Step 3. Determine RMR: 500 + 22(70)
= 2,040 kilocalories

Thermic Effect of Activity

The events of skeletal muscle activity are extremely costly from an ATP standpoint. Sarcomere contraction and relaxation requires the hydrolysis of ATP and myosin ATPase activity that powers the "power stroke" of sliding filaments and Ca^{2+} pumping across the sarcoplasmic reticulum and plasma membranes accounts for most of the energy expenditure. The **thermic effect of activity (TEA)** includes not only skeletal muscle activity during obvious movements, such as walking, running, bicycling, climbing stairs, or vacuuming the floor but also skeletal muscle activity associated with the maintenance of position and posture. Although the contribution of the latter skeletal muscle effort may seem minor, sitting on a stool without back support increases heat production by 3 to 5%. The increase in metabolism is even greater when standing.

TEA is often subdivided into nonexercise activity thermogenesis (NEAT) and exercise. NEAT includes the activities associated with daily living, such as showering, driving, chores, and occupational activities. Meanwhile, exercise includes planned, structured physical activity for improved health and fitness or physical performance. That strategy is particularly useful for evaluating athletes as well as for demonstrating the benefit of school physical education programs and the inclusion of regular exercise in weight control regimens.

To account for TEA, RMR (or BMR) can be multiplied by a specific physical activity level (PAL) factor (**TABLE 8.3**). For example, a person with a sedentary lifestyle would multiply his or her RMR by 1.25, accounting for BMR, TEF, and NEAT. Meanwhile, a very active person would multiply his or her RMR by 2.2, which would also include energy expenditure for exercise. Generally, the PAL is based on the ratio of TEE to RMR. Meanwhile, the thermal effect of a specific activity, such as running, cycling, or weight training, can also be assessed (**TABLE 8.4**). For individuals engaged in serious training whereby skeletal muscle and/or the cardiovascular system undergo physical and physiologic adaptations, the incremental energy expenditure associated with adaptation is assessed as part of BMR or RMR. For instance, intense resistance training can result in the expenditure of a couple hundred kilocalories during an intense training session. However, energy expenditure by skeletal muscle can remain elevated for several hours after the intense session as the tissue repairs and remodels itself (adapts).

Thermic Effect of Food

The **thermic effect of food (TEF)** is the increase in energy expenditure associated with food; it is also known as the specific dynamic action (SDA) of food and as diet-induced thermogenesis (DIT). It represents an augmentation in metabolism attributable to the digestion, absorption, processing, and storage of food and its components. TEF increases metabolism above BMR by 5 to 15%, depending on the size and composition of a meal. Generally, TEF is estimated as 10% of total energy intake during a particular period. For instance, TEF can be estimated at 250 kilocalories for an individual who ingests a mixed diet containing 2,500 kilocalories over a 24-hour period. However, based on differences in internal processing of the energy nutrients, protein is predictably more thermogenic than carbohydrates, and unsaturated fatty acids are more thermogenic than saturated fatty acids.

TEF can even begin prior to the digestion and absorption of food. As mentioned previously, the mere thought, sight, smell, and taste of food results in a cephalic phase of digestion. This cephalic phase, which is mediated autonomically, can result in several secretory and motile operations. TEF appears to peak approximately 1 hour after ingestion of the meal and wanes after 3 to 5 hours. The events include smooth muscle operations, active-transport release of various digestive and endocrine secretions, active transport at the apical and basolateral membranes of enterocytes, and processing and storage of absorbed substances.

Adaptive Thermogenesis

Changes in environmental temperature and radiant energy (e.g., solar radiation) can influence metabolic

TABLE 8.3 Physical Activity Level (PAL) Categories and Walking Equivalence

			Walking Equivalence (miles/day at 3–4 mph)		
PAL Category	PAL Range	Average PAL	Light-Weight Individual (44 kg/97 lb person)	Middle-Weight Individual (70 kg/154 lb person)	Heavy-Weight Individual (120 kg/265 lb person)
Sedentary	1.0–1.39	1.25	~0	~0	~0
Low active	1.4–1.59	1.5	~2.9 miles 43–58 min	~2.2 miles 33–44 min	~1.5 miles 22–30 min
Active	1.6–1.89	1.75	~9.9 miles 148–198 min	~7.3 miles 109–146 min	~5.3 miles 79–106 min
Very active	1.9–2.5	2.2	~22.5 miles 337–450 min	~16.7 miles 250–337 min	~12.3 miles 184–246 min

Note: Walking equivalence decreases as body weight increases. This means that a heavier person needs to walk a shorter distance and for less time to expend the same energy as a lighter person.

Data from Institute of Medicine, Food and Nutrition Board. *Dietary Reference Intakes for Energy, Carbohydrate, Fiber, Fat, Fatty Acids, Cholesterol, Protein, and Amino Acids (Macronutrients).* Washington, DC: National Academy of Sciences; 2005.

TABLE 8.4 Kilocalories per Minute Expended During Various Activities and Body Weight

	Weight in Pounds					
Activity	100	120	140	160	180	200
Bicycling						
5 mph	1.9	2.3	2.7	3.1	3.5	3.9
10 mph	4.2	5.1	5.9	6.8	7.6	8.5
15 mph	7.3	8.7	10.0	11.6	13.1	14.5
20 mph	10.7	12.8	14.9	17.1	19.2	21.3
Running						
6 mph	7.2	8.7	10.2	11.7	13.1	14.6
7 mph	8.5	10.2	11.9	13.6	15.4	17.1
8 mph	9.7	11.6	13.6	15.6	17.6	19.5
9 mph	10.8	12.9	15.1	17.3	19.5	21.7
Skiing (cross country)						
2.5 mph	5.0	6.0	7.0	8.0	9.0	10.0
4.0 mph	6.5	7.8	9.2	10.5	11.9	13.2
5.0 mph	7.7	9.2	10.8	12.3	13.9	15.4
Skiing (downhill)	6.5	7.8	9.2	10.5	11.9	13.2
Soccer	5.9	7.2	8.4	9.6	10.8	12.0
Tennis	5.0	6.0	7.0	8.0	9.0	10.0
Walking						
7 mph	2.7	3.3	3.8	4.4	4.9	5.4
4 mph	4.2	5.1	5.9	6.8	7.6	8.5
5 mph	5.4	6.5	7.7	8.7	9.8	10.9
Weight training	5.2	6.0	7.3	8.3	9.4	10.5

rate. A homeostatic objective of man is to maintain constant or near constant **core body temperature**, because several aspects of human physiology are temperature based, such as the activity of enzymes.

Thermal sensors are located both at the level of the skin and deeper toward the body core, mainly in the spinal cord, the abdominal viscera, and in and around the great veins. Both skin and deep receptors are more sensitive to cold than to warmth. Most actions that regulate body core temperature are initiated in the posterior hypothalamus. Under more comfortable temperatures, radiation and convection can account for as much as 60 and 15% of heat loss, respectively. Evaporation accounts for the majority of the remaining heat loss, and conduction accounts for only about 2 to 3%.

As environmental temperature increases, heat production decreases until a lower critical temperature is reached. As environmental temperature continues to rise, metabolic heat production demonstrates a plateau until an upper critical environmental temperature is reached. Despite a reduction in the energy gradient for convection and radiation losses in a hotter environment, the body is still able to maintain the core temperature by increasing evaporative loss. The upper critical temperature is the point at which core body temperature begins to rise and the well-being of the body is thus placed in jeopardy. Here, metabolic heat production increases in a survival effort to increase cardiac output and circulation to the periphery for heat removal. The upper critical environmental temperature is lower in more humid and sunny environments.

In contrast, as environmental temperature decreases, heat-conserving and heat-producing operations are increased. Less blood is circulated to the periphery, as regulated by the hypothalamus, thereby reducing heat by conduction, convection, and radiation. There is also a decrease in the production of sweat for evaporation. At the same time, piloerection (the standing on end of body hair) occurs. This has very little impact in humans, but in other animals, it allows for the creation of a layer of insulating air close to the skin. In humans, body temperature can be maintained as environmental temperature continues to fall, but only to a point. This point, called the summit metabolism, is defined as the maximal rate of metabolism that occurs in response to cold without a decline in body temperature. Increases in metabolism are accounted for by either shivering or nonshivering (chemical) thermogenesis. Shivering is the visible contraction and generated tension of subcutaneous skeletal muscle. ATP is hydrolyzed, and heat is liberated.

Nonshivering thermogenesis (NST) may result from epinephrine- or norepinephrine-promoted uncoupling of oxidative phosphorylation in certain cells, such as brown adipose tissue. The mitochondria in those cells are designed to perform this operation. This mechanism is more significant in infants. By adulthood, only negligible amounts of brown adipose tissue remain,

and NST by that means is minimal. In addition, thyroid hormone secretion is increased by a series of steps as follows. The cooling of the body leads to a release of thyrotropin-releasing hormone (TRH) from the hypothalamus, which then stimulates the anterior pituitary gland to release thyroid-stimulating hormone (TSH), which, in turn, stimulates the release of thyroid hormone from the thyroid gland. Thyroid hormone increases the general metabolic rate of many cells. However, this response may be more significant with chronic exposure to cold and not necessarily an acute response to cold.

● BEFORE YOU GO ON . . .

1. What are the principles of each of the three methods used to determine BMR?

2. What is total energy metabolism, and what techniques are employed to measure it?

3. What are the key components that contribute to basal metabolism?

4. What impact does consuming food have on body metabolism, and do different energy nutrients have the same impact on TEF?

5. What impact do physical activity and exercise have on energy expenditure, and what role does body weight play?

6. Can environmental temperature influence metabolism and energy expenditure, and is this a consideration in the real world?

▶ Metabolic States and Integrated Energy Metabolism

Over the course of the day, the body's metabolism fluctuates. Typically, those fluctuations are the result of eating or not eating and of physical activity and exercise. During those times, energy metabolism in different tissue is influenced by substrate availability as well as by hormones (**FIGURE 8.5** and **TABLE 8.5**). For ATP to be available, cells must have a constant supply of energy substrates. Carbohydrates, proteins (amino acids), fat, and ethanol, as well as intermediate molecules of their metabolism (e.g., pyruvate, lactate), are broken down within metabolic pathways, and their inherent energy is transferred to the high-energy bonds of ATP and, to a lesser degree, to GTP. Those energy substrates can be derived directly from the diet during

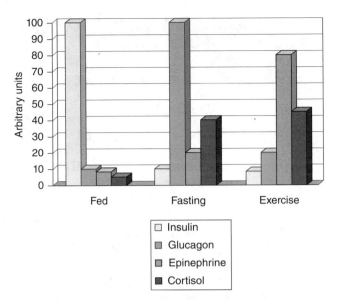

FIGURE 8.5 Hormone Levels During Different Metabolic States. Relative levels of the major metabolic hormones during and right after a meal (fed), more than 8 to 12 hours after a meal (fasting), and during sustained moderate- to higher-intensity exercise. (Glucagon levels may increase during exercise if blood glucose levels decline.)

a fed state (external eating) or from endogenous stores of carbohydrate, protein, and fat (internal eating) during a fasting period. Hormonal and neurological factors, as well as the availability of those substrates, are involved in the utilization of the different sources and are briefly reviewed in this section.

Cellular and Tissue Metabolism

The utilization of energy substrates varies among cell type based on availability, cellular design, the presence of hormones, and the physiologic state (**TABLE 8.6**). The consumption of substrates in some cell types is limited to a single nutrient, as is the case with glucose in red blood cells. Many other cells, such as hepatocytes and skeletal muscle fibers, can use different energy nutrients over the course of a day, as influenced by nutrient availability, hormones, the presence of mitochondria, the rate of expression of enzymes and transporters, allosteric influences, and the energy and redox state of the cell. Still, other cell types have the ability to adapt in more extreme metabolic scenarios to use

TABLE 8.5 Actions of Insulin, Glucagon, Cortisol, and Epinephrine in General Energy Metabolic Systems

Metabolic Process	Insulin	Glucagon	Cortisol	Epinephrine
Glycolysis in cells	✓			
Glycogen synthesis in liver and skeletal muscle[a]	✓		✓	
Glycogenolysis in liver and skeletal muscle[b]		✓		✓
Gluconeogenesis in liver (and kidneys)[c]		✓	✓	
Fat breakdown in adipose tissue		✓	✓	✓
β-oxidation in skeletal muscle, liver, and adipose tissue		✓	✓	✓
Fatty acid synthesis in liver and adipose tissue	✓			
Protein synthesis in skeletal muscle and liver	✓			
Protein breakdown in skeletal muscle and liver[d]			✓	
Ketone body formation in liver		✓	✓	
Ketone body utilization in the brain		✓	✓	

Checked boxes indicate a regulatory role of the metabolic hormone.

[a]Cortisol promotes liver glycogen synthesis in the liver (not muscle).
[b]Muscle cells do not have glucagon receptors, so glucagon promotes glycogen breakdown in the liver.
[c]Gluconeogenesis in the kidneys serves as a glucose source for other renal cells.
[d]Insulin decreases muscle protein breakdown in skeletal muscle, thus promoting a net protein production.

TABLE 8.6 Fuel Sources for Select Organs and Tissue

Tissue or Cell Type	Energy Substrate	Metabolic or Cellular Considerations[a]
Erythrocytes (RBCs)	Glucose	▪ Lack mitochondria ▪ Obligatory glucose use ▪ Obligatory lactate production
Hepatocytes	Glucose, fatty acids, amino acids, lactate, fructose, galactose, ethanol	▪ Primary site of ketone body synthesis ▪ Primary site of fatty acid synthesis ▪ Primary site of gluconeogenesis
Skeletal muscle	Glucose, fatty acids, certain amino acids, ketone bodies, some fructose	▪ Availability of substrate ▪ Metabolic state
Cardiac muscle	Glucose, fatty acids, certain amino acids, ketone bodies, lactate	▪ Availability of substrate ▪ Metabolic state
Smooth muscle	Primarily glucose	▪ Produces some lactate
GI tract	Primarily glucose, certain amino acids (especially glutamine)	▪ Produces some lactate
Retina	Primarily glucose	▪ Produces some lactate
Kidneys	Primarily glucose, some lactate, glycerol, and ketone bodies	▪ Produces some glucose
Central nervous system	Glucose, lactate, ketone bodies during starvation	▪ Ketone bodies during fasting and diet-induced ketogenesis
Adipose tissue	Glucose, fatty acids, some fructose	▪ Metabolic state

[a]Metabolic conditions are regulated by hormones. Availability of nutrients, such as glucose, fatty acids, amino acids, and glycerol will influence what some cells use for fuel.

alternative substrates, such as the brain's use of ketone bodies during starvation.

Nutritional state is the most influential factor in determining general energy nutrient use. The major organs involved in the processing of energy molecules in the human body are the liver, adipose tissue, and skeletal muscle; however, the heart should also be recognized. Those organs accommodate energy intake in excess of current need by creating energy stores. Other tissue can also do this, but not to the extent of the liver, skeletal muscle, and adipose tissue.

Obligate Glucose Utilization

Red blood cells (RBCs) are considered obligate glucose users because they derive all of their energy from glucose all of the time. The brain uses glucose in very high proportions under normal circumstances. Because the brain and RBCs require a constant supply of glucose (as certain parts of the renal tubule system might), one of the primary metabolic objectives during fluctuating daily nutritional states is the maintenance of blood glucose levels (euglycemia). Moreover, during extended fasting periods lasting several days, euglycemia is viewed as perhaps the most important objective. However, as starvation continues, the preservation of body protein becomes a strong consideration as well.

Transitional Metabolic States

One final factor must be considered with regard to metabolic states. Although it is often easier to discuss metabolic states as distinct, there are transitional periods during which opposing influences overlap. The molar concentration of insulin to glucagon and the residual effects of those hormones is a significant factor. For example, during the first hour or so after eating a meal, some of the residual effects of fasting still linger; conversely, the transition from a fed to a fasting state is not easily defined.

Metabolic Crossroads

The fact that several intermediates of energy pathways sit at metabolic crossroads provides coordination of energy pathways. Therefore, although the energy pathways are often thought of as if they were discrete processes, they can also be viewed as feeding in and out from each other. For instance, acetyl CoA, which can be formed by β-oxidation or from pyruvate, can be used to make ketone bodies or citrate, which can continue through the Krebs cycle for immediate energy use or used in fatty acid synthesis. Pyruvate is another crossroad intermediate. It can be produced via glycolysis or from lactate and the catabolism of certain amino acids. Pyruvate can be used to produce acetyl CoA or oxaloacetate in mitochondria or to synthesize alanine or lactate in the cytosol.

Fed State

Although the size of a meal and its composition are influential, the following discussion assumes a typical mixed diet containing carbohydrate, protein, and fat. Ingestion of food leads to the absorption of energy molecules into both the hepatic portal vein (amino acids, monoglycerides, glycerol, shorter-chain-length fatty acids, and medium-chain triglycerides) and the lymphatic circulation (chylomicron-endowed triglycerides). Both of those circulations eventually flow into the systemic circulation after perfusing the liver and passing through the thoracic duct, respectively.

The liver removes more than half of the absorbed amino acids and glucose and nearly all of the galactose and fructose during the first pass (**FIGURE 8.6**). The remaining amino acids and glucose serve to increase the levels of those energy sources in the blood. The increased levels of circulating glucose and amino acids become the primary stimuli for insulin release, and the resulting increase in the insulin-to-glucagon ratio dictates the majority of the ensuing metabolic events (see Figure 8.5). The release of insulin, as strongly stimulated by glucose and less strongly by amino acids, is actually primed or amplified,

or both, by circulating digestion-related hormones such as gastrin, cholecystokinin, secretin, and gastrin inhibitory polypeptide. Insulin promotes the translocation of GLUT4 receptors to the plasma membrane of muscle and adipose tissue (see Figure 8.6). Additionally, insulin promotes the increased uptake of glucose in the liver and decreases the breakdown of muscle protein.

Early Refeeding

During the period of early refeeding, the liver is still engaged in gluconeogenic operations that will linger for some time. Thus, some of the glycogen synthesized in hepatocytes in early refeeding is actually derived from gluconeogenic precursors, such as amino acids and lactate from muscle (**FIGURE 8.7**). Dietary glucose is phosphorylated to glucose-6-phosphate, and, along with glucose-6-phosphate derived from gluconeogenesis, is used to synthesize glycogen. Some glucose-6-phosphate will also continue through glycolysis as glycolytic enzymes become activated by the increasing insulin-to-glucagon ratio. However, glucose flux through glycolysis in early refeeding is not as great as perhaps would be expected. The primary reason is that the gluconeogenic and lipolytic effects of fasting are still prevalent, yet waning, and hepatocytes are still oxidizing fatty acids. As a result, increased quantities of acetyl CoA are available in the cell and inhibit pyruvate dehydrogenase, thereby favoring gluconeogenesis and slowing glycolysis upstream.

Some diet-derived amino acids, as well as amino acids delivered to hepatocytes during fasting, are also used to produce glucose-6-phosphate and, subsequently, glycogen. This notion is supported by experimental findings that liver glycogen monomers are derived from the carbon skeletons of amino acids. Thus, in the liver, gluconeogenic and glycolytic operations coexist for a brief period of time as the former wanes and the latter predominates. The slowing of glycolysis in early refeeding allows for more glucose-6-phosphate to be used as a reactant for the pentose phosphate pathway. The primary significance of this operation for energy metabolism is that the oxidative reactions of the pentose phosphate pathway produce NADPH, which is necessary for subsequent fatty acid synthesis.

In the early refeeding state, fatty acid oxidation continues in skeletal muscle and wanes slowly with time. Again, pyruvate dehydrogenase is inactivated by increased levels of mitochondrial acetyl CoA and ATP, as well as relatively higher amounts of NADH:NAD$^+$.

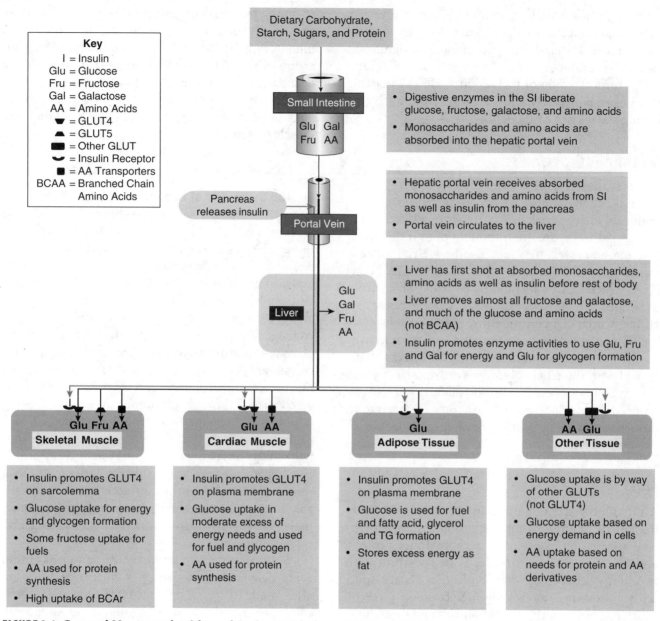

FIGURE 8.6 General Monosaccharide and Amino Acid Absorption and Uptake. Monosaccharides and amino acids are absorbed from the small intestine (SI) into the hepatic portal vein, which, along with insulin from the pancreas, circulate to the liver first. Most of the fructose and galactose and much of the glucose and amino acids are taken up by the liver during the first pass. Branched-chain amino acids (BCAA) are preferentially taken up by skeletal muscle.

Therefore, some of the pyruvate generated from glycolysis is converted to lactate. This lactate can diffuse from the cell, circulate to the liver, and be used in gluconeogenesis or other operations. Additionally, muscle cell glucose-6-phosphate is used to resynthesize glycogen within muscle cells. The pentose phosphate pathway is not a consideration in muscle, primarily because of its lack of fatty acid and steroid synthesis.

Although small amounts of glycogen exist in adipose cells, most of the glucose entering those cells is oxidized for energy and to begin the generation of glyceraldehyde-3-phosphate, which is metabolized to citrate and then acetyl CoA for fatty acid synthesis (**FIGURE 8.8**). Those fatty acids, along with fatty acids delivered from the blood, are available for synthesis of triglyceride. Therefore, those cells use the increased intracellular pool of glucose-6-phosphate to synthesize fatty acids and a little glycogen as well as to provide energy to drive the synthetic and homeostatic operations within those cells during early refeeding.

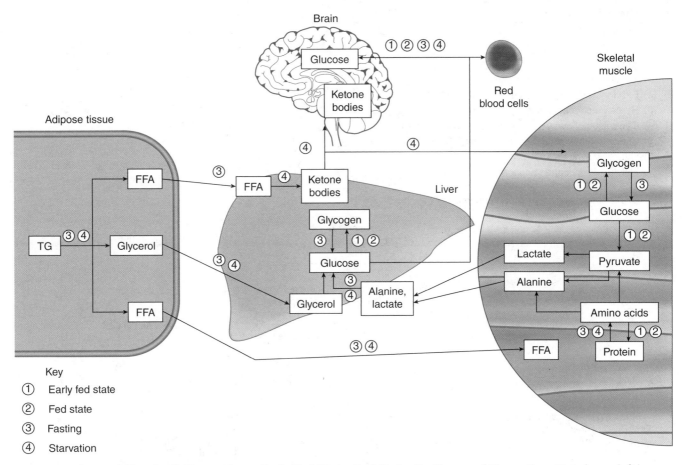

FIGURE 8.7 General Metabolic Events in an Early Fed State, Fed State, Fasting, and Starvation. Note lower left key that indicates either usage or production of metabolic compounds in adipose tissue, liver, and skeletal muscle as a function of fed and caloric restricted states.

Intermediate to Longer Fed State

As the fed state continues, the anabolic effects of the elevated insulin-to-glucagon ratio dominate. Gluconeogenesis in hepatocytes is now inhibited in the liver, and fatty acid oxidation trickles to a stop. At this time, glucose becomes the primary source of fuel in skeletal muscle cells, which are also fully engaged in glycogen synthesis (see Figure 8.7). The extent to which muscle cells will take up glucose from the blood is strongly influenced by their ability to store glucose as glycogen as well as their ability to metabolize glucose as an energy source. Because skeletal muscle will not synthesize fatty acids, the skeletal muscle triglyceride pool available for triglyceride production and storage is largely derived from lipoproteins (via lipoprotein lipase [LPL]) and circulating fatty acids loosely bound to albumin.

Most other cell types oxidize glucose in the fed state, which is a mixture of premeal circulating glucose and absorbed glucose. The net effect is a reduction in circulatory glucose as promoted by a relatively high molar ratio of insulin to glucagon. Glucose levels can decrease from over 140 milligrams per deciliter (100 milliliters) of blood in a fed state to under 100 milligrams per deciliter during the transition to a fasting state.

Fasting

After several hours, depending on the size and composition of the meal, the metabolic state of the human body slowly slips into early fasting. Here, the anabolic effects of insulin linger, while the catabolic effects of glucagon begin to become more prominent. As less and less absorbed glucose enters the circulation, allowing the concentration of glucose to normalize and move in the direction of hypoglycemia, more glucagon is secreted. Homeostatic efforts swing in favor of providing glucose to the blood from energy stores, while, at the same time, making other energy substrates available to reduce glucose use in tissue throughout the body. The central nervous system and RBCs alone can

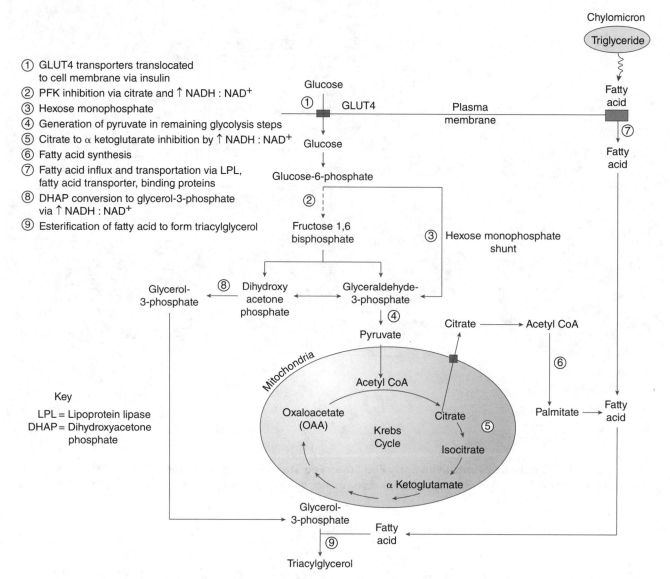

① GLUT4 transporters translocated to cell membrane via insulin
② PFK inhibition via citrate and ↑ NADH : NAD$^+$
③ Hexose monophosphate
④ Generation of pyruvate in remaining glycolysis steps
⑤ Citrate to α ketoglutarate inhibition by ↑ NADH : NAD$^+$
⑥ Fatty acid synthesis
⑦ Fatty acid influx and transportation via LPL, fatty acid transporter, binding proteins
⑧ DHAP conversion to glycerol-3-phosphate via ↑ NADH : NAD$^+$
⑨ Esterification of fatty acid to form triacylglycerol

Key

LPL = Lipoprotein lipase
DHAP = Dihydroxyacetone phosphate

FIGURE 8.8 Glucose Uptake and Utilization in Adipocytes. Glucose entering adipocytes is oxidized for energy and used to generate glyceraldehyde-3-phosphate, which is metabolized to citrate and then acetyl CoA for fatty acid synthesis. Fatty acids can be made or derived from circulation to make triglycerides.

consume about 100 to 125 grams and 45 to 50 grams of glucose daily, respectively, in an adult. Those high requirements continue in early fasting but decrease if fasting becomes protracted.

When the blood glucose level is low, elevated glucagon levels activate phosphorylase in liver cells and diminished insulin levels relieve the suppression of phosphorylase (**FIGURE 8.9**). At the same time, hepatic glucokinase activity is suppressed by the presence of glucagon and the absence of insulin. Also, insulin's positive influence on the glycogen synthase system's enzymes decreases. The net effect of those activities is that glucose entry into hepatocytes is minimized and glycogen stores are liberated. At the same time, glucose-6-phosphatase is induced by glucagon, which

liberates glucose from glucose-6-phosphate derived from glycogen and gluconeogenesis. The substrates for gluconeogenesis include circulating lactate from muscle and glycerol from triglyceride breakdown in adipose tissue.

Perhaps, the most significant source of substrate for gluconeogenesis is amino acids, primarily alanine from skeletal muscle. Cortisol is the principal stimulus for the catabolism of muscle protein, and pyruvate serves as the recipient of transaminated nitrogen to form alanine. Interestingly, increased circulating alanine levels serve as a stimulus of glucagon release; in turn, glucagon promotes gluconeogenesis in the liver. Once in hepatocytes, pyruvate is reformed and enters mitochondria. Pyruvate

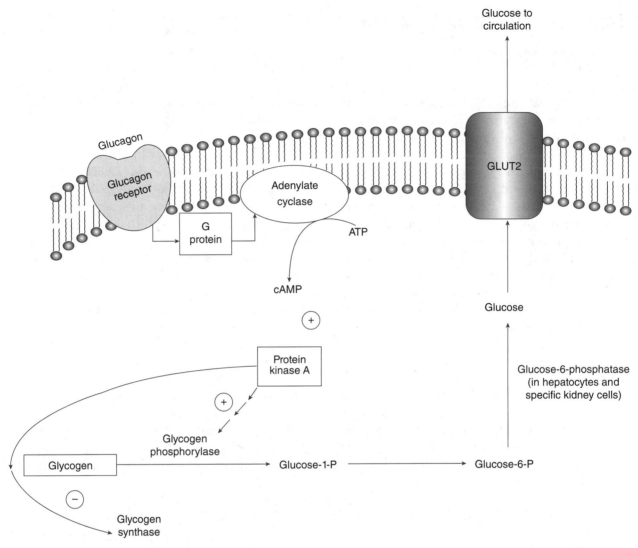

FIGURE 8.9 Glucagon and Glycogen Breakdown. Glucagon via protein kinase A promotes the activation of glycogen phosphorylase and inhibition of glycogen synthase to produce glucose-1-phosphate from glycogen. Glucose-1-phosphate is converted to glucose-6-phosphate, which can be dephosphorylated to glucose in hepatocytes.

carboxylase converts much of the pyruvate to oxalo-acetate, some of which condenses with acetyl CoA (derived from β-oxidation) to satisfy hepatocyte energy demands. The remaining pyruvate is available for gluconeogenesis.

Starvation

As starvation continues beyond 1 day, several events take place. First, hepatic glycogen stores become exhausted within the first 24 to 36 hours (see Figure 8.7). Thus, reliance upon skeletal muscle amino acids and other gluconeogenic precursors increases. Second, the production of ketone bodies increases as more and more fatty acids are mobilized and oxidized in the liver. And finally, as fasting continues for many days to weeks, tissues in the body adapt to use more ketone bodies in an effort to spare body protein.

◆ BEFORE YOU GO ON . . .

1. What is the fuel source for red blood cells and other major tissue types, such as skeletal muscle, liver, and heart?

2. What is the metabolic scenario during early refeeding, and which hormones are involved?

3. What impact will a higher ratio of insulin to glucagon (e.g., during a fed state) have on glycogenolysis, lipogenesis, and protein synthesis in different tissue?

4. Describe the metabolic events that take place in different tissue during early fasting and indicate which hormones are involved.

5. During a starvation state, what are the major gluconeogenic precursors, and what is the role of ketone bodies?

▶ Body Weight and Composition

Body weight is an important concern for many, if not most, people today. Many adults and teens step on and off scales on a daily basis, which, in turn, can lead to the initiation or sustainment of diet efforts. Although body weight is the measure of interest and concern for many people, fitness and health professionals understand that body composition needs to be an important consideration as well. **Body weight** is the total mass of a person and is expressed in pounds (lb) or kilograms (kg); **body composition** refers to the relative contributions to a person's mass made by different substances or tissues that make up the body. Body composition can be broken down to the level of molecules and elements or to major tissue classes such as fat mass and fat-free mass. This section looks more closely at the components of body composition as well as the relationships among body weight, body composition, and health.

Body Weight and Health

Body weight has long been used as a predictor of health because of its association with body composition, especially for inactive people. Generally speaking, heavier people tend to have greater amounts and percentages of fat. Likewise, inactivity in individuals is a reasonable predictor of body fat levels. As the amount of body fat increases above desirable levels, the risk of certain diseases (such as heart disease) rises in a related manner. With this in mind, weight standards have been developed to determine body weight ranges that can be used to characterize a population and be used in health promotion. For instance, the Department of Health and Human Services published the *2015–2020 Dietary Guidelines for Americans*, which includes healthy body weight ranges based on height (**FIGURE 8.10**).

The concept of a **healthy weight** was developed to identify a body weight specific to an individual's gender, height, and frame size for which there is a strong association with good health and longevity. A person is deemed overweight if his or her body weight falls above this healthy weight range, or ideal body weight (IBW). When a person's body weight increases above or falls below the IBW range, he or she is at greater risk of illness. **TABLE 8.7** presents simple formulas for estimating IBW.

In 1943, the Metropolitan Life Insurance Company developed its weight and height tables, which were modified in 1983 and are still used as references today. Those tables present weight ranges for a given height for adults that were developed as part of a system for setting premiums for insurance policies. Standards, such as IBW, have been used for estimating obesity as well. For instance, the threshold for estimating obesity

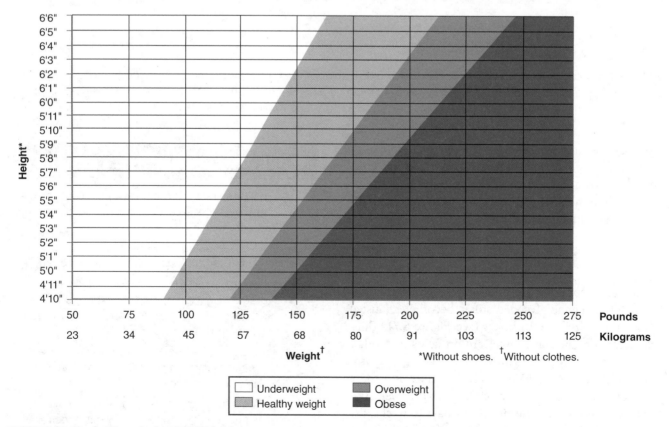

FIGURE 8.10 Body Mass Index (BMI) Table.

Data from: *Nutrition and Your Health: Dietary Guidelines for Americans*, 8th ed. Washington, DC: U.S. Departments of Health and Human Services and Agriculture; 2015-2020. Retrieved March 16, 2017, from http://www.health.gov/dietaryguidelines.

TABLE 8.7 Estimated Ideal Body Weight Formulas

Broca's index	
Men	Weight (kg) = Height (cm) − 100 ± 10%
Women	Weight (kg) = Height (cm) − 100 ± 15%
Hamwi equation (rule of thumb)	
Men	106 lb for the first 5 ft and 6 lb for each additional inch
Women	100 lb for the first 5 ft and 5 lb for each additional inch
Devine formula	
Men	Ideal body weight (kg) = 50 + 2.3 kg per inch over 5 ft
Women	Ideal body weight (kg) = 45.5 + 2.3 kg per inch over 5 ft
Robinson formula	
Men	Ideal body weight (kg) = 52 kg + 1.9 kg for each inch over 5 ft
Women	Ideal body weight (kg) = 49 kg + 1.7 kg for each inch over 5 ft
Miller formula	
Men	Ideal body weight (kg) = 56.2 kg + 1.41 kg for each inch over 5 ft
Women	Ideal body weight (kg) = 53.1 kg + 1.36 kg for each inch over 5 ft
Deurenberg formula	
Child	Body fat % = (1.51 × BMI) − (0.70 × Age) − (3.6 × Sex) + 1.4
Adult	Body fat % = (1.20 × BMI) + (0.23 × Age) − (10.8 × Sex) − 5.4 Note: Sex is 1 for males and 0 for females.

from height for the general population is set at more than 120% of an IBW for a particular gender and height.

Some of the major criticisms of simple IBW formulas are that they are not sensitive to age and physical condition. Furthermore, the values suggested by the Devine formula for women of shorter stature are unrealistically low. On the other hand, some formulas might be unrealistic for taller men. In general, IBW formulas remain as commonly used, simple methods for assessing general body weight status. However, those formulas are not considered to be a true sensitive indicator of health risk and are not as accepted as body mass index and more definitive measures of body composition and biochemical indices.

Body Mass Index

Body mass index (BMI) is a more modern method used to express body size and is calculated by dividing weight by the squared height:

$$\text{BMI} = \frac{\text{Weight (kg)}}{\text{Height}^2 \ (\text{m}^2)} \text{ or } \text{BMI} = 730 \times \frac{\text{Weight (lb)}}{\text{Height}^2 \ (\text{in}^2)}$$

Although different estimates exist, a BMI of between 18.5 and 24.9 is considered normal for a member of the general population, whereas a BMI of between 25 and 29.9 is considered overweight and a BMI of 30 or more is considered to indicate obesity (see Figure 8.10). As BMI increases above 25, the risk of disease increases, as does the rate of mortality. For instance, an adult with a BMI of 37 has double the risk of all-cause mortality of a person with a BMI of 23. In this situation, the increase in body weight is believed to play a direct role in the development of diseases that increase mortality. Because BMI is suggestive of body fat levels, researchers have attempted to generate conversion equations from BMI to body fat in adults and children (see Table 8.7). When BMI falls below 20, the risk of disease and mortality also increases. Here, the relationship is not as clear-cut as it is with a higher BMI, because a lower body weight is often a manifestation of a preexisting disease process.

Active People, Body Weight, and Health

Body weight alone cannot be used to estimate health risk for more active people and athletes because many athletes engaged in strength- and power-oriented sports maintain greater muscle mass than the generally inactive population at large. Thus, those people would be characterized as overweight or even obese by general standards, yet, they may have a relatively low body fat level and, therefore, a desirable body composition and low health risk. For example, a 5-foot, 10-inch, 225-pound bodybuilder would have a BMI of 32 and would be classified as obese. However, no one in real life would likely consider him as such. Therefore, body weight and BMI are practical estimators of body size and overweight and obesity in the general population, but they are not as useful for more active populations.

Body Composition
Elements and Molecules

Body composition can be assessed several ways, beginning at the level of elements. Here, oxygen, hydrogen, carbon, and nitrogen are recognized as the greatest contributors to human mass. This is easily understandable because those four elements are the primary atomic building blocks for key organic molecules and water. Next, human body composition can be assessed at the molecular level, with minerals grouped together to represent that which is not molecular. For instance, in a lean adult male, water can account for roughly 60% (56 to 64%) of his body mass, and protein and fat each account for roughly 15 to 16% of his total mass. About 4 to 6% of human mass can be attributed to minerals, and the remaining 1% or so is attributable to substances such as carbohydrates and nucleic acids.

Body fat shows the greatest degree of fluctuation because it can contribute from as little as 5% of mass in excessively lean adult males to as much as 65 to 70% of the total mass in excessively (morbidly) obese individuals. Adipose tissue is approximately 86% triglyceride. The remaining 14% of adipose tissue mass is largely water, protein, carbohydrate, and minerals. Those substances are associated with the intracellular and extracellular fluids, connective tissue, and enzymes as well as structural cell components, such as membranes. Because of the disproportion of major substances found in adipose tissue, as an individual accumulates larger fat stores, his or her body fat percentage increases while the percentage of the other substances, such as water, protein, carbohydrate, and minerals, decreases.

Fat Mass and Fat-Free Mass

Typically, body composition is assessed to determine the percentage of body fat and of **lean body mass (LBM)** or **fat-free mass (FFM)** (**TABLE 8.8**). Although FFM and LBM are often used interchangeably, LBM includes not only all nonfat portions of the human body but also essential fat depots. **Essential fat** is found associated with bone marrow, the central nervous system, and internal organs. Women also have essential body fat associated with the mammary glands and the pelvic region. Essential body fat for a normal adult male and female may be 3 to 5% and 10 to 13% of their body weight, respectively. **FIGURE 8.11** presents the percentage of contributions of fat, muscle, bone, and organs to total body mass for a reference man and woman. **FIGURE 8.12** presents the relative contributions to total body mass made by fat, muscle, bone, and organs in a leaner vs an obese man.

Factors such as age, gender, stature, heredity, and pregnancy influence body composition. At birth and during infancy and early childhood, minimal but evident differences exist between males and females with regard to body composition. Boys tend to have a little more total body mass and a slightly higher percentage of FFM. However, at the onset of puberty, boys experience an increase in the development of FFM, whereas girls tend to experience an increase in body fat accumulation. At about 10 years of age, a boy may have a body fat percentage of 13%, compared with 19% in a girl of the same age. Throughout adolescence and into early adulthood, the percentage of body fat typically increases for both genders, particularly for girls. In early adulthood, men possess approximately 15 to 16% of fat mass, compared with 22 to 24% for women. Also, females tend to achieve their maximal FFM by age 18, whereas males tend to demonstrate increases in FFM into their early 20s. That does not factor in the initiation of an exercise program that could allow for accretion of FFM for both males and females past those ages.

TABLE 8.8 Components of Body Composition

Component	Characteristics of Component
Fat mass (FM)	Mass of body fat (fat is defined as any lipid material that would be soluble and extractable in ether)
% Body fat (%BF)	Percentage of total body mass that is fat mass
Fat-free mass (FFM)	Mass of body substances that are not fat, including water, protein, and minerals, as found in organs, muscle, bone
Lean body mass (LBM)	Mass of FFM plus essential body fat
Total body water (TBW)	Total of intracellular and extracellular water
Bone mineral mass (BMM)	Mass of mineral content of bone based on estimators of bone density

Body Water

The contribution made by water to body weight is never higher than at birth. Approximately, 73% of a term newborn's weight is water, and even higher body water percentages—as much as 83%—are possible in premature infants. During the first year of life, an infant's body water content decreases slightly as more body fat accumulates. However, during the next 5 to 6 years, a child's body water percentage increases only slightly and then demonstrates a minor decline during the ensuing 2 to 3 years. By about the age of 10 years old, a child's body water content is still roughly 62 to 65%. At this point, boys generally possess a slightly higher percentage of body water than girls, mostly due to a changing muscle-to-fat ratio. By adulthood, body water content is generally 56 to 64%. Because the water content of the extracellular fluid is, by and large, controlled hormonally, the greatest influence on tissue water content remains the ratio of skeletal muscle to adipose tissue.

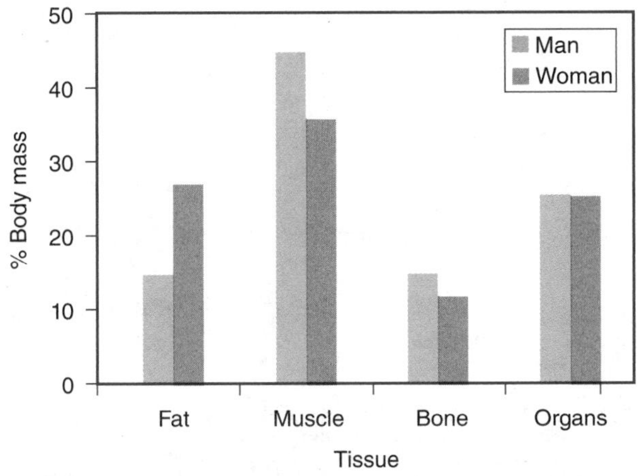

Minerals (Ash)

Whereas body water content seems to decrease as a percentage of total mass from birth to adulthood, the opposite appears to be true for mineral content or ash percentage. A typical term newborn is about 3.2% mineral, whereas an adult is 4 to 6% minerals by mass. Although many general statements can be made regarding body composition, gender, and aging, it is very likely that heredity plays a role as well and might extend to body mineral content. For example, African Americans tend to have greater total body calcium content, which is an indirect result of having more FFM and denser bones than European Americans.

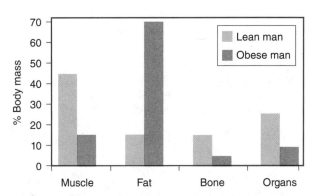

FIGURE 8.11 Theoretical Contributors to Body Weight for a Lean Man and Woman. Lean males have higher muscle mass and lower fat mass compared to lean females. Bone and organ mass does not change by sex.

FIGURE 8.12 Body Composition of a Lean and a Morbidly Obese Man. Note how the increased mass of adipose tissue "dilutes" the percentage contribution of fat-free mass components.

▶ Assessment of Body Composition

Modern techniques for the assessment of body composition range from simple use of calipers to measure skinfold (fatfold) thickness to the use of complex instrumentation, such as **computerized axial tomography (CAT)**, **dual-energy x-ray absorptiometry (DEXA or DXA)**, and **magnetic resonance imaging (MRI)**. This section focuses on three of the more common methods, and **TABLE 8.9** describes the advantages and shortcomings of several of the techniques.

Body Densitometry

The Greek mathematician Archimedes is often credited with the original concept of **densitometry**, which is the basis for hydrostatic or **underwater weighing (UWW)** (**FIGURE 8.13**). He concluded that the volume of an object submerged in water was equal to the volume of water displaced by the object. He also hypothesized that an object's density can be calculated simply by dividing the object's weight on land by its loss of weight submerged in water. This concept can be applied to humans; however, to do so, the residual lung air and gases in the lumen of the gut must be accounted for.

TABLE 8.9 Select Techniques for Body Composition Assessment

Technique	Advantages	Disadvantages
Anthropometry (skinfold thickness and circumferences)	▪ Inexpensive ▪ Estimates total body fat and regional muscle	▪ Inaccuracy increases with obesity and for individuals with firm subcutaneous tissue
CT scan	▪ Assesses organ size, fat distribution, and bone size	▪ Expensive equipment ▪ Limited availability ▪ Small radiation exposure
Bioelectrical impedance analysis (BIA)	▪ Estimates LBM via total body water ▪ Inexpensive equipment ▪ Nonhazardous	▪ Several prediction formulas ▪ Fluid and electrolyte inconsistencies can produce error
Creatinine excretion	▪ Provides estimation of muscle mass ▪ Nonhazardous	▪ Influenced by diet ▪ Several factors can decrease accuracy ▪ Participant cooperation is vital
Densitometry (Underwater weighing)	▪ Provides estimation of FM and FFM simultaneously ▪ Generally nonhazardous	▪ Participant cooperation is vital ▪ Unsuitable for children and elderly individuals ▪ Intestinal gas may induce element of error
Dual-energy x-ray absorptiometry (DXA)	▪ Provides estimate of total body FFM and FM ▪ Can provide bone mineral estimation	▪ Expensive equipment ▪ Limited availability ▪ Radiation (x-ray) exposure
Infrared interactance	▪ Safe ▪ Noninvasive ▪ Fast	▪ Overestimates body fat in very lean individuals ▪ Underestimates body fat in very obese individuals
Magnetic resonance imaging (MRI)	▪ Provides estimation of organ sizes, muscle, fat, fat distribution, total body water	▪ Expensive equipment ▪ Limited availability
Total body potassium (TBK)	▪ Nonhazardous ▪ Minimal participant cooperation necessary	▪ Expensive equipment ▪ Limited availability ▪ Potassium imbalances affect accuracy

CT, computed tomography; LBM, lean body mass; FM, fat mass; FFM, fat-free mass

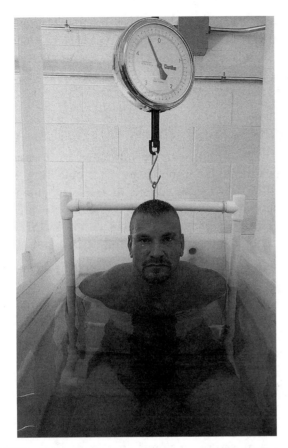

FIGURE 8.13 Hydrostatic or Underwater Weighing Tank Used for Assessment of Body Composition. Water volume displaced by a person submerged is equal to the volume of an object submerged in water. A person's weight on land divided by loss of weight in water by that submerged person is the person's density.

Body density can then be estimated using the following calculation:

$$\text{Body density} = \frac{\text{Body weight (BW) on land}}{\dfrac{\text{BW (land)} - \text{BW (submerged)}}{\text{Density of water}} - \text{Lung gas} - \text{GI gas}}$$

Residual lung gas is estimated to be approximately 24% of vital lung capacity, and the residual gas in the gastrointestinal tract is typically 50 to 300 milliliters. Some researchers choose to either ignore residual gastrointestinal gas or simply use 100 milliliters. Also, the temperature of the water needs to be known and taken into account when calculating the density of water.

Underwater weighing is considered a noninvasive tool for assessing body fat. The error of estimation of body fat by this means is about ± 2.7% for adults and ± 4.5% for children and adolescents. Estimations of body density are based on assumptions that the density of body fat is 0.9 gram per cubic centimeter and that of fat-free mass is 1.1 grams per cubic centimeter. Also, it is assumed that fat-free mass is cumulatively composed of 20.5% protein, 72.4% water, and 7.1% mineral.

Once body density is known, the percentage of body fat and total fat and lean body mass can be estimated using equation A in the following table. The percentage of body fat can then be used to estimate FM and FFM using calculations B and C.

A. %Fat mass (%FM) = $\dfrac{495}{\text{Body density}} - 450$

B. Fat mass (FM) = Total body mass × % FM = FM

C. Fat-free mass (FFM) = Total body mass − FM

Plethysmography

Like UWW, air displacement **plethysmography** applies density in estimating body composition. The technique uses a sealed chamber of known volume, commonly known as the BOD POD (**FIGURE 8.14**). An individual sits in the chamber in thin, tight clothing (e.g., a bathing suit and cap) and breathes normally. The concept is similar to underwater weighing; however, air is displaced instead of water in determining volume. The BOD POD is considered a precise tool for body composition, and estimates of %BF using this technique are similar to those obtained by UWW. Additionally, air displacement plethysmography is considered a more comfortable and more practical procedure than UWW. Methodologic considerations include transient variations in body surface unrelated to changes in body composition, such as abdominal bloating after a large meal.

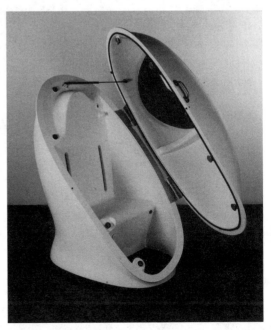

FIGURE 8.14 BOD POD Used for Plethysmography Assessment of Body Composition. Technique is similar to underwater weighing except air displacement using normal breathing is used to estimate body composition.
Courtesy of COSMED USA, Inc.

Dual-Energy X-Ray Absorptiometry

Dual-energy x-ray absorptiometry (DEXA or DXA) allows for a more comprehensive assessment of body composition because it quantifies three compartments: FM, FFM (soft tissue), and bone mineral mass (BMM). Thus, FFM is separated into bone and nonbone components. DXA also allows for regional body tissue assessment, which includes bone density for osteoporosis risk assessment. DXA assessment times are short (10 to 20 minutes) and comfortable; an individual lies on the machine table as shown in **FIGURE 8.15**. In addition, DXA

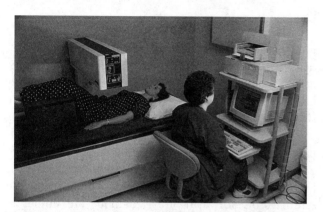

FIGURE 8.15 Dual-Energy X-Ray Absorptiometry Used for Assessment of Body Composition and Bone Mineral Density. Low dose x-rays used to determine fat mass, fat-free mass, and bone mineral mass.
© Photodisc/Getty.

is generally believed to be safe because the radiation dose is 800 to 2,000 times lower than a typical chest x-ray. The most significant factors limiting the use of DXA equipment are its size and cost. Therefore, DXA is primarily found in clinical institutions and research facilities.

Skinfold Assessment

Body composition can be estimated by measuring various limb circumferences and obtaining skinfold thickness measurements to assess subcutaneous fat deposition. This method is commonly used by dietitians and personal trainers. Skinfold thickness estimation of body fat uses the following assumptions:

- A direct relationship exists between the quantity of fat deposited just below the skin and total body fat and does not vary within or between individuals
- The thickness of the skin and **subcutaneous** adipose tissue has a constant compressibility throughout
- The thickness of skin is negligible and is a constant fraction of skinfold measurements. Skin thickness tends to vary between 0.5 and 2.0 millimeters.

Skinfold thickness measurements are obtained with calipers at several anatomic locations. Primary sites of measurement are the triceps, abdomen, subscapular, thigh, and suprailiac (**TABLE 8.10**). Secondary sites include the chest, midaxillary, and the medial calf. The

TABLE 8.10 Sites of Skinfold Measurements

Location	Measurement Technique
Tricep	Vertical skinfold measurement on the back of the arm at the midpoint between the tip of the shoulder or lateral process of the acromion and the tip of the elbow or the olecranon process of the ulna
Subscapular	Oblique skinfold measurement made just beneath the tip of the scapula or inferior angle of the scapula bone
Abdominal	Vertical skinfold measurement made approximately 7 centimeters to the right and 1 centimeter below the midpoint of the umbilicus or navel
Suprailiac	Slightly oblique skinfold measurement just above the iliac crest at the midaxillary line
Thigh	Anterior vertical fold measured at the midpoint between the superior border of the patella bone or knee cap and the inguinal crease
Pectoral (chest)	Skinfold measurement made as high as possible, just beneath the fingers, along the line from the anterior axillary fold to the nipple
Medial calf	Subject sits with the right leg flexed approximately 90° at the knee; vertical skinfold measurement made at the medial region of maximum calf circumference
Midaxillary	Skinfold measurement made at the right midaxillary line at the level of the superior aspect of the xiphoid process

use of skinfold calipers requires training and precision in measurement technique. Several factors must be taken into consideration. When a caliper is initially applied to a skinfold, a brief period of time is necessary prior to reading the thickness. About 4 seconds will allow the tips of the caliper to appropriately compress the skinfold. The reading tends to become smaller with time as the calipers compress the skinfold and fluids are forced out of the area. This increases error in the measurement. Therefore, if an accurate measurement is not obtained after 4 to 5 seconds, the skinfold should be released and measurement should be attempted again momentarily. Error is also typically introduced when different individuals perform the skinfold measurements.

It should not matter from which side of the body skinfold measurements are obtained. However, it seems that many North American investigators prefer the right side, whereas many European investigators prefer the left. It is recommended that inexperienced skinfold technicians mark the subject's body at the points of measurement, especially if tape measures are used to locate midpoints. For instance, the midpoint of the tricep can be located and marked at the midpoint between the acromiale (lateral edge of the acromial process, i.e., bony tip of shoulder) and the radiale (proximal and lateral border of the radius bone, at the elbow joint) on the posterior surface of the arm.

The caliper is most easily used by holding it in the right hand so that the dial is exposed for reading during measurement. The caliper tips should be placed 1 centimeter (approximately half an inch) distal to the fingers holding the skin (**FIGURE 8.16**).

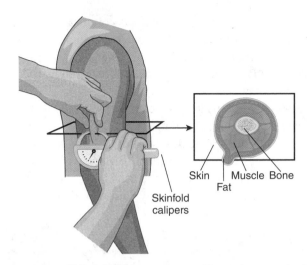

FIGURE 8.16 Skinfold Measurement. Several anatomical sites are measured for skinfold thickness using calipers. Tables and equations have been developed to estimate body composition using such measures.

Bioelectrical Impedance Analysis

Bioelectrical impedance analysis (BIA) and total body electrical conductivity (TOBEC) assessments are based on the conductive properties of an electrolyte-based medium. For clinical assessment using BIA, typically, an individual rests in a supine position with electrodes on peripheral extremities (hands and feet). A weak electrical current is then passed through the body that moves from one electrode to the next (**FIGURE 8.17**). The current is painless, and the rate of conductivity represents proportions of LBM and fat mass. LBM has more water and associated electrolytes and, therefore,

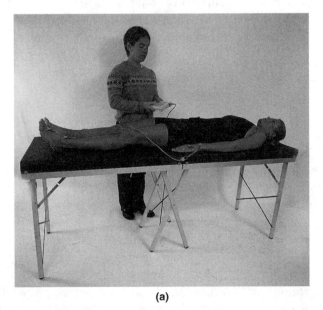
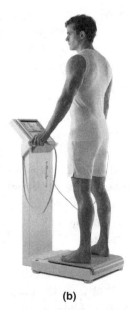

(a) (b)

FIGURE 8.17 Bioelectrical Impedance Analysis (BIA) or Total Body Electrical Conductivity (TOBEC). Assessment is based on the conductivity properties of an electrolyte-based medium. (a) supine BIA measurement; (b) standing on unit BIA measurement.

(b) © 2017 InBody Co., Ltd. www.inbody.com.

will demonstrate greater electric conductivity. Hand-held BIA devices exist, and some bathroom scales have built-in BIA systems, while more advanced systems have been validated for accuracy and precision to be used in research studies. Meanwhile, TOBEC devices tend to be larger, and thus less available to the public, than BIA devices. The subject lies in a cylinder that generates a weak electromagnetic field, and TOBEC makes 10 conductivity readings that estimate LBM in less than a minute. The strength of the field depends on the electrolytes found in the participant's body fluids and tissue.

● BEFORE YOU GO ON . . .

1. What are the major tissue components of the human body?
2. What are the different ways that body composition can be assessed?
3. What are the general procedures and assumptions of body densitometry?
4. What are the steps involved in skinfold measurement?
5. What is the basic principle of bioelectrical impedance assessment?

▶ Regulation of Energy Intake, Storage, and Expenditure

With the exception of a limited amount of energy stored as glycogen, it is clear that fat is the means by which excessive energy is stored in the human body. The first law of thermodynamics, when applied to humans, states that the amount of energy stored is equal to the amount of energy in excess of that which is used for metabolic operations. Although subtle homeostatic mechanisms attempt to keep minimal imbalances close to zero, even a small imbalance over time can thus result in significant gains in body weight. For instance, a healthy, nonobese adult may ingest as many as 900,000 kilocalories during a year and not experience a change in body weight. However, in theory, if energy intake exceeds expenditure by as little as 2% daily, this imbalance can result in an accumulation of approximately 2.3 kilograms (5 pounds) of fat over that same year's time.

At least two assumptions are being made here. First, it is assumed that 0.45 kilogram (1 pound) of fat uniformly contains 3,500 kilocalories, and, second, that an increase in energy storage results only in an expansion of fat volume in adipocytes. With respect to the latter assumption, it is clear that not all of the mass accumulated during an increase in body weight is actually triglyceride. Adipocyte **hypertrophy**, and perhaps, hyperplasia, has to allow for an expansion of the plasma membrane and nonfat cellular components as well. Furthermore, increases in bone density, muscle, and associated connective tissue occur to physically support a greater mass against the force of gravity. Thus, the average 9.1 kilograms of body weight increase that Americans between the age of 25 and 55 experience would only represent an average daily imbalance of 0.3% of kilocalories; once nonfat gains are taken into consideration, the imbalance would become smaller still.

Contrary to scientific and medical hope, the physiology associated with feeding is complex and involves numerous factors. The hypothalamus, and more specifically, local hypothalamic regions, is responsible for food intake and body weight regulation. Those regions include the paraventricular nucleus in the dorsomedial region; the arcuate nucleus, suprachiasmatic nucleus, ventromedial nucleus, and medial eminence in the basomedial region; and the medial preoptic area just anterior to the paraventricular nucleus. Those regions form the primary components of a system that integrates information regarding body composition and energy intake and expenditure. Information via vagal and catecholaminergic impulses and hormonal factors, such as cholecystokinin, leptin, glucocorticoids, and insulin, is received by the hypothalamus. The hypothalamus can then release peptide factors and initiate efferent signals that influence food intake and energy deposition. In addition, autonomic impulses influence energy expenditure and insulin release. Experimental lesions within the ventromedial hypothalamus are known to result in hyperinsulinemia, hyperphagia, and hypometabolism in animals.

Futile Cycle Systems

Animals, such as the rat, have metabolic futile cycling systems that regulate energy expenditure to allow for weight maintenance despite fluctuations in energy intake. **Brown adipose tissue (BAT)** is a specialized form of adipose tissue that is highly vascularized, which accounts for its darker color relative to white adipose tissue (WAT). It is innervated by the sympathetic nervous system. BAT is present in other animals and in human neonates and, to a lesser extent, in human adults. When stimulated, BAT activates thermogenesis via an uncoupling of the oxidative and phosphorylative activities of the electron transport chain. The mitochondrial protein involved is called **thermogenin**, or uncoupling protein 1 (UCP1), which allows electrons to move down their concentration gradient across the inner mitochondrial membrane without coupling the liberated energy with ATP generation. The net result is an increased flux of energy nutrients through oxidative pathways without the associated generation of ATP. Thus, there is a continuation of an ADP-to-ATP ratio that favors further oxidation and a continued generation of heat. Typically, the BAT content in humans decreases with age, and the significance of this futile cycle in adults has long been believed to be negligible. However, there is some evidence that, albeit small, demonstrates a difference in UCP1-expressing adipocytes in lean and obese adults, suggesting a potential role in obesity development protection or difficulty in management.

Brown adipocytes are located in dedicated depots and express constitutively high levels of thermogenic genes, whereas inducible "brown-like" adipocytes, also known as beige cells, develop in white fat in response to various activators. Precursor cells for brown and beige adipocytes appear to be different and they express differences in activity as well. Further research will help us better understand the role of brown and beige adipocytes in human obesity prevention and potential treatment.

Chemical Mediators of Energy Homeostasis

Several chemical mediators of energy homeostasis exist, including hormones, such as insulin, cholecystokinin (CCK), and leptin. Many chemical mediators were discussed in Chapter 2, but only a few of the major ones will be discussed in greater depth here. Research is ongoing to better understand those factors and how they fit together and play roles in weight control.

Insulin

The level of circulating insulin is typically proportionate to the volume of adipose tissue. In addition to its effect on energy substrate metabolism, insulin influences appetite and food intake. Insulin is able to cross the blood–brain barrier by way of a saturable transport system and may reduce feeding by inhibiting the expression of neuropeptide Y (NPY), enhancing the effects of CCK and inhibiting neuronal norepinephrine reuptake. Thus, the correlation between adiposity and plasma insulin levels may be an adaptive mechanism to support decreased energy consumption. Interestingly, the influence of insulin on NPY expression is not seen in the genetically obese Zucker (*fa/fa*) rat. Because the *fa* gene codes for the leptin receptor, it is likely that some of the effects of insulin regarding reducing appetite are leptin mediated.

Ghrelin

Ghrelin is a hormone produced mainly by the stomach and pancreas and is involved in the stimulation of hunger. Ghrelin levels increase before meals and decrease after meals, and it is considered to be in opposition to leptin. Ghrelin tends to increase food intake and increase fat mass by an action exerted at the level of the hypothalamus, which is also sensitive to the counterbalancing actions of leptin and insulin. Ghrelin is encoded by the same gene as **obestatin** Obestatin is a hormone produced by stomach cells and is thought to promote an anorectic response, thus having an effect opposite to Ghrelin.

Cholecystokinin

Cholecystokinin is secreted by mucosal cells of the proximal small intestine in response to the presence of food components. Postprandial circulating CCK levels are related to satiety and feeding in humans. There are two types of CCK receptors (A and B), and both may be involved in regulating food intake. CCK-A receptors are present within the gastrointestinal system, whereas CCK-B receptors are present in the brain. Via interaction with CCK-A receptors in the pylorus, CCK promotes contraction of the pyloric sphincter, which increases gastric distention. This initiates vagal afferents from the stomach that terminate in the nucleus of the solitary tract within the brain stem. Impulses are then transmitted to the parabrachial nucleus and then connected to the ventromedial hypothalamus, resulting in decreased food intake. This mechanism is diminished by vagotomy.

Although CCK-B receptors are found in the brain, CCK circulating in the systemic circulation doesn't seem to cross the blood–brain barrier. Therefore, it has been suggested that because the brain can also produce some CCK, afferent neural signals may result in the release of CCK in the cerebral spinal fluid, which binds with CCK-B receptors and decreases feeding.

Leptin

Leptin is a protein chain of 167 amino acids and the product of the obese (*ob*) gene. The name *leptin* is derived from the Greek word *leptos*, meaning "thin." In obese hyperphagic homozygote *ob/ob* mice, two prominent mutations have been identified that either lead to a lack of mRNA expression or to production of an ineffective protein. Leptin has been shown to reduce food intake and increase energy expenditure in both obese and lean animals. In humans, adipose cells also synthesize and secrete leptin relative to the amount of body fat stores. Leptin receptors have been found in various body organ tissues, such as the kidneys, liver, heart, skeletal muscle, hypothalamus, pancreas, and anterior pituitary. Leptin receptors found in the arcuate nucleus of the hypothalamus have led researchers to hypothesize that leptin plays a significant role in regulating satiety. Leptin appears to also decrease NPY synthesis and release from the arcuate nucleus as well as increase corticotropin-releasing factor (CRF) expression and release from the hypothalamus.

It is possible that serum leptin levels are elevated in some obese subjects due to the receptor's resistance to leptin's action. This is supported by another model of genetic obesity in mice. The so-called obese diabetic mouse has a mutation in the diabetes (db) gene. It is typical for those mice to have a 10-fold greater level of leptin compared with lean control mice. Because there does not seem to be an anomaly in the ob gene in those animals, a defect in the receptor remains suspect. Some human cross-sectional studies have revealed that obese individuals may also have elevated levels of leptin; however, recent efforts have not found a defect in the hypothalamic leptin receptor in those individuals. It is speculated that there may be leptin resistance, although the mechanism has not been resolved.

The presence of receptors in the pancreas has led researchers to hypothesize that serum leptin may play a regulatory role in insulin metabolism. However, in vitro studies have demonstrated that leptin alters neither uptake of glucose in the absence of insulin nor glucose sensitivity to insulin. Meanwhile, other studies appear to strongly correlate a counter-regulatory effect of leptin with insulin resistance.

Leptin may also play a role in energy substrate metabolism; some studies demonstrate an inverse correlation between leptin and energy intake, fat intake, resting energy expenditure, carbohydrate oxidation, and respiratory quotient (RQ). Therefore, individuals resistant to leptin may encounter two metabolic obstacles: (1) a disturbed link between the central nervous system and appetite regulation and (2) decreased resting energy expenditure with resulting weight gain. There is also evidence to suggest that leptin levels decrease in response to weight loss and remain decreased as long as the weight loss is maintained. Furthermore, increased levels of leptin have been found in normal-weight and obese women compared with their male counterparts as well as in female-patterned obesity (or peripheral fat stores). This is an expected finding because females have a greater percentage of body fat mass.

Neuropeptide Y

Neuropeptide Y is a peptide synthesized and secreted by the neurons of the arcuate nucleus of the hypothalamus. Increased activity of those neurons has been demonstrated in animal studies during periods of energy deficit, and; therefore, obesity may develop in response to abnormal increased production. NPY stimulates food intake, especially of carbohydrate-rich foods. The paraventricular nucleus is particularly sensitive to NPY. Interestingly, NPY is also synthesized and released into the circulation by the adrenal glands and sympathetic nerves; however, it does not cross the blood–brain barrier.

When NPY is injected directly into the medial hypothalamus of satiated animals, feeding is stimulated. Furthermore, there is a preference for carbohydrates. NPY seems to increase respiratory quotient (RQ) while simultaneously reducing energy expenditure. It is believed that the NPY-induced, increased utilization of carbohydrate allows for the production of more acetyl CoA for lipogenesis. NPY also seems to support fat storage in white adipose tissue, while decreasing BAT activity. Interestingly, NPY may have a stimulatory effect on the secretion of insulin, vasopressin, and leuteinizing hormone.

Galanin

Galanin is a neuropeptide factor that has a greater tissue concentration and number of receptors in the hypothalamus. Galanin increases feeding, especially of carbohydrate and fat. Although galanin does not appear to affect the respiratory exchange ratio (RER), it is associated with a reduction in energy expenditure because it inhibits sympathetic nervous system activity. Two subclasses of receptors have been identified in rats, but only one in humans. Unlike leptin and NPY, plasma galanin concentrations and activity do not appear to be regulated by body weight. It has an inhibitory effect on insulin secretion, and synthesis of galanin is inhibited in response to increased serum insulin.

● BEFORE YOU GO ON . . .

1. What are the major hormones involved in regulating metabolism and body weight?

2. What is leptin, and how is it related to hunger and satiety?

3. What are metabolic futile cycles, and what impact do they have on human metabolism?

4. What parts of the brain are involved in energy intake?

5. What are NPY and galanin, and do they promote feeding or reducing appetite?

SPECIAL FEATURE 8.1

Obesity

Obesity is a worldwide epidemic. Populations in European nations (e.g., Finland, Greece, The Netherlands, and Spain), the Pacific and Indian Ocean islands, Canada, and the United States have witnessed an increase in the prevalence of obesity over the past few decades. Results from two recent surveys by the Centers for Disease Control and Prevention (CDC): the National Health and Nutrition Examination Survey (NHANES), and the National Health Examination Survey stated that for adults (aged 20 years and over) in the United States (**FIGURE 1**):

- More than 70.2% of adults are considered to be overweight or obese
- More than 37.7% of adults are considered to be obese (including extreme obesity)
- More than 7.7% are extremely obese
- Almost 74% are considered to be overweight or obese compared to 67% for women
- The prevalence of obesity in men is slightly lower in men (35%) compared to women (40.4%)
- Approximately 10% of women are considered extremely obese, whereas the figure for men was lower at 5.5% .

Meanwhile, among young people aged 2 to 19 years, obesity and extreme obesity remains a significant public health problem.

- Among children and adolescents aged 2 to 19 years, about 17.2% were considered obese, and about 6% were considered extremely obese.
- Young children aged 2 to 5 years had a lower prevalence of obesity than older youth, which was about 9.4%. Less than 2% of young children were considered extremely obese.
- Among children and youth aged 6 to 11 years, about 17.4% were considered to be obese, and about 4.3% were considered to extremely obese.
- Among adolescents, aged 12 to 19 years, about 20.6% were considered obese, and about 9.1% were considered extremely obese.

A number of ideas have been proposed to explain this increased weight gain. Researchers continue to debate the role of dietary fat in the development and maintenance of obesity. A body of current literature suggests that under isoenergetic conditions, the proportion of kilocalories from dietary fat neither influences the development of obesity nor corrects the problem. However, health professionals are generally in agreement that excess energy intake relative to energy expenditure promotes weight gain and increasing adiposity. The term energy gap has recently been coined to describe this imbalance. **FIGURE 2** presents scales that show the different general components of energy balance. "Energy in" includes all kilocalorie-containing substances (food), and "energy out" includes the components of TEE described in this chapter.

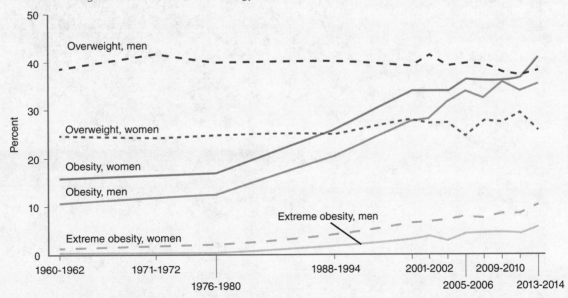

FIGURE 1 **Trends in adult overweight, obesity, and extreme obesity among men and women aged 20–74: United States, 1960–1962 through 2013–2014.**

(continues)

SPECIAL FEATURE 8.1 (*continued*)

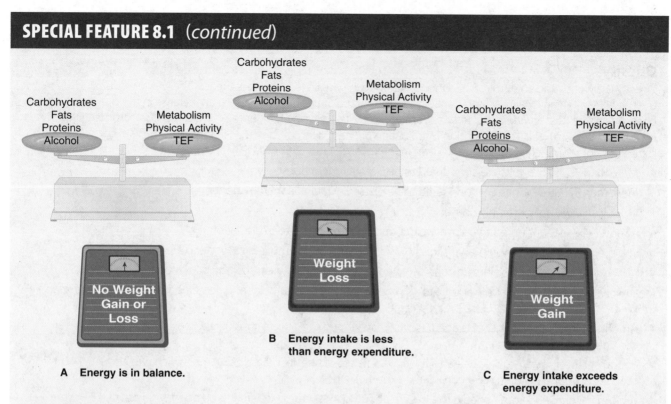

FIGURE 2 Energy Balance Scale. (TEF = thermic effect of food)

An increased occurrence of disease accompanies the rising obesity rate. A positive correlation between obesity and mortality has been well established by large American cohort studies, such as the Framingham Heart Study, NHANES, the Epidemiologic Follow-up Study, and the Nurses' Health Study. Many ailments, such as hypertension, dyslipidemia, diabetes mellitus, osteoarthritis, gastrointestinal disorders, and respiratory anomalies, occur secondarily to obesity (**TABLE 1**).

The many social and psychological aspects related to appetite also seem to influence weight gain and the efficacy of weight loss efforts. The general availability of food in developed countries in modern times has allowed for the consumption of food for reasons other than the relief of hunger. For many individuals, food enhances celebration or

TABLE 1 Disorders and Diseases Associated with Obesity

Tissue or Physiologic System	Pathology or Disorder
Cardiovascular system	<ul><li>Hypertension</li><li>Atherosclerosis</li></ul>
Hormonal/metabolic systems	<ul><li>Diabetes (type 2)</li><li>Hypercholesterolemia</li><li>Hypertriglyceridemia</li><li>Gout</li></ul>
Joints and connective tissue	<ul><li>Arthritis of knees and hips</li><li>Bone spurs</li></ul>
Respiratory systems	<ul><li>Obstructive sleep apnea</li></ul>
Psychological state	<ul><li>Depression</li><li>Social isolation</li></ul>
General physical state	<ul><li>Decreased mobility</li><li>Decreased vitality</li></ul>

entertainment, suppresses stress or anxiety, and alleviates boredom. Also, convenient and efficient meals are extremely popular in today's Western society.

Financial Impact of Obesity

Overweight (BMI 25 to 29.9) and obesity (BMI greater than 30) and their associated health problems have a significant economic impact, both direct and indirect, on the healthcare system in the United States and in other countries. Direct medical costs may include preventive, diagnostic, and treatment services. Meanwhile, indirect costs include those that are morbidity related, such as the value of income lost from decreased productivity, restricted activity, absenteeism, and bed days. Estimates of the cost of obesity in the United States are roughly $150 billion (e.g., $147 billion in 2008). Pharmaceutical companies annually invest millions of research dollars into developing drugs (primarily appetite regulators) that will combat obesity. From a consumer's perspective, the American population spends billions of dollars yearly on exercise equipment and facilities and on dietary supplements that claim to prevent obesity or promote weight loss.

History of Obesity

Evidence of obesity exists as far back as 25,000 years ago. Drawings and artifacts from the Paleolithic period (the early Stone Age) depict stout women and primarily female-pattern (gynoid) obesity. Treatment for obesity can be traced back as early as the fifth century BC. Hippocrates prescribed the following therapy for obese individuals in his day:

> Obese people and those desiring to lose weight should perform hard work before food. Meals should be taken after exertion and while still panting from fatigue and with no other refreshments before meals except only wine, diluted and slightly cold. Their meals should be prepared with a sesame or seasoning and other similar substances and be of a fatty nature as people get thus, satiated with food. They should, moreover, eat only once a day and take no baths and sleep on a hard bed and walk naked as long as possible.

An indication that obesity has been on the rise since the 18th century exists in a monograph written by Thomas Short: "I believe no age did ever afford more instances of corpulence than our own." Various diets have been published throughout history, with fad diets and diet books in general publication since the 1850s. Data from NHANES have documented this century's obesity explosion, at least in the United States. In modern times, numerous books on dieting are available to the population at large. At least one book of this nature could be found on the *New York Times* best seller lists for at least four decades now.

Although some early scientists expressed medical concern, society at large viewed obesity as a sign of wealth and prosperity. Even current perceptions of ideal body weight vary by culture. As the study of obesity, adipose tissue, and metabolism increased with the advent of modern medicine in the 20th century, concern arose regarding obesity and disease risk. Research funding for studies on obesity has increased in the past 50 years, with a greater amount invested in determining genetic influences on its onset and mechanisms of appetite regulation.

Definition of Obesity and Prevalence

Obesity has been defined in several manners. The truest definition is also perhaps the most simple. Obesity is a physical state of excessive body fat, or overfatness. Here, body fatness is best estimated by underwater weighing or one of the other techniques mentioned in this chapter. The term *overweight* specifies excess mass of all body tissue: FM and FFM. Therefore, an individual is overweight but not obese if, for example, excess muscle mass is present. This is often the situation for body builders and muscular, yet lean, athletes. However, numeric classifications, such as BMI and IBW ranges, of obesity often define overweight as a condition preceding obesity, or the terms are often used interchangeably.

The more common and accurate determinant of obesity based on body weight is the body mass index (BMI; kilograms body weight/meters of height^2). Classification of obesity by this method varies, depending on the referenced standards and definitions. Although a universal cutoff point does not exist, a BMI of 30 or more is a common indicator of obesity, and a BMI of 25 to 29.9 defines overweight; those definitions are supported by U.S. agencies as well as the World Health Organization.

Distribution of Fat Mass in Obesity

Two patterns of obesity exist: **android** and **gynoid**. Android obesity, in which excess fat stores accumulate in the torso area, is more associated with males. This type of obesity is a public health concern because of its association with disease states such as hypertension, insulin resistance, breast cancer, stroke, diabetes, and cardiovascular disease. Gynoid obesity, in which excess fat stores accumulate in the periphery, especially the hips and thighs, is more associated with females. Peripheral fat stores seem to release free fatty acids more readily than truncal fat stores. Throughout history, women have relied upon the accessibility of those fat stores during pregnancy and lactation.

The location of adipose tissue relative to other body tissue is also a health risk concern. Fat tissue located just beneath the skin tissue is subcutaneous fat. Adipose tissue within muscle and associated with organ tissue is visceral fat. Fat is located in both areas; however, visceral fat obesity, which is highly correlated with android obesity, is a greater

(continues)

SPECIAL FEATURE 8.1 (continued)

health concern. Because of its association with impaired glucose metabolism, dyslipidemia, and hypertension, increased accumulation of visceral fat is considered a risk factor for heart disease.

Distribution of adipose tissue is assessed by calculating the waist-to-hip ratio. The waist-to-hip ratio represents the relationship between the circumference of the waist at its narrowest point and the circumference of the hips at their widest point, including the buttocks. Abdominal obesity and increased risk of heart disease are indicated by a larger ratio. **TABLE 2** depicts the rating scale for health risks associated with waist-to-hip ratio measurements. Meanwhile, waist circumference alone is often regarded as a more accurate predictor of health risk (**TABLE 3**).

Adipocyte Regulation in Energy Balance

Classically viewed as relatively simple and inert containers of stored energy, adipocytes are now appreciated as complex cells with endocrine functions that regulate energy homeostasis. Because adipose tissue is the most adaptable human tissue from an energy perspective, it only makes sense that this tissue would function as a gauge for energy storage. For some very lean individuals, body fat represents as little as 5 to 10% of body mass, whereas in morbidly obese individuals, it accounts for as much as 65 to 70% of body mass. Although not all body fat is found within adipocytes, the majority of it is, and thus increases in human body fat occur by expansion of adipose tissue mass.

TABLE 2 Waist-to-Hip Ratio Ratings for Increased Health Risk

Risk	Men	Women
Highest	>0.95	>0.85
Moderate	0.90–0.95	0.80–0.85
Lowest	<0.90	<0.80

TABLE 3 Classification of Overweight and Obesity by BMI, Waist Circumference, and Associated Disease Risk

	BMI (kg/m^2)	Obesity Class	Disease Risk[a] Relative to Normal Weight and Waist Circumference[b]	
			Men 102 cm (40 in) or less Women 88 cm (35 in) or less	Men > 102 cm (40 in) Women < 88 cm (35 in)
Underweight	<18.5		—	—
Normal	18.5–24.9		—	—
Overweight	25.0–29.9		Increased	High
Obesity	30.0–34.9	I	High	Very high
	35.0–39.9	II	Very high	Very high
Extreme obesity	40.0 +	III	Extremely high	Extremely high

[a]Disease risk for type 2 diabetes, hypertension, and CVD.

[b]Increased waist circumference also can be a marker for increased risk, even in persons of normal weight.

Reproduced from National Heart, Lung, and Blood Institute, National Institutes of Health, U.S. Department of Health and Human Services. Available at: http://www.nhlbi.nih.gov/health/public/heart/obesity/lose_wt/bmi_dis.htm. Accessed November 11, 2010.

The notion that adipocytes play a role in human energy homeostasis, via secretion of endocrine factors, probably dates back to the 1950s. At that time, it was proposed that adipocytes possessed the capability of registering excessive energy stores and responded by secreting an endocrine factor, called adipostat, which would limit food intake. However, interest waned in the years that followed and was not reawakened for several decades. In the 1980s, a serine protease called adipsin was reported to be secreted by cultured adipocytes. Because subsequent investigations revealed that adipsin secretion was markedly reduced in various obese rodent models, scientists speculated that this chemical might be the underlying factor involved in human obesity. However, it was soon determined that adipsin is not reduced in obese humans and thus could not be the causative factor. As researchers continued to investigate the endocrine properties of adipocytes, they discovered that this tissue could secrete a variety of interesting factors, including angiotensinogen and tumor necrosis factor α (TNF-α). TNF-α is a cytokine expressed in cell types, such as macrophages. Subsequent investigations determined that TNF-α is overexpressed in obese animals and humans. Furthermore, leptin may also be involved in the development of obesity-linked insulin resistance.

Adipocyte Hypertrophy vs. Hyperplasia

Adipose tissue can expand by both hypertrophy and hyperplasia. Once an adipocyte has matured and thus is terminally differentiated, it has minimal capacity for cell division. Therefore, the potential for hyperplasia must reside in precursor forms of adipocytes. This means that the majority of adipose tissue expansion by mild energy imbalance occurs by hypertrophy of mature, terminally differentiated adipocytes. However, since the presence of new adipocytes has been observed as adiposity increases significantly, those new adipocytes will store more fat as the ability of existing adipocytes nears capacity.

Within adipose tissue, there appear to be pockets of fibroblast-like adipocyte precursor or stem cells that can reproduce and differentiate into adipocytes. More than likely, growth factors regulate the process of adipocyte development from the early commitment of stem cells to the terminal stages of differentiation (**FIGURE 3**).

Although the genetic factors involved in committing the stem cells to the adipocyte lineage are still elusive, some potential clues have been discovered. For instance, a lipid-activated transcription factor called PPARγ2, where PPAR is an abbreviation for **P**eroxisome **P**roliferator **A**ctivator **R**eceptor, may be involved. The expression of this factor may be unique to adipocytes. Another factor, called preadipocyte factor-1 (Pref-1), may also be involved in adipocyte stem cell commitment. Pref-1 is expressed only in proliferating preadipocytes.

Insulin-like growth factors (IGFs) have also been shown to be involved in the proliferation and differentiation of adipocyte stem cells. For instance, in chicks, both IGF-I and IGF-II stimulate stem cell proliferation. IGFs may function in an autocrine, paracrine, or endocrine fashion. IGF-I is expressed in chick adipocyte precursor cells as well as those of certain mammals. The involvement of IGFs is probably regulated via the expression of IGF-binding proteins. To make the events of adipocyte stem cell proliferation and differentiation even more complicated, several other factors appear to be involved, including a number of fibroblast growth factors (FGFs) and their receptors, transforming growth factors α and β (TGF-α and

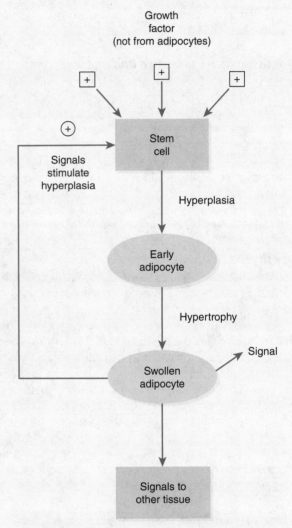

FIGURE 3 Hypertrophy and Hyperplasia of Adipose Tissue. Fat is accumulated in existing adipocytes, which release growth factors as they swell (hypertrophy) that stimulate production of new adipocytes (hyperplasia).

Reproduced from National Heart, Lung, and Blood Institute, National Institutes of Health, U.S. Department of Health and Human Services. Available at: www.nhlbi.nih.gov/health/public/heart/obesity/lose_wt/bmi_dis.htm. Accessed November 11, 2010.

(continues)

SPECIAL FEATURE 8.1 *(continued)*

TGF-β), and epidermal growth factor (EGF). More likely than not, those various growth factors work synergistically in the complicated process of adipogenesis.

Genetic Influences on Obesity

Is obesity the result genes? This is an interesting question and one without a simple answer. Studies involving identical twins, adoptees, and families as well as obese vs leaner populations indicate that both heredity and environment play a role in the development of obesity. One of the most commonly discussed explanations of the modern epidemic of obesity is the mismatch between today's environment and "energy-thrifty genes." According to the thrifty genotype hypothesis, the same genes that aided our ancestors in survival during periods when food was scarce are now working against us in environments in which food is plentiful year round. However, thrifty genes are probably only part of the genetic influence on obesity development in modern times. For instance, researchers are addressing the role of genetics in inactivity, regional adipose tissue deposition, resting metabolic rate, lipolysis, energy metabolism in response to overeating, food preferences, lipoprotein lipase activity, maximal insulin-stimulated lipogenesis, and various aspects of eating behavior.

Obesity in Men vs. Women and Age

Obesity affects women to a greater extent than men. This was seemingly even the case during the Paleolithic period: discovered artifacts and sketches representing obese humans depicted only women. Since the beginning of time, women have relied on fat stores more than men for reproduction. In women, essential body fat may account for 12% of total body weight, vs 3% for men. So, how does obesity prevalence break down against gender? Based on recent estimates, more than 35% of U.S. men and women are obese, however, in general, there was no significant difference in prevalence between men and women at any age. Almost 41 million women and more than 37 million men aged 20 and over were obese in 2009–2010. Overall, adults aged 60 years and over were more likely to be obese than younger adults. Looking more closely at gender and different age groups, there was no significant difference in obesity prevalence by age for men while 42.3% of women aged 60 years and over were obese compared with 31.9% of women aged 20–39 years.

Obesity in Children

Obesity is not just an adult issue: the prevalence of obesity among children aged 6 to 11 years has more than doubled in the past 25 years. Among children and adolescents aged 2–19 years, more than 5 million girls and approximately 7 million boys were obese in 2009. The prevalence of obesity was higher among boys than girls (18.6% of boys and 15.0% of girls were obese). The prevalence of obesity among boys increased from 14.0% in 2000 to 18.6% in 2009. There was no significant change among girls: the prevalence was 13.8% in 2000 and 15.0% in 2009. Children and adolescents are commonly measured using growth charts by pediatricians; however, BMI is a more consistent and accurate predictor of adiposity.

As children approach puberty, the percentage of adipose tissue changes, but in different ways for males and females. As mentioned previously, while the fat percentage decreases in males, females begin to deposit fat in preparation for reproduction and lactation. Although a natural growth pattern for young girls, this increased fat deposition contradicts the "American ideal" and often enhances preoccupation with body image.

Decreased physical activity is evident among today's youth. In an effort to increase physical activity among children, the Centers for Disease Control and Prevention in the United States has championed a set of guidelines for schools and community programs to encourage physical activity among children as a means to help prevent childhood obesity and, later, adulthood obesity.

Obesity and Related Diseases

Dyslipidemia

Excessive accumulation of body fat, especially fat deposited within the abdominal region, has an adverse effect on blood lipids. The dyslipidemia associated with obesity is characterized by elevated fasting plasma triglycerides, decreased HDL-cholesterol, and moderate elevations in total cholesterol and LDL-cholesterol. Fat deposition in the abdominal region appears to present more atherogenic lipid profiles than excessive fat accumulation in the gluteofemoral region. Lifestyle modifications, such as exercise and hypocaloric diet therapy, are effective strategies not only for promoting weight loss and decreases in body fat percentage but also for causing favorable changes in plasma lipid profiles. Numerous research efforts have indicated that lower-fat diets are effective in reducing serum concentrations of total cholesterol and LDL-cholesterol, irrespective of calorie level. However, reductions in total cholesterol and LDL-cholesterol are typically accompanied by reductions in HDL-cholesterol as well. Therefore, exercise is an important component of a lower-fat, weight-loss program to improve HDL-cholesterol levels.

Hypertension

As many as one in three adult Americans have hypertension. Obesity is perhaps the most important controllable risk factor in the development and maintenance of hypertension. Obesity is correlated not only with the risk of new-onset hypertension but also with the severity of existing hypertension. The development of obesity-related hypertension is often coupled with the development of other risk factors for heart disease, such as dyslipidemia. Weight loss results in rapid reductions in blood pressure that can be maintained with a stabilized lower body weight. More than 80% of obese adolescents have elevated blood pressure; most have at least one additional cardiovascular disease risk factor. Much of the problem is related to the high-fat, high saturated–fat, and high-cholesterol diet and reduced physical activity common to obese adolescents in comparison with nonobese adolescents.

The mechanisms underlying obesity-related hypertension are multifactorial. Potential factors involved in the pathogenesis of obesity-related hypertension can be separated into volume-related factors, neurohumoral factors, and others. Volume-related factors include increased sodium sensitivity, renal sodium reabsorption, and plasma volume. Neurohumoral factors include insulin resistance syndrome, elevated sympathetic activity, and elevated levels of hormones such as aldosterone and norepinephrine and the enzyme renin. Obesity-related hypertension may also result from left ventricular hypertrophy (independent of blood pressure) and sleep apnea.

Diabetes Mellitus

According to the American Diabetes Association, more than 23 million individuals in the United States have diabetes, of which only approximately 18 million cases have been diagnosed. In addition, 57 million people are believed to have prediabetes. Each year, 1.6 million new cases of diabetes are diagnosed in people aged 20 years and older.

Of those adults with diabetes, approximately 90% have type 2 diabetes mellitus, and of those individuals, as many as 80% to 90% are overweight or obese. The risk of developing type 2 diabetes mellitus is relative to the severity and duration of the obesity and is further amplified by the centralized (visceral) adiposity. Thus, managing obesity is a first-line therapy for diabetes mellitus. It has been well established that even modest reductions in weight can reduce hyperglycemia in type 2 diabetes mellitus.

Several physiologic mechanisms are involved in the improved glycemic control that results from weight loss. Perhaps one of the clearest effects is a reduction in hepatic glucose production. Hepatic glucose production is associated with the level of hyperglycemia in type 2 diabetes mellitus; in fact, hepatic glucose production is one of the most significant supportive factors in hyperglycemia. Perhaps as significant as the reduction of hepatic glucose production is the return of insulin sensitivity in skeletal muscle and adipose tissue. Again, the severity of insulin resistance is directly related to the severity of the obesity; furthermore, there is evidence that centralized visceral obesity is a correlate of insulin resistance in type 2 diabetes mellitus. This effect of reduced body weight and fat is paramount because insulin resistance is at the hub of interrelated cardiovascular risk factors, such as dyslipidemia, hypertension, and impaired fibrinolysis. One of the cellular mechanisms involved in the improvement in insulin resistance induced by weight loss is improved tyrosine kinase activity of the transmembrane insulin receptor. It is believed that tyrosine kinase activity in insulin-resistant type 2 diabetes mellitus is only half of that found in obese nondiabetic individuals.

Metabolic Syndrome

The above issues associated with obesity often do not occur in an isolated fashion but in combination with one another. In the last 15 to 20 years, the term **metabolic syndrome**, sometimes referred to as *Syndrome X*, has been of interest due to deleterious clinical outcomes and increased incidence in western cultures. Metabolic syndrome is simply a set of blood and anthropometric conditions that increase the risk of diseases, in particular, cardiovascular disease and Type 2 diabetes. In fact, several organizations have developed standards of identified variables in diagnosing metabolic syndrome (e.g., National Cholesterol Education Program and International Diabetes Federation). Research has suggested that key variables collectively identify who has metabolic syndrome. Some researchers have stated that those with metabolic syndrome are in a constant state of inflammation and that obesity is an inflammatory disorder. A key observation, though, is increased body fat, in particular, in the abdominal area (android), which has been linked to increased incidence of cardiovascular disease and Type 2 diabetes. Body mass index in itself does not define metabolic syndrome. Waist circumference, blood levels of triglycerides, reduced blood HDL cholesterol levels, increased blood pressure, and raised fasting blood glucose levels are key variables in identifying metabolic syndrome. Current thinking is that metabolic syndrome is a combination of genetic and lifestyle conditions. Moreover, early life events have a strong predictive likelihood of developing metabolic syndrome in adult life. Infant undernutrition and/or poor in utero

(continues)

SPECIAL FEATURE 8.1 *(continued)*

nutrition may have a higher incidence of metabolic syndrome if exposed to the type of western diets commonly consumed in combination with physical inactivity.

Waist circumference, not BMI, is strongly predictive of metabolic syndrome, as defined earlier, for obesity. Men with a waist circumference of 40 in (102 cm) or more, and women with 35 in (88 cm) or more were more likely to develop metabolic syndrome. The National Cholesterol Education Program requires that the waist circumference value and three of the following variables be present as a diagnosis of metabolic syndrome: raised triglycerides above 150 mg/dL, increased blood pressure approximately 130/85 mmHg, low HDL-Cholesterol, 40 mg/dL for men and 50 mg/dL for women, and raised fasting blood glucose above 110 mg/dL. The International Diabetes Federation has more stringent criteria for defining metabolic syndrome in terms of blood values but requires that waist circumference does not exceed 37 in (94 cm) in men and 32 in (80 cm) in women. Two of the above variables are required for metabolic syndrome to be diagnosed. The treatment of metabolic syndrome first and foremost focuses on waist circumference by using a healthy diet and enhancing physical activity. Decreasing waist circumference through adoption of a healthy diet of fruits and vegetables and increased physical activity are still the best options presently available to reverse the syndrome short of bariatric surgery.

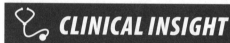
CLINICAL INSIGHT

Ketogenesis

In addition to prolonged fasting, ketone bodies can be produced if carbohydrate, particularly starch and sugar, are limited in the diet, despite what could be adequate energy consumption. Diet-induced thermogenesis has long been practiced in certain medical conditions, particularly to help control seizures in some people with epilepsy. However, ketogenic diets have been popularized for people attempting to manage their weight and disease risk. In order to produce ketone bodies (β-hydroxybutyrate (BHB), acetoacetate, and acetone), diet carbohydrate is maintained low (e.g., < 50–70g daily or 5% energy) and protein is also maintained at a moderate intake level (e.g., 20–25% calories). That leaves the remaining 70-75% of the calories to be derived from fat sources.

Humans seem to be relatively unique when it comes to ketogenesis. As newborns, ketogenesis can support energy needs in the first days of life. Humans seem to be the most significant animal when it comes to ketogenesis and the reason is because the higher brain:body weight ratio and perhaps, even more so, the brain REE relative to total REE, which is roughly 20–25%. During starvation-driven ketogenesis, the brain can derive roughly half of its energy from ketones, which, in turn, spares body proteolysis and prolongs survival. This occurs to a similar degree in a caloric–adequate (or hypocaloric) state as well.

The potential application of ketogenesis is being explored in numerous scenarios, including management of blood lipids, neurologic issues, migraines, and cancer. While some favorable metabolic outcomes have been reported, time will tell whether some people can derive greater benefit and its sustainability. Additionally, while the presence of ketones has classically been driven by very low carbohydrate diets, researchers are also looking into the potential therapeutic application of supplemental, gram-dosed ketones (e.g., beta hydroxybutyrate BHB).

▶ Here's What You Have Learned

1. Metabolism is a general term referring to internal reactions that occur in cells and tissues throughout the body. It includes the production of new molecules and cells powering membrane-associated pumps as well as the energy expended in physical movement and exercise.

2. Total energy metabolism includes basal or resting metabolic rate, the thermic effect of food, physical activity, and adaptive thermogenesis. All of those components can be manipulated to affect final total energy expenditure (TEE); however, physical activity is the most potent means to immediately increase TEE.

3. Metabolism is measured directly via heat release from the body (direct calorimetry) or indirectly via gas exchange. Oxygen use and carbon dioxide production can be used to assess metabolism as well as estimate the relative contributions of different fuel sources because fat oxidation requires more oxygen than carbohydrate oxidation.

4. Cellular metabolism of energy nutrients is regulated by hormones such as insulin, epinephrine, glucagon, and cortisol, which can have complementing, synergizing, or competing influences. Insulin is an anabolic hormone that promotes glucose uptake and the production of glycogen and fat stores and supports net protein production, whereas glucagon, epinephrine, and cortisol lead to a breakdown in energy stores and the release of glucose into the blood from the liver.

5. Metabolic states change throughout the day and include fasting, fed, and exercising states. They are regulated by hormones, such as insulin, glucagon, epinephrine, and cortisol, which regulate circulating and cellular energy nutrient availability.

6. Body weight control is primarily influenced by the level of kilocalories consumed chronically. Protein and unsaturated fatty acids tend to have higher thermic effects (i.e., are more thermogenic) than carbohydrate and saturated fat, respectively. However, it remains to be proven that manipulating the ratio of macronutrients can effectively and predictably affect body weight and weight control.

7. Body composition can be assessed at the level of elements and molecules (e.g., water, protein, carbohydrate), specific tissue (e.g., muscle, adipose tissue, organs), or major tissue groups (e.g., fat mass, fat-free mass).

8. Densitometry can be used to predict body composition via underwater (hydrostatic) weighing and air displacement plethysmography. Densitometry is considered a gold standard for body composition assessment.

9. DXA, BIA, and skinfold assessments are all used to predict body composition and have different strengths and disadvantages. Among the key factors to consider are the predicted errors for BIA and skinfold assessments and the availability and cost for DXA.

10. Obesity is a major concern in the United States and many other countries. Excessive body fat is linked to diabetes, hypertension, elevated cholesterol, and reduced self-efficacy. Currently, over 30% of American adults are classified as obese based on a body mass index (BMI) measurement of 30 or above.

11. Metabolic syndrome is a condition used to describe the combination of those variables that are abnormal and associated with increased waist circumference.

▶ Suggested Reading

Alberti KG, Zimmet P, Shaw J. Metabolic syndrome—a new worldwide definition. A consensus statement from the International Diabetes Federation. *Diabet Med* 2006;23(5):469–480.

Astrup A, Buemann B, Christensen NJ, et al. The contribution of body composition, substrates, and hormones to the variability in energy expenditure and substrate utilization in premenopausal women. *J Clin Endocrinol Metab.* 1992;74(2):279–286.

Biaggi RR, Vollman MW, Nies MA, et al. Comparison of air-displacement plethysmography with hydrostatic weighing and bioelectrical impedance analysis for the assessment of body composition in healthy adults. *Am J Clin Nutr.* 1999;69(5):898–903.

Campbell WW, Crim MC, Young VR, Evans WJ. Increased energy requirements and changes in body composition with resistance training in older adults. *Am J Clin Nutr.* 1994;60(2):167–175.

Cunningham JC. Body composition as a determinant of energy expenditure: a synthetic review and a proposed general prediction equation. *Am J Clin Nutr.* 1991;54(6):963–969.

Cypess AM, Kahn CR. Brown fat as a therapy for obesity and diabetes. *Curr Opin Endocrinol Diabetes Obes.* 2010;17(2):143–149.

Deurenberg P, Weststrate J, Seidell J. Body mass index as a measure of body fatness: age- and sex-specific prediction formulas. *Brit J Nutr.* 1991;65(2):105–114.

Drolet R, Richard C, Sniderman AD, et al. Hypertrophy and hyperplasia of abdominal adipose tissues in women. *Int J Obes (Lond).* 2008;32(2):283–291.

Farooqi IS, O'Rahilly S. Genetic factors in human obesity. *Obes Rev.* 2007;8(suppl 1):37–40.

Finkelstein EA, Fiebelkorn IC, Wang G. National medical spending attributable to overweight and obesity: how much, and who's paying? *Health Aff (Millwood).* 2003;W3:219–226.

Finkelstein EA, Fiebelkorn IC, Wang G. State-level estimates of annual medical expenditures attributable to obesity. *Obes Res.* 2004;12(1):18–24.

Grabacka M, Pierzchalska M, Dean M, Reiss K. Regulation of ketone body metabolism and the role of PPARα. *Int J Mol Sci.* 2016. 17(12). pii: E2093.

Han TS, Lean ME. A clinical perspective of obesity, metabolic syndrome and cardiovascular disease. *JRSM Cardiovasc Dis.* 2016;5:1–13.

Harms M, Seale P. Brown and beige fat: development, function and therapeutic potential. *Nat Med.* 2013;19(10):1252–1263.

Hill JO, Peters JC, Wyatt HR. Using the energy gap to address obesity: a commentary. *J Am Diet Assoc.* 2009;109(11):1848–1853.

Houston DK, Nicklas BJ, Zizza CA. Weighty concerns: the growing prevalence of obesity among older adults. *J Am Diet Assoc.* 2009;109(11):1886–1895.

Illner K, Brinkmann G, Heller M, Bosy-Westphal A, Müller MJ. Metabolically active components of fat free mass and resting energy expenditure in nonobese adults. *Am J Physiol Endocrinol Metab.* 2000;278(2):E308–E315.

McCrory MA, Molé PA, Gomez TD, Dewey KG, Bernauer EM. Body composition by air-displacement plethysmography by using predicted and measured thoracic gas volumes. *J Appl Physiol.* 1998;84(4):1475–1479.

National Cholesterol Education Program (NCEP) Expert Panel on Detection, Evaluation, and Treatment of High Blood Cholesterol in Adults (Adult Treatment Panel III). Third report of the National Cholesterol Education Program (NCEP) Expert Panel on detection, evaluation, and treatment of high blood cholesterol in adults (adult treatment panel III) final report. *Circulation* 2002;106(25):3143–3421.

Nelson KM, Weinsier RL, Long CL, Schutz Y. Prediction of resting energy expenditure from fat-free mass and fat mass. *Am J Clin Nutr.* 1992;56(5):848–856.

Nielsen S, Hensrud DD, Romanski S, Levine JA, Burguera B, Jensen MD. Body composition and resting energy expenditure in humans: role of fat, fat-free mass and extracellular fluid. *Int J Obes Relat Metabol Disord.* 2000;24(9):1153–1157.

Puchalska P, Crawford PA. Multi-dimensional roles of ketone bodies in fuel metabolism, signaling, and therapeutics. *Cell Metab.* 2017;25(2):262–284.

Ogden CL, Carroll MD, Flegal KM. High body mass index for age among US children and adolescents, 2003–2006. *JAMA.* 2008;299(20):2401–2405.

Sparti A, DeLany JP, de la Bretonne JA, Sander GE, Bray GA. Relationship between resting metabolic rate and the composition of the fat-free mass. *Metabolism.* 1997;46(10):1225–1230.

Wang Z, Ying Z, Bosy-Westphal A, et al. Evaluation of specific metabolic rates of major organs and tissues: comparison between nonobese and obese women. *Obesity* (Silver Spring). 2012;20(1):95–100.

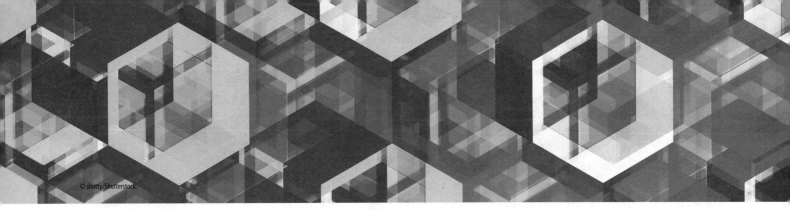

CHAPTER 9

Nutrition, Exercise, and Athletic Performance

← HERE'S WHERE YOU HAVE BEEN

1. Trillions of cells operate independently and combine in a synergistic fashion to create the tissue that forms the very basis of the human body. Nourishment of the body depends on efficient digestion of foods, which involves a complex synergy of physical actions of chewing, mixing, and moving and the chemical actions of saliva, enzymes, and emulsifiers.
2. Carbohydrates include sugars, starches, fibers, and related molecules, such as glycosaminoglycans (amino sugars) that, in general, are more abundant in plant-based foods than animal sources (with the exception of mammalian milk).
3. Proteins are key structural molecules in cells and tissue that function as enzymes and hormones and are involved in blood clotting, transport, cell signaling, and more. Proteins consist of amino acids and vary in size, shape, and function.
4. Fats are composed of glycerol and one to three fatty acids and serve as a key energy source for many cells in the body. In addition, certain fatty acids can play a regulatory role in the body by serving as precursors for eicosanoids.
5. Human energy expenditure, or metabolism, is the extraction of energy from food and body stores to drive internal operations; it is measured directly as heat release or indirectly via gas exchange with the air. The body is composed of fat mass and fat-free mass, such as muscle, organs, and bone.

HERE'S WHERE YOU ARE GOING →

1. Physical activity refers to any movement that engages the skeletal muscular system, whereas exercise is a voluntary, planned physical activity, often having a desired goal or associated benefit or physical outcome.
2. Exercise training refers to targeted and specific physical activity designed to enhance an individual's performance of one or more activities or sports.
3. Carbohydrate and fat from intramuscular stores as well as from circulation from other sources provide the majority of the energy that fuels exercise.
4. Depletion of glycogen stores in muscle and dehydration are the most critical factors in determining fatigue. One effect of regular training is an increase in the concentration of muscle glycogen levels.
5. Sport drinks provide an effective way to maintain hydration while providing fuel for muscle and electrolytes for the body, a need that becomes more important during prolonged activity.

▸ Introduction

Exercise and exercise training demand the involvement of several organ systems not only to support acute bouts of activity but also to adapt in response to training, thus providing an improvement of performance. The skeletomuscular system, under the command of the motor cortex of the brain, provides the human body's locomotion. The coordinated and concerted contraction of skeletal muscle cells pulls on bones to provide movement. Contraction of skeletal muscle cells is powered by ATP, which is generated via the breakdown of carbohydrate, fat, and amino acids derived from several endogenous stores (e.g., glycogen, intramuscular lipid droplets, and adipocytes) as well as from exogenous sources (e.g., recently consumed food and beverages). The cardiovascular system transports hormones, nutrients, and oxygen to support an exercise bout while also providing an avenue for the removal of CO_2, lactate, and heat from muscle. Hormones, such as epinephrine, glucagon, cortisol, thyroid hormone, and growth hormone work to support activity and maintain homeostasis. The exocrine activity of sweating allows for excessive heat removal, and the **renal system** helps regulate fluid and electrolyte balance as well as blood pressure.

The increase in total energy expenditure (TEE) during and after exercise is mostly attributable to an increased metabolism within working muscles themselves. For example, the basal oxygen (O_2) consumption rate for a sedentary adult is roughly 250 milliliters per minute; however, oxygen consumption for an elite marathon runner might approximate 5,000 milliliters per minute during a race. This increase in oxygen utilization is often expressed in metabolic equivalent (MET) units or multiples of an individual's resting oxygen consumption. One MET is defined as a rate of oxygen consumption of 3.5 milliliters of oxygen per kilogram of body weight per minute (O_2/kg/min) in adults. One MET is considered the resting metabolic rate (RMR) measured during quiet sitting. Meanwhile, sleeping would have a MET value of 0.9, whereas running at a pace of 10 minutes per mile would have a MET value of about 10. Additionally, the associated increase in metabolism during exercise can be expressed as PAL (physical activity level), which is the ratio of TEE to the basal metabolic rate (BMR). See **TABLE 9.1** for a listing of METs and PALs for different exercise activities.

TABLE 9.1 Metabolic Equivalent (Met) Impact of Various Exercise on Physical Activity Level (PAL) In Adults[a]

Activity	METs[b]	ΔPAL/10min[c]
Volleyball (noncompetitive)	2.9	0.018
Walking (2 mph)	2.5	0.014
Calisthenics (no weight)	4.0	0.029
Cycling (leisurely)	3.5	0.024
Golf (without cart)	4.4	0.032
Cycling (moderately)	5.7	0.045
Jogging (10-minute miles)	10.2	0.088
Ice skating	5.5	0.043
Roller skating	6.5	0.052
Skiing (water or downhill)	6.8	0.055
Surfing	6.0	0.048
Swimming	7.0	0.057

[a]PAL (physical activity level) is the ratio of total energy expenditure (TEE) to the basal metabolic rate (BMR).
[b]METS are multiples of resting oxygen uptake and are set for adults at an O_2 consumption of 3.5 milliliters of O_2 per minute per kilogram body weight.
[c]The presented PAL factors is the residual effect of physical activity after completion as well as thermic effect of food.
Data from Institute of Medicine, Food and Nutrition Board. *Dietary Reference Intakes for Energy, Carbohydrate, Fiber, Fat, Fatty Acids, Cholesterol, Protein, and Amino Acids.* Washington, DC: National Academy of Sciences; 2005. Original table adapted from Fletcher, G. F., et al. Exercise standards for testing and training: a statement for healthcare professionals from the American Heart Association. *Circulation.* 2001;104:1694–1740.

▸ Muscle and Exercise Basics

The body contains over 215 pairs of skeletal muscle, which constitute approximately 40% of human mass, more so for leaner, more muscular athletes. The principal function of muscle is to contract, which, in turn, leads to movement. Muscle actions are coordinated to allow for motion, thereby allowing the human body to complete physical tasks. Planned movement with a desired outcome is called exercise with exercise training being the means to achieve benefits.

Muscle and Neuromuscular Junctions

Muscles vary in size and in their origin and insertion (**FIGURE 9.1**). All skeletal muscle is composed of numerous skeletal muscle cells (myocytes or muscle fibers) that range from 10 to 80 micrometers in diameter and generally extend the length of the muscle (**FIGURE 9.2**). Almost all muscle fibers are innervated by only one nerve fiber or motor neuron. The motor neuron terminates at the neuromuscular endplate or junction, typically located in the central region of the muscle fiber (**FIGURE 9.3**). Conversely, a single motor neuron can innervate several muscle fibers. A motor neuron plus all of the muscle fibers it innervates are called a **motor unit**. The nature of movement generally defines the number of muscle fibers innervated by a single motor neuron. For example, motor units of extraocular muscle controlling the fine movement of the eyes have a fairly low motor neuron-to-muscle fiber innervation ratio (1:15). Conversely, motor units associated with the gastrocnemius and tibialis anterior muscles of the legs and controlling gross movement have an innervation ratio as high as 1:2,000.

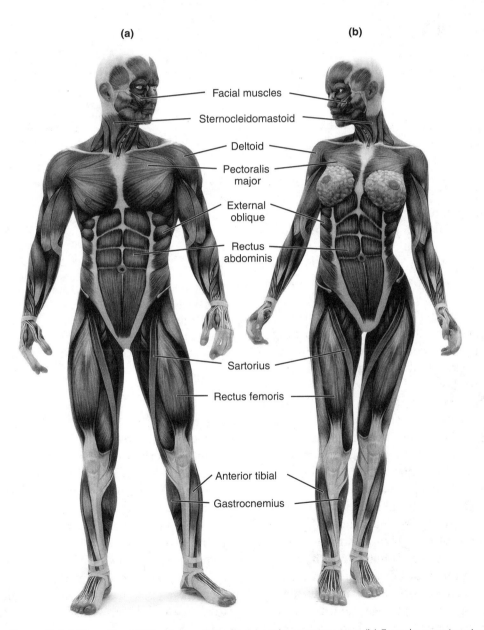

(a) (b)

FIGURE 9.1 Major Superficial Muscles of the Human Body. (a) Male anterior view. (b) Female anterior view.

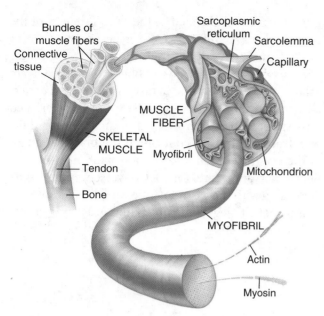

FIGURE 9.2 Structure of Muscle. Muscle cells or fibers are wrapped in connective tissue and bundled together. Muscle attaches to bone via tendons.

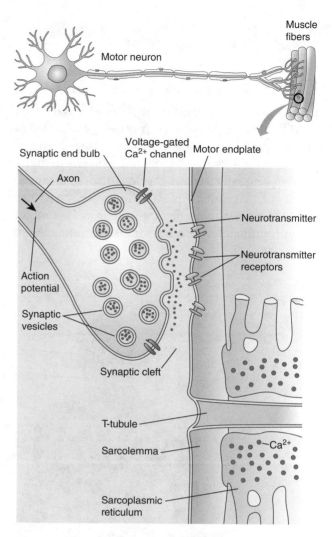

FIGURE 9.3 Neuromuscular Junction with Acetylcholine as the Neurotransmitter. Motor neurons terminate adjacent to the sarcolemma and release acetylcholine, which binds with its receptor and initiates the action potential on the sarcolemma.

Muscle Action Potentials

Acetylcholine is a neurotransmitter released by motor neurons into the synaptic gap at **neuromuscular junctions** (see Figure 9.3). Acetylcholine then elicits the firing of an action potential, which radiates uniformly outward along the **sarcolemma (plasma membrane)** of the muscle fiber. Acetylcholine initiates the action potential by evoking the opening of acetylcholine-gated protein channels. The opening of specific channels allows sodium to traverse the sarcolemma from the extracellular fluid and depolarize the membrane to threshold.

Muscle fibers contain several unique features that are supportive of muscle contraction. First, muscle fibers are excitable, as indicated previously. Quite simply, they can respond to a specific stimulus by initiating an action potential and then propagating the action potential along the sarcolemma. This sets in motion the activities that ultimately allow muscle fiber contraction. Second, from a structural perspective, skeletal muscle fibers contain contractile fibrils, a relatively rich compartment of mitochondria, specialized endoplasmic reticulum called the sarcoplasmic reticulum, a T-tubule system that invaginates the sarcolemma, and augmented glycogen and triglyceride stores. They also contain creatine phosphate, which helps maintain optimal levels of ATP during the first seconds of intense exercise (**FIGURE 9.4**).

Sarcomeres and Contraction

Excited (stimulated) muscle cells are flooded with calcium, primarily from the sarcoplasmic reticulum and, to a lesser degree, from the interstitial space. Calcium evokes muscle fiber contraction by allowing sarcomeres to contract. Sarcomere**s** are the smallest contractile unit of muscle fibers; each one is composed of overlapping thick (myosin) and thin (actin) filaments (see Figure 9.2). Sarcomeres are arranged in series (side by side) that make up myofibrils. Actin filaments are attached at both ends of the sarcomeres and extend toward the center. Myosin is positioned between actin fibers in parallel. In a nonstimulated (resting or relaxed) state, binding sites for myosin on actin fibrils are obscured by a long filamentous protein called

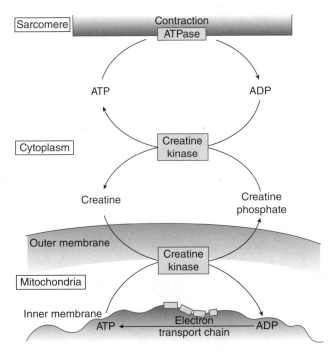

FIGURE 9.4 Creatine Phosphate System. Creatine phosphate is used to regenerate ATP within the cytoplasm and is regenerated via ATP in mitochondria.

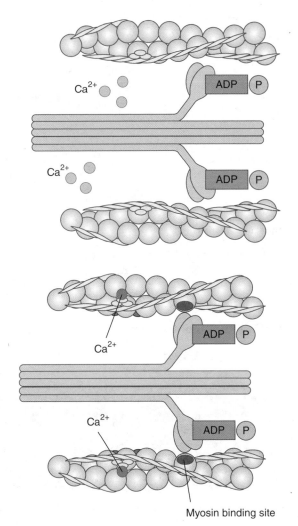

FIGURE 9.5 Role of Calcium, Troponins, and Tropomyosin in Muscle Fiber Contraction. Binding of calcium to troponin promotes movement of tropomyosin and the exposure of the myosin binding site.

tropomyosin. Also associated with actin and tropomyosin is a complex of proteins called troponin. When a muscle fiber is stimulated and the intracellular calcium concentration increases, calcium binds with the troponin complex; this interaction moves tropomyosin away from myosin binding sites on actin fibers (**FIGURE 9.5**). Once myosin binds to actin, it pulls actin toward the center of the sarcomere, contributing to the shortening of the myofibril, which, in turn, contributes to the shortening of the myofiber as a whole (**FIGURE 9.6**).

Muscle Fiber Type

Human muscle fibers can be separated into two primary classes, which are distinguished by their rate of tension development. Type I fibers take approximately 110 milliseconds to generate peak tension, whereas type II fibers can generate peak tension in about 50 milliseconds. With respect to this relative difference, type II fibers are also referred to as fast-twitch (FT) fibers and type I fibers as slow-twitch (ST) fibers. The difference in the rate of tension development is largely attributable to the expression of different myosin ATPase **isozymes**. Type II fibers produce a more rapid form of myosin ATPase, in comparison with type I fibers (**TABLE 9.2**). Thus, type II fibers can split ATP more rapidly and generate tension at a faster rate.

There is only one recognized type of type I fiber, whereas there are three types of type II fibers (types II_a,

II_x, and II_b). On average, most muscles contain about 50% type II fibers: 25% type II_a, 22 to 25% type II_x, and 1 to 3% type II_b. Motor units contain similar muscle fiber types. For example, if a certain motor unit innervates 100 muscle fibers, all 100 of the fibers will be of the same type.

Motor Unit Recruitment

When a muscle is stimulated, the percentage of contained muscle fibers actually contracting largely depends on the force necessary to perform a specific movement. The motor cortex calls on, or recruits, more and more motor units to contract a muscle, depending on the perceived necessary force. There appears to be a fixed order of recruitment of motor neurons, which may be associated with the size of motor neurons. For example, assuming a muscle contains 200 motor units, those units may be

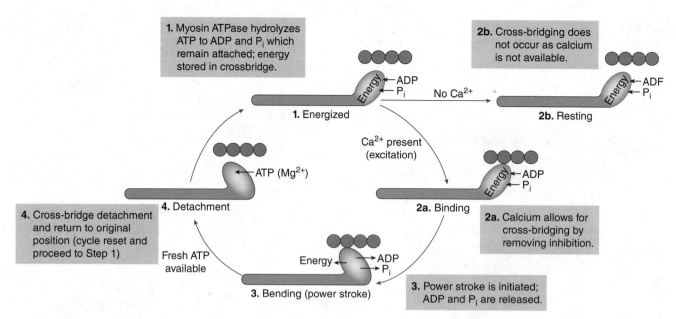

FIGURE 9.6 Muscle Contraction. (a) Cross-bridge cycle. (b) Changes in banding patterns during contraction.

TABLE 9.2 Characteristics of Muscle Fiber Types

	Type I	Type II$_a$	Type II$_x$	Type II$_b$
Performance aspects				
Twitch rate	Slow	Moderately fast	Fast	Very fast
Force production rate	Slow	Fast	Fast	Fast
Fatigue resistance	High	Moderately high	Moderately low	Low
Structural aspects				
Mitochondrial density	Very high	High	Moderate	Low
Capillary density	High	Moderate	Low	Low
Myoglobin content	High	Moderate	Low	Low
Energy systems				
Creatine phosphate	Low	Moderately high	High	High
Glycogen stores	Low	High	High	High
Triglycerides stores	High	Moderate	Low	Low
Glycolytic activity	Low	High	High	High
Oxidative activity	High	High	Moderate	Low

Data from Wildman REC, Miller BS, Wilborn C. *Sports and Fitness Nutrition*. Belmont, CA: Wadsworth; 2014.

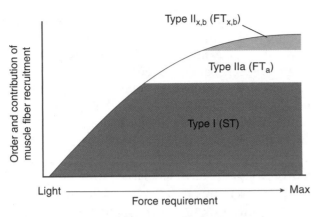

FIGURE 9.7 Order of Motor Unit Recruitment. Motor units containing type I fibers are always recruited first, followed by motor units containing type II fibers.

designated 1 through 200. Motor unit 1 would always be recruited first and 200 recruited last. Because type I fibers tend to be innervated by smaller motor neurons, they will predominate in those motor units recruited first (**FIGURE 9.7**). Thus, for muscular movements requiring lesser amounts of force, slow-twitch muscle fibers provide most of the contraction.

Beyond the rate of tension development, types I and II fibers can also be distinguished by other intracellular features, as well as some extracellular features (see Table 9.2). Type I fibers have a relatively higher blood flow capacity, greater capillary density, and a relatively greater mitochondrial and myoglobin content. Type I muscle fibers produce most of their ATP via the oxidation of energy substrates, such as fatty acids and glycolysis-derived pyruvate in what is often referred to as aerobic metabolism. If blood flow is sufficient, type I fibers are generally resistant to fatigue. In contrast, type II fibers are much more glycolytic and prone to early fatigue. Although still inferior to type I muscle fibers in their oxidative capabilities, type II_a fibers have more mitochondria, myoglobin, and associated vascularization than the other type II fibers.

Exercise and Training Components

Exercise bouts challenge muscle to perform muscle actions with purpose, including sport/athletic specific training adaptation and competition. Because exercise bouts tend to occur daily or almost daily, each training session is linked to the previous and ensuing bout. Put differently, recovery and adaptation processes associated with a training bout today can overlap with the preparation period prior to a similar workout on the next day. That might be more common in endurance-oriented sports, such as running, cycling, or sports, such as soccer.

Pretraining or preworkout is typically broken into the 30 to 60 minutes prior to exercise and up to 4 hours whereby carbohydrate stores can be enhanced and other nutrients, such as caffeine, can be used strategically. Meanwhile, the recovery period from exercise can endure for even longer. Here, exercise recovery is inclusive of the period of time after a bout of muscular work whereby physiologic processes work to achieve homeostasis by reestablishing baseline metabolic, neuroendocrine, and performance aspects of muscle and connective tissue. Assessments can include changes in measures of muscle tissue damage, immunological response, protein balance, performance, range of motion, and perceived soreness and exertion.

Muscle Adaptation to Strength Training

Muscle fiber hypertrophy, not hyperplasia, appears to be the primary cause of muscle enlargement produced by strength training. The increase in skeletal muscle mass developed during strength training is attributable to comparable increases in the cross-sectional area of both type I and II muscle fibers, with a disproportionate increase in the latter. The hypertrophy is primarily the result of an augmentation of the number of myofibrils and supportive structural components. In addition, the mechanical actions, hormonal actions, and immune system responses promote the differentiation of satellite cells that fuse with existing and trained muscle fibers to increase the number of nuclei in an enlarging muscle fiber (**FIGURE 9.8**). In general, the events associated with myofibril hypertrophy are coordinated and channeled through signaling systems, such as mTOR (mammalian target of

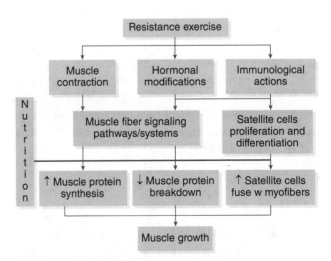

FIGURE 9.8 Exercise-Related Events That Support Muscle Hypertrophy. This scheme details various events that lead to muscle growth as a result of resistance exercise.

rapamycin). The role of those pathways is to integrate multiple signals derived from nutritional, mechanical, hormonal, and immune systems.

Muscle fiber hypertrophy is associated with gains in strength. However, increments in strength gain exceed what can be accounted for by increased muscle fiber area. For instance, strength training may result in a gain in force generation of 30 to 40% above what can be accounted for by muscle hypertrophy alone. Thus, neuromuscular energy and physical systems also become more efficient. Additionally, the hypertrophic process associated with strength training may be complemented by a shift in myosin isoforms from the slower to faster isoform.

Muscle Adaptation to Endurance Exercise

The primary adaptations resulting from endurance training are metabolic and cardiovascular. Endurance training increases the ability of muscle cells to oxidize fatty acids and conserve carbohydrates. Mitochondrial protein, as well as the oxidative activity of muscle, increases twofold after endurance training. Furthermore, adaptation in the storage, transport, mobilization, and endogenous production of energy molecules occurs because of endurance training.

Endurance training elicits changes in muscle vasculature content as well as circulatory dynamics. The vascular density (capillary-to-muscle fiber ratio) may increase by 5 to 10% as a result of endurance training. The augmentation in capillary density increases the opportunity for nutrient and gas exchange between blood and muscle fibers. At low-intensity levels of exercise, blood flow to muscle may remain unchanged from flow prior to training. However, at higher intensities, active muscle blood flow is greater than at pretraining levels. Furthermore, endurance training results in a precise redistribution of blood flow within active muscle. More oxidative portions of active muscle receive an increased portion of blood flow compared with more glycolytic regions. This occurs both in anticipation of and during an exercise bout.

Muscle Fiber Type and Endurance Adaptation

The ability of muscle cells to adapt to endurance training by augmentation of the mitochondrial compartment is observed in both type I and II fibers. However, in order for a muscle fiber to adapt, it must be recruited. Because type I fibers demonstrate an

earlier recruitment, they will adapt at lower-intensity training levels, whereas both type I and II fibers will adapt at higher intensities. Furthermore, training duration (weeks) and the relationship between training intensity and duration influence adaptations in muscle fiber mitochondrial content. For instance, the greatest increase in mitochondrial content might be observed at higher intensities, such as training bouts of 15 minutes at 100% maximum oxygen uptake (**VO$_2$max**) performed regularly for several weeks. However, training at a level approximating 85% VO$_2$max for 30 minutes will result in similar mitochondrial increases as training at a level approximating 70% VO$_2$max for 90 minutes. At lower intensities, such as 50% VO$_2$max for 90 minutes, mitochondrial content can increase linearly; however, it is likely to plateau at a level less than training at 70% VO$_2$max for the same length of time. Finally, exercising at a level of 30 to 40% VO$_2$max results in only minimal adaptation of mitochondrial content.

Conversely, detraining (nonuse) of muscle reduces the level of trained muscle fiber mitochondria. In muscle fibers that have been trained to reach a steady state of mitochondrial content, significant reductions in training gains can be expected in a week or so. Retraining of that muscle will allow a reestablishment of the steady-state mitochondrial content; however, the time involved will be longer than the detraining interval.

Hormonal Adaptation to Acute and Chronic Exercise

In a healthy human, exercise is arguably the most significant acute physiologic perturbation. The endocrine system must adapt not only to support the increased metabolic demands of exercising muscle but also to maintain euglycemia and other aspects of homeostasis. The endocrine factors that are modified during a single bout of exercise—and that potentially adapt as an effect of training—include catecholamines, insulin, glucagon, adrenocorticotropic hormone (ACTH), cortisol, growth hormone (GH), and endorphins (**TABLE 9.3**). Those circulating factors greatly dictate energy nutrient metabolism during exercise as well as during recovery and adaptation.

Catecholamines

The circulating concentrations of epinephrine and norepinephrine increase during exercise according to intensity and duration. However, catecholamine release from the adrenal glands during a bout of exercise

TABLE 9.3 General Hormonal Responses to Endurance Exercise

Hormone	Response	Reason or Purpose
Insulin	↓	Response to specific glucose level tends to decrease above 50% VO_2 max
Glucagon	↔	Response during exercise is dependent on glucose level, not directly on exercise intensity (like insulin)
Epinephrine	↑	Increases relative to intensity; increases heart rate, blood pressure; dilates bronchioles, increases glycogen and fat breakdown
Norepinephrine	↑	Increases relative to intensity; increases heart rate, blood pressure; dilates bronchioles, increases glycogen and fat breakdown
Cortisol	↑	Maintenance of blood glucose through gluconeogenesis and indirectly via fat breakdown and mobilization
Adrenocorticotropin hormone (ACTH)	↑	Increases during prolonged moderate intensity or higher intensity, shorter duration endurance exercise
Testosterone	↑	Increase is relative to exercise stress; might abate during consistent training
Estrogen	↑	Increases with exercise levels (levels influenced by menstrual phase)
Growth hormone	↑	Supports muscle protein production (mainly connective tissue) and adaptation through IGF-1 and other factors; supports fat breakdown and maintenance of blood glucose
Insulin-like growth factor-1 (IGF-1)	↑	Supports muscle protein synthesis in response to exercise
Thyroid-stimulating hormone (TSH)	↑	Increases release of T_3 and T_4 during exercise
Triiodothyronine (T_3)	↑	Increases during exercise, supports cardiovascular function and activity of other hormones
Thyroxine (T_4)	↑	Less-active thyroid hormone; increases during exercise, supports cardiovascular function and activity of other hormones
Antidiuretic hormone (ADH)	↑	Increases at > 60% VO_2 max to conserve water and maintain blood volume
Aldosterone	↑	Maintenance of plasma sodium and potassium to preserve performance and blood volume
Endorphins	↑	Increases with long-duration exercise

can be dampened by elevated blood glucose levels. This is especially true for norepinephrine. For example, a fasting individual will experience a greater catecholamine increase than an individual who consumed a carbohydrate-containing pre-event meal or supplement. The presence of elevated concentrations of epinephrine stimulates glycogen breakdown in muscle fibers and hepatocytes as well as triglyceride breakdown in adipocytes and muscle fibers. Epinephrine appears to be a much more potent stimulator of muscle glycogenolysis and probably muscle fiber lipolysis than norepinephrine. Meanwhile, both epinephrine and norepinephrine are potent stimulators of lipolysis in adipocytes.

SPECIAL FEATURE 9.1

Caffeine and Athletic Performance

Athletes continually look for means to enhance their performance. Although many practices certainly have merit, sadly there are many others that do not. Among the most efficacious practices is the use of caffeine. Caffeine (1,3,7-trimethylxanthine) occurs naturally in plant sources, such as the coffee bean, tea leaf, kola nut, and cacao seed. The average cup of coffee contains 50 to 150 milligrams of caffeine, tea has about 50 milligrams per cup, and caffeinated cola drinks contain about 35 milligrams per 12 ounces. Although chocolate contains some caffeine, most of its methylxanthine is in the form of theobromine; teas contain most of their methylxanthine as theophylline. The term *caffeine* is used in a general sense in this discussion and is inclusive of other methylxanthines (e.g., theobromine, theophylline).

Actions of Caffeine

After absorption, caffeine is taken up by most tissues in the body. However, the brain appears to be most sensitive to caffeine. Wakefulness and sleep latency are probably two of the most common effects of consumption. Caffeine appears to antagonize adenosine, which has more of a relaxing effect. Caffeine and adenosine are structurally similar and, therefore, compete for the same binding sites. However, with time, more adenosine receptors are produced, and, in turn, more caffeine must be consumed to effectively compete. It also seems that if caffeine ingestion is discontinued, adenosine interaction with receptors goes unchallenged and can be more potent because of the augmentation in receptors. This probably accounts for many of the side effects associated with caffeine withdrawal. Finally, some of the effects of caffeine may be indirect. For example, caffeine ingestion is typically associated with increases in plasma epinephrine levels.

Caffeine also appears to have a direct stimulatory effect on neurons and can influence chloride channel actions. Caffeine can inhibit phosphodiesterase, the enzyme that produces the second messenger cyclic AMP (cAMP). Thus, caffeine could prolong the influence of ligands using cAMP as a second messenger (e.g., glucagon and epinephrine).

Caffeine and Performance

Theoretically, caffeine has the potential to be an ergogenic aid for at least three reasons. First, caffeine and related substances have a central nervous system stimulatory effect. Second, caffeine may have direct action on skeletal muscle and increase its performance. It has been speculated from in vitro studies that caffeine may positively influence calcium transport and key enzymes in metabolic pathways (e.g., glycogenolysis). Third, caffeine may increase the availability and thus the utilization of fatty acids and potentially decrease carbohydrate utilization and possibly prolong glycogen stores.

Caffeine exerts a greater ergogenic effect when consumed in an anhydrous state compared with coffee. Caffeine is effective for enhancing sport performance in trained athletes when consumed in low to moderate dosages (approximately 3 to 6 milligrams per kilogram body weight; overall, it does not result in further enhancement in performance when consumed in higher dosages (≥ 9 milligrams per kilogram body weight). Caffeine supplementation is beneficial for high-intensity exercise, including team sports, such as soccer and rugby, which are characterized by intermittent activity within a period of prolonged duration. However, within any sport, there will be athletes who are more responsive than others. Also, at this time, research is not supportive of the notion that caffeine-induced diuresis during exercise negatively affects performance.

Caffeine as a Doping Agent?

At one time, the International Olympic Committee considered caffeine to be a doping agent when ingestion of caffeine leads to urinary levels greater than 12 micrograms per milliliter. However, caffeine is listed as part of the 2017 Monitoring Program and is not considered a prohibited substance. Meanwhile, caffeine is a banned substance by the NCAA when an athelete's urinary caffeine concentration exceeds 15 micrograms per milliliter, which corresponds to ingesting about 500 milligrams, the equivalent of six to eight cups of brewed coffee, two to three hours before competition testing.

Regular cardiovascular exercise can lead to slight reductions in epinephrine, which might occur simultaneously with a slight increase in parasympathetic drive. Those two changes combined can lead to a lower resting heart rate. Meanwhile, some studies indicate that the resting plasma epinephrine levels of individuals who have been engaged in endurance training for several years are higher than those in untrained individuals. Conversely, even though catecholamine levels are increased during exercise relative to intensity levels, they initially appear to be reduced at a given workload as the result of endurance training. That effect can begin within the first week of routine training and may be complete within 30 to 60 days. It is likely that as muscle adapts, the physiologic intensity at which an activity is performed decreases to achieve the same workload. Moreover, with long-term (years of) strenuous endurance training, the reduction in circulating catecholamine response at a given workload actually becomes similar to or even greater than that in untrained levels.

Insulin and Glucagon

Circulating insulin levels decrease during exercise of higher intensities (> 50% of VO_2max). This is largely attributable to α-adrenergic inhibition of insulin release from the pancreas. Moreover, exercise training also can enhance insulin sensitivity (see Table 9.3). Thus, despite a reduction in the insulin response to a given glucose level, **glucose tolerance** can actually be improved with training due to a significant increase in GLUT4 presence in muscle cell plasma membranes, independent of insulin. Meanwhile, resting insulin levels can decrease as a result of endurance training. Glucagon secretion, however, does not seem to be influenced strongly by adrenergic activity. This makes circulatory glucose concentration the primary regulator of glucagon secretion during exercise.

Cortisol, Growth Hormone, and ACTH

Circulatory levels of growth hormone and cortisol also can increase during exercise, and elevated levels are associated with the intensity of exercise. Although the exact mechanisms regulating the secretion of those hormones during exercise are unclear, it appears likely that there is central command. Whether endurance training alters resting levels of other hormones, such as ACTH and cortisol, has not been firmly established. Whereas some researchers have found that training decreases resting levels of those hormones, others have reported no change. ACTH, glucagon, and growth hormone have been reported to decrease at a given workload after periods of training.

● BEFORE YOU GO ON . . .

1. What is exercise, and how is it different from regular daily activity?
2. What are the structural and functional characteristics of muscle that allow for its unique function?
3. What are the different types of muscle fibers, and how are they different?
4. What is the order of muscle fiber recruitment, and what is the reason?
5. Which hormones are principally involved in exercise, and what are their effects?

▶ Energy, Supportive Nutrients, and Exercise

ATP is the energy currency spent during muscular activity. The hydrolysis of ATP not only fuels muscle fiber contraction but also allows for relaxation, postexercise recovery, and adaptation. Skeletal muscle fibers possess three principal ATP-regenerative mechanisms (**FIGURE 9.9**):

- The creatine phosphate (ATP-CP) system
- Anaerobic ATP generation (e.g., lactic acid system)
- Aerobic ATP production

TABLE 9.4 provides a look at the levels of ATP, creatine phosphate, and glycogen levels in type I and II muscle fibers. Intensity and duration of exercise are primary factors in determining the relative contribution to total energy needs. As shown in **FIGURE 9.10**, the anaerobic systems—the ATP-CP system and lactic acid system—contribute most of the energy during the first seconds to minutes of moderate- to higher-intensity exercise.

Creatine Phosphate

Certain cell types, chiefly muscle and brain, are endowed with an accessory means of rapid regeneration of ATP, namely, creatine phosphate. Briefly, creatine phosphate is similar to adenosine triphosphate in that the phosphate bond has high energy potential. Hydrolysis

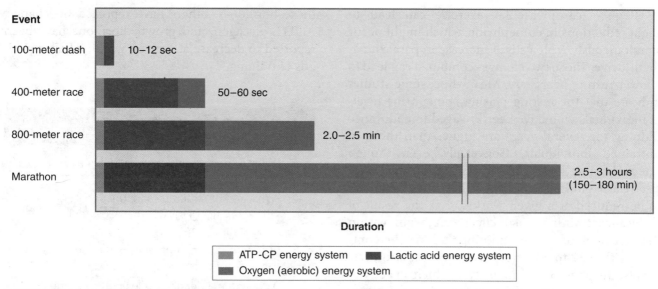

FIGURE 9.9 Primary Energy Systems in Muscle. The relative involvement of each of the 3 sources of ATP production is dependent on time and intensity of the exercise performed.

TABLE 9.4 Approximate ATP, Creatine Phosphate, and Glycogen Content of Skeletal Muscle

ATP mmol/kg[a]		Creatine Phosphate mmol/kg[a]		Glycogen mmol/kg[a]	
Type I	Type II	Type I	Type II	Type I	Type II
25	26	75	85	385	470

[a]Skeletal muscle tissue dry weight. Units for ATP, creatine phosphate, and glycogen levels are millimoles per kilogram (mmol/kg) dry tissue.

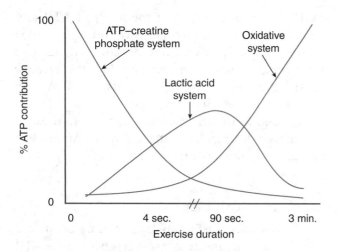

FIGURE 9.10 Contribution to ATP During Early Exercise. General contribution of different energy systems to ATP production during the first few minutes of moderate submaximal endurance exercise.

of the phosphate bond liberates sufficient energy to reattach phosphate to ADP, reforming ATP (see Figure 9.4). Creatine phosphate and glycogen are the primary fuels for weight training exercises and higher-intensity aerobic exercise within the first minute (see Figures 9.9 and 9.10).

Carbohydrate Metabolism and Exercise

Fuel sources for working muscle are derived from stores within muscle fibers and circulating carbohydrate, fat, and amino acids (**FIGURE 9.11**). Ingestion of energy nutrients, such as glucose, glucose polymers, fructose, fat, and certain amino acids, can become an important source of fuel to support an exercise bout as well as preparation for and recovery from exercise. After accounting for water, the major mass of the human body can be viewed as an energy reserve, much

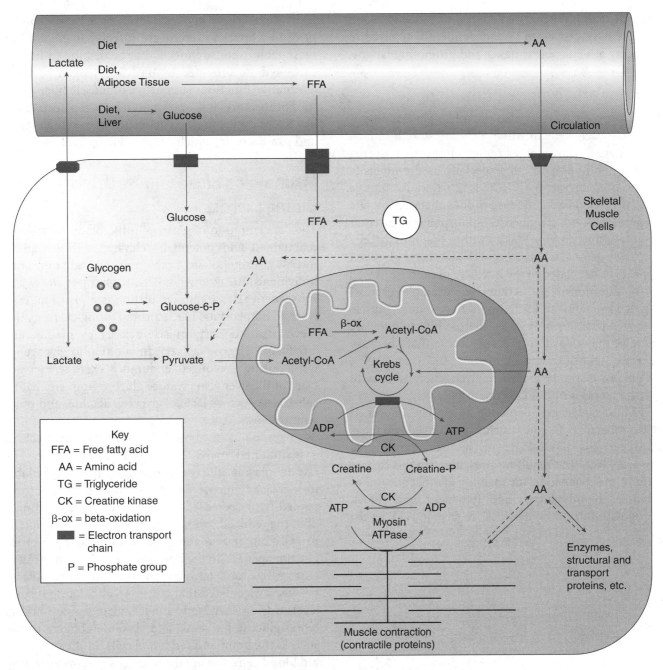

FIGURE 9.11 **Metabolic Aspects of Muscle Fibers.** Muscle has multiple metabolic pathways that allow it to store circulation-derived carbohydrate, fat, and protein at rest (nonexercise) and to use those nutrients from storage and circulation during exercise. Note: The different shapes on the sarcolemma indicate different types of transporters. The dotted lines indicate less significant pathways, except during prolonged fasting and endurance exercise.

of which is available to support physical activity. This notion is based on the relatively high contribution of adipose tissue, triglyceride, and skeletal muscle-based protein to human mass.

Carbohydrate stores in the form of glycogen are largely found in liver hepatocytes and muscle fibers. Typically, glycogen accounts for roughly 7 to 8% and 1 to 2% of the mass of the liver and muscle, respectively. Muscle glycogen levels tend to be 10 to 25%

higher in type II versus type I muscle fibers. Cumulatively, hepatic tissue contains approximately 100 grams of carbohydrate, and skeletal muscle tissue in totality contains between 300 and 400 grams of carbohydrate. In addition, approximately 5 grams of carbohydrate circulates freely in the blood in the form of glucose. Thus, the total carbohydrate reserve in a typical man may be about 500 grams, or about 2,000 kilocalories. As discussed later in this chapter, both muscle glycogen depletion and reduced blood glucose have proved to be independently involved in reducing athletic performance and promoting fatigue.

Muscle Carbohydrate Utilization

Muscle glycogen stores also provide a glucose source for the muscle cells in which they are stored. In fact, that energy source is extremely important during training and competition, especially as the intensity of the bout increases (**FIGURE 9.12**). Because muscle cells do not possess glucose-6-phosphatase, the fate of glycogen-derived glucose-6-phosphate is to enter glycolysis and provide energy within that muscle cell.

The rate of catabolism of skeletal muscle glycogen appears to be related to the intensity of exercise as well as the duration of the activity. For example, exercising at low intensity for 2 hours may reduce muscle glycogen levels by only 20%, whereas higher-intensity exercise may deplete pre-event stores. That's because exercise intensities approximating 50, 75, and 100% VO_2max can produce muscle glycogenolysis rates of 0.7, 1.4, and 3.4 mmol/kg/min, respectively.

Muscle glycogen depletion is closely associated with muscular fatigue during prolonged exercise. However, the physiologic mechanisms responsible are less clear. The resulting muscular fatigue cannot simply be explained by the inability of other substrates (such as blood glucose and free fatty acid [FFA], along with intramuscular FFA) to sustain ATP levels.

Individuals whose glycogen levels have been depleted prior to a bout of exercise are still able to engage in a reasonable exercise effort. It may be that the additional carbohydrate provided by muscle glycogen provides alternative functions supportive of muscle fiber activity. For instance, it is important for the replacement of key Krebs cycle intermediates, such as α-ketoglutarate and oxaloacetate, which are lost during exercise.

Maintaining Blood Glucose Levels During Exercise

The concentration of glucose in the blood is typically maintained and potentially elevated during higher-intensity exercise in both trained and untrained individuals. Breakdown of hepatic glycogen stores and subsequent release into circulation is a principal euglycemic homeostatic mechanism. During exercise, this mechanism supports muscle activity by maintaining circulatory glucose delivery. In addition to glycogenolysis, during prolonged endurance exercise, hepatocytes of the liver also produce glucose from circulating substrates, such as lactate, glycerol, alanine, and other amino acids.

Exercise at or above 50% VO_2max can result in a maintained increase in circulatory glucose. The rise in plasma glucose concentration is attributable to increased glucose production by the liver, accompanied by a decreased secretion of insulin. Not only does the reduced insulin level decrease glucose uptake in cells but it also removes its inhibitory effect on gluconeogenesis in the liver, glycogenolysis in the liver and muscle, and fat breakdown in adipose tissue. It has been speculated that a drop in circulating insulin levels during exercise is a mechanism for conserving blood glucose for semi- and absolute obligate tissue, such as the brain and red blood cells. In the brain and red blood cells, the uptake of glucose is concentration driven, not insulin driven.

Cori Cycle

Lactate produced by glycolysis in active skeletal muscle tissue increases during exercise in a manner relative to intensity; it is an important mechanism for maintaining blood glucose levels during prolonged exercise. In skeletal muscle, lactate is mostly produced by type II fibers via glucose derived from glycogen stores. Lactate can diffuse into circulation and circulate to the liver, where it is oxidized back to pyruvate, which is a substrate for gluconeogenesis. This new glucose molecule can then enter circulation and be used by skeletal muscle in a cyclic manner. This cycle has been called the **Cori cycle** or lactic

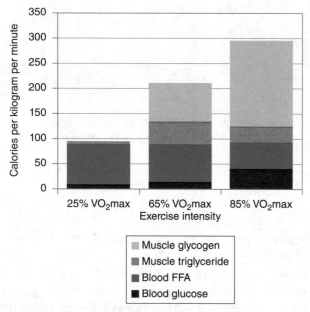

FIGURE 9.12 Contribution of Different Fuel Sources to Cycling Exercise (Prefasted) at Three Submaximal Intensities. Here, FFA is free fatty acid.

Data from Romijn JA, Coyle EF, Sidossis LS, et al. Regulation of endogenous fat and carbohydrate metabolism in relation to exercise intensity and duration. *Am J Physiol.* 1993;265:E380–E391.

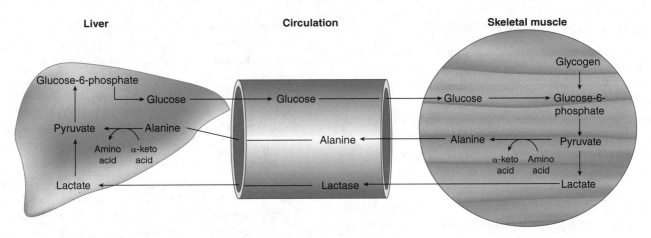

FIGURE 9.13 Alanine (via Amino Acid Catabolism) and Lactate (via Glycolysis) Are Primary Sources for Glucose Production During Endurance Exercise. Once glucose is created in the liver, it can circulate back to muscle and be used as fuel.

acid cycle (**FIGURE 9.13**). However, only a portion of the lactate produced by working skeletal muscle engages in the Cori cycle. Lactate is also available to other skeletal muscle fibers, especially those with greater oxidative capacity, such as type I fibers. Additionally, cardiac muscle cells use more and more lactate during exercise.

Alanine Cycle

Alanine is involved in a cyclic operation as well. Alanine derived from the skeletal muscle amino acid pool, as well as from the catabolism of muscle protein and transamination reactions, can diffuse into the blood and circulate to the liver. Once inside hepatocytes, alanine can be converted to pyruvate (via transamination) and hence become a substrate for gluconeogenesis. Alanine-derived glucose can diffuse into the blood and circulate to working muscle. This operation has sometimes been referred to as the alanine cycle or the **alanine–glucose cycle** (see Figure 9.13).

Carbohydrate Oxidation During Exercise

During exercise, the utilization of carbohydrate increases in relation to the intensity of the exercise (**FIGURE 9.14**). Moreover, muscle glycogen provides the principal carbohydrate during exercise, in an intensity-related manner. At the same time, glucose entry into muscle fibers is enhanced to support muscle glycogen. Keeping in mind that circulating insulin levels are typically decreased during exercise intensity above 50% VO_2max, exercise must independently stimulate the translocation of GLUT4 transporters to the sarcolemma. Many other factors influence how much carbohydrate is used during exercise, including an athlete's general diet, the timing and composition of the most recent meal, and the consumption of a sport beverage during exercise.

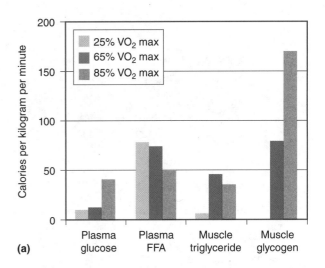

(a)

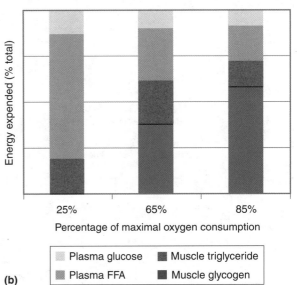

(b)

FIGURE 9.14 Utilization of Different Fuel Sources During Exercise. Quantity (**a**) and percentage contribution (**b**) to total energy expended made by carbohydrate and fat sources after 30 minutes of cycling (prefasted) exercising at low (25% VO_2max), moderate (65% VO_2max), and higher (85% VO_2max) submaximal intensities.

Glycogen Stores and Exercise

As exercise is prolonged, the use of muscle glycogen decreases for both endurance and intermittent activity, such as ice hockey and multiple-set weight training (**FIGURES 9.15** and **9.16**). Initial muscle glycogen stores are also very important in allowing an individual to sustain prolonged moderate to heavy exercise. For example, in a classic study, an initial glycogen content of 1.75 grams per 100 grams of wet muscle allowed individuals to tolerate a standard workload for 114 minutes, whereas an initial glycogen content of 0.63 and 3.31 grams per 100 grams wet muscle allowed for 57 minutes and 167 minutes, respectively, at that same

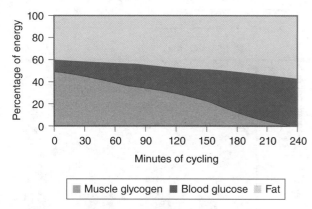

FIGURE 9.15 Energy Sources During Endurance Exercise. Levels are based on cycling at 65% VO₂max for 4 hours by young males without food or caloric beverage before or during the ride.

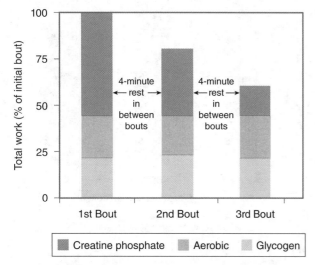

FIGURE 9.16 Expected General Fuel Contributions by Aerobic Systems, Glycogen, and Creatine Phosphate. The contribution made by glycogen becomes progressively lower during the second and third bouts, which accounts for the reduction in work output during those bouts.

workload. Muscle glycogen levels can be increased as an adaptation to moderate- to higher-intensity training, thus allowing muscle to perform longer prior to fatigue.

Once glycogen is depleted, the time frame for repletion can be significant. Only about 5% of muscle glycogen is replaced per hour. Thus, glycogen repletion may take place over the course of 24 hours after a glycogen-exhaustive exercise bout if dietary carbohydrate intake levels of 8 grams of carbohydrate per kilogram body weight per day are achieved. This is an important concept, especially for multistage endurance athletes, such as cyclists (e.g., during the Tour de France) that perform over several sequential days. Meanwhile, while repeated sets of resistance exercise can reduce acute resistance performance (e.g., rep number), most people will not completely deplete glycogen in trained muscle within a targeted muscle.

Carbohydrate Consumption Before, During, and After Exercise

The status of muscle glycogen stores at the onset of exercise is one of the most significant factors influencing the duration of endurance performance. It is generally agreed that a pre-event meal containing carbohydrate is beneficial in maximizing those stores. However, the timing of the meal requires some consideration. The general recommendation for carbohydrate intake for an adult 3 to 4 hours prior to strenuous endurance exercise is 1 to 4 grams per kilogram of body weight. That would be appropriate to raise glycogen stores at the onset of exercise and, potentially, to enhance performance, especially if there had been an extended fasting period previously (e.g., during sleep). In addition, athletes should choose foods that they tolerate well and that have minimal indigestible material, such as fiber. This meal should be lower in fat and fiber to allow for an optimal rate of gastric emptying, and fluids should be consumed to optimize hydration status.

However, it has been speculated that consuming carbohydrate within 1 hour prior to an event may be a detriment to performance. The assumed concept is that an individual can experience the effects of hyperinsulinemia at the onset of activity, resulting in a period of transient hypoglycemia early in the exercise session. This concept has not been substantiated; in fact, many studies have indicated that consumption of carbohydrate within 1 hour prior to cycling or running at higher intensities is beneficial or not a factor.

During endurance exercise bouts lasting < 45 minutes, exogenous carbohydrate may not be necessary in general. For bouts lasting 45 to75 minutes, small amounts can be consumed along with a mouth rinse with carbohydrate beverages. For longer duration bouts, including intermittent high-intensity sports, athletes should strive to ingest 30 to 60 grams of carbohydrate per hour of performance for 1 to 2.5 hours and 60 to 90 grams/hour for even longer events or training.

Accordingly, a practical recommendation for most athletes engaged in sports and general endurance training/competition is to consume 600 to 1,200 milliliters of a 6 to 8% carbohydrate sport drink per hour. It is generally stated that the maximal uptake of glucose for endurance athletes is approximately 1g/min; however, researchers have reported benefit to co-ingestion of glucose and fructose based on utilization of different absorption transport systems.

Endurance and other glycogen depleting sport athletes should consume at least 1 to 1.2 grams of carbohydrate per kilogram of body weight as soon as possible after training or competition for the first 4 hours and resume recommended carbohydrate intake. Maximal glycogen levels can be restored within 24 hours at dietary carbohydrate intake levels of above 8 grams of carbohydrate per kilogram body weight per day. Failing to ingest carbohydrate for a couple of hours after strenuous exercise will dramatically reduce the rate of glycogen recovery. In general, a carbohydrate intake of 8 to 10 grams per kilogram per day is suggested for athletes who are completing intense endurance exercise bouts on consecutive days. However, for athletes performing strength training over consecutive days but who are training varied muscle groups, such a high daily carbohydrate target is not necessary and should be gauged against workout performance and general weight management and health goals.

Carbohydrate Supercompensation (Glycogen Loading)

Glycogen loading is a means of maximizing muscle glycogen stores and is used to enhance endurance performance. Because muscular fatigue is closely associated with depletion of muscle glycogen stores, augmentation of those stores can theoretically allow an individual to perform at a moderate- to higher-intensity level for a longer period of time before exhaustion. Exercise activities that demonstrate benefit from glycogen loading include soccer, marathons, triathlons, ultramarathons, ultra-endurance events, cross-country skiing, long-distance swimming, and cycling.

The classic method of glycogen loading involved depleting muscle tissue of its glycogen over a 3-day period of exhaustive exercise and a low-carbohydrate diet followed by 3 days of a very high carbohydrate diet (> 90% of kilocalories). However, many participants experienced hypoglycemia, irritability, and fatigue during the first half of this protocol and demonstrated poor compliance during the latter half of the protocol. More modern approaches to glycogen loading are very tolerable and effective in maximizing glycogen stores. For instance, tapering down exercise during the 6 days prior to an event while, at the same time, increasing or ensuring higher carbohydrate intake (**TABLE 9.5**). More recently, enhanced glycogen levels have been assessed in even shorter periods of time, such as all training for 48 hours while maintaining a high carbohydrate training diet. Here, athletes are encouraged to consume roughly 10 to 12 grams per kilogram of body weight for 36 to 48 hours prior to events lasting greater than 90 minutes. For shorter events, 7 to 12 grams per kilogram of body weight is a good guideline.

Triglyceride and Fatty Acid Metabolism and Exercise

Fat and, more specifically, fatty acids, and glycerol are important energy sources during exercise (see Figure 9.14). Adipocyte triglyceride stores provide FFAs as well as glycerol, both of which can be used during exercise. Hormone-sensitive lipase in adipocytes hydrolyzes the ester bonds between glycerol and fatty acids in triglyceride molecules. FFAs liberated from adipocytes circulate to muscle loosely bound to albumin (**FIGURE 9.17**). Glycerol liberated from adipocytes dissolves into the blood and circulates to the liver, where it can be used for gluconeogenesis. Hormone-sensitive lipase (HSL), which is stimulated by catabolic hormones, such as epinephrine, glucagon, and cortisol, liberates fatty acids from the adipocyte triglyceride pool. Furthermore, a lipase enzyme similar to liver HSL has been isolated in muscle. This enzyme appears to be epinephrine sensitive in both skeletal and cardiac muscle and is responsible for liberating fatty acids from muscle fiber triglyceride for use in those cells. That means that skeletal and cardiac muscle both have HSL as well as lipoprotein lipase (LPL), which is responsible for liberating fatty acids from lipoproteins.

Fat Stores and Exercise

A 70-kilogram man with 15% body fat theoretically has approximately 10,500 grams of triglyceride contributing to his mass. This could be viewed as 94,500 kilocalories of potential energy. Although not all of this triglyceride is readily available, much of it is.

TABLE 9.5 Seven-Day Glycogen-Loading Protocol

Time Prior to Competition	Intensity and Duration of Training	Diet Protocol
6 days	90 minutes at intensity, approximating 70 to 75% VO$_2$ max	Target 50% of energy as carbohydrate or 4 to 5 grams per kilogram of body weight
5 days	40 minutes at intensity, approximating 70 to 75% VO$_2$ max	Target 50% of energy as carbohydrate or 4 to 5 grams per kilogram of body weight
4 days	40 minutes at intensity, approximating 70 to 75% VO$_2$ max	Target 50% of energy as carbohydrate or 4 to 5 grams per kilogram of body weight
3 days	20 minutes at intensity, approximating 70 to 75% VO$_2$ max; rest muscle while not training	Target greater than 60% of total energy as carbohydrate or 10 grams per kilogram of body weight
2 days	20 minutes at intensity, approximating 70 to 75% VO$_2$ max	Greater than 60% of total energy as carbohydrate or 10 grams per kilogram of body weight
1 day (the day before)	Rest muscle	Greater than 60% of total energy as carbohydrate or 10 grams per kilogram of body weight
Competition	Rest muscle before event	Depending on the time of day, consume carbohydrate as appropriate

Note: Athletes need to experiment with glycogen-loading protocols during training periods to find what works best for them. It is very important that athletes also consume appropriate levels of water.

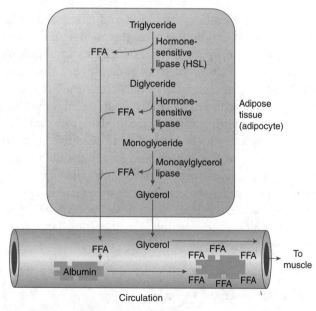

FIGURE 9.17 The Breakdown of Triglycerides in Adipose Tissue During Exercise. Hormone-sensitive lipase (HSL) is activated by epinephrine. Fatty acids bind to albumin for circulation. FFA, free fatty acid.

Thus, the stored energy potential of fat far exceeds that of carbohydrate and protein. Most of the triglyceride in the human body is stored in adipocytes, whereas a relatively minor portion of human body fat is found within muscle tissue. However, skeletal muscle triglyceride is extremely significant as an energy contributor for that tissue, especially during exercise.

Electron microscopy has revealed the presence of tiny triglyceride-rich droplets typically situated near mitochondria. Also, muscle contains some adipose tissue. Skeletal muscle may contain 7 to 25 micromoles of triglyceride per gram of tissue and may collectively contain 150 to 200 grams of triglyceride. Training enhances the concentration of lipid droplets in muscle fibers, especially type I fibers, which makes sense based on their oxidative nature. Moreover, aerobic training can enhance the triglyceride content of type I fibers roughly twofold after a couple of months, thereby enhancing its availability during physical activity.

Because skeletal muscle cells do not make fatty acids, the balance of fatty acids within the muscle triglyceride pool is attributable to circulating FFA. Diet-derived chylomicrons as well as VLDL from the liver provide most of the fatty acids to muscle. Lipoprotein lipase is the enzyme complex responsible for the breakdown of fat in lipoproteins, allowing fatty acids to move into muscle cells, which can then be incorporated in a triglyceride molecule for assimilation into a droplet. In addition, some FFAs that circulate to muscle bound to albumin can contribute to TG droplets in muscle fibers.

Fatty Acid Oxidation in Muscle

Fatty acids are an important source of energy during exercise (see Figure 9.11). Regardless of their source, FFAs must first be activated within muscle cells prior to oxidation for energy. Acyl CoA is formed from longer-chain fatty acids in the cytosol, whereas shorter-chain fatty acids become activated within mitochondria. Once in the mitochondrial matrix, fatty acids undergo β-oxidation, producing NADH and $FADH_2$, which transfer electrons to the electron transport chain for ATP generation. In addition, the end product of most fatty acid oxidation, acetyl CoA, is available to the Krebs cycle. Thus, the energy potential of fatty acid oxidation is great. For instance, when all factors are considered, the oxidation of palmitate (16:0) yields 129 ATP molecules.

Muscle biopsies quantifying the actual muscle fiber triglyceride content, as well as measurements of blood glycerol content, are indicative of intramuscular triglyceride utilization during exercise. As discussed below, the relative contribution of intramuscular fat to total energy utilization in muscle fibers depends on the intensity of the exercise as well as the duration. Intramuscular triglyceride may provide as much as half of the total fat used during an exercise bout, and, as mentioned earlier, endurance training enhances the ability of muscle fibers to use intramuscular stores of triglyceride. For example, the contribution of intramuscular triglyceride-derived fatty acids to total fat used during an exercise bout can increase from approximately 35 to 57% in a trained state.

Exercise and Fat Utilization

Chronic endurance training enhances the fatty acid oxidation potential of trained fibers. Major factors associated with this adaptation include an increase in the number and size of mitochondria along with an accompanying enhancement in the activity of 3-OH-acyl-CoA dehydrogenase, a principal enzyme in β-oxidation, as well as enzymes in the Krebs cycle.

The increase in mitochondria is especially apparent in type I fibers, but it also occurs in recruited type II fibers that undergo training adaptation. The increased vascularization allows for increased oxygen and nutrient delivery and a decrease in the diffusion distance for the exchange of substances between muscle fibers and circulation.

As mentioned previously, training enhances the concentration of intramuscular triglyceride stores, especially in type I fibers. What's more, aerobic training can further enhance the concentration of triglyceride in type I fibers. The fatty acids released from this intramuscular pool appear to be a very important energy source during exercise (see Figure 9.14). Meanwhile, liberated glycerol diffuses into the blood and is available for gluconeogenesis in the liver.

Fat Utilization After Exercise

Bouts of endurance exercise increase the clearance rate of circulating triglycerides for several hours after the event. This is attributable to LPL activity, which can increase two- to threefold as a result of an exercise bout and remains elevated for several hours thereafter. This increased activity, which is most significant in type I fibers, not only allows for greater fatty acid utilization during activity but also for repletion of triglyceride stores. Furthermore, as an adaptation to endurance training, the clearance rate of circulating triglycerides can increase, therefore, allowing more fatty acids to be available for skeletal muscle storage and oxidation in upcoming exercise. This effect is largely due to higher resting LPL activity in trained muscle.

Protein and Amino Acid Metabolism and Exercise

Skeletal muscle protein-derived amino acids are a potential energy source during exercise. Consuming protein-rich or amino acid-rich foods/supplements or sports drinks during training or competition is not as common as consuming carbohydrate-containing resources; however, more protein- and amino acid-endowed products are appearing on the market. For instance, supplements containing branched-chain amino acids (BCAAs) are marketed to support muscle protein synthesis and recovery. However, amino acids used during exercise in an individual not receiving amino acids or protein before or during the bout are principally derived from skeletal muscle proteins and amino acid pools, with the latter only amounting to 0.5 to 1.0% of total body amino acids.

A 70-kilogram man with about 40% skeletal muscle has about 5,000 to 6,000 grams of body protein in skeletal muscle alone. That estimate is based on the idea that human skeletal muscle is approximately 22% protein by weight (>80% dry weight). However, it is generally believed that no more than 3 to 4% of the body's protein is engaged in turnover at any given time, thereby limiting the availability of amino acids. Although their utilization during weight training is limited, amino acids typically supply only 5 to 10% of energy turnover during prolonged endurance exercise.

Protein turnover is determined by the net balance between protein synthesis and breakdown. As shown in **FIGURES 9.18** and **9.19**, an imbalance in muscle protein turnover can be the result of contrasting directional fluctuations in both synthesis and breakdown, or perhaps of an augmentation of either while the other remains the same.

$$\frac{\text{Net Muscle}}{\text{Protein Balance}} = \frac{\text{Muscle Protein}}{\text{Synthesis (MPS)}} - \frac{\text{Muscle Protein}}{\text{Breakdown (MPB)}}$$

Effect of Resistance Exercise and Postworkout Nutrition on Net Muscle Protein Turnover

Exercise induces changes in muscle protein turnover. For instance, muscle protein synthesis (MPS) remains

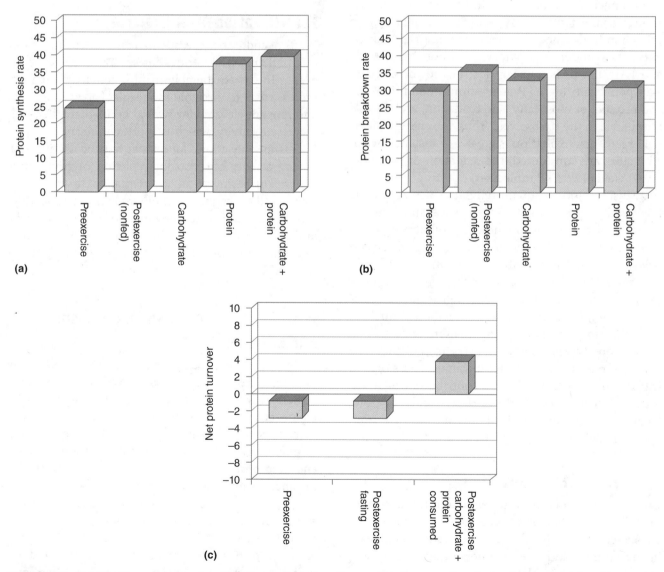

(a)

(b)

(c)

FIGURE 9.18 **Protein Turnover During Resistance Exercise.** Expected influence of bout of weight training on (a) muscle protein synthesis, (b) protein breakdown, and (c) net protein turnover 3 to 4 hours after training and while fasting (postexercise) or when carbohydrate, protein, or both carbohydrate and protein were provided immediately after training. Pre-exercise was a fasting state, and units are arbitrary.

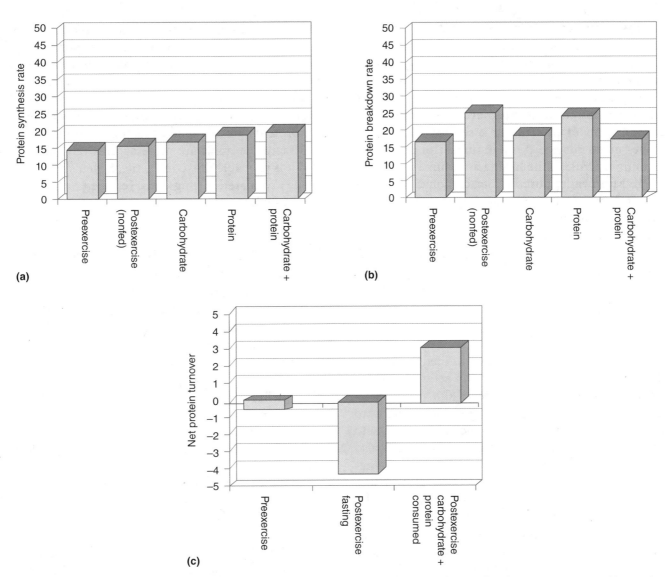

FIGURE 9.19 Protein Turnover During Endurance Exercise. Expected influence of bout of endurance training on (a) muscle protein synthesis, (b) protein breakdown, and (c) net protein turnover 3 to 4 hours after training and while fasting (postexercise) or when carbohydrate, essential amino acids, or both carbohydrate and essential amino acids were provided immediately after training. Pre-exercise was a fasting state, and units are arbitrary.

unchanged or even decreases during resistance training, whereas it is ramped up for several hours after training stops (see Figure 9.18). Meanwhile, muscle protein breakdown (MPB) remains unchanged during resistance training and then increases after cessation of exercise. Eating immediately or soon after completion of exercise modulates the effect of resistance exercise on the degree of MPS and MPB and thus, on net muscle protein turnover. For instance, consumption of protein (or essential amino acids) at appropriate levels (e.g., more than 20 grams of protein or more than 6 grams of EAA) augments the positive impact of resistance training on MPS while having a minimal impact on MPB. Meanwhile, postexercise carbohydrate raises insulin levels, which, in turn, dampen

or minimize MPB while having only a mild, permissive effect, if any, on enhancing MPS. Based on those concepts, it appears that in order to maximize muscle development gains from resistance training, a person should consume carbohydrate and protein after strenuous exercise, especially if a meal was not consumed prior to exercise.

Effect of Endurance Exercise and Postworkout Nutrition on Net Muscle Protein Turnover

As shown in Figure 9.19, MPS decreases during endurance training and then tends to increase after completion of the training. Meanwhile, MPB increases during training and tends to continue after completion in an unfed state. As is the case with resistance training, eating immediately or soon after completion of endurance exercise modulates the effect of the session on MPS and MPB and thus, affects net muscle protein turnover. For instance, the consumption of protein (or essential amino acids alone) augments the positive impact of endurance training on MPS while having a minimal impact on MPB. Meanwhile, postworkout carbohydrate raises insulin levels, which, in turn, dampen or minimize MPB while having only a little or mild effect on MPS. Based on those concepts, it seems vital to maximize muscle performance adaptations from endurance training.

Muscle Amino Acid Metabolism During Exercise

Muscle tissue itself is somewhat limited in its ability to completely metabolize amino acids for energy. However, relative to hepatocytes of the liver, skeletal muscle cells demonstrate a greater capacity to metabolize the BCAAs via branched-chain α-keto acid dehydrogenase. Skeletal muscle cells are also able to synthesize glutamine via glutamine synthetase. During longer-duration exercise, alanine and glutamine are released from muscle into circulation in amounts greater than what can be accounted for by their concentration in muscle protein (see Figure 9.13). This demonstrates that amino acid metabolism is indeed occurring during exercise.

The BCAA transaminase reaction that removes the amino group from valine, leucine, and isoleucine appears to have a relatively high K_m. That means that it will operate most productively when those amino acids become most available, such as during exercise. Furthermore, a significant portion of the nitrogen used for the transamination of pyruvate in exercising muscle is derived from BCAAs, which collectively make up approximately one-third of the essential amino acids in muscle protein. In conjunction, the availability of pyruvate in muscle fibers is dramatically increased during exercise because it is derived from intracellular glycogen stores via glycolysis. In addition, the carbon skeletons derived from BCAAs are ultimately metabolized to succinyl CoA and acetyl CoA, which help fuel working muscle fibers.

During maximal-intensity exercise of very brief duration, the contribution of muscle protein to the production of ATP is negligible. However, as exercise is prolonged or repeated, the catabolism of muscle protein (partly due to increases in circulating cortisol) and the contribution of muscle-derived amino acids to energy expenditure increase. For instance, during endurance exercise at 70% VO_2max, the concentration of alanine increases by over 50% in muscle cells. Furthermore, not all muscle proteins are catabolized at the same rate. Noncontractile proteins are more aggressively targeted, and it is probable that contractile proteins in muscle tissue are spared during exercise based on need for continued activity.

General Protein Recommendations

Protein recommendations for both endurance and strength/power athletes are 1.4 to 2.0 grams a day, or 15 to 20% of the energy needed for weight maintenance. A higher percentage can be seen in some weight management strategies. Consuming a postexercise meal containing both carbohydrate and protein maximizes the positive effects of the exercise on muscle protein turnover; however, it is the protein that is more important for MPS and both can play a role in reducing MPB.

In general, athletes should strive for at least 0.3g/kg (20–30 grams) of a targeted athletic body weight, either immediately before or after training. Protein intakes of 40 grams have shown incremental MPS above 20 grams in a whole body training model for previously fasted males. Research suggests that the level of protein necessary to evoke a similar MPS response is higher in older individuals. This is supportive of a growing awareness that protein minimum recommendations for older individuals (e.g., > 50 years old) should be greater than younger adults.

The importance of protein immediately after training to help maximize the benefits on net muscle protein balance (e.g., "anabolic window") is strongly influenced by the timing of protein-rich meals prior to exercise and when the ensuing meal would occur. However, it is vital for an individual who is fasting prior to exercise. In general, athletes should strive to ensure that they are meeting daily protein recommendations as well as pay special attention to the meals flanking training to ensure adequate protein.

Protein supplementation is not necessary if diet protein levels (and some timing aspects) and energy intake are appropriate. However, some can find this challenging if they are focused more heavily on carbohydrate (endurance athletes), have long or multiple daily training schedules, or engage in sports that limit pre-exercise meals, etc. Meanwhile, during weight reduction periods for some sports, protein-based products might be advantageous.

Furthermore, protein intake and muscle and body balance should be viewed on a 24-hour basis. Protein digestion and absorption, as well as body and muscle tissue MPS occur during sleep in the same manner and intensity as during waking hours. That establishes an opportunity for nighttime protein to be used strategically to meet daily protein goals. Furthermore, protein prior to bed does not seem to disrupt typical fat breakdown and oxidation during sleep, which is helpful for those resistant to using a prebed protein strategy.

Water and Exercise

Plasma volume tends to decrease during exercise. This is due to increased sweating as well as a redistribution of water from the vascular compartment into the interstitial spaces (and within muscle cells). The loss of water via the former mechanism during a bout of activity is enhanced by the intensity of the bout and the ambient temperature and humidity. It is estimated that plasma volume can decrease by as much as 2.4% for each 1% loss in body weight during the increased sweating associated with training or competition. About 0.58 kilocalorie of heat can be removed from the human body in every milliliter of water, or about 580 kilocalories per liter of sweat.

The shift of water from the vascular to interstitial space is initiated within the first minute or so of exercise. This redistribution is due to elevated blood pressure, which results in increased hydrostatic pressure in capillaries and increased oncotic pressure in the interstitial space. The movement of protein from the capillaries into the interstitial space is responsible for the increased osmotic (oncotic) pressure in that compartment.

Dehydration and Performance

Hypohydration of the plasma, or hypovolemia, can result in significant reductions in athletic performance. For instance, as little as a 2 to 3% loss in body weight as water can result in detectable decreases in performance (**TABLE 9.6**). When trained runners were dehydrated by 2% of their body weight via a diuretic, their running speeds in 5,000- and 10,000-meter races decreased. As more water is lost, the more the impact on physiologic function and athletic performance intensifies. Every liter of water lost increases heart rate by as much as 8 beats per

TABLE 9.6 Effects of Body Water Loss on Physiologic Performance

Percentage Body Weight Loss as Water	Physiologic Effect
1–2	Thirst is evoked; some fatigue; possible reductions in strength
3–4	Maximal aerobic power and endurance reduced; plasma volume reductions can increase heart rate; thermoregulation can become compromised
5–6	Decreased concentration/focus; headache; increased breathing; reduced thermoregulation; reduced cardiac output; chills; nausea; rapid pulse
7–10	Dizziness; exhaustion; muscle spasms; poor body balance; delirium; critically reduced blood volume; potential cardiogenic shock

minute, and cardiac output declines by about 1 liter per minute (**FIGURE 9.20**).

One of the most critical of the homeostatic functions that is compromised by a reduction in plasma volume is the ability to appropriately dissipate heat from the body (see Table 9.6). For every liter of water lost, core temperature can increase by 0.3°C. Increased core temperature, coupled with hampered blood flow to extremities for heat removal, can lead to heat exhaustion at losses of approximately 5% body weight as water. Furthermore, a 7% reduction can result in hallucinations and dehydration beyond 9 to 10% body weight is associated with heat stroke, coma, and, eventually, death.

Water Recommendations for Athletic Performance

It is generally recommended that individuals consume approximately 400 to 600 milliliters of water or water-based fluid approximately 2 hours prior to a bout of

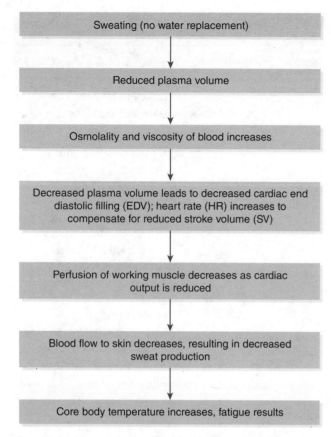

FIGURE 9.20 Physiologic Effects of Reduced Plasma Volume. Dehydration can lead to increased heart rate and decreased cardiac output. This results in decreased sweating and an increase in core body temperature.

activity. That will allow for rehydration, if needed, and excretion of residual water. Larger athletes and athletes who sweat more can experiment with higher levels. Furthermore, it has become apparent that ingestion of fluid within an hour of exercise may result in a slightly lower core body temperature and heart rate at the onset and during exercise. This is considered beneficial because it reduces some of the physiologic stress associated with exercise. The importance of preworkout exercise or precompetition water consumption cannot be overemphasized, especially for individuals in warmer climates.

Regular water intake becomes more critical with the duration of the effort, both in training and competition. It is recommended that for efforts such as a 10,000-meter (10-kilometer) run or longer, 150 to 350 milliliters (5 to 12 ounces) of fluid be consumed every 15 to 20 minutes. For shorter events, such as those that conclude within 1 hour, pure water can provide

maximal benefit; however, during longer endurance events, water replacement may be most beneficial in the form of a sport drink composite.

Vitamins, Minerals, and Exercise

The influence of vitamin status on exercise performance cannot be overstated. Several vitamins and minerals are directly involved in the metabolism of energy that fuels exercise as well as recovery and adaptive processes. At the same time, various vitamins and minerals are involved in protein and connective tissue turnover, neurologic function, erythrocyte production, and immune and antioxidant functions. Therefore, an imbalance in one or more vitamins and/or minerals can markedly affect performance. Furthermore, it is likely that chronic training increases the daily requirement for some of those nutrients, particularly the B vitamins. One reason for that is that the DRI recommendations (AI and RDA) do not take into consideration athletic performance, enhanced energy and protein needs, or tissue repair and recovery from training and competition.

The idea that athletes have higher vitamin and mineral needs appears to be recognized by athletes. For instance, survey data of college athletes routinely suggest that they know they need more vitamins than their nonathletic peers. Furthermore, vitamins are one of the most commonly consumed ergogenic aids. Conversely, the intake of some vitamins, including B_6, A, C, and B_{12}, has been reported to be low for some athletes. **TABLE 9.7** lists factors that can influence vitamin and mineral intake, absorption, and excretion for athletes.

● BEFORE YOU GO ON . . .

1. What are the sources of fuel during exercise?
2. How do exercise intensity and duration affect fuel utilization?
3. What are the principal factors involved in fatigue during exercise?
4. How does exercise training affect muscle stores of carbohydrate and fat?
5. What are some of the reasons why vitamins and minerals should be important considerations for athletes?

TABLE 9.7 Factors That Could Influence Vitamin and Mineral Needs Related to Exercise

Factors	Comments
Changes in eating patterns or volumes	■ Athletes may focus on altering the macronutrient ratio or the involvement of particular foods or food groups ■ Athletes may engage in chronic restrictive food intake to manipulate body weight and composition
Changes in nutrient absorption	■ Decreased status, via increased metabolism and/or excretion related to exercise, can increase the efficiency of absorption from the digestive tract
Greater metabolic requirements	■ Increased energy metabolism, oxidative stress, and recovery and adaptive efforts could increase the requirement for specific vitamins and minerals. This could be enhanced muscle tissue, oxidative systems, antioxidant systems, enhanced myoglobin and hemoglobin, or increased connective tissue.
Changes in nutrient metabolism and excretion	■ May increase or decrease urinary loss of vitamins and minerals ■ May increase loss of nutrients in sweat (e.g., sodium, chloride, potassium, calcium, iron)

CLINICAL INSIGHT

Exercise Recommendations and Health Benefits

There are numerous benefits of physical activity and planned exercise for people of all ages. Benefits can include increased self-esteem, strength, flexibility and reduced risk of injury as well as cardiorespiratory health and weight management. In addition, physical activity and sound nutrition practices can help reduce the risk of chronic degenerative diseases, such as heart disease, osteoporosis, and sarcopenia. While we have discussed the benefits of nutrition, dietitians and nutritionists should also give advice on exercise as those factors are interdependent upon one another.

A recent position stand by the American College of Sports Medicine provided scientific evidence-based recommendations to health and fitness professionals in the development of individualized exercise prescriptions for healthy adults of all ages. ACSM's overall recommendation is for most adults to engage in at least 150 minutes of moderate-intensity exercise each week. The basic recommendations—categorized by cardiorespiratory exercise, resistance exercise, flexibility exercise, and neuromotor exercise—are as follows:

Cardiorespiratory Exercise
■ Adults should get at least 150 minutes of moderate-intensity exercise per week
■ Exercise recommendations can be met through 30 to 60 minutes of moderate-intensity exercise (5 days per week) or 20 to 60 minutes of vigorous-intensity exercise (3 days per week)
■ One continual session and multiple shorter sessions (of at least 10 minutes) are both acceptable to accumulate desired amount of daily exercise
■ Gradual progression of exercise time, frequency, and intensity is recommended for best adherence and least injury risk
■ People unable to meet those minimums can still benefit from some activity

Resistance Exercise
■ Adults should train each major muscle group 2 or 3 days each week using a variety of exercises and equipment
■ Very light or light intensity is best for older persons or previously sedentary adults starting exercise
■ Two to four sets of each exercise will help adults improve strength and power
■ For each exercise, 8 to 12 repetitions improve strength and power, 10 to 15 repetitions improve strength in middle age and older persons starting exercise, and 15 to 20 repetitions improve muscular endurance
■ Adults should wait at least 48 hours between resistance training sessions

(continues)

CLINICAL INSIGHT (continued)

Flexibility Exercise

- Adults should do flexibility exercises at least 2 or 3 days each week to improve range of motion
- Each stretch should be held for 10 to 30 seconds to the point of tightness or slight discomfort
- Repeat each stretch two to four times, accumulating 60 seconds per stretch
- Static, dynamic, ballistic, and PNF stretches are all effective
- Flexibility exercise is most effective when the muscle is warm. Try light aerobic activity or a hot bath to warm the muscles before stretching.

Neuromotor Exercise

- Neuromotor exercise (sometimes called "functional fitness training") is recommended for 2 or 3 days per week
- Exercises should involve motor skills (balance, agility, coordination, and gait), proprioceptive exercise training, and multifaceted activities (tai ji and yoga) to improve physical function and prevent falls in older adults
- Twenty to 30 minutes per day is appropriate for neuromotor exercise

▶ Here's What You Have Learned

1. Muscle is activated by the CNS and muscle contraction is the result of contraction of muscle sarcomeres. Type I muscle fibers are recruited first and Type II fibers are recruited based on incremental needs for force generation.

2. Contraction of skeletal muscle cells is powered by ATP, which itself is generated via carbohydrate, fat, and amino acids derived from several endogenous storage facilities (e.g., glycogen, intramuscular lipid droplets, and adipocytes) as well as from exogenous resources (e.g., food and beverages).

3. Muscle glycogen stores become an increasingly important fuel source as exercise intensity increases. More strenuous training can increase muscle glycogen stores in trained muscle fibers. Exhaustion of muscle glycogen stores and dehydration are the most significant factors that determine muscular fatigue. Meanwhile, reduction in blood glucose concentration is a principal cause of fatigue.

4. Protein turnover is determined by the balance between protein synthesis and degradation; exercise type and duration can influence the rates of either or both protein synthesis and breakdown during and after exercise.

5. Protein recommendations for both endurance and strength/power athletes are 1.4 to 2.0 grams a day, or 15 to 20% of energy needed for weight maintenance. Consuming a postexercise meal containing both carbohydrate and protein maximizes the positive effects of the exercise on muscle protein turnover.

6. Fat is an important energy source during exercise. It is the primary fuel during lower-intensity exercise and becomes increasingly important as more strenuous activity is prolonged and glycogen levels wane. Exercise training can increase the concentration of fat in muscle cells, particularly type I fibers.

7. Plasma volume tends to decrease during a bout of exercise. This is the consequence of increased sweating as well as a redistribution of water from the vascular compartment to the interstitial spaces (and within muscle cells). Sweating can exceed 2 liters per hour for some athletes.

8. Vitamins and minerals are heavily involved in exercise performance because they are directly involved in the metabolism of energy that fuels both exercise as well as recovery and adaptive processes. At the same time, various vitamins and minerals are involved in protein and connective tissue turnover, neurologic function, erythrocyte production, and immune and antioxidant functions.

9. Caffeine is an effective ergogenic nutrition supplement when consumed in low to moderate doses (approximately 3 to 6 milligrams per kilogram of body weight). In general, it is not more effective when consumed at higher dosages (≥ 9 milligrams per kilogram of body weight).

10. Sport drinks are an effective means of maintaining hydration and providing energy and electrolytes during exercise. Volume consumption recommendations match hydration needs, which can be estimated via sweat losses.

▶ Suggested Reading

Beaudart C, Dawson A, Shaw SC, et al. Nutrition and physical activity in the prevention and treatment of sarcopenia: systematic review. *Osteoporos Int.* 2017;28(6):1817–1833.

Bergström J, Hultman E. A study of the glycogen metabolism during exercise in man. *Scand J Clin Lab Invest.* 1967;19(3):218–228.

Black CD, Waddell DE, Gonglach AR. Caffeine's ergogenic effects on cycling: neuromuscular and perceptual factors. *Med Sci Sports Exerc.* 2015;47(6):1145–1158.

Coggan AR, Coyle EF. Reversal of fatigue during prolonged exercise by carbohydrate infusion or ingestion. *J Appl Physiol.* 1987;63(6):2388–2395.

Constantin-Teodosiu D, Cederblad G, Hultman E. PDC activity and acetyl group accumulation in skeletal muscle during prolonged exercise. *J Appl Physiol.* 1992;73(6):2403–2407.

Coyle EF, Coggan AR, Hemmert MK, Ivy JL. Muscle glycogen utilization during prolonged strenuous exercise when fed carbohydrate. *J Appl Physiol.* 1986;61(1):165–172.

Duncan MJ, Thake CD, Downs PJ. Effect of caffeine ingestion on torque and muscle activity during resistance exercise in men. *Muscle Nerve.* 2014;50(4):523–527.

Garber CE, Blissmer B, Deschenes MR, et al. American College of Sports Medicine position stand. Quantity and quality of exercise for developing and maintaining cardiorespiratory, musculoskeletal, and neuromotor fitness in apparently healthy adults: guidance for prescribing exercise. *Med Sci Sports Exerc.* 2011;43(7):1334–1359.

Greenhaff PL, Ren JM, Söderlund K, Hultman E. Energy metabolism in single human muscle fibers during contraction without and with epinephrine infusion. *Am J Physiol.* 1991;260(5 pt 1):E713–E718.

Greenhaff PL, Soderlund K, Ren JM, Hultman E. Energy metabolism in single human muscle fibres during intermittent contraction with occluded circulation. *J Physiol.* 1993;460:443–453.

Hurley BF, Nemeth PM, Martin WH, Hagberg JM, Dalsky GP, Holloszy JO. Muscle triglyceride utilization during exercise: effect of training. *J Appl Physiol.* 1986;60(2):562–567.

Keizer HA, Kuipers H, van Kranenburg G, Geurten P. Influence of liquid and solid meals on muscle glycogen resynthesis, plasma fuel hormone response, and maximal physical working capacity. *Int J Sports Med.* 1987;8(2):99–104.

Kerksick C, Harvey T, Stout J, et al. International Society of Sports Nutrition position stand: nutrient timing. *J Int Soc Sports Nutr.* 2008;5:17.

Kim IY, Schutzler S, Schrader A, et al. The anabolic response to a meal containing different amounts of protein is not limited by the maximal stimulation of protein synthesis in healthy young adults. *Am J Physiol Endocrinol Metab.* 2016;310(1):E73–E80.

MacNaughton LS, Wardle SL, Witard OC, et al. The response of muscle protein synthesis following whole-body resistance exercise is greater following 40 g than 20 g of ingested whey protein. *Physiol Rep.* 2016;4(15):e12893.

Moore DR, Robinson MJ, Fry JL,, et al. Ingested protein dose response of muscle and albumin protein synthesis after resistance exercise in young men. *Am J Clin Nutr.* 2009;89(1):161–168.

Myers J, McAuley P, Lavie CJ, Despres JP, Arena R, Kokkinos P. Physical activity and cardiorespiratory fitness as major markers of cardiovascular risk: their independent and interwoven importance to health status. *Prog Cardiovasc Dis.* 2015;57(4):306–314.

Phillips SM. A brief review of critical processes in exercise-induced muscular hypertrophy. *Sports Med.* 2014;44 (suppl 1):S71–S77.

Rennie MJ, Tipton KD. Protein and amino acid metabolism during and after exercise and the effects of nutrition. *Annu Rev Nutr.* 2000;20:457–483.

Romijn JA, Coyle EF, Sidossis LS, et al. Regulation of endogenous fat and carbohydrate metabolism in relation to exercise intensity and duration. *Am J Physiol.* 1993;265(3 pt 1): E380–E391.

Saltin B, Gollnick PD. Fuel for muscular exercise: role of carbohydrate. In: Horton ES, Terjung RL, eds. *Exercise, Nutrition and Energy Metabolism.* New York: Macmillan; 1988:45–71.

Sawka MN, Pandolf KB. Effects of body water loss on physiological function and exercise performance. In: Gisolfi CV, Lamb DR, eds. *Perspectives in Exercise Science and Sports Medicine, Vol. 3: Fluid Homeostasis During Exercise.* Indianapolis, IN: Benchmark Press; 1990:1–30.

Schrauwen P, van Aggel-Leijssen DP, Hul G, et al. The effect of a 3-month low-intensity endurance training program on fat oxidation and acetyl-CoA carboxylase-2 expression. *Diabetes.* 2002;51(7):2220–2226.

Seip RL, Semenkovich CF. Skeletal muscle lipoprotein lipase: molecular regulation and physiological effects in relation to exercise. *Exerc Sport Sci Rev.* 1998;26:191–218.

Söderlund K, Greenhaff PL, Hultman E. Energy metabolism in type I and type II human muscle fibres during short term electrical stimulation at different frequencies. *Acta Physiol Scand.* 1992;144(1):15–22.

Schoenfeld BJ, Aragon AA, Krieger JW. The effect of protein timing on muscle strength and hypertrophy: a meta-analysis. *J Int Soc Sports Nutr.* 2013;10(1):53.

Spriet LL, Lindinger MI, McKelvie RS, Heigenhauser GJ, Jones NL. Muscle glycogenolysis and H⁺ concentration during maximal intermittent cycling. *J Appl Physiol.* 1989;66(1):8–13.

Tipton KD, Wolfe RR. Exercise, protein metabolism, and muscle growth. *Int J Sport Nutr Exerc Metab.* 2001;11(1):109–132.

Thomas DT, Erdman KA, Burke LM. Position of the Academy of Nutrition and Dietetics, Dietitians of Canada, and the American College of Sports Medicine: Nutrition and Athletic Performance. *J Acad Nutr Diet.* 2016;116(3):501–528.

Timmins TD, Saunders DH. Effect of caffeine ingestion on maximal voluntary contraction strength in upper- and lower-body muscle groups. *J Strength Cond Res.* 2014;28(11):3239–3244.

Witard OC, Jackman SR, Breen L, Smith K, Selby A, Tipton KD. Myofibrillar muscle protein synthesis rates subsequent to a meal in response to increasing doses of whey protein at rest and after resistance exercise. *Am J Clin Nutr.* 2014; 99(1):86–95.

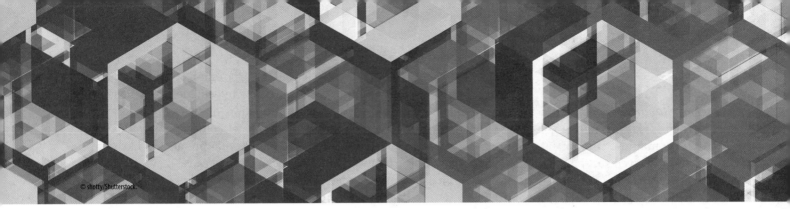

CHAPTER 10
Fat-Soluble Vitamins

← HERE'S WHERE YOU HAVE BEEN

1. The major metabolic pathways involved with energy metabolism and with body growth and maintenance have been presented.
2. The digestion and absorption of macronutrients are unique for each class and subclass of the energy-yielding macronutrients and involve specific enzymes and absorption processes.
3. Physical activity and exercise may affect energy metabolism significantly as well as have a profound impact on body composition.
4. Water does not supply energy but comprises the majority by weight of living organisms. The effects of deficiency set in much quicker for water than for other nutrients.
5. Endocrine and other factors greatly affect how energy-yielding macronutrients and water are metabolized and used.

HERE'S WHERE YOU ARE GOING →

1. Vitamin A may be found in the diet as preformed or provitamin A; or previtamin A in the form of carotenoids and xanthophylls.
2. Vitamin D is often considered a hormone as well as a vitamin as it can be synthesized by the body through a reaction with ultraviolet rays from sunlight and circulates to target tissue where it elicits a response by binding to a receptor.
3. The fat-soluble vitamins A, D, and E, can regulate body functions at the gene level.
4. Vitamin E is a strong antioxidant vitamin, whereas vitamin K has a reputation as the blood-clotting vitamin.
5. Fat-soluble vitamins, particularly vitamin E, may delay the onset and progression of Alzheimer's disease.

▶ Introduction

The term *vitamine* was coined in the early 1900s by the biochemist Casimir Funk to describe a vital amine (nitrogen)-containing component of food. Newly discovered food-derived substances thought to be vital to human operation were subsequently also called vitamines. However, as scientists observed that many of those substances did not contain nitrogen, the "e" was dropped from the word *vitamine*, converting it to the more familiar term **vitamin**.

For a substance to be recognized as a vitamin, it must be organic and be an essential player in at least one necessary chemical reaction or process in the human body. Also, a vitamin cannot be made in the human body, either at all or in sufficient quantities, to meet the body's needs. Vitamins that fall into the latter category include niacin and vitamin D, which can be made in the human body, and two others, vitamin K and biotin, which can be made by bacteria inhabiting the large intestine. Vitamins are noncaloric substances and are required in very small amounts—microgram to milligram quantities.

Water and Fat Solubility

Because water is the principal component of the human body—forming part of blood (transport), digestive juices (absorption), and urine (primary metabolic excretion route)—vitamins are broadly classified based on their water solubility (**TABLE 10.1**). Many general statements can be made about the water-soluble and fat-soluble vitamins with regard to digestion and absorption, transport from the intestines, plasma circulatory mechanisms, storage, and the timing to onset of deficiency and toxicity. This chapter discusses the fat-soluble vitamins.

The fat-soluble vitamins depend on the processes of normal lipid digestion and absorption, such as the presence of bile and incorporation into chylomicrons in the intestinal mucosa. Any situation in which there is decreased bile production or delivery to the small intestine greatly decreases fat-soluble vitamin digestion and absorption. Fat-soluble vitamins are less likely to be removed by urinary excretion because they are typically transported aboard lipoproteins or in association with a transport protein or complex. In general, it requires relatively longer periods of time to bring about deficiency states of fat-soluble vitamins than of water-soluble vitamins. The most outstanding exception is vitamin K.

▶ Vitamin A

Vitamin A, or **preformed vitamin A** (also known as provitamin A), was first identified in 1914 and its structure was elucidated in 1930. It has three primary forms: retinol (an alcohol form), retinal (an aldehyde form), and retinoic acid (an acid form that is derived from retinal). Vitamin A consists of a ring structure attached to a hydrocarbon tail that terminates with a variable chemical group—either an alcohol, aldehyde, or acid (**FIGURE 10.1**). Palmitic

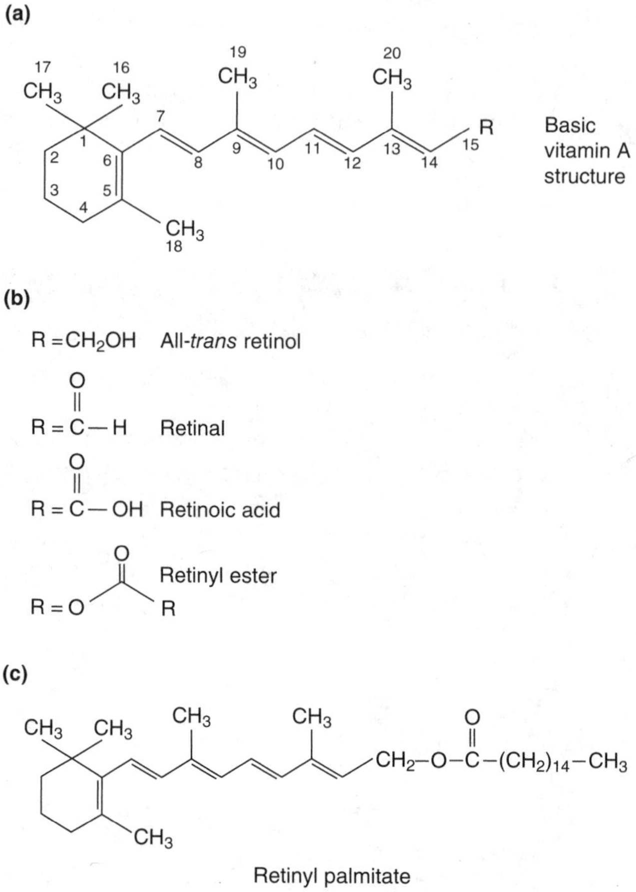

TABLE 10.1	Vitamins	
Water-Soluble Vitamins		**Fat-Soluble Vitamins**
Vitamin C	Folate	Vitamin A
Thiamin	Biotin	Vitamin D
Riboflavin	Niacin	Vitamin E
Vitamin B$_6$	Pantothenic acid	Vitamin K
Vitamin B$_{12}$	Choline[a]	

[a]Not a strict vitamin.

FIGURE 10.1 Basic Structures of Vitamin A Compounds. (a) Basic backbone structure. (b) Various vitamin A isomers. (c) Retinyl palmitate form, which is found in blood and tissues.

acid can bind to vitamin A to transport it in blood and tissues. The nature of the double bonds in the hydrocarbon tail can vary between *cis* and *trans* configurations. For instance, retinol, which is regarded as the vitamin A parent compound, is all-*trans* retinol. The form of vitamin A vital to vision is 11-*cis* retinal, whereas 13-*cis* retinoic acid is used to treat cystic acne (**FIGURE 10.2**).

Previtamin A refers to carotenoid structures, which include the carotenes and xanthophylls. Carotenes and xanthophylls differ slightly in that true carotenes (e.g., lycopene, α-carotene, β-carotene, γ-carotene) are pure hydrocarbon molecules. In contrast, the xanthophylls (e.g., lutein, capsanthin, cryptoxanthin, zeaxanthin, astaxanthin) contain oxygen in the form of a hydroxyl, methoxyl, carboxyl, keto, or epoxy group. Carotenoids have the potential to be converted into retinol within human cells. The most obvious carotenoid in foods is β-carotene; however, other forms, such as α-carotene and γ-carotene, are nutritionally significant as well. **FIGURE 10.3** presents the structures of various carotenoids.

α-Carotene and β-carotene differ in the location of a double bond in a ring, whereas one side of what would be a ring in γ-carotene is actually open (see Figure 10.3). Those differences influence the carotene's efficiency of conversion to vitamin A. Hundreds of carotenoids are found in nature; however, only about 50 or so demonstrate the ability to be converted to vitamin A. Of those carotenoids, only a half dozen or so are found in the diet in appreciable amounts. β-Carotene is perhaps the most potent in its ability to be converted to vitamin A, whereas α-carotene, γ-carotene, and cryptoxanthin have approximately 40 to 60% of the potency of β-carotene. Other carotenoids, such as xanthophyll, zeaxanthin, and lycopene, have virtually no vitamin A potency.

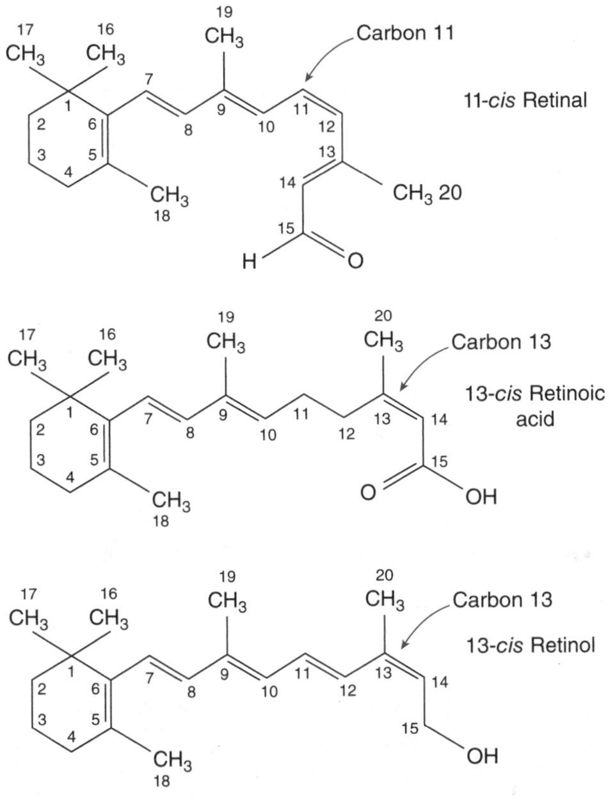

Dietary Sources of Vitamin A and Carotenoids

All-*trans* retinol is generally found in foods esterified to fatty acids. Retinyl palmitate is among the most abundant forms. Retinyl esters are found only in certain animal products, such as liver, fish liver oils, egg yolks, milk, and butter. Vitamin A-fortified milk and milk products are among the major contributors of vitamin A in certain countries. Vitamin A in the previtamin A carotenoid form is found in plant sources, mainly in orange and dark green vegetables (such as squash, carrots, spinach, broccoli, papaya, sweet potatoes, and pumpkin) and in some fruits (such as cantaloupe and apricots). **TABLE 10.2** lists food sources of vitamin A.

Digestion and Absorption of Vitamin A and Carotenoids

Retinyl esters and carotenoids complexed with proteins must be liberated prior to absorption. This is accomplished mainly by pepsin and proteases. Pepsin functions in this manner in the stomach, and proteases do so in the small intestine (**FIGURE 10.4**). Removal of the fatty acids of retinyl esters is accomplished by pancreatic lipase and cholesterol esterase as well as other intestinal esterases rather than having a specific esterase dedicated to this task. Free carotenoids and retinols integrate into micelles and most likely traverse the enterocyte plasma membrane by passive diffusion. As much as 70 to 90% of the retinol is absorbed. In contrast, the efficiency of carotenoid absorption varies tremendously and probably decreases as the concentration of the carotenoid increases in the intestinal lumen. For example, the absorption of β-carotene may be 20 to 50%, whereas the absorption of other carotenoids may be as low as 3 to 10%. The intake of carotenoids in America is typically around 1 to 3 milligrams per day; in other countries, where the inhabitants eat

FIGURE 10.2 Other Isomers of Vitamin A. Vitamin A may exist in the *cis* configuration. The *cis* configuration occurs around carbon 11 for retinal and carbon 13 for retinoic acid and retinol.

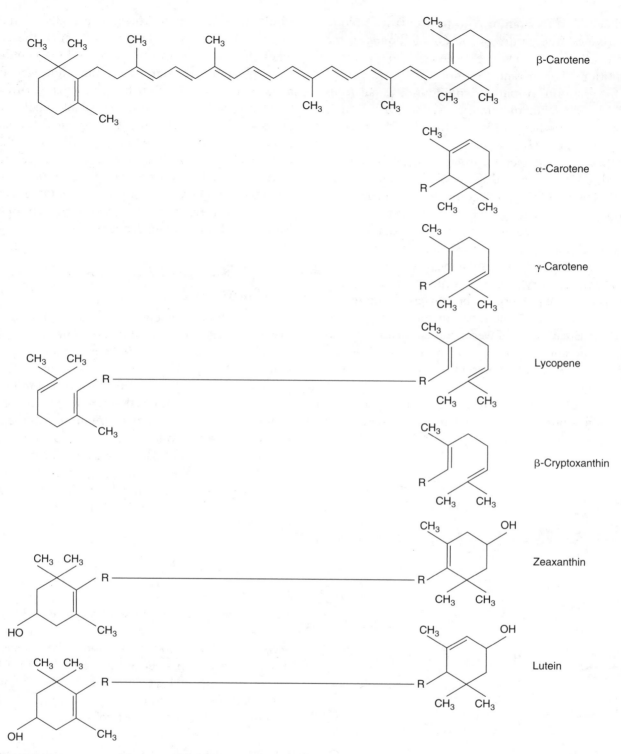

FIGURE 10.3 Structures of Carotenoids Having Vitamin A Activity. R, hydrocarbon plus ring structure; R—R, hydrocarbon only. The activity of each carotenoid varies by structure.

more fruits and vegetables, this amount is increased. Dietary fat is important for the digestion and absorption of both pre- and pro-vitamin A forms; however, the presence of bile salts may be even more critical for carotenoids.

Within an enterocyte, some of the β-carotene (all-*trans*) and other carotenoids can be converted to

retinol by cleavage at the central double bond by β-carotene 15,15′-monooxygenase (NOTE: some journals refer to this enzyme as dioxygenase but it is the same enzyme). In the case of β-carotene, enzymatic cleavage yields two molecules of retinal. The conversion of carotenoids to vitamin A depends on the activity of this enzyme, which itself is dependent on the

TABLE 10.2 Vitamin A Content of Select Foods	
Food	**Vitamin A (μg)**
Vegetables	
Pumpkin, canned (½ cup)	953
Sweet potato, canned (½ cup)	555
Carrots, raw (½ cup)	538
Spinach, cooked (½ cup)	472
Broccoli, cooked (½ cup)	114
Winter squash (½ cup)	269
Green peppers (½ cup)	14
Fruits	
Cantaloupe (½ cup)	150
Apricots, canned (½ cup)	80
Nectarine (½ cup)	12
Watermelon (½ cup)	17
Peaches, canned (½ cup)	22
Papaya (½ cup)	39
Meats	
Liver (3 oz)	6,311
Salmon (3 oz)	50
Tuna (2 oz)	10
Eggs	
Egg (1 whole)	91
Milk and milk products	
Milk, skim (1 cup)	149
Milk, 2% (1 cup)	139
Cheese, American (1 oz)	45
Cheese, Swiss (1 oz)	62
Fats	
Margarine, fortified (1 tbsp)	116
Butter (1 tbsp)	97

structure of the carotenoid as well as the efficiency of the enzymatic cleavage. The retinal that is formed can subsequently be converted to retinol by retinaldehyde reductase. This reaction requires NADH for its reducing equivalent. The central acting enzyme can also convert 9-*cis* β-carotene to a mixture of 9-*cis* and all-*trans* retinals. Some retinol is also converted to retinoic acid through oxidation.

Retinal formed in enterocytes can associate with a protein called cellular retinoid-binding protein (CRBP) type II and be subsequently reduced to retinol and then esterified to a long-chain fatty acid. The enzyme responsible for the esterification is lecithin retinol acyl transferase (LRAT). Phosphatidylcholine (lecithin) is the primary provider of fatty acids, and acyl CoA is the secondary provider.

Retinyl esters, retinol, and carotenoids (carotenes and xanthophylls) are packaged into chylomicrons, which are released from enterocytes and enter the lymphatic circulation. Because the long-chain fatty acids esterified to retinol are derived primarily from lecithin, the fatty acid composition of lymph retinyl esters is independent of the fatty acid composition of the associated meal. Retinyl palmitate usually constitutes approximately 50% of the retinyl esters, retinyl stearate constitutes about 20 to 30%, and retinyl oleate and retinyl linoleate make relatively smaller contributions. Vitamin A and carotenoids are taken up primarily by hepatocytes as components of chylomicron remnants. Retinoic acid is absorbed into the portal system, where it is transported to the liver bound to albumin in the blood.

Implications of β-Carotene Cleavage and Associated Enzymes

As noted above, in the enterocyte, β-carotene 15, 15′-monooxygenase converts β-carotene into two molecules of retinol (**FIGURE 10.5**). The gene that encodes this enzyme is abbreviated as BCMO1. However, carotenoids can also be cleaved in an eccentric manner to produce different products. The enzyme is β-carotene-9′, 10-oxygenase 2 and the gene that encodes this enzyme is referred to as BCO2. The products of this reaction are β-ionone and β-10′-apocarotenal. It can also metabolize lutein and other xanthophylls. The end products of those enzymes are not as relevant as the genes that encode those enzymes. There are different intracellular locations for these two enzymes. β-carotene 15, 15′-monooxygenase (BCMO1) is located in the cytoplasm and β-carotene-9′, 10-oxygenase 2 (BCO2) is located in the mitochondria.

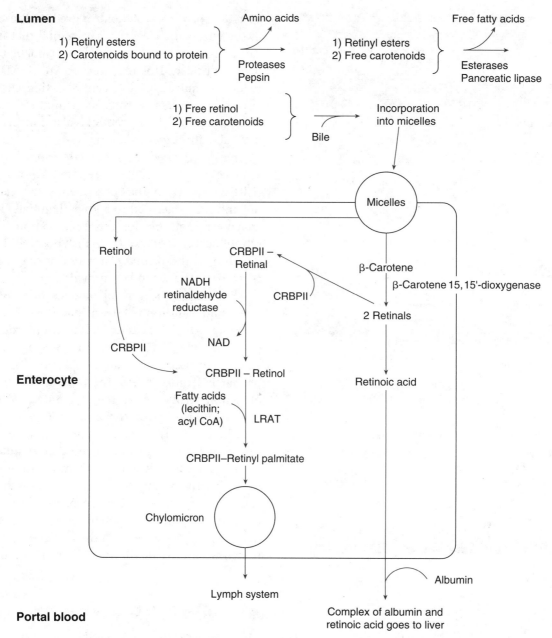

FIGURE 10.4 Digestion, Absorption, and Processing of Vitamin A and Carotenoid Compounds in the Enterocyte.
CRBP, cellular retinoid-binding protein; LRAT, lecithin retinol acyl transferase.

Studies have revealed that mutations in the BCO2 gene can lead to a variety of disease states. In animals, such as sheep, cows, and chickens, a mutation in this enzyme results in the accumulation of carotenoids in adipose tissue, resulting in the tissue turning a yellow color. In humans, single nucleotide polymorphisms (SNPs) of BCO2 resulted in a strong correlation of the proinflammatory IL-18 cytokine. The exact mechanism that causes the SNPs to increase IL-18 is not known. However, the cytokine is associated with atherosclerosis, cardiovascular disease, and type 2 diabetes. As that enzyme is located within the mitochondria, a defect leads to accumulation of β-carotene and reduces

respiration. In the eye, those with SNPs for BCO2 had a greater incidence of age-related macular degenerative disease. Other mutations have led to anemia, increased oxidative stress, and hepatic steatosis.

Plasma Transport of Vitamin A and Carotenoids

In the liver, vitamin A (as all-*trans* retinol) complexes with retinol-binding protein (RBP), forming **holo-RBP**, which circulates in the plasma. The synthesis of RBP by hepatocytes is regulated by vitamin A status. The normal serum retinol concentration is 45 to 65 micrograms

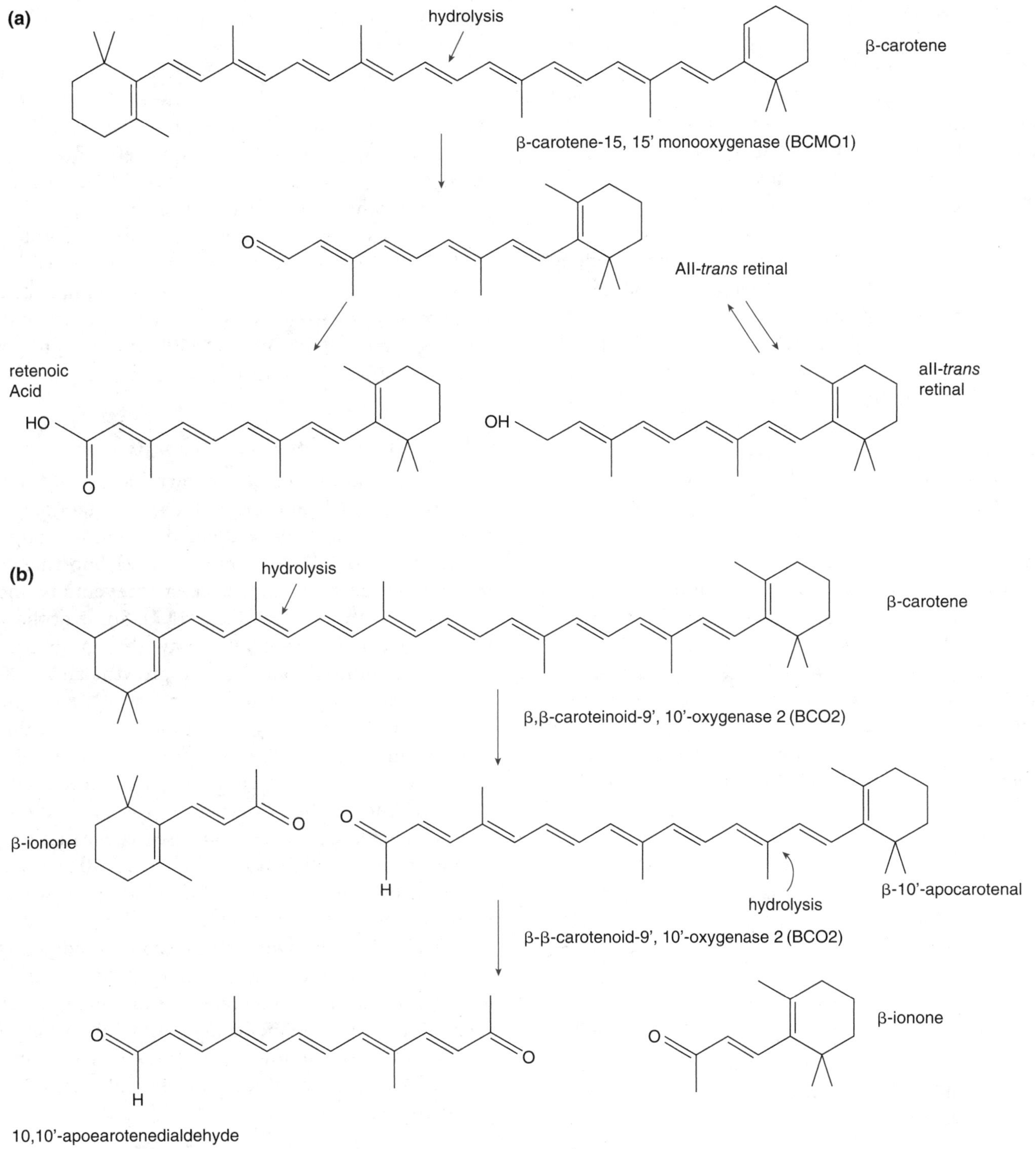

(a)

hydrolysis

β-carotene

β-carotene-15, 15' monooxygenase (BCMO1)

All-*trans* retinal

retenoic
Acid

all-*trans*
retinal

(b)

hydrolysis

β-carotene

β,β-caroteinoid-9', 10'-oxygenase 2 (BCO2)

β-ionone

β-10'-apocarotenal

hydrolysis

β-β-carotenoid-9', 10'-oxygenase 2 (BCO2)

β-ionone

10,10'-apoearotenedialdehyde

FIGURE 10.5 Hydrolysis of β-carotene. There are two pathways for the hydrolysis of β-carotene. (a) by either β-carotene-15, 15' monooxygenase (BCMO1) or (b) β, β- carotenoid-9', 10'-oxygenase 2 (BCO2). BCMO1 results in two molecules of retinol whereas BCO2 results in β-ionone and β-10'-apocarotenal. BCMO1 is located in the cytoplasm and BCO2 is located in mitochondria.

per 100 milliliters for adults. Other vitamin A forms—such as retinoic acid, retinyl ester, and retinoyl β-glucuronide—are also transported in the plasma, but in much lower amounts. The carotenoids circulate as components of lipoproteins, with the principal ones being α-carotene, β-carotene, lycopene, cryptoxanthin, lutein, and zeaxanthin. The hydrocarbon carotenes appear to associate more with LDL, whereas the xanthophylls are found in both LDL and HDL. Although the specific and relative concentrations of different carotenoids vary with dietary intake, β-carotene typically represents 15 to 30% of plasma carotenoids.

Storage of Vitamin A and Cell Binding Proteins

Vitamin A is stored very well, with more than 90% being found in the liver and distributed between two liver cell types. Liver parenchymal cells (hepatocytes) contain mostly retinyl esters derived from chylomicron remnants. In addition, those cells synthesize RBP. **Stellate cells**, which constitute 5 to 15% of total liver cells, are distinct from parenchymal cells in that they are relatively small, nonphagocytic, fat-storing cells. As much as 80% of a healthy adult's vitamin A store may be stored in lipid globules within these cells. Stellate cells are found associated with other tissue. Stellate cells can also store vitamin A in this extrahepatic tissue, but to a much smaller extent than in the liver.

Carotenoids can be irreversibly converted to retinal. Retinal itself can be reversibly reduced to retinol (**FIGURE 10.6**). The conversion of retinal to retinol occurs in many tissue. Retinol can be reversibly converted to retinyl phosphate (minor pathway), retinyl esters, and retinyl β-glucuronide, as well as irreversibly converted to retinoic acid. Retinoic acid can be irreversibly converted to retinoyl coenzyme A (minor pathway) and retinoyl β-glucuronide or can be irreversibly converted to inactive structures, such as 4-hydroxy-retinoic acid, 4-oxo-retinoic acid, or other metabolites. In addition, vitamin A structures can undergo isomerization reactions to convert *trans* to *cis* configurations and vice versa.

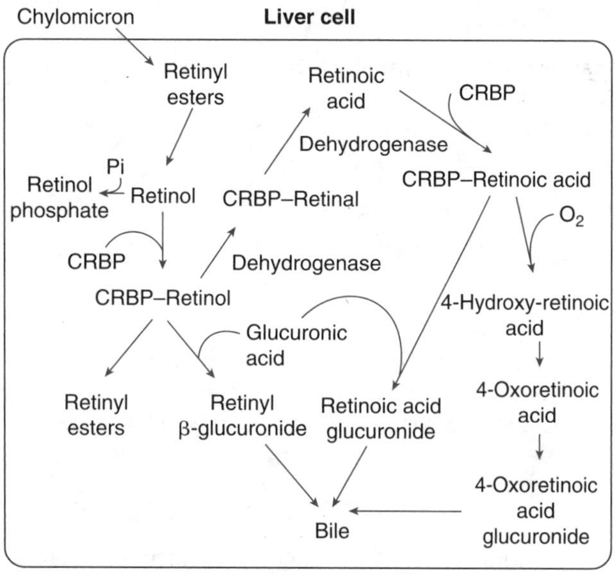

Within cells, retinol, retinoic acid, and retinal associate with CRBPs (see Figure 10.6). As mentioned earlier, retinal binds with CRBP type II in enterocytes, where it is converted to retinol. Retinol, in many other cell types, binds to CRBP, whereas in the interphotoreceptor space of the eye, it binds to interphotoreceptor (interstitial)-binding protein (IRBP). Retinal in the eye associates with cellular retinal-binding protein (CRALBP) and retinoic acid in several tissues binds to cellular retinoic acid-binding protein (CRABP). CRABP type II is present in many tissues of newborns.

Functions of Vitamin A and Carotenoids

There are a number of well-known biological functions of vitamin A and carotenoids. The functions of those compounds may be divided into four groups: 1) treatment of disease conditions; 2) boosting of immune function; 3) cancer chemoprevention; and 4) prevention of disease (**TABLE 10.3**). Some of those biological activities are related to the antioxidant properties, inhibition of tumor growth, and ability to induce apoptosis among the carotenoids and vitamin A. Epidemiological studies have revealed that a number of diseases are decreased with increased diet intake of vitamin A and carotenoids. Examples include breast, cervical, ovarian, and colorectal cancers; cardiovascular disease; eye diseases; osteoporosis; and diabetes. However, not all research is consistent with a prevention of those diseases with increased vitamin A and β-carotene. Some of the mechanisms by which those compounds exert their effects included, but are not limited to, their antioxidant capacity, increased immune response, regression of malignant lesions, and inhibition of mutagenesis. The following sections discuss some of the biological activities, or roles, of vitamin A and carotenoids.

Vision

The most recognizable function of vitamin A is its involvement with the eye and normal vision. After *all*-trans retinol (bound to RBP) binds with specific receptors on retinal pigment epithelial cells of the eye, retinol enters the cells and becomes bound to CRBP. It is isomerized to 11-*cis* retinol. 11-*cis* retinol undergoes oxidative conversion to 11-*cis* retinal. It is then transferred to the photoreceptor and associates with a specific lysine residue in the membrane protein, **opsin**, forming **rhodopsin**, as depicted in

FIGURE 10.6 Vitamin A Metabolism in Liver Parenchymal Cells. CRBP, cellular retinoid-binding protein. In liver metabolism of vitamin A, retinol, retinoic acid, and retinal are associated with CRBPs as they are being metabolized.

TABLE 10.3 Biological Activity or Roles of Vitamin A and Carotenoids

Treatment of disease

a. Malaria

b. Brain injury

c. Age-related macular degeneration

d. Depression

Immune function

a. Decrease proinflammatory cytokine expression

b. Suppression of NFκB

c. Induction of lymphocyte proliferation

d. Promotion of Nκ-Cell cytotoxicity

e. Inhibition of inducible nitric oxide synthase and cyclooxygenase-2

Chemoprevention

a. Neuroblastoma

b. Colon cancer

c. Prostate cancer

d. Breast cancer

e. Liver cancer

f. Lung cancer

Prevention

a. Alzheimer's disease

b. Leukemia

c. Infectious disease

d. Eye disease

e. Cardiovascular disease

FIGURE 10.7. When exposed to light, the 11-*cis* retinal component of rhodopsin isomerizes, causing a series of conformational changes in the protein. An intermediate form of the changing rhodopsin, called metarhodopsin, interacts with the G-protein transducin. Guanosine diphosphate (GDP) is subsequently replaced on transducin with guanosine triphosphate (GTP), which activates phosphodiesterase, which then hydrolyzes cyclic guanosine monophosphate (cGMP) to guanosine monophosphate (GMP).

Because cGMP is involved in maintaining rod sodium channels in an open position, the decrease in rod cell cGMP concentration results in a reduction in sodium flux through the channel, which allows for hyperpolarization of the membrane potential and the generation of an action potential. Neural impulses are then transmitted to the optic center of the brain. In the process of interacting with transducin, metarhodopsin is split to all-*trans* retinal and opsin, which can then form another complex with available 11-*cis* retinal.

Cell Differentiation

Perhaps, the second most recognized function of vitamin A is its involvement in favoring cell differentiation, its antiproliferative properties, and its ability to induce apoptosis. The effect that vitamin A has at the molecular level, including cell differentiation, involves nuclear receptors. There are two sets of nuclear retinoic acid receptors (RXR and RAR), both with subgroups designated α, β, and γ. RXR specifically binds 9-*cis* retinoic acid, whereas RAR binds either 9-*cis* retinoic acid or all-*trans* retinoic acid. After binding vitamin A, both RAR and RXR form dimer complexes (**FIGURE 10.8**). The term **dimerization** refers to an event in which two molecular complexes specifically interact and proceed to perform a purposeful function. RAR complexes with RXR, whereas RXR can also complex with either vitamin D receptors, triiodothyronine (T_3) receptors, or various PPARs. Typically, those dimeric interactions lead to activation of specific gene expression. However, if RAR dimerizes with *jun* (a nuclear transcription factor), the result can be inhibitory on gene expression. Typically, *jun* complexes with *fos*, another transcription factor, and the result is stimulatory with regard to cell proliferation. The activity of the RXR and RAR nuclear receptors favor pathways that promote cell differentiation in particular. Retinoic acid may also form retinoylated proteins that approximate the size of nuclear receptors. Scientists speculate that this may influence cell

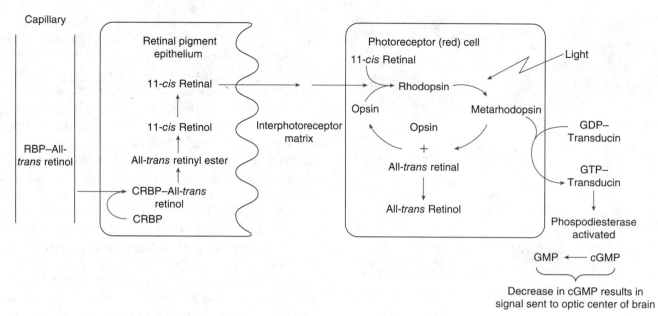

FIGURE 10.7 Role of Vitamin A, as *cis*-Retinal, in Vision. Reactions of all trans retinols is converted to 11-*cis* retinal in the retinal pigment epithelium and transferred to photoreceptors. Rhodopsin is formed, which initiates a series of reactions whereby GMP is eventually produced. This leads to neural impulses to the optic center of the brain.

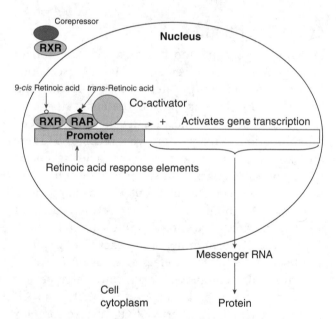

FIGURE 10.8 The Interaction of the Retinoic Acid Receptors and Vitamin A on Gene Expression.
Retinoic acid receptor action at the gene level favors cell differentiation and inhibition of cell proliferation. Additionally, RXR may interact with either vitamin D receptor or tri-iodothyronine receptor to alter expression of other genes.

proliferative activities as well. In addition, retinoic acid may be involved in the expression of *hox* genes, which appear to be involved in the sequential development of embryonic tissue.

Cancer

It is the role of vitamin A in promoting epithelial cell differentiation that has been the basis of interest in its possible link with cancer. A wide variety of studies have examined whether vitamin A affords a protective role in the development or treatment of cancer. Some of those studies have shown promising results with using retinoids to treat cancers, such as head and neck cancer and promyelocytic leukemia. For instance, some studies have demonstrated inverse relationships between dietary vitamin A intake and blood vitamin A levels with risk of cervical cancer. The association was maintained for dietary retinol, β-carotene, and other carotenoids and for blood levels of retinol and β-carotene.

However, retinoids may not be as effective in the prevention and treatment of lung cancer. It is common for lung cancer patients to use complementary medicine, including consumption of vitamin A-containing products. With respect to lung cancer, vitamin A has been used in the treatment of the disease despite the lack of evidence as to whether it is effective. Lung cancer is the most common type of cancer with a high mortality. Because lung tissue is composed of epithelial tissue, the role of vitamin A in protecting against cancer via promoting cell differentiation is not unreasonable. One study examined the impact of retinol and β-carotene on over 18,000 subjects who had a history of smoking or asbestos exposure (the β-Carotene and Retinol Efficacy Trial, or CARET).

The study had to be terminated early due to the increased lung cancer risk and mortality risk that resulted in subjects consuming β-carotene and retinol compared with controls. Another study in Finland (Alpha-Tocopherol, Beta-Carotene trial, or ATBC), conducted in more than 29,000 male smokers, reported an increased incidence of 16% of lung cancers in participants supplemented with β-carotene. A systematic review of the literature does not support the idea that any of the retinoids are effective in either the prevention or treatment of lung cancer. However, in the case of β-carotene, the impact on lung cancer risk is detrimental. It should be noted that those findings are specific for lung cancer. Overall, the evidence on the role of vitamin A and cancer suggests that specific types of cancers may benefit from vitamin A, but not lung cancer.

Glycoproteins

Vitamin A may also be involved in the synthesis of certain glycoproteins that are key components of the plasma membrane. Glycoproteins are important for cell communication, recognition, aggregation, and adhesion. Interestingly, here the impact of vitamin A may not be at the nuclear level. It is speculated that retinyl phosphate is converted to retinyl phosphomannose, which, in turn, can transfer mannose to an accepting glycoprotein. This is another possible mechanism for the involvement of vitamin A in cell proliferation and differentiation.

Reproduction

Another fundamental role of vitamin A is with reproductive processes. Part of this is due to the role of vitamin A in maintaining epithelial tissue. In vitamin A-deficient rodents, both male and female reproductive systems are affected. In males, many reproductive tissues are of epithelial origin. In male rodents that are deficient in vitamin A, keratinized epithelium may build up in the epididymis, seminal vesicles, and prostate. Additionally, the ability to produce sperm ceases. Apparently, this occurs early in the process of sperm development where the undifferentiated spermatogonia A in the seminiferous tubules are differentiated into spermatogonia A1. This transition from an undifferentiated cell into a differentiated cell requires vitamin A. Spermatogonia A1 eventually become sperm through a series of steps that involves both mitosis and meiosis. A fundamental issue here is the role of RAR, specifically RARγ. Males lacking this receptor are sterile, and the epithelial cells become thickened in the seminal vesicles and prostate. RARα is also thought to play a role in the development of sperm through the various cell stages of development.

In female rodents, the impact of vitamin A deficiency depends on when the deficiency occurs. If severe vitamin A deficiency is present before mating, implantation of the fertilized egg, or oocyte, does not occur. The vitamin A-deficient females ovulate, but the eggs are likely to degenerate in the fallopian tubes. With a mild vitamin A deficiency, fertilization and implantation occur, but the embryo may die at midgestation. In most cases, a mild vitamin A deficiency in a pregnant animal will likely result in fetal resorption.

Vitamin A is also needed for the proper development of the placenta for humans and other animals. A mild vitamin A deficiency may lead to necrosis of the placenta. If the fetus from a mildly vitamin A-deficient female survives to birth, a number of abnormalities may be present. It is important to note that those abnormalities may affect almost every organ system because vitamin A plays such a fundamental role in cell growth and maintenance of almost all cell types. Defects in lungs, eyes, skeleton, kidney, heart, and glands; increased diaphragmatic hernia; a less-developed nasal region; and underdeveloped ureter are examples of some of the problems that may result from mild vitamin A deficiency during pregnancy.

Antioxidant Capacity

The antioxidant function of vitamin A is relegated specifically to the carotenoids and not the preformed vitamin A. Carotenoids appear to function as antioxidants because they possess the ability to squelch free radical substances. For example, β-carotene and lycopene are able to interact with singlet oxygen radicals, and β-carotene can also squelch peroxyl radicals (O_{-2}^2). The ability of carotenoids to squelch free radicals is attributed to their double-bond system.

Other Functions

Vitamin A also plays important roles in bone development and maintenance and immune system function. The mechanisms for vitamin A involvement in those operations remain unclear at present. With respect to cardiovascular disease, the impact of vitamin A and carotenoid intake has had mixed results, both from epidemiological and animal studies, and in some instances, data have suggested increased cardiovascular risk. Lycopene appears to be one possible exception as it may inhibit cholesterol synthesis and enhance LDL degradation.

Nutrient Relationships for Vitamin A and Carotenoids

Vitamin A appears to have significant relationships with vitamins E and K, protein, and the minerals zinc and iron. Vitamin E appears to be necessary for the cleavage of β-carotene to retinal, and a greater consumption of vitamin E (more than 10 times the RDA) may reduce β-carotene absorption or conversion to retinol in enterocytes, or both. Excessive intake of vitamin A seems to interfere with vitamin K absorption.

Protein malnutrition can result in a reduced synthesis of RBP. A zinc deficiency can also reduce RBP production as well as reduce the mobilization of retinyl esters from storage in hepatocytes. Vitamin A also seems to be involved in iron metabolism, because a deficiency results in a microcytic **anemia** characteristic of iron deficiency. It is unclear whether vitamin A is influencing iron metabolism, iron storage, or key differentiation steps in red blood cell formation.

Excretion of Vitamin A and Carotenoids

Oxidized products of vitamin A are conjugated to glucuronide and excreted as a component of bile (see Figure 10.6). This accounts for approximately 70% of vitamin A losses. Carotenoid metabolites are also added to bile for excretion. The remaining 30% of vitamin A metabolites are voided in the urine.

Recommended Levels of Vitamin A Intake

The Dietary Reference Intake (DRI) for vitamin A is expressed as a Recommended Dietary Allowance (RDA), except for infants, where it is expressed as an Adequate Intake (AI). The RDA for vitamin A is 900 micrograms per day for adult men and 700 micrograms per day for adult women. The requirements for children are lower. Breastfeeding women have increased vitamin A requirements, with 1,200 to 1,300 micrograms of vitamin A per day being required, depending on the woman's age. Infants have an AI of 400 micrograms per day for up to 6 months of age, and 500 micrograms per day for 6 to 12 months of age. The units by which β-carotene and other precursors (such as other carotenoids) are quantified are **retinol activity equivalents (RAE)**. About 12 micrograms of β-carotene equals 1 microgram of retinol; thus, a person needs 12 times as much β-carotene to get the same benefit as 1 microgram of retinol.

Vitamin A Deficiency

Vitamin A deficiency is perhaps the leading cause of nonaccidental blindness in children worldwide. It has been estimated that as many as half a million school age children go blind each year due to vitamin A deficiency. Common signs of deficiency include night blindness and **xerophthalmia**. The eye's cornea consists of conjunctiva; in xerophthalmia, the conjunctiva becomes dry and the eye is no longer able to form tears. The conjunctiva becomes thickened and wrinkled and the cornea can become ulcerated, which can lead to blindness. As discussed with the reproductive system, a vitamin A deficiency in cells can lead to keratinization of cells, and that is what is occurring with the conjunctiva. **Bitot spots** on the eyes of young children are used as a diagnostic indicator. Bitot spots appear as foamy, whitish accumulations appearing in the conjunctiva of the eye.

Xerophthalmia is one of the leading causes of blindness in the world, and it is completely preventable. Those most at risk are children from birth to 5 years of age. The mortality rate and the incidence of xerophthalmia appear to be declining with increased food fortification, improved access to vitamin A-containing foods, and the availability of vitamin A supplements. Prior to those measures, a 25% mortality rate for children within this age range was common in impoverished areas of the world.

Vitamin A Toxicity

At doses approximating 10 times the RDA (slightly less than 10 grams per day), signs of hypervitaminosis may develop, including decreased appetite; dry, itchy, flaky skin; headache; hair loss; bone and muscle pain; ataxia; nausea and vomiting; dry mouth; and eye irritation and conjunctivitis. Resorption of a fetus, abortion, and the development of birth defects are the most serious side effects of hypervitaminosis. At higher intakes, yet not high enough to cause physical deformities, learning disabilities in progeny have been observed. Serum retinol levels may be augmented fourfold (> 200 micrograms per 100 milliliters) as more and more retinol is incorporated into lipoproteins. The delivery of retinol to peripheral tissue in lipoproteins, and not as an RBP complex, has been suggested to be a factor in the development of toxicity.

One form of vitamin A—11-*cis* retinoic acid (isotretinoin, or Accutane)—is used to treat severe cystic acne. Accutane is typically taken orally at doses between 0.5 and 1.0 milligram per kilogram of body weight per day, with a maximum of 2 milligrams per kilogram of body weight per day. The dose is split and taken twice daily with food for 15 to 20 weeks, with 2-month intermissions between 20-week treatments. The side effects of Accutane are those of vitamin A toxicity described earlier; clinical signs include proteinuria, hematuria, hyperuricemia, hypertriglyceridemia, and hyperglycemia. Because of the high risk of physical abnormalities associated with vitamin A toxicity, women of childbearing years using Accutane should use proper contraception.

Carotenoid toxicity does not appear to be a significant concern. Carotenoid overload causes carotenosis of the skin, which is not a serious health concern but might be cosmetically undesirable. Carotenosis is a condition in which the skin turns an orange color, which may look unnatural to some people. However, large doses of carotene are sold as sun tanning pills due to this property. The complexion resulting from high doses may be a personal one in terms of cosmetic appearance.

⬢ BEFORE YOU GO ON . . .

1. What are the similarities and differences between preformed vitamin A and previtamin A? Give examples of each form.

2. Discuss how β-carotene becomes vitamin A and how it leaves the enterocyte for the blood circulation. Include the enzymes involved and the relevance of each.

3. Diagram how vitamin A metabolites help with night vision.

4. How does vitamin A play an important role in regulating gene expression with respect to cell differentiation?

5. Discuss the possible role that vitamin A may have in the prevention or treatment of cancer.

6. What impact does a vitamin A deficiency have upon the reproductive system?

▶ Vitamin D

Although long known for its fundamental role in calcium and phosphorus metabolism, vitamin D is now recognized to be involved in numerous aspects of human physiology. Vitamin D has been regarded as having questionable status as a vitamin for two reasons. First, vitamin D can be synthesized in the human body in adequate quantities provided that there is sufficient exposure to sunlight and proper associated organ (skin, liver, and kidney) function; second, it functions more like a hormone than a vitamin because its activity is dependent on first interacting with a receptor.

The chemical structures for vitamin D were determined in the 1930s. Vitamin D_2 (ergocalciferol) was produced via ultraviolet irradiation of ergosterol. Vitamin D_3 (cholecalciferol) was produced by irradiating 7-dehydrocholesterol. **FIGURE 10.9** shows the molecular structures of those vitamin D-related molecules. Whereas 7-dehydrocholesterol and ergosterol carry the four-ring structure that is characteristic of a steroid, vitamins D_2 and D_3 are actually secosteroids because one of their rings is broken. Both of those structures will be referred to in this chapter as vitamin D.

Sources of Vitamin D

In humans, as in most higher mammals, vitamin D_3 is created photochemically as ultraviolet light converts the precursor sterol 7-dehydrocholesterol to cholecalciferol. That reaction takes place as sebaceous oil glands secrete 7-dehydrocholesterol onto the skin's surface. Cholecalciferol can then be reabsorbed to varying depths within the skin. Double bonds present at the fifth and seventh carbons in the B ring structure are necessary for this conversion, which, in essence, opens the B ring. As long as humans receive adequate exposure to sunlight, dietary vitamin D may not be needed. However, because adequate exposure to sunlight is not possible in some geographic regions and seasons, and because reduced exposure to sunlight is recommended to decrease the risk of skin cancer, dietary vitamin D is still deemed essential.

Dietary vitamin D is derived mostly from foods of animal origin. Eggs, liver, fatty fish, and butter are the best natural sources. The fortification of milk has greatly improved its vitamin D content, augmenting it from between approximately 0.03 and 0.13 to 1.0 microgram per 100 grams. Therefore, fortified milk and dairy products made from fortified milk are among the better sources of vitamin D and certainly are the major contributors in the human diet. Margarine has also been fortified to contain approximately 11 micrograms of vitamin D per 100 grams. **TABLE 10.4** lists foods and their vitamin D content.

Absorption and Transport of Dietary Vitamin D

Vitamin D becomes incorporated into micelles in the small intestine and enters mucosal enterocytes by passive diffusion. Approximately half of vitamin D is absorbed along the length of the small intestine, with the majority absorbed in the more distal aspects. Once within enterocytes, vitamin D is incorporated

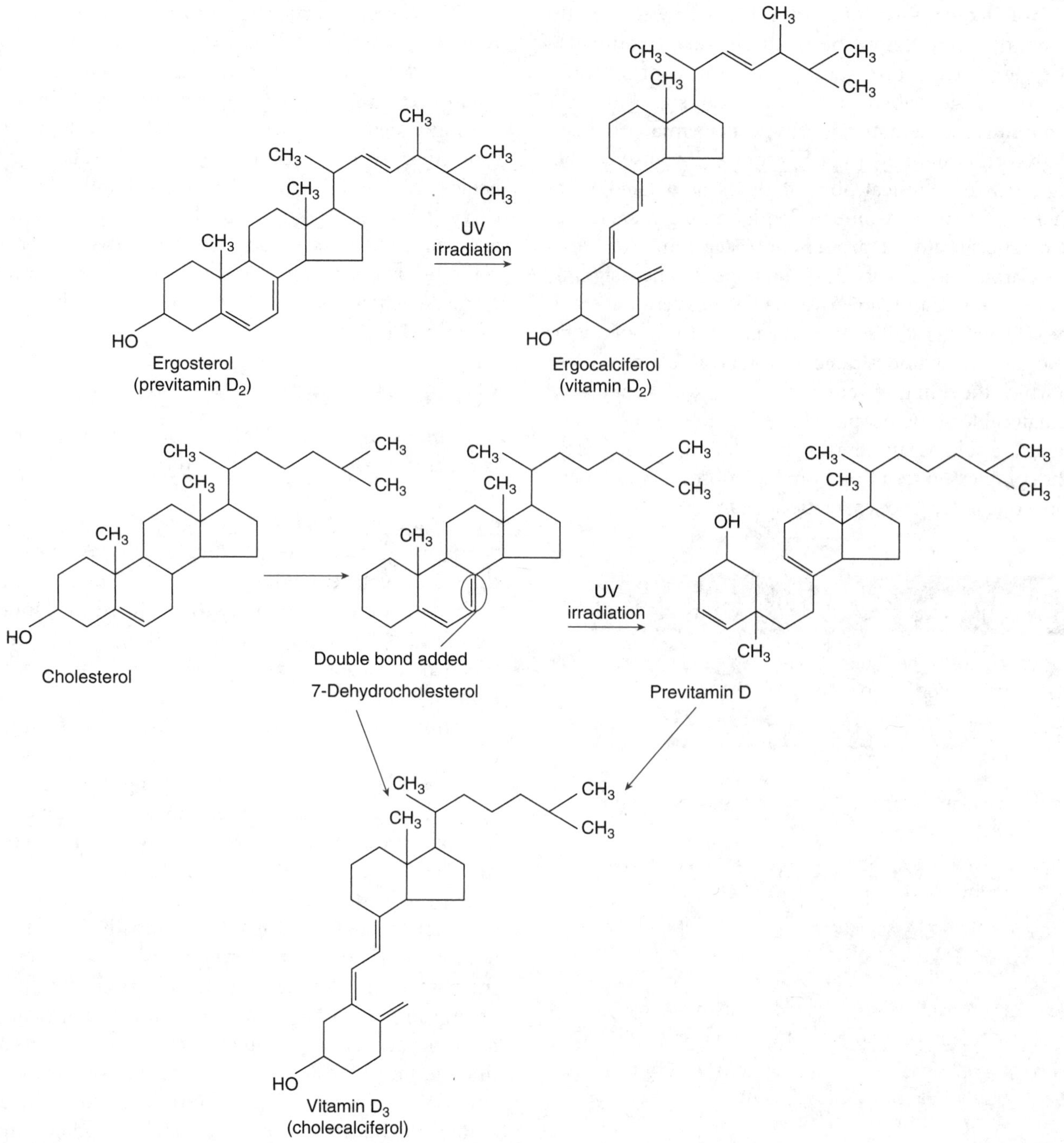

FIGURE 10.9 Production of Ergocalciferol and Cholecalciferol. Ergosterol and 7-dehydrocholesterol have a four-ring structure, but ergocalciferol (vitamin D₂) and cholcalciferol (vitamin D₃) have a three-ring structure with one ring broken.

into chylomicrons that reach the systemic circulation via the lymphatic circulation. Some of the vitamin D is actually transferred from plasma chylomicrons to circulating vitamin D-binding protein (DBP). Vitamin D carried aboard chylomicrons will be taken into hepatocytes as chylomicron remnants are removed. Meanwhile, the vitamin D transported by DBP can be delivered to extrahepatic tissue, such as skeletal muscle and adipocytes. DBP also picks up cholecalciferol

created in the skin. About 40% of circulating vitamin D is transported by chylomicrons; the remaining 60% is transported by DBP.

Metabolism of Vitamin D

Vitamin D is, in effect, a prohormone. First, its activity requires an interaction with a vitamin D receptor (VDR). Furthermore, the efficiency of vitamin D

TABLE 10.4 Vitamin D Content of Select Foods

Food	Vitamin D (μg)
Milk	
Milk, all (1 cup)	2.5
Fish and seafood	
Salmon (3 oz)	9.6
Tuna (3 oz)	5.7
Shrimp (3 oz)	0.1
Meats	
Beef liver (3 oz)	1.0
Eggs	
Egg (1 whole)	1.0

binding is tremendously increased after two hydroxylations to its molecular form (**FIGURE 10.10**). Upon reaching the liver, either by chylomicron remnant removal or by transport by DBP, vitamin D is hydroxylated at carbon 25 by 25-hydroxylase. The status of existing active vitamin D is fundamental for the efficiency of this enzyme: when vitamin D status is low, efficiency increases. Vitamin D is converted to 25-hydroxycholecalciferol, or, more simply, 25-(OH)D$_3$.

The enzyme 1α-hydroxylase (1α-OHase) catalyzes the conversion of 25-(OH)D$_3$ to 1,25-(OH)$_2$D$_3$, the most potent metabolite of vitamin D. This enzyme is found in renal cells lining the proximal tubule. The activity of the enzyme is enhanced by parathyroid hormone (PTH) and insulin-like growth factor-I (IGF-I) and inhibited by calcium and phosphorus. 1α-OHase is part of the enzyme systems associated with cytochrome P450. What controls PTH secretion by the parathyroid glands? As demonstrated in **FIGURE 10.11**, low blood calcium levels will trigger PTH release from the parathyroid glands. PTH will stimulate the release of calcium from bone. Furthermore, PTH will have two effects on the kidneys: (1) it will stimulate 1α-hydroxylase to produce 1,25(OH)$_2$D$_3$, and (2) it will stimulate the reabsorption of calcium by the kidney tubules. The 1,25(OH)$_2$D$_3$ will be released to the blood and target the small intestinal cells to stimulate the production of calbindin, which is a calcium-uptake protein. Collectively, all of those reactions will raise blood calcium levels to a normal physiologic range. The molecular perspectives of those reactions are described below.

Vitamin D Receptor and non-Genomic Functions

Vitamin D exerts most of its effects via binding to a Vitamin D Receptor (VDR) that interacts with DNA. The vitamin D receptor is a member of the superfamily of nuclear receptors that regulate gene expression. The gene coding for VDR was first cloned in the 1980s. The gene for VDR is located on chromosome 12 and has characteristics similar to other nuclear receptor genes, both in the structure of its heteronuclear RNA and posttranscriptional processing. VDR is expressed in bone, intestines, and kidneys as well as in the stomach, heart, brain, and other tissue.

VDR exerts its influence once it is associated with a specific ligand, namely 1,25-(OH)$_2$D$_3$. The VDR/1,25-(OH)$_2$D$_3$ complex controls specific gene expression by first associating with vitamin A/retinoid X receptor (RXR) to form a dimer and then interacting with specific vitamin D-responsive elements (VDREs) in target genes (**FIGURE 10.12**). VDREs are short sequences of DNA and are found in DNA regions associated with 1,25-(OH)$_2$D$_3$-activated genes, such as osteocalcin, osteopontin (expressed in osteoblasts), β_3 integrin (found in osteoclasts and macrophages), 24-OHase, and calbindin D (kidney).

Active vitamin D, via VDR association, affects calcium and phosphate homeostasis. As already indicated, hypocalcemia results in the secretion of PTH, which increases 1α-OHase activity in the kidneys. In turn, this increases the quantity of 1,25-(OH)$_2$D$_3$ (see Figure 10.10). Vitamin D stimulates calcium and phosphate absorption from the gut, bone calcium and phosphate resorption, and renal calcium and phosphate reabsorption. The net effect of those activities is to increase circulatory levels of calcium. In the intestines, VDR/1,25-(OH)$_2$D$_3$ induces the expression of key proteins involved in calcium and phosphorus absorption. Calbindin and intracellular membrane calcium-binding protein (IMCBP), both calcium-binding proteins in the intestinal mucosa, are synthesized in response to VDR/1,25-(OH)$_2$D$_3$. VDR/1,25-(OH)$_2$D$_3$ is believed to also increase the activity of brush border alkaline phosphatase, which increases the availability of phosphorus for absorption by cleaving phosphate ester bonds with other molecules. VDR can increase the transient receptor potential cation channel, subfamily V, member 6 (TRPV6) and calcium-binding protein D$_{9K}$ (calbindin D$_{9K}$).

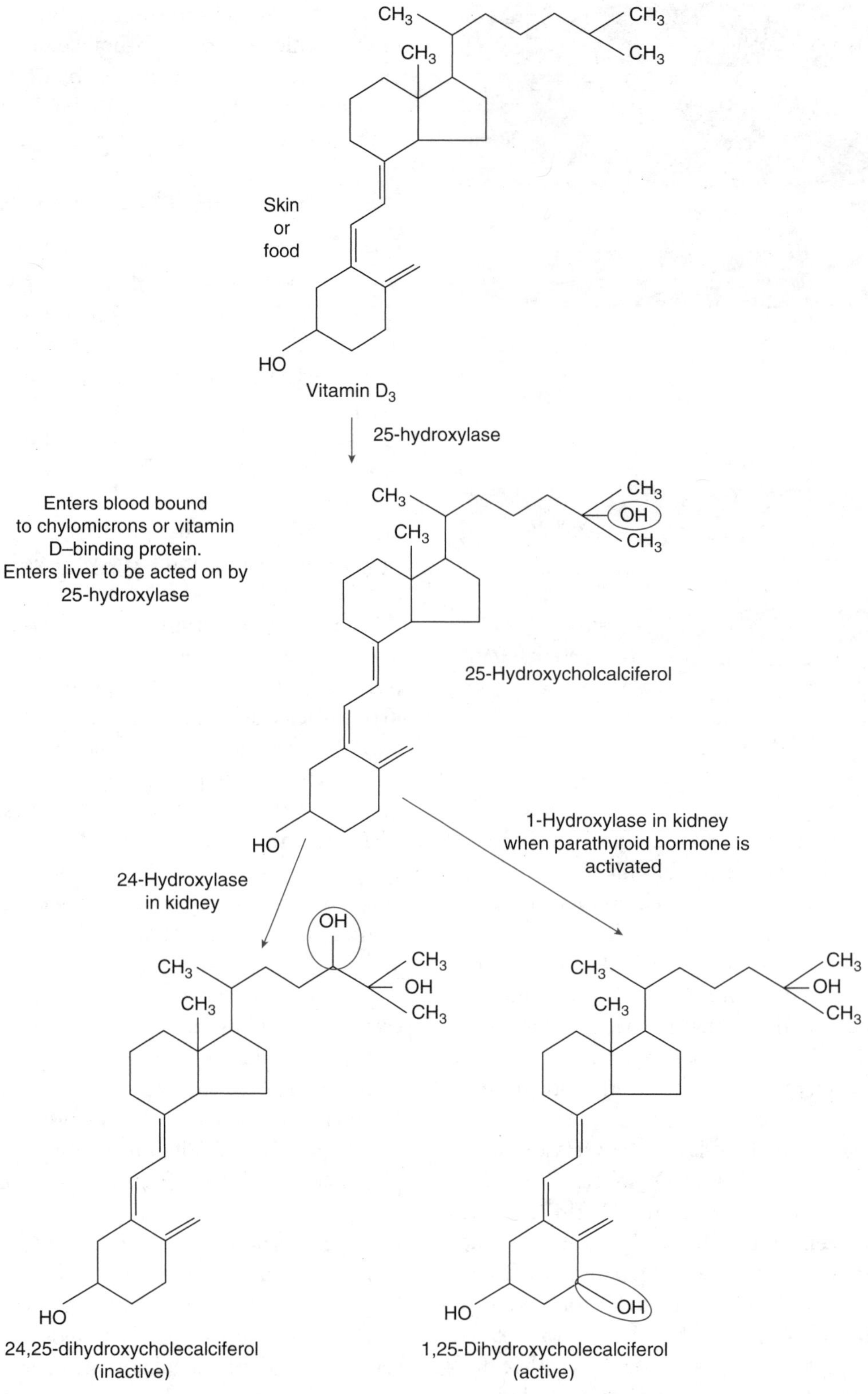

FIGURE 10.10 Hydroxylation Reactions of Vitamin D of Biological Significance. Vitamin D_3 is a prohormone. It is not until hydroxylation at C-25 in the liver and C-1 in the renal cells lining the proximal tubule that the active form of vitamin D, 1,25-dihydroxycholcalciferol is produced.

Deletion of VDR in mice leads to a decrease in intestinal calcium absorption efficiency (> 70%) and reduced expression of the molecular markers of intestinal calcium absorption, such as calbindin D_{9K} (down 55%) and TRPV6 (down 90%). In addition, VDR/1,25-$(OH)_2D_3$ may modulate the quantity of brush border phosphate carriers. In bone tissue, VDR/1,25-$(OH)_2D_3$ is probably involved in the differentiation of stem cells into osteoclasts, which mediate bone resorption and the mobilization of calcium and phosphate into the blood.

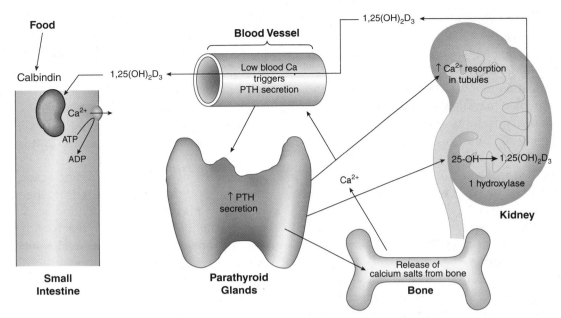

FIGURE 10.11 Role of Parathyroid Hormone in the Homeostatic Control of Calcium Through Interaction with Vitamin D Metabolism. Low blood calcium increases secretion of PTH. PTH stimulates (1) calcium release from bone; (2) 1 α-hydroxylase to produce 1,25 $(OH)_2D_3$ and (3) the reabsorption of calcium by the kidney tubules. 1,25 $(OH)_2$ will enhance calcium absorption by stimulating small intestinal cells to produce the calcium uptake protein, calbindin. These series of reactions maintain calcium levels within a normal range.

VDR/1,25-$(OH)_2D_3$ may regulate the differentiation of hair follicles. VDR knockout mice develop alopecia. The alopecia persists even after mice are provided a rescue diet consisting of relatively high amounts of lactose, calcium, and phosphate, which corrects PTH levels and normalizes bone mineralization. VDR/1,25-$(OH)_2D_3$ is also likely to be involved in the differentiation of skin epidermal cells.

The VDR/1,25-$(OH)_2D_3$ complex plays a pivotal role in feedback regulation of the level of 1,25-$(OH)_2D_3$ produced by renal tubular cells. Thus, VDR/1,25-$(OH)_2D_3$ is involved in the turnover of one of its own constituents. The 24-OHase enzyme is markedly enhanced by 1,25-$(OH)_2D_3$ in a VDR-dependent manner. This occurs in both renal tissue and all vitamin D target tissue. Both 1,25-$(OH)_2D_3$ and 25-$(OH)D_3$ serve as substrates for 24-OHase. In the past, it was believed that 24-hydroxylated D metabolites were not functional; however, it may be that they are involved in some aspect of bone metabolism or bone formation via an uncharacterized receptor.

A major aspect of Vitamin D and VDR is that it has extensive health implications. There are a multitude of tissues that contain VDR: bone, pancreatic β cells, parathyroid glands, brain, skin, prostate and testes, heart and skeletal muscle tissues, breast, liver, lung, intestine, kidneys, adipose tissue and immune response cells, such as macrophages, dendritic cells, and activated B and T cells.

The vitamin D receptor and vitamin D have been suggested as perhaps having an important role in

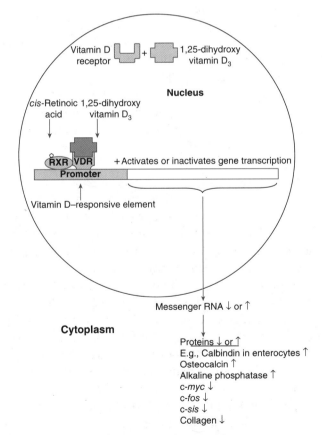

FIGURE 10.12 How Vitamin D Exerts Its Actions on Genes. The vitamin D receptor (VDR) acts in partnership with the retinoic acid receptors (RXR) and binds to nucleotide base pairs called the vitamin D–responsive elements (VDRE) to control gene expression. *Cis*-retinoic acid and 1,25-dihydroxycholecalciferol are ligands that must be present to control gene expression.

cancer prevention. Part of this comes from the fact that the complexed nuclear receptor and vitamin D binds to gene promoters that favor cell differentiation and inhibit proliferation. Moreover, the complex may induce termination of a variety of normal and tumor cells. The complex may alter the transcription of cell growth regulatory factors, such as c-*myc*, c-*fos*, and c-*cis* (see Figure 10.12). Also, one cannot rule out that in some cases, the vitamin D receptor may be defective. It is known that vitamin D itself may be useful in treatment of some types of proliferative disorders. For instance, topical or oral 1,25-dihydroxycholecalciferol is useful for hyperproliferative skin disorders (e.g., psoriasis). The drug calcipotriene (Dovonex) is marketed for this purpose.

As suggested earlier, a defect in the vitamin D receptor may lead to increased cancer risk. Polymorphism in the vitamin D receptor gene increases the risk of prostate cancer 2 to 2.5 times. Breast cancer was not linked to vitamin D receptor polymorphism in one study, but another study showed a 20 to 89% reduction of risk for breast cancer in women with a particular type of vitamin D receptor polymorphism. Other studies suggest that certain polymorphisms in the vitamin D genotype increase bladder cancer. Another study suggests that dietary vitamin D may be effective in treating colon cancer at levels of 4,000 IU per day. In summary, with respect to cancer, vitamin D has been implicated in the following cancer types: colon, prostate, breast, pancreatic, leukemia, ovarian, gastric, esophageal, and gall bladder.

Apparently, the role of Vitamin D in health and disease is not limited to its impact on bone and cancer. There is evidence that it may play an important role in autoimmune diseases, such as multiple sclerosis, Type 1 diabetes, inflammatory bowel disease (ulcerative colitis and Crohn's disease), and rheumatoid arthritis. It has been demonstrated to be effective in preventing psoriasis. There has been much attention paid as to whether it may play a protective role against cardiovascular disease, including vascular integrity, cardiac hypertrophy, and hypertension. Studies on various cell types composing the cardiovascular system have demonstrated decreased potential for atherosclerosis, thrombogenicity, hypertension, cardiac hypertrophy, and heart failure. Epidemiology studies suggest that low levels of vitamin D can produce increased incidence of coronary heart disease and mortality. Some studies have not revealed an association. Currently, there is no conclusive or consistent evidence to suggest that vitamin D supplementation to control cardiovascular disease exists. An issue in

some studies is that clinical trials have compared those with low vitamin D status and placed subjects on supplements at the RDA level of vitamin D, which is a level known to prevent rickets. With other diseases, a conventional wisdom is that larger doses are possibly needed to conclusively suggest a benefit.

Vitamin D has nongenomic functions where it exerts its effects within a cell's cytoplasm. In the cytoplasm, Vitamin D has a key role in calcium flux, particularly involving a signaling cascade that eventually releases stored calcium into the cytoplasm. Vitamin D may interact with endoplasmic reticulum stress protein 57. This protein reacts with G-protein, which produces a cascade of biochemical reactions leading to the release of calcium within the cell. That process requires VDR, but does not require it to bind to DNA.

Recommended Levels of Vitamin D Intake

Infants up to 1 year of age have an RDA of 10 micrograms per day (400 IU/day). The RDA for those 1 to 70 years of age is 15 micrograms per day (600 IU/day); those older than 70 years have an RDA of 20 micrograms per day (800 IU/day). The latter were increased in older adults because of their reduced sun exposure, reduced skin biosynthesis efficiency, and lower renal hydroxylase activity. The upper tolerable level for vitamin D is 50 micrograms per day. The RDAs for vitamin D are controversial. The vitamin D RDAs in essence have been set with implications on bone health. It is now known that vitamin D has many roles beyond bone and the requirements for these other roles may result in a need for greater intake.

On a practical level, a person can avoid a vitamin D deficiency simply by getting approximately 15 minutes of exposure to sunlight each day. However, the latitude where an individual lives is important for meeting this requirement. Those individuals living in the southern portion of the United States have more exposure to sunlight in the winter months than those living in the northern portion of the country. In Boston, Massachusetts, little vitamin D is produced after 1 hour of being outside from November through February. In Los Angeles, California, in contrast, a reasonable conversion can occur in January after 1 hour of being outside. During the winter months, the ultraviolet radiation hits the ozone layer above Boston at an oblique angle and is deflected. In the spring, summer, and fall, the ultraviolet radiation can penetrate the ozone layer.

Vitamin D Deficiency

In children, vitamin D deficiency results in a syndrome called **rickets,** in which the associated characteristics result from a failure of growing bone to mineralize. As the epiphyseal cartilage of bone continues to grow, it is not properly replaced with matrix and hydroxyapatite. This results in a bowing of longer weight-bearing bones, such as the femur, tibia, and fibula, deformations of the knee region, and curvature of the spine.

Vitamin D deficiency during adulthood reduces calcium and phosphate absorption. As bone turnover occurs, the matrix is preserved; however, bone progressively loses its mineralization. Loss of mineral resulting in decreased bone density is referred to as **osteomalacia.** Vitamin D deficiency, despite poor dietary intake, can be avoided by adequate exposure to sunlight.

People with lighter skin color require only about 10 to 15 minutes of summer sun exposure to make adequate amounts of vitamin D; the necessary

SPECIAL FEATURE 10.1

Are Americans Suffering from Vitamin D Deficiency?

Much debate has arisen among nutritionists and pediatricians over whether the recommended intake of vitamin D for children, adolescents, and adults should be increased above the current levels set by the Food and Nutrition Board. Why all the controversy? Although some believe that measuring serum levels of 1,25-dihydoxycholecalciferol is the method of choice, because 1,25-dihydoxycholecalciferol is the bioactive and physiologically active form, those levels are tightly regulated by endocrine mechanisms. It turns out that the best method of assessing vitamin D status in humans is the level of 25-hydroxycholecalciferol. Using this as a guide, the cutoff for defining vitamin D deficiency has varied among various sources, but a typical cutoff value is 12 nanograms per milliliter. Below this level in infants, there is a risk for vitamin D deficiency that can lead to rickets. For older individuals, 12 to 20 nanograms per milliliter is also considered inadequate for bone and overall health. A concentration of 20 nanograms per milliliter or greater is the target level set for overall health. It should be pointed out that some sources may have slight variations to those levels.

The cutoff for adequate vitamin D status in adults has been considered to be 32 nanograms per milliliter. Using this level of adequacy and applying it to children and adolescents can result in a greater number of cases of vitamin D deficiency in this age group. Although vitamin D can be made via cutaneous routes and exposure to sunlight, it is widely accepted that dietary sources of this nutrient are needed to ensure adequacy. Some variation in the ability to produce vitamin D arises from where populations live: those living in northern latitudes have less exposure to sunlight during winter months. Those with greater skin pigmentation are less efficient in the production of vitamin D. Whereas light-skinned people may only require 5 to 10 minutes of sunlight exposure in the spring, summer, and fall, darker-skinned people need 5 to 10 times more sunlight exposure to obtain equivalent conversions to vitamin D endogenously. The ability to synthesize vitamin D also decreases as a person ages.

A Boston, Massachusetts, study reported that 65% of neonates were vitamin D deficient (below 12 nanograms per milliliter) when sampled during the winter months. A larger study in Pittsburgh, Pennsylvania, reported that 10% of white neonates and 46% of black neonates were vitamin D deficient (defined as less than 15 nanograms per milliliter), thereby illustrating racial differences. In children, the same results may be observed. A study conducted in Philadelphia, Pennsylvania, examined children aged 6 to 21 years; the researchers found that 68% of white children and 94% of black children were vitamin D deficient. Another study among girls aged 12 to 18 years in Cleveland, Ohio, revealed that black adolescents were many more times likely to be vitamin D deficient than white adolescents.

What should be done about this prevalence of vitamin D deficiency? One solution is that people can be educated about the benefits of getting more sunlight exposure. However, many medical groups warn against too much sun exposure because of the risk of ultraviolet radiation, which can lead to skin cancer. Another avenue is to increase intake of vitamin D through the diet.

The American Academy of Pediatrics (AAP) recommends that "breastfed and partially breastfed infants should be supplemented with 400 IU/day of vitamin D in the first few days of life." The group went further and essentially recommended 400 IU per day for all nonbreastfed infants and older children consuming less than 1 liter of milk per day. Adolescents who do not obtain 400 IU of vitamin D per day from milk should take vitamin D supplements. The AAP also addressed the issue of what constitutes sufficient vitamin D status. For children and infants, the recommended minimum level is 20 nanograms per milliliter of 25-hydroxycholcalciferol. Children may need even higher levels of vitamin D than 400 IU per day if they have malabsorption issues. The RDA is now set at 15 micrograms, or 600 IU, per day.

exposure time for people with darker skin color seems to increase relative to the degree of skin color. Also, the ability to make vitamin D appears to be stronger in youth and decreases relative to age.

● **BEFORE YOU GO ON . . .**

1. How is vitamin D transported in the blood?
2. How is vitamin D involved in the regulation of gene products?
3. List the key hydroxylation reactions of vitamin D_3 in terms of the carbons at which they occur, their location in the body, and their activity.
4. Why is the retinoic acid receptor, and, therefore, vitamin A, important in the function of vitamin D?
5. How does vitamin D_3 increase calcium absorption in the small intestine?
6. In addition to maintaining bone health, what other health benefits are possible with an adequate vitamin D status?
7. Discuss how vitamin D may affect cancer development or prevention?

▶ **Vitamin E**

Like many other vitamins, vitamin E is not a single molecule but a class of related molecules possessing similar activity. There are eight or so vitamin E molecules, which can be subdivided into two major classes: **tocopherols** (α, β, γ, and δ) and **tocotrienols** (α, β, γ, and δ). Structurally, the tocotrienols have unsaturated phytyl side chains, whereas tocopherols have saturated side chains. The α, β, γ, and δ forms of tocopherols and tocotrienols are based on the number and position of the methyl groups attached to the chromanol ring. **FIGURE 10.13** shows the structures of various isomers of vitamin E. All-rac α-tocopheryl acetate is used in the fortification of food. This is a synthetic form of vitamin E derived from petroleum products. It contains eight isomers in this mixture. The acetate group allows the vitamin greater stability in food compared with the naturally occurring α-tocopherol.

Food Sources of Vitamin E

The best sources of vitamin E include plant oils (e.g., cottonseed, corn, sunflower, safflower, soybean, and palm oils) and oil-derived products such as margarine,

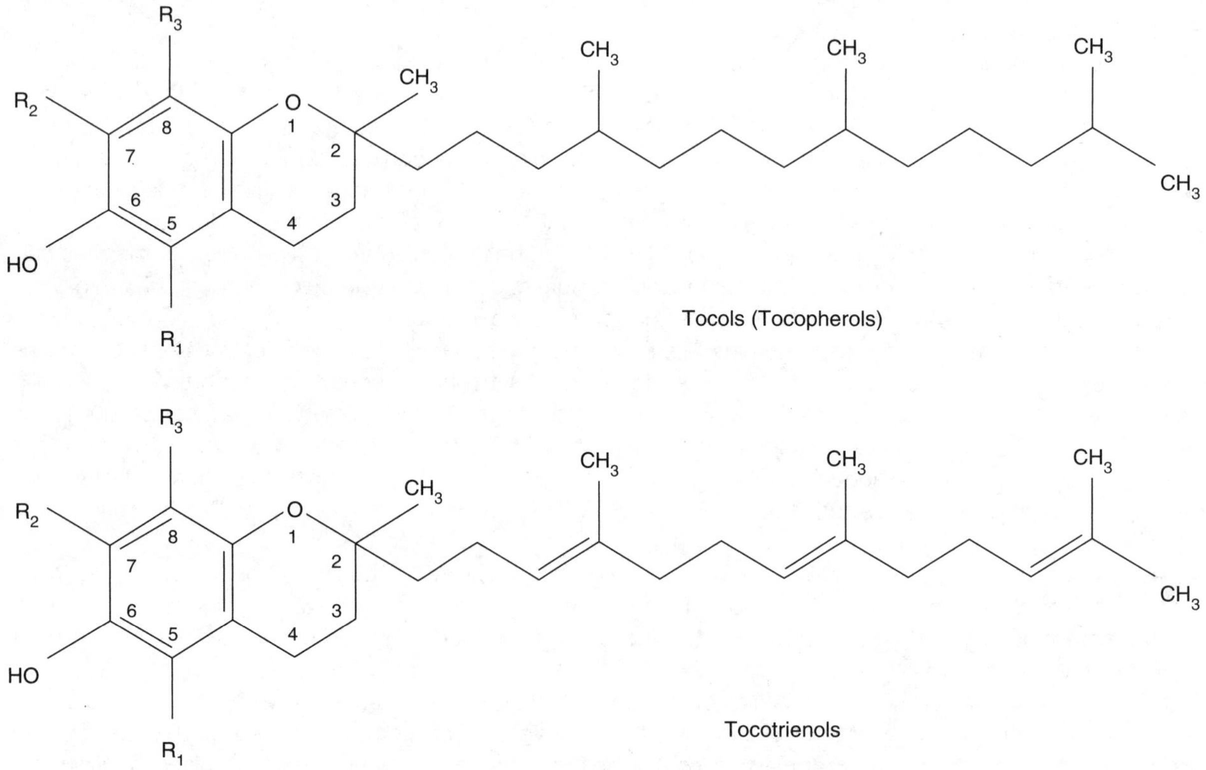

α-Tocopherol or tocotrienol: R_1, R_2, R_3 = CH$_3$
β-Tocopherol or tocotrienol: R_1, R_3 = CH$_3$; R_2 = H
γ-Tocopherol or tocotrienol: R_2, R_3 = CH$_3$; R_1 = H
δ-Tocopherol or tocotrienol: R_3 = CH$_3$; R_1, R_2 = H

FIGURE 10.13 Vitamin E Isomers. There are 8 vitamin E molecules that are divided into two classes: tocopherols and tocotrienols.

shortenings, and mayonnaise. Wheat germ (and its oil) and nuts are also rich sources. Some fruits and vegetables, such as peaches and asparagus, are fair sources, and meats and fish contain appreciable amounts (**TABLE 10.5**). The tocopherols are more widely distributed in nature than the tocotrienols and, therefore, are more nutritionally significant. α-Tocopherol is the most prevalent form as well as the most potent. For this reason, the RDA for vitamin E is given as milligrams of α-tocopherol. That value for adults is 15 milligrams per day.

Vitamin E Absorption and Transport

The absorption efficiency of vitamin E is approximately 20 to 50%. However, as the dose increases, the efficiency of absorption decreases. For example, at doses approximating 200 milligrams or higher, the efficiency of absorption falls to 10% and below. With respect to its lipid nature, vitamin E must first be solubilized into micelles within the lumen of the small intestine. Esterases produced by the pancreas and intestinal mucosa digest vitamin E esters. Free vitamin E then appears to penetrate enterocytes via passive diffusion and is incorporated into chylomicrons for export into the lymphatic circulation. Once chylomicrons reach the systemic circulation, their triglyceride is progressively translocated into peripheral tissue by lipoprotein lipase, and some vitamin E can enter the tissue as well. Some vitamin E can also translocate into circulating HDL. However, the majority of absorbed vitamin E remains in chylomicron remnants and is released in hepatocytes as the remnants are removed and catabolized.

In liver cells, vitamin E binds to a cytosolic protein called hepatic tocopherol transfer protein (HTTP), which preferentially interacts with α-tocopherol. HTTP releases vitamin E into VLDL under construction in the endoplasmic reticulum or Golgi apparatus. Intuitively, then, the predominant form of vitamin E in the plasma will be α-tocopherol. α-Tocopherol contained in VLDL can remain in VLDL during its lipolytic transformation to LDL and then circulate within LDL. Some vitamin E can also translocate into HDL. Typically, the plasma content of α-tocopherol is 5 to 20 micrograms per milliliter in adults. It is lower in children and infants, especially in preterm infants. There are cases in which genetic defects within HTTP can occur. This results in vitamin E deficiency as it cannot be secreted by the liver into the circulation. Within enterocytes and other cells, vitamin E is bound to a protein. ATP-binding cassette (ABC) A1 is involved in intracellular distribution and cell efflux of vitamin E.

TABLE 10.5 Vitamin E Content of Select Foods

Food	Vitamin E Content (mg α-Tocopherol)
Oils	
Oils (1 tbsp)	1.9
Margarine (1 tbsp)	1.6
Nuts and seeds	
Sunflower seeds, dry roasted (¼ cup)	8.4
Almonds (¼ cup)	6.2
Peanuts (¼ cup)	2.5
Cashews (1 tbsp)	0.15
Vegetables	
Sweet potato, baked without skin (½ cup)	1.5
Collard greens, boiled (½ cup)	0.8
Asparagus, boiled (½ cup)	1.4
Spinach, raw (½ cup)	0.24
Grains	
Wheat germ (1 cup)	18.0
Bread, whole wheat (1 slice)	0.09
Bread, white (1 slice)	0.08
Seafood	
Crab, cooked (3 oz)	1.6
Shrimp, boiled (3 oz)	1.2

Vitamin E Storage and Excretion

Vitamin E is found in tissue throughout the body, such as the adrenals, heart, lungs, and brain, but perhaps the most significant sites of storage are the liver, adipose tissue, skeletal muscle, and lipoproteins. The liver represents a more transient site of storage because turnover or rate of release is very rapid. Therefore, the hepatic vitamin E concentration does not increase significantly under normal conditions. This is largely attributable to the delivery of vitamin E to VLDL construction sites by HTTP. Adipose tissue, in contrast, accumulates vitamin E slowly, and the rate of turnover is also very slow. Vitamin E is found largely within the lipid droplet compartment of adipocytes or associated with membranes. Whereas the concentration of vitamin E remains somewhat constant in most other tissue, the vitamin E concentration in adipose tissue increases linearly with dietary intake. Because of its large contribution to human mass, skeletal muscle is considered a significant store of vitamin E as well. In cells, vitamin E is likely stored in cell, mitochondria, and microsomal membranes. Finally, lipoproteins are the principal transport vehicle for vitamin E in the blood. During a fasting state, most of the α-tocopherol in the body can be found in LDL in males and in HDL in females.

Vitamin E is excreted from the body by several mechanisms. The major route of α-tocopherol excretion is as a component of bile and subsequent incorporation into feces. Fecal vitamin E is also derived from enterocyte-secreted vitamin E and sloughed-off enterocytes. Some vitamin E may be excreted from the body as a component of skin secretions and dermal exfoliation. Two metabolites of α-tocopherol have been identified in the urine. α-Tocopheronic acid and α-tocopheronolactone can both be conjugated to glucuronic acid and excreted into the urine or they can enter the bile, which will be released into the small intestine and end up in the feces (**FIGURE 10.14**). Although those metabolites are typically present to a minimal degree, their concentration in the urine rises in proportion to increased vitamin E intake.

Function of Vitamin E

Without question, the predominant function of vitamin E is that of an antioxidant necessary for the maintenance of cellular membrane integrity. It is often referred to as a chain-breaking antioxidant. Vitamin E prevents the oxidation (peroxidation) of the unsaturated fatty acid component of membrane phospholipids. There are differences in the concentration of unsaturated fatty acids between the plasma membrane and membranes of the various organelles as well as between the same membranes in different tissue. For instance, the membranes of the mitochondria and endoplasmic reticulum contain a higher concentration of unsaturated fatty acids and are, therefore, at greater risk of free radical peroxidation. Tissue membranes with a relatively higher risk of lipid peroxidation include lungs, brain, and red blood cells due to their higher degree of unsaturation, metabolism, and oxygen presence.

Free radicals are either taken into the human body or created within cells. They are atoms or molecules with one or more unpaired electrons, which renders them unbalanced and highly reactive. Many free radicals are oxygen related, such as the superoxide radical (O_2^-), peroxyl radical (O_2^{2-}), hydroxyl radical (OH^-), and peroxide (H_2O_2). Within cells, free radicals can be generated by the reduction of oxygen, such as occurs in the endoplasmic reticulum via the cytochrome P450 system and in mitochondria via the electron transport chain. In the process of interacting with a free radical, tocopherol molecules are oxidized to form a tocopheroxyl radical, which can then be re-reduced to tocopherol by vitamin C, glutathione, and, perhaps, ubiquinone.

Some studies suggest that vitamin E may exert its effect at the gene level. Supplemental vitamin E given to old mice may influence gene expression of cell-cycle proteins. Also, vitamin E may regulate antioxidant gene expression. Hyperthyroidism induced in rats by thyroxine administration reduced copper, zinc superoxide dismutase, and catalase mRNA levels. However, vitamin E supplementation can normalize and thus prevent the decrease in those transcripts.

Regarding the role that vitamin E may play in disease prevention, there is evidence to suggest that vitamin E could be effective in combating heart disease and the development of atherosclerotic plaque in blood vessels. Individuals in one study were reported to have a 35% reduction in the likelihood of heart disease mortality if they consumed 7 milligrams of α-tocopherol daily. Other studies suggest that doses of approximately 70 milligrams of α-tocopherol per day result in reduced risk of cardiovascular disease in both genders. Another disease that may demonstrate a link with vitamin E is dementia. Supplementing with 900 milligrams of α-tocopherol daily slowed Alzheimer disease progression over a 2-year period in one study; however, not all studies have been as promising. Other studies tend to suggest that other types of dementia may be linked to vitamin E.

Recommended Levels of Vitamin E Intake

Previous editions of recommendations used α-tocopherol equivalents; those units have now been abandoned. The different isomers differ in their activity.

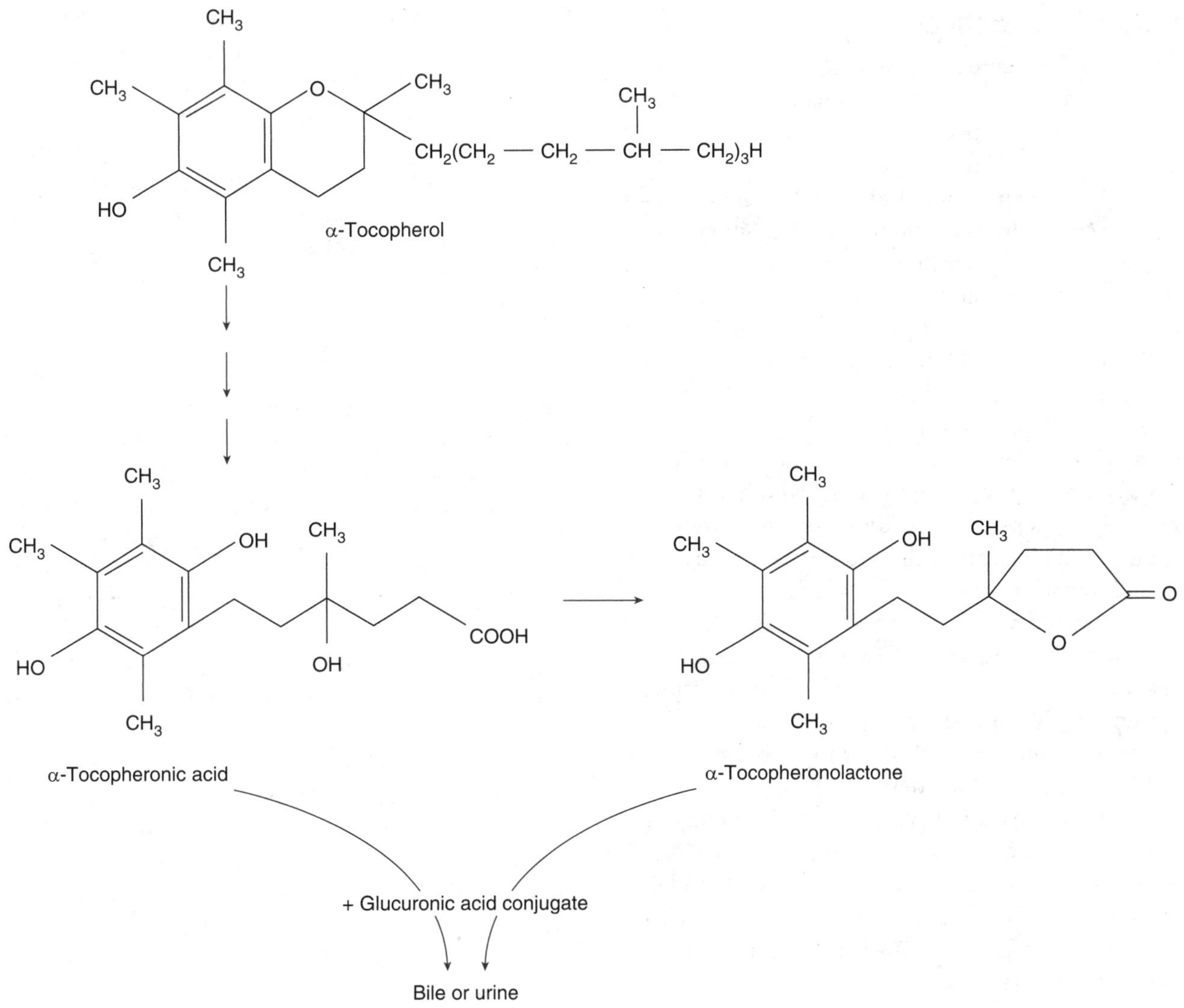

FIGURE 10.14 Excretory Pathway for Tocopherol. The breakdown products, α-tocopheronic acid and α-tocopheronolactone, are conjugated to glucuronic acid and subsequently excreted by the urine or they may enter bile, which will be released into the feces.

β-Tocopherol has only about 25 to 50% of the bioactivity as α-tocopherol, γ-tocopherol has only approximately 10 to 30%, and α-tocotrienol about 25 to 30% the bioactivity. The new recommendations are based simply on milligrams of α-tocopherol. Other isomers, although they have some vitamin E activity, are not included in the contribution toward a daily dietary value.

The intake of vitamin E is based on what dietary level is needed to maintain a certain blood level of the vitamin. It was determined that an estimated average requirement (EAR) of 12 milligrams per day is needed to attain and maintain a plasma level of 12 micromoles per day, a level thought to maintain adequate health. Based, in part, on the EAR, the DRI for vitamin E is listed as an RDA: 15 milligrams a day for adults of both genders, using α-tocopherol as the reference isomer. Pregnancy and lactation increase the recommendations to 15 and 19 milligrams, respectively. For infants, an AI is given and not an RDA. The AI is 4 milligrams for infants from birth to 6 months and 5 milligrams for those aged 6 months to 1 year. For children aged 1 to 3 years, the RDA is 6 milligrams; for those aged 4 to 8 years, it is 7 milligrams; and for those aged 9 to 13 years, it is 11 milligrams per day. However, for adults of both genders, some recent reports suggest that the RDA for vitamin E may be too high and, in fact, could be lower. It has been suggested that an RDA of 10 milligrams per day, instead of the current 15 milligrams per day, would be sufficient to maintain the target blood level of vitamin E at 12 micromoles per day.

Vitamin E Deficiency

Because of the general availability of vitamin E in popular foods, deficiency related to inadequate intake is rare. However, conditions resulting in maldigestion of lipids, such as cystic fibrosis, celiac disease (nontropical sprue), and hepatic and biliary insufficiencies, can result in a compromised vitamin E status. Situations in which enterocyte lipoprotein production is impaired, such as abetalipoproteinemia, can also compromise vitamin E status. **Abetalipoproteinemia** is a rare genetic anomaly in which an individual fails to produce apoprotein B, which is necessary for chylomicron and VLDL formation.

The time to onset of vitamin E deficiency signs and symptoms is very long in adults who had normal vitamin E stores prior to the development of a maldigestion or malabsorption situation. It may take a year or so before plasma vitamin E levels fall to the critical levels associated with deficiency signs. Furthermore, it may take as long as a decade before neurologic signs of deficiency appear. In infants and children experiencing hepatic or biliary insufficiencies, the onset to deficiency is much more rapid because their stores have not been fully developed.

Manifestations of a vitamin E deficiency are assumed to have their origins in the degeneration of cellular membranes. The destruction of red blood cell membranes can result in hemolytic anemia. Degeneration of neuronal and muscular membranes may result in cerebellar ataxia and muscular weakness. Retinal degeneration has also been reported.

Vitamin E and Other Fat Soluble Vitamins in the Development of Alzheimer's Disease

A deficiency of vitamin E has been implicated in the acceleration of Alzheimer's disease. However, other fat-soluble vitamins also play a role and thus separating them out under each vitamin is not a simple feat. Vitamin E deficiency is perhaps the most important of the vitamins that impact this disease, albeit the others cannot be ignored. Thus, we have chosen to discuss the impact of those nutrients under the vitamin E section.

It is important to understand the pathogenesis of this neurological disease. The incidence of the disease appears to be increasing as people are living longer. The rate appears to be doubling for every 20 years of life extension. Almost 50 million people worldwide have this disease. There is a loss of synapses and neurons within two major areas of the brain: the cortex

and the hippocampus. Also, in those areas, there is the presence of what is termed neurotic plaques and intracellular neurofibrillary tangles. The critical part of the disease appears to be the production of the plaques that are termed **amyloid-β peptides**. The neurofibrillary tangles contain an abnormal protein termed **tau**. For our discussion we will focus on amyloid-β peptides. Those peptides have a precursor protein called **amyloid precursor protein**. A set of reactions occurs in the amyloid precursor protein to eventually produce amyloid-β protein (**FIGURE 10.15**). A number of enzymes termed secretases (α, β, and γ) hydrolyze amyloid precursor protein to produce the amyloid-β protein. The resulting amyloid-β protein aggregates are thought responsible for neurotoxicity. From a nutrition perspective, it appears that fat-soluble vitamins, in particular, can modulate the β and γ secretases indirectly. Lipids, such as cholesterol, polyunsaturated fatty acids, and trans fatty acids, are risk factors for Alzheimer's disease. Some lipids, such as polyunsaturated fatty acids, can produce reactive oxygen species that can increase amyloid-β protein pathology. While docosahexaenoic acid can be oxidized, the unoxidized form can decrease amyloid-β protein. The antioxidant activity can decrease the oxidation of amyloid-β protein, which is favorable to slowing down the damage the protein may exert. More important, though, is that vitamin E can impair the synthesis of cholesterol. This is important in that cholesterol enhances the enzymatic activities of the secretases that produce the

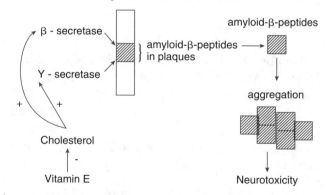

FIGURE 10.15 Production of Amyloid-β Peptide That Forms Plaques in Brains of Alzheimer Patients. Amyloid-β peptides are toxic to the brain. Cholesterol may enhance the production of enzymes that favor the production of these peptides. Vitamin E will impair cholesterol synthesis, leading to decreased levels of amyloid-β peptides. Vitamin E is an antioxidant and can prevent the oxidation of amyloid-β peptide, which will slow down the disease progression.

amyloid-β proteins; vitamin E decreases the amount of cholesterol produced. Thus vitamin E can block the negative impact of protein-β protein in two ways: 1) as an antioxidant, and 2) decreased cholesterol biosynthesis.

The remaining three fat-soluble vitamins are also known to dampen the onset and progression of Alzheimer's disease. In all cases, those afflicted with Alzheimer's disease have lower blood levels of fat-soluble vitamins. As reviewed previously, vitamin A through the various receptors regulate gene expression and that includes neuronal differentiation and neurotransmitter release. Also, its role as an antioxidant is well known. Vitamin D also has antioxidant functions along with anti-inflammatory actions. A notable role is its ability to phagocytize, clear, and enzymatically degrade amyloid-β peptides. Low levels of vitamin K are present in Alzheimer patients but their role is less well known. One notion is that Vitamin K is involved with sphingolipid homeostasis. Ceramides are converted to sulfatides in sphingolipid metabolism. In Alzheimer's disease patients, sulfatides and vitamin K are lower in their brains. One mechanism is that there could be decreased clearance of amyloid-β peptides in patients as sulfatides have been hypothesized to reduce amyloid-β peptides. Collectively, for those either at risk for Alzheimer's disease or those who have any early onset, many healthcare professionals are advocating for additional clinical trials on the impact that fat-soluble vitamins, especially vitamin E, may have on the progression of that disease.

Vitamin E Toxicity

Compared with the fat-soluble vitamins discussed previously, vitamin E is relatively nontoxic. In fact, vitamin E is recognized as one of the least toxic of all of the vitamins. Intakes as high as 500 to 800 milligrams of α-tocopherol for several months to years have not resulted in significant effects. However, gram doses may result in fatigue, muscle weakness, and gastrointestinal distress. Infants, especially preterm infants, may be more sensitive to relatively higher doses of vitamin E. The tolerable upper intake level is 1,000 milligrams of α-tocopherol.

Although toxic effects from supplementation of vitamin E are not a large concern, it is important to understand that the practice of megadosing may affect the absorption and function of other fat-soluble vitamins. For instance, gram doses of vitamin E appear to hinder vitamin K absorption. Furthermore, gram doses of vitamin E may impede the involvement of vitamin K in blood clotting while also increasing the effect of oral anticoagulant drugs, such as coumarin, which can lead to increased bleeding tendencies in some individuals. Vitamin D's involvement in bone mineralization may be altered by excessive vitamin E intake, and the absorption of β-carotene, as well as its conversion to vitamin A, may be hindered as well.

> ● **BEFORE YOU GO ON . . .**
>
> 1. What are the two major classes of vitamin E, and how do they differ chemically?
> 2. Once vitamin E is absorbed and is transferred to the liver, how is it processed for export to other tissues?
> 3. How is vitamin E excreted from the body?
> 4. Although dietary vitamin E deficiency is not likely to occur, compromised vitamin E status may occur. List the ways in which an individual's vitamin E status may become compromised.
> 5. How does the toxicity of vitamin E compare with the fat-soluble vitamins A and D?
> 6. Explain how vitamin E may impact Alzheimer's disease?

▶ Vitamin K

First recognized in the 1930s, vitamin K is a group of naturally occurring or synthetically created 2-methyl-1,4-naphthoquinones with a hydrophobic substitution at the number 3 position of the structure (**FIGURE 10.16**). The form of vitamin K naturally occurring in green plants is phylloquinone, which has a phytyl group at the number 3 position. Bacteria produce a number of forms of vitamin K called menaquinones, which have an unsaturated multiprenyl group at the number 3 position. The most common menaquinones are those with 6 to 10 isoprenoid groups, which are abbreviated as MK6 to MK10. Menadione is the synthetic version of vitamin K, which is primarily used in animal feeds.

Sources of Vitamin K

In the human diet, vitamin K is largely provided by plant foods; however, the vitamin K content of many foods has yet to be determined. Good sources appear to be spinach, broccoli, Brussels sprouts, cabbage, lettuce, and kale; some vitamin K is also provided by cereals, meats, nuts, legumes, dairy products, and fruits. Vitamin K may also be derived from bacteria in the human colon, primarily anaerobes, such as *Escherichia coli* and *Bacillus fragilis*.

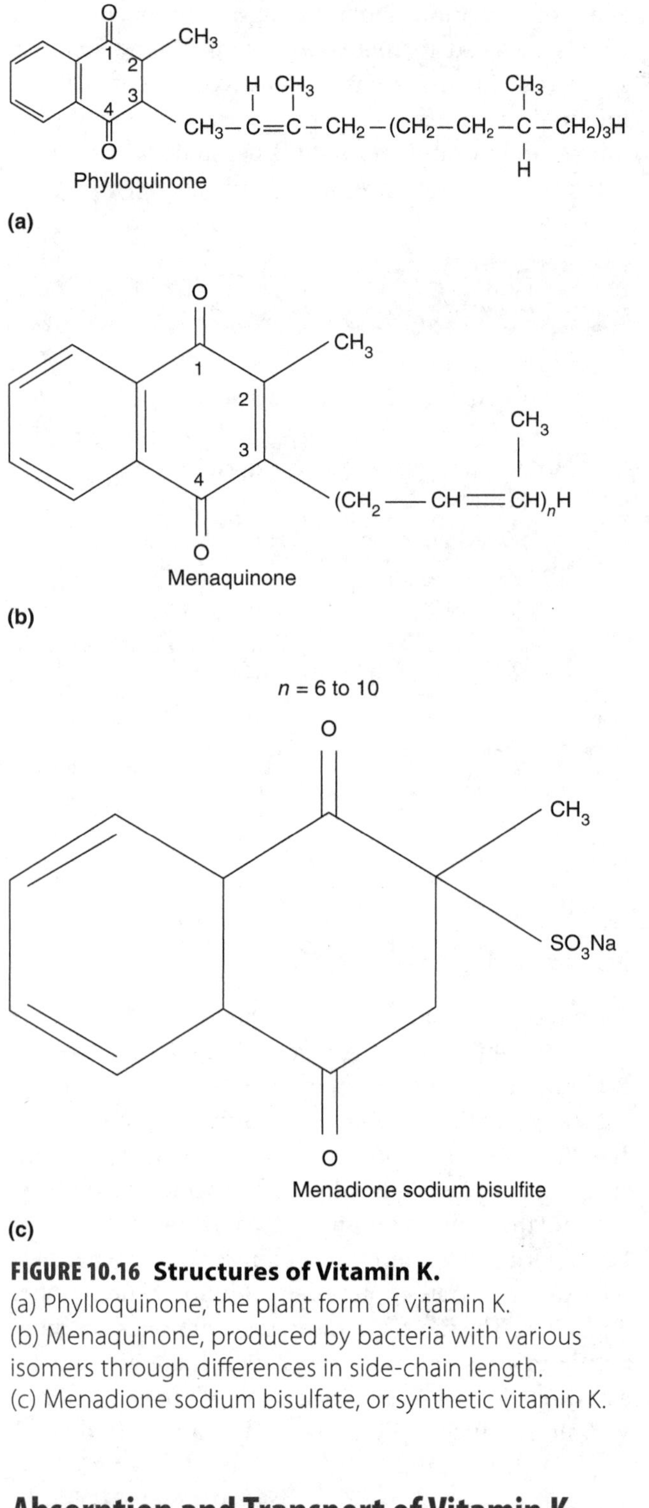

(a)

n = 6 to 10

(b)

(c)

FIGURE 10.16 Structures of Vitamin K.
(a) Phylloquinone, the plant form of vitamin K.
(b) Menaquinone, produced by bacteria with various isomers through differences in side-chain length.
(c) Menadione sodium bisulfate, or synthetic vitamin K.

Absorption and Transport of Vitamin K

Phylloquinone appears to be taken into enterocytes in the small intestine via an active, saturable process. This primarily takes place in the duodenum and jejunum, with the latter being the primary site of absorption. Conversely, menaquinones and menadione seem to cross the wall of the intestine via passive diffusion, which occurs mostly in the distal small intestine and in the colon. That allows the menaquinones synthesized by bacteria in the colon to be absorbed, although

the extent to which this occurs is still unclear. The absorption of vitamin K in the small intestine is positively influenced by the presence of pancreatic and biliary secretions, especially bile acids.

Vitamin K entering mucosal cells is incorporated into chylomicrons, which enter the lymphatic circulation and, in turn, the systemic circulation. As chylomicron remnants are removed from circulation, vitamin K enters hepatocytes. Once in the liver, vitamin K can be metabolized and then incorporated into VLDL for export. The plasma concentration of phylloquinone is about 0.14 to 1.17 nanograms per milliliter. The duration of diet-derived vitamin K in the liver is not very long; thus, the liver is not considered a significant site of storage for this vitamin. Typically, the vitamin K content of the liver is less than 20 to 25 nanograms per gram of liver tissue. However, it should be recognized that hepatic turnover of menaquinones is much slower than that of phylloquinones, allowing for a large concentration difference (10-fold or more) in the liver.

Functions of Vitamin K

The fact that vitamin K is essential for proper clotting of the blood in response to a hemorrhage has been known for at least 60 years. For the several decades that followed, it was assumed that assistance in blood clotting might be the only physiologic role of vitamin K. However, newer information about the roles of vitamin K has emerged since then. Vitamin K influences physiologic processes, such as blood clotting, by post-translation carboxylation of glutamic acid residues to form γ-carboxyglutamic acid in key proteins. The enzyme responsible for this reaction is vitamin K-dependent gamma-glutamyl carboxylase. With respect to vitamin K, this enzyme is referred to as **vitamin K carboxylase. FIGURE 10.17** gives an example of this reaction in the production of prothrombin. When γ-carboxyglutamic acid forms, calcium is

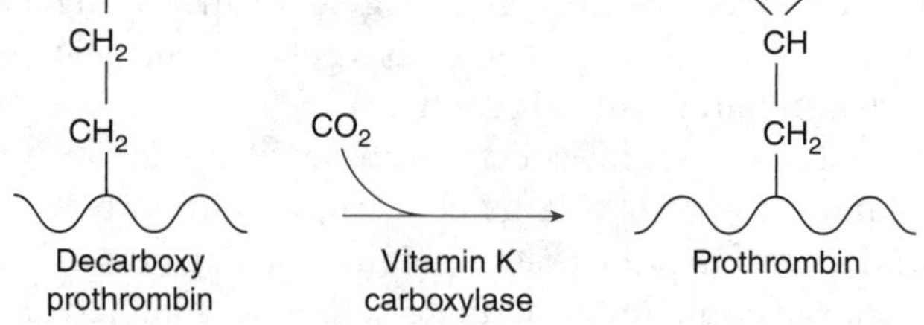

FIGURE 10.17 Vitamin K Carboxylase Reaction. The production of one blood clotting factor, prothrombin, is one example of the role of vitamin K-dependent gamma-glutamyl carboxylase, or vitamin K carboxylase, in this example.

able to bind with proteins that contain those residues, which also allows those proteins to interact with phospholipids. There are many other reactions requiring vitamin K carboxylase in addition to the reaction presented here.

The coagulation of blood requires a series of activation reactions involving clotting factors synthesized in the blood (**FIGURE 10.18**). The final reaction in the series is proteolytic activation of fibrinogen to fibrin, which forms the structural basis of an insoluble fibrous network at the site of a hemorrhage. The enzyme that

catalyzes this reaction is thrombin, which itself circulates as an inactive enzyme (zymogen) called prothrombin or clotting factor II. Four clotting factors, including prothrombin, are dependent on vitamin K for normal function.

Factor X is vitamin K dependent and is responsible for activating prothrombin to thrombin. Factor X is activated by one of two means. First, it can become functional via a series of activation reactions beginning with factor XII and involving factors XI and IX, the latter of which is also vitamin D

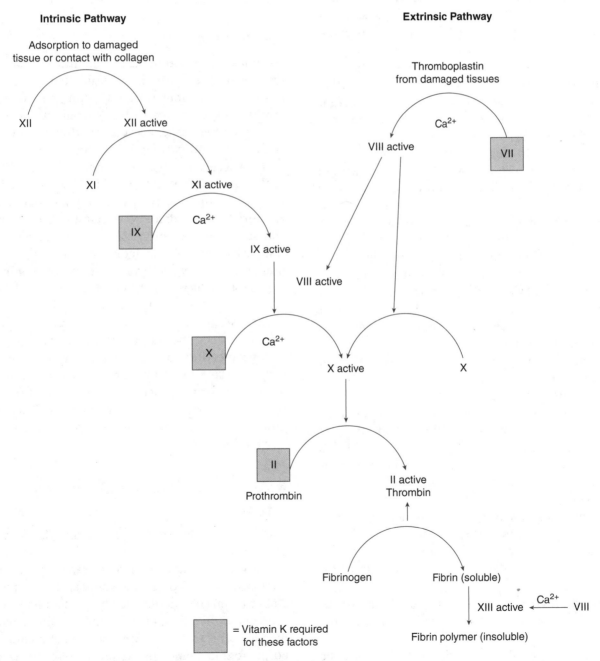

FIGURE 10.18. Vitamin K-Dependent Blood Coagulation Process. Cascade of events leading to the activation of insoluble fibrin to form a blood clot.

dependent. The initial reaction occurs as the inactive form of factor XII interacts with exposed collagen fibers at the site of a hemorrhage. Collagen fibers would normally not be exposed to the blood because they are part of the interstitial connective tissue (i.e., basal laminae) of endothelial cells and local tissue. However, rupture of the endothelial lining exposes the underlying connective tissue. This series of events leading to activation of prothrombin is called the **intrinsic pathway**.

The second mechanism leading to the activation of prothrombin tissue is called the **extrinsic pathway**. Here, clotting factor VII, one of the vitamin D-dependent proteins, is activated by a tissue factor called **thromboplastin**. Activated factor VII then activates factor X, which activates prothrombin. Because both the intrinsic and extrinsic pathways involve clotting factors dependent on vitamin K post-translational modification, the proper coagulation of blood is sensitive to vitamin K status. Anticoagulant drugs, such as coumarin and warfarin, inhibit the action of vitamin K.

In addition to the clotting factors already discussed, four other proteins (C, M, S, and Z) involved in the regulation of blood clotting appear to be vitamin K dependent. Protein C is a protease that appears to inhibit coagulation, whereas protein S appears to promote the breakdown of the fibrin network and thus, the clot. Meanwhile, protein M may be involved in the conversion of thrombin from prothrombin. The blood clotting factors VII, IX, and X and proteins C, S, and Z require vitamin K so that they can be carboxylated. Prothrombin also requires vitamin K carboxylase.

Other vitamin K-dependent proteins have been identified in tissue, such as bone and kidneys. In bone, two proteins—bone Gla protein (BGP, or osteocalcin) and matrix Gla protein (MGP)—are modified post-translationally by carboxylation of specific glutamic acid residues involving vitamin K. "Gla" refers to glutamic acid; carboxylated glutamic acid residues are able to bind calcium. Osteocalcin, which is expressed under the influence of vitamin D, is produced in osteoblasts in bone and the dentin of teeth. MGP is associated with the matrix of bone, dentin, and cartilage. The specific roles of those proteins are still being investigated, but MGP may be an inhibitor of calcification.

In addition, another protein has been identified in the renal cortex that is dependent on post-translational modification involving vitamin K. Here again, the modification is carboxylation of specific glutamic acid residues. This protein is referred to as kidney Gla protein (KGP); its physiologic significance is under investigation.

There is much debate as to what role vitamin K plays in osteoporosis. As noted, vitamin K plays a role in two bone proteins. A finding from the Nurses' Health Study suggests that those nurses in the bottom fifth of vitamin K diet intake had a 30% increased likelihood of a bone fracture compared with others. Reports from the Framingham study revealed that women and men in the top 25% of dietary vitamin K intake had a 65% risk reduction in hip fractures compared with those consuming lower doses.

The Vitamin K Cycle

Gamma-carboxylation via the vitamin K carboxylase reaction occurs within the liver, and more specifically, in the rough endoplasmic reticulum, where protein synthesis occurs along with post-translational modification. Other tissues also contain this enzyme, especially bone and cartilage. For the carboxylation to occur, a series of reactions is required that is known as the **vitamin K cycle** (**FIGURE 10.19**). The reduced form of vitamin K (hydroquinone) is oxidized to vitamin K 2,3-epoxide via vitamin K carboxylase and subsequent carboxylation of the glutamic acid residues of various proteins, including the reduction of decarboxy prothrombin to prothrombin. The regeneration of the hydroquinone form of vitamin K begins by the reduction of vitamin K 2,3-epoxide in the presence of thiol groups; the reducing equivalents produce the quinone form of vitamin K via the enzyme vitamin K epoxide reductase. The latter enzyme is inhibited by warfarin. Once the hydroquinone is formed, there is another reduction reaction via quinone reductase with NADPH and thiol groups to finally regenerate the hydroquinone form of vitamin K.

Recommended Levels of Vitamin K Intake

The DRI for vitamin K is set as an AI: 90 micrograms per day for adult women and 120 micrograms per day for adult men. No tolerable upper intake level is specified. For infants younger than 6 months, 2 micrograms of vitamin K daily is recommended; for those older than 6 months, 2.5 micrograms is recommended. The AI for children ranges between 30 and 60 micrograms, and the AI for adolescents aged 14

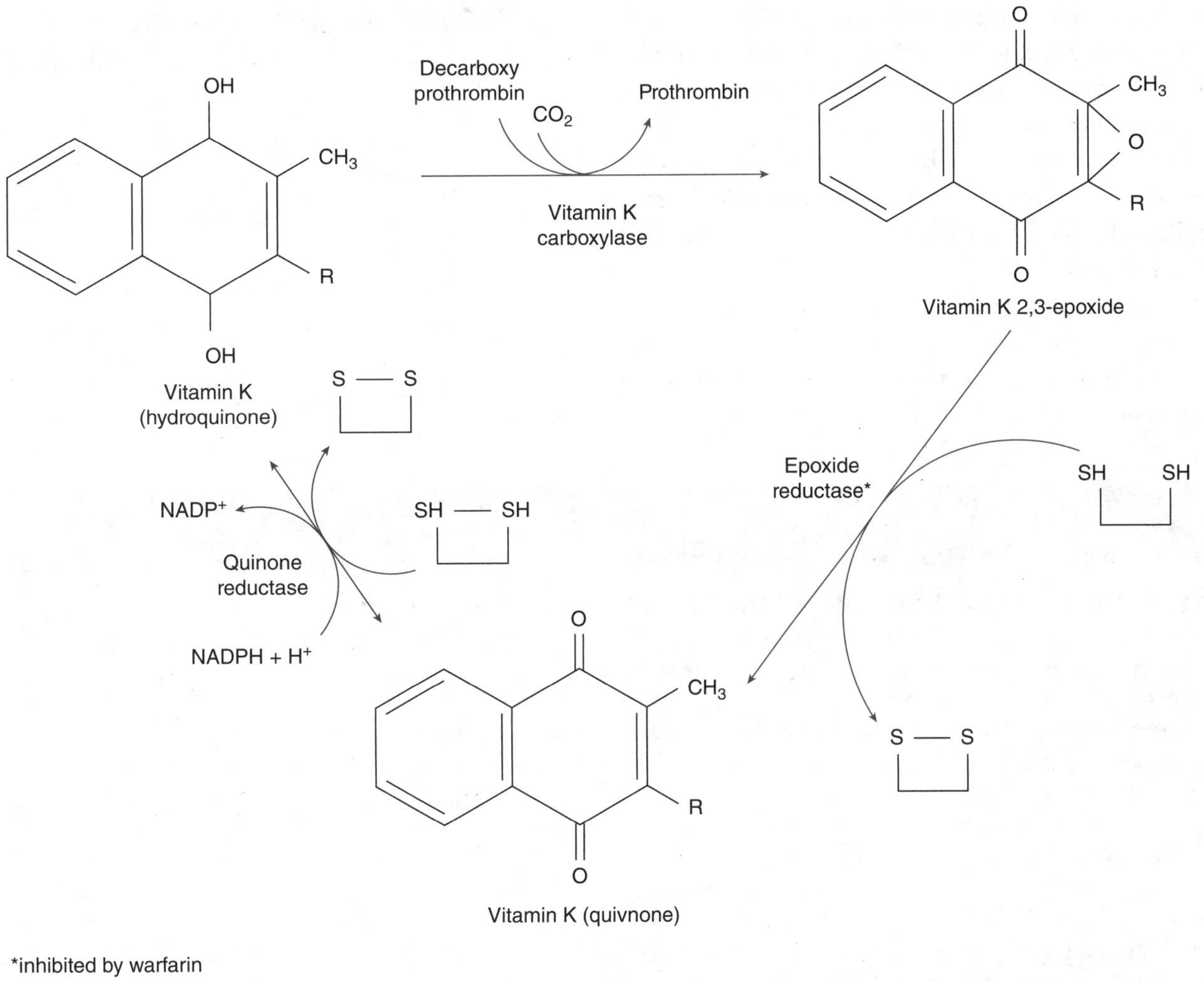

FIGURE 10.19 The Vitamin K Cycle. The cycle is a series of reactions that require carboxylation. Reduced vitamin K or hydroquinone is central to this cycle. Reduced vitamin K is oxidized to vitamin K 2,3-epoxide by vitamin K carboxylase. This allows for carboxylation of other proteins that contain glutamic acid. For this reaction to continue, the cycle regenerates additional reduced vitamin K for subsequent carboxylation reactions.

to 18 years of age is 75 micrograms per day for both genders. Pregnancy and lactation do not increase the vitamin K recommendation above the highest level for women (90 micrograms). Vitamin K should be given to all newborns as a single, intramuscular dose of 0.5 to 1.0 milligram.

Vitamin K Deficiency and Toxicity

Unlike other fat-soluble vitamins, vitamin K is not stored well in human tissue, and appreciable amounts are lost in the urine and feces daily. This presents a theoretical opportunity for a rapid onset to deficiency. However, vitamin K is relatively abundant in the diet, and respectable amounts are also absorbed from intestinal bacterial synthesis, thereby making vitamin K deficiency uncommon in adults.

The typical American adult may actually eat five to six times the DRI.

Opportunities for vitamin K deficiency do arise in infancy. There does not seem to be an appreciable transfer of vitamin K from the mother to the fetus. Therefore, newborns have very limited stores. Furthermore, a newborn's digestive tract is sterile and will not develop a mature bacterial population for months. Additionally, maternal breast milk is not a good source of vitamin K. All of those factors place infants at greater risk for developing a vitamin K deficiency, which can lead to poor blood clotting and hemorrhage, among other considerations. With those concerns in mind, many pediatricians routinely treat newborns with vitamin K.

One other situation may raise concerns regarding the development of a vitamin K deficiency. Those individuals using antibiotics for long periods of time are at a greater risk for vitamin K deficiency. Certain antibiotics can remove vitamin K-producing bacteria from the colon, which puts a person at a greater risk for deficiency, especially if he or she is consuming a diet low in vitamin K or is experiencing problems with lipid digestion. The combination of those factors is rare, however.

Vitamin K is relatively nontoxic in natural forms; however, there have been cases of toxicity from the chronic use of excessive vitamin K in the synthetic menadione form.

● BEFORE YOU GO ON . . .

1. List the different forms of vitamin K, and state whether their absorption occurs via passive or active transport.
2. Distinguish between the intrinsic and extrinsic pathways involved with blood clotting.
3. How is vitamin K related to bone metabolism?
4. Although a deficiency of vitamin K is rare, under what conditions may it occur in humans?
5. How does vitamin K assist with blood clotting?

🩺 CLINICAL INSIGHT

Malabsorption of Fat-Soluble Vitamins in Primary Biliary Cirrhosis

It is not uncommon to have patients afflicted with primary biliary cirrhosis. The name of this disease has been changed to primary biliary cholangitis in some areas as the term cirrhosis is a late-stage disease and intervention is actually done at the early stages of the disease.

Primary biliary cirrhosis is considered a cholestatic disease, meaning that there is an obstruction of some type, which prevents bile from flowing from the liver to the small intestine (duodenum). There is some consideration that primary biliary cirrhosis is an autoimmune disease. This results in the backup of bile in the liver and can lead to permanent damage, such as fibrosis of the liver. Gallstones and cancer can lead to obstruction of the bile duct, which can lead to liver fibrosis. A consequence of this results in decreased bile salts or acids in the digestive tract in which to emulsify lipids prior to enzymatic digestion by lipases that are available in the small intestine. It is not unusual to have more than 60 grams of fat excreted per day by individuals, thereby creating steatorrhea. A challenge in such cases is that without emulsification, fat-soluble substances, the fat-soluble vitamins included cannot be solubilized into the aqueous environment of the small intestine for subsequent enterocyte absorption. Jaundice, pruritus or itching, fatigue, and dry eyes and mouth can be some of the symptoms. The presence of edema in the lower extremities is not uncommon. A clinical check will determine if there is an antibody to mitochondria in the blood.

There is a treatment for the disease, if caught soon enough. The drug ursodeoxycholic acid can facilitate the movement of bile from the liver to the small intestine. If that treatment is started too late, often, a liver transplant becomes the only option.

With respect to the fat-soluble vitamins, it suggests that a decrease in absorption is theoretically possible. Several studies have been conducted over the years to determine if primary biliary cirrhosis leads to compromised fat-soluble vitamin status. A number of studies indicate that the status of vitamins A and D are mostly affected and that vitamins E and K are affected to a lesser extent. The recommendations on fat-soluble vitamin supplementation are mixed, but the consensus is that if there is evidence of compromised status in either of those vitamins, supplementation is warranted.

▶ Here's What You Have Learned

1. Vitamin A may be divided into preformed and previtamin A. Preformed vitamin A includes retinol, retinal, and retinoic acid. Previtamin A includes a group of compounds collectively referred to as carotenoids. Previtamin A compounds have the potential to be converted to retinol within human cells. Both forms of vitamin A are absorbed by passive diffusion. Vitamin A and carotenoids are packaged into chylomicrons, enter the lymphatic circulation, and are eventually taken up by the liver. BCMO1 can cleave β-carotene into 2 molecules of retinol whereas BCO2 has an eccentric cleavage pattern to produce β-ionone and β-10′-apocarotenal. Mutations in BCO2 can lead to a variety of disease conditions.

2. Vitamin A plays important roles in night vision, cell differentiation, bone development, immune function, and reproduction. Vitamin A functions by binding with nuclear receptors that bind

to gene promoters. The retinoic acid receptors (RXR and RAR) are a group of vitamin A receptors involved in gene regulation. Vitamin A may act as a chemopreventive agent for some cancer types, but not for others, such as lung cancer.

3. Vitamin D has many functions, most of which are associated with calcium absorption and bone mineralization. Like vitamin A, some of its functions are at the gene level, where vitamin D binds to a nuclear receptor called the vitamin D receptor (VDR). The complex binds to the promoter of a gene along with the retinoic acid receptor and turns gene function on or off. Deficiency of vitamin D results in rickets in children, which is associated with poor mineralization of growing bone. Vitamin D receptor is found in a plethora of tissues and has been implicated in a significant number of different types of diseases, especially a fundamental role in cancer prevention.

4. Vitamin E is known as an antioxidant and serves to protect the cell membrane and oxidation of unsaturated fatty acids. There are eight isomers of vitamin E (the tocopherols). Vitamin E deficiency is rare, but can occur in a genetic abnormality called abetalipoproteinemia in which chylomicrons and VLDL formation are compromised, limiting vitamin E absorption and transport. If deficiency in the diet does occur, it may take a year or more to develop deficiency signs, which include hemolytic anemia, neuronal degeneration, muscular weakness, and cerebellar ataxia.

5. Vitamin E and other fat-soluble vitamin levels are often inversely related to those with Alzheimer's disease. The major impact that those vitamins appear to have upon the disease is a lowering of amyloid-β peptides.

6. Vitamin K is the anticoagulant vitamin. It is found in a variety of foods and can also be produced by the microflora of the gut. It is absorbed via active transport and reaches the bloodstream via chylomicrons, like other fat-soluble vitamins. Once in the liver, it can be packaged into VLDL to be transported to other tissues. Vitamin K plays a role in anticoagulation at several points in the cascade reactions for blood clots. Vitamin K also plays a role in the synthesis of two bone proteins: Gla protein (osteocalcin) and matrix Gla protein (MGP).

▶ Suggested Reading

Booth SL, Tucker KL, Chen H, et al. Dietary vitamin K intakes are associated with hip fracture but not with bone mineral density in elderly men and women. *Am J Clin Nutr.* 2000;71(5):1201–1208.

Carlberg C, Seuter S. A genomic perspective on vitamin D signaling. *Anticancer Res.* 2009;29(9):3485–3493.

Clagett-Dame M, Knutson D. Vitamin A in reproduction and development. *Nutrients.* 2011;3(4):385–428.

Combs GF. *The Vitamins.* San Diego: Academic Press; 1992.

DiRenzo J, Söderstrom M, Kurokawa R, et al. Peroxisome proliferator-activated receptors and retinoic acid receptors differentially control the interactions of retinoid X receptor heterodimers with ligands, coactivators, and corepressors. *Mol Cell Biol.* 1997;17(4):2166–2176.

Dong LM, Ulrich CM, Hsu L, et al. Vitamin D related genes, CYP24A1 and CYP27B1, and colon cancer risk. *Cancer Epidemiol Biomarkers Prev.* 2009;18(9):2540–2548.

Feskanich D, Weber P, Willett WC, Rockett H, Booth SL, Colditz GA. Vitamin K intake and hip fractures in women: a prospective study. *Am J Clin Nutr.* 1999;69(1):74–79.

Fritz H, Kennedy D, Fergusson D, et al. Vitamin A and retinoid derivatives for lung cancer: a systematic review and meta analysis. *PLoS One.* 2011;6(6):e21107.

Grimm MO, Mett J, Hartmann T. The impact of vitamin E and other fat-soluble vitamins on Alzheimer's disease. *Int J Mol Sci.* 2016;17(11):E1785.

Gropper SS, Smith JL, Groff JL. *Advanced Nutrition and Human Metabolism.* Belmont, CA: Wadsworth; 2005.

Hans SN, Pang E, Zingg JM, Meydani SN, Meydani M, Azzi A. Differential effects of natural and synthetic vitamin E on gene transcription in murine T lymphocytes. *Arch Biochem Biophys.* 2010;495(1):49–55.

Harkness L, Cromer B. Low levels of 25-hydroxy vitamin D are associated with elevated parathyroid hormone in healthy adolescent females. *Osteoporos Int.* 2005;16(1):109–113.

Harkness LS, Cromer BA. Vitamin D deficiency in adolescent females. *J Adolesc Health.* 2005;37(1):75.

Heathcote EJ. Management of primary biliary cirrhosis. The American Association for the Study of Liver Diseases practice guidelines. *Hepatology.* 2000;31(4):1005–1013.

Ingraham BA, Bragdon B, Nohe A. Molecular basis of the potential of vitamin D to prevent cancer. *Curr Med Res Opin.* 2008;24(1):139–149.

Knekt P, Reunanen A, Järvinen R, Seppanen R, Heliövaara M, Aromaa A. Antioxidant vitamin intake and coronary mortality in a longitudinal population study. *Am J Epidemiol.* 1994;139(12):1180–1189.

Köstner K, Denzer N, Müller CS, Klein R, Tilgen W, Reichrath J. The relevance of vitamin D receptor (VDR) gene polymorphisms for cancer: a review of the literature. *Anticancer Res.* 2009;29(9):3511–3536.

Kushi LH, Folsom AR, Prineas RJ, Mink PJ, Wu Y, Bostick RM. Dietary antioxidant vitamins and death from coronary heart disease in postmenopausal women. *N Engl J Med.* 1996;334(18):1156–1162.

Lee JM, Smith JR, Phillipp BL, Chen TC, Mathieu J, Holick MF. Vitamin D deficiency in a healthy group of mothers and newborn infants. *Clin Pediatr (Phila).* 2007;46(1):42–44.

Marcason W. Vitamin D: are children and adolescents at risk for deficiency? *J Am Diet Assoc.* 2009;109(5):952.

Masaki KH, Losonczy KG, Izmirlian G, et al. Association of vitamin E and C supplement use with cognitive function and dementia in elderly men. *Neurology.* 2000;54(6):1265–1272.

Milani A, Basirneiad M, Shahbazi S, Bolhassani A. Carotenoids: biochemistry, pharmacology and treatment. *Br J Pharmacol.* 2017; 174(11):1290–1324.

Moukayed M, Grant WB. Molecular link between vitamin D and cancer prevention. *Nutrients.* 2013;5(10):3993–4021.

Norman PE, Powell JT. Vitamin D and cardiovascular disease. *Circ Res.* 2014;114(2):379–393.

Novotny JA, Fadel JG, Holstege DM, Furr HC, Clifford AJ. This kinetic, bioavailability, and metabolism study of RRR-α-tocopherol in healthy adults suggests lower intake requirements than previous estimates. *J Nutr.* 2012;142(12):2105–2111.

Peterlik M, Grant WB, Cross HS. Calcium, vitamin D and cancer. *Anticancer Res.* 2009;29(9):3687–3698.

Phillips JR, Angulo P, Petterson T, Lindor KD. Fat-soluble vitamin levels in patients with primary biliary cirrhosis. *Am J Gastroenterol.* 2001;96(9):2745–2750.

Ragsdale SW. Catalysis of methyl group transfers involving tetrahydrofolate and B(12). *Vitam Horm.* 2008;79:293–324.

Rimm EB, Stampfer MJ, Ascherio A, Giovannucci E, Colditz GA, Willett WC. Vitamin E consumption and the risk of coronary heart disease in men. *N Engl J Med.* 1993;328(20):1450–1456.

Rovner AJ, O'Brien KO. Hypovitaminosis D among healthy children in the United States: a review of the current evidence. *Arch Pediatr Adolesc Med.* 2008;162(6):513–519.

Samuel S, Sitrin MD. Vitamin D's role in cell proliferation and differentiation. *Nutr Rev.* 2008;66(10 suppl 2): S116– S124.

Sano M, Ernesto C, Thomas RG, et al. A controlled trial of selegiline, alpha-tocopherol, or both as treatment for Alzheimer's disease. The Alzheimer's Disease Cooperative Study. *N Engl J Med.* 1997;336(17):1216–1222.

Sherwin JC, Reacher MH, Dean WH, Ngondi J. Epidemiology of vitamin A deficiency and xerophthalmia in at-risk populations. *Trans R Soc Trop Med Hyg.* 2012;106(4):205–214.

Stampfer MJ, Hennekens CH, Manson JE, Colditz GA, Rosner B, Willett WC. Vitamin E consumption and the risk of coronary disease in women. *N Engl J Med.* 1993;328(20):1444–1449.

Subudhi U, Chainy GB. Expression of hepatic antioxidant genes in I-thyroxine-induced hyperthyroid rats: regulation by vitamin E and curcumin. *Chem Biol Interact.* 2010;183(2):304–316.

Thorne J, Campbell MJ. The vitamin D receptor in cancer. *Proc Nutr Soc.* 2008;67(2):115–127.

Weng FL, Shults J, Leonard MB, Stallings VA, Zemel BS. Risk factors for low serum 25-hydroxyvitamin D concentrations in otherwise healthy children and adolescents. *Am J Clin Nutr.* 2007;86(1):150–158.

Willis CM, Laing EM, Hall DB, Hausman DB, Lewis RD. A prospective analysis of plasma 25-hydoxyvitamin D concentrations in white and black prepubertal females in the southeastern United States. *Am J Clin Nutr.* 2007;85(1):124–130.

Wolf G. Retinoic acid as cause of cell proliferation or cell growth inhibition depending on activation of one of two different nuclear receptors. *Nutr Rev.* 2008;66(1):55–59.

Wu L, Guo X, Wang W, Medeiros DM, Clarke SL, Lucas EA, Smith BJ, Lin D. Molecular aspects of β, β-carotene-9', 10'-oxygenase 2 in carotenoid metabolism and diseases. *Exp Bio Med.* 2016; 241:1879–1887.

Xue Y, Fleet JC. Intestinal vitamin D receptor is required for normal calcium and bone metabolism in mice. *Gastroenterology.* 2009;136(4):1317–1327.

Yin M, Wei S, Wei Q. Vitamin D receptor genetic polymorphisms and prostate cancer risk: a meta-analysis of 36 published studies. *Int J Clin Exp Med.* 2009;2(2):159–175.

Zhang X, Dai B, Zhang B, Wang A. Vitamin A and risk of cervical cancer: a meta-analysis. *Gynecol Oncol.* 2012;124(2):366–373.

Ziegler EE, Filer LJ, eds. *Present Knowledge in Nutrition.* Washington, DC: ILSI Press; 1996.

Ziouzenkova O, Plutzky J. Retinoid metabolism and nuclear receptor responses: new insights into coordinated regulation of the PPAR-RXR complex. *FEBS Lett.* 2008;582(1):32–38.

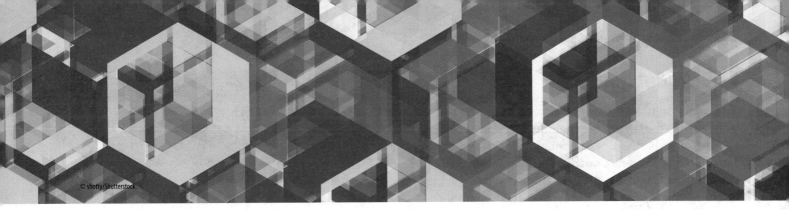

CHAPTER 11

Water-Soluble Vitamins

← HERE'S WHERE YOU HAVE BEEN

1. The fat-soluble vitamins are stored for a longer period of time than water-soluble vitamins and require some fat in the diet for absorption.
2. Two of the fat-soluble vitamins, A and D, exert much of their effects at the gene level.
3. There are several biochemical forms of the fat-soluble vitamins, which differ in their activity; some can be metabolized further.
4. The dietary requirements for many of the fat-soluble vitamins are continually being updated as new functions and understandings are uncovered.
5. Although the fat-soluble vitamins can be stored, there is concern that some population groups have insufficient reserves and are deficient.

HERE'S WHERE YOU ARE GOING →

1. The water-soluble vitamins can result in deficiency signs more quickly than the fat-soluble vitamins if they are not provided in adequate amounts in diets.
2. Several of the water-soluble vitamins act as cofactors in key enzymatic pathways of macronutrient metabolism, but some have roles beyond coenzyme activities.
3. Deficiencies of many water-soluble vitamins were at one time common in Western societies.
4. Folate and vitamin B_{12} play critical roles in cell proliferation.
5. Most of the water-soluble vitamins have specific membrane transporters to aid in both intestinal absorption and cell uptake by a wide variety of tissues.

▶ Introduction

The water-soluble vitamins encompass more compounds than the fat-soluble vitamins. The class includes the so-called B vitamins and vitamin C. Whereas the fat-soluble vitamins are not directly involved in energy metabolism, one characteristic of most water-soluble vitamins is a direct involvement in such operations. This involvement is largely in the form of coenzymatic activity associated with metabolic pathways for carbohydrates, protein (amino acids), fat, and ethanol. Notable exceptions are vitamins C and B_{12} and folic acid. Although those three water-soluble vitamins are not coenzymes in energy pathways, they are coenzymes for other key operations. Therefore, coenzyme function is the most salient characteristic of this class of vitamins. In the last several years, we have learned that these vitamins play more than a coenzyme role. They may exert gene expression. Also, a significant number of transporters have been identified and characterized for these vitamins. In some cases, there are genetic defects in the transporters leading to deficiencies and other metabolic anomalies. **TABLE 11.1** lists the transporters for the specific vitamins indicated and will be referred to frequently throughout this chapter.

Although much has been said pertaining to the fat-soluble vitamins' potential for toxicity because of their longer storage time in tissue, water-soluble vitamins are also toxic in large quantities, although the amounts must be far greater than those observed for the fat-soluble vitamins.

▶ Vitamin C (Ascorbic Acid)

Vitamin C has long been a controversial and popular vitamin among scientists and the general public. Deficiency of vitamin C, or ascorbate, results in one of the most famous nutrition-related diseases—**scurvy**. Scurvy was prevalent until the mid-18th century and was the scourge of sailors who were at sea for extended periods. It was not unusual to observe fleets of ships return with 90% of the crew either dead or incapacitated as a result of scurvy. In 1754, the British navy hired the physician James Lind to investigate the disease. He became aware that the disease was not of microbial origin, but rather, was associated with the diet. Eventually, he determined that the juice from one sour lime would protect individuals from the disease. As a result of his findings, the British navy, at the suggestion of Captain James Cook, required ships to carry sufficient citrus fruits for each man for the estimated time of the voyage. British sailors' practice of sucking the juice of limes resulted in the nickname "Limeys." It

TABLE 11.1 Select Water Soluble Vitamin Transporters

Vitamin	Transporter Name	Abbreviation
Vitamin C		
Ascorbate	Sodium-Ascorbate Co-Transporter	SVCT1, SVCT2
Dehydroascorbic acid	Glucose Transporter	GLUT1-4
B-Vitamins		
Thiamin	Thiamin Transporter	THTR1, THTR2
Riboflavin	Riboflavin Transporter	RFVT1, RFVT2, RFVT3
Folate	Reduced Folate Transporter	RFT
	Proton-Coupled Folate Transporter	PCFT
Biotin	Sodium-Dependent Multivitamin Transporter	SMVT
Pantothenic Acid	Sodium-Dependent Multivitamin Transporter	SMVT

wasn't until 1933 that the Hungarian scientist Albert Szent-Györgyi isolated the active component from his native Hungarian green peppers. Following the isolation of ascorbate, he and Norman Haworth, a carbohydrate chemist, worked out its structure. Szent-Györgyi received the Nobel Prize in 1936 for his work on vitamin C.

Ascorbate is a derivative of glucose. Through a series of reactions shown in **FIGURE 11.1**, glucose is converted to glucuronate and then L-gulonolactone; the latter compound is oxidized via L-gulonolactone oxidase to yield ascorbate. Unfortunately, humans are unable to carry out this latter reaction because they lack L-gulonolactone oxidase. The guinea pig, primates, bats, and some fish (e.g., catfish) are unable to synthesize ascorbate. In contrast, many other animals, such as rats and chickens, are able to synthesize vitamin C.

A biochemically useful property of vitamin C is that it can both donate and accept hydrogen

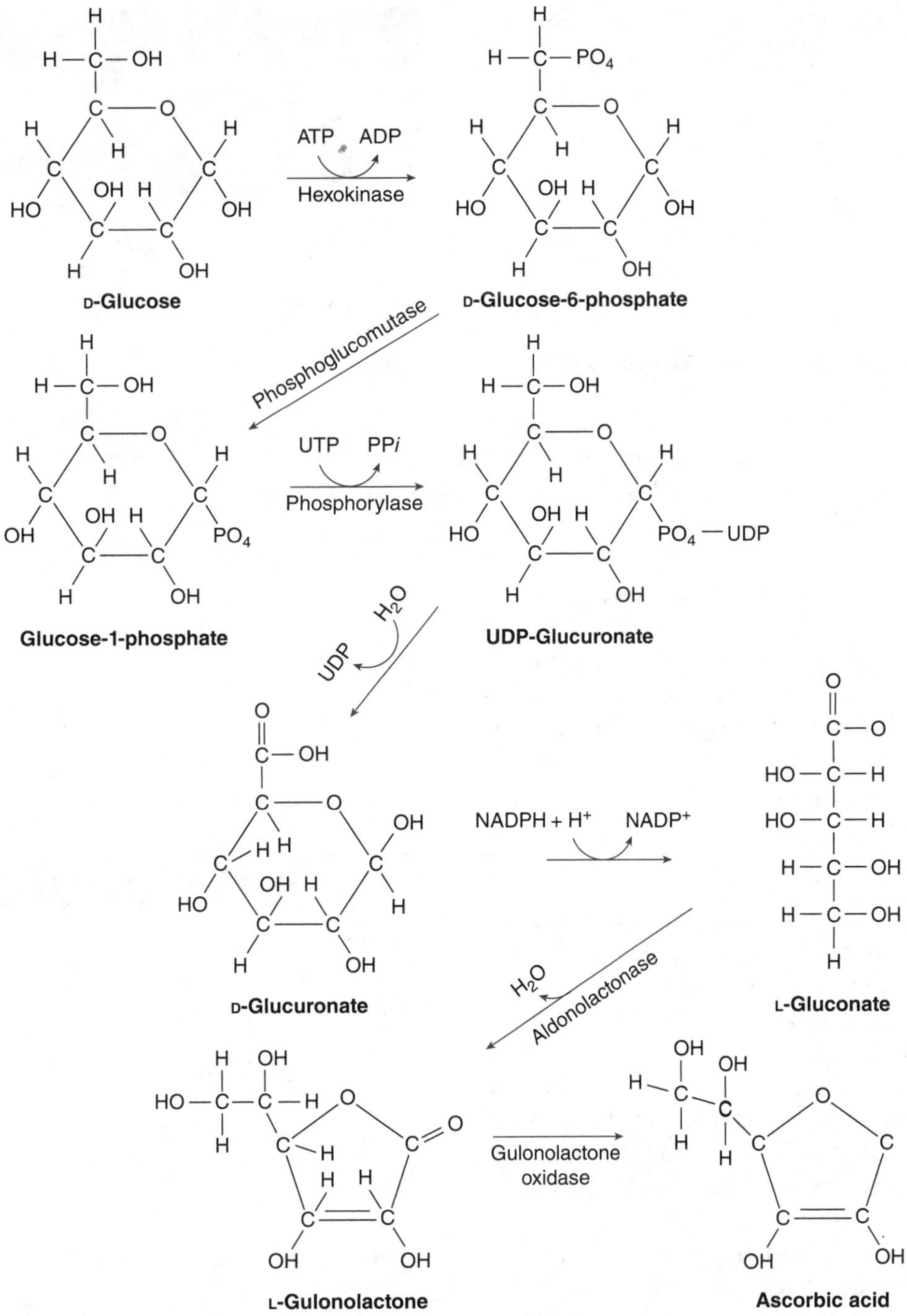

FIGURE 11.1 Biosynthesis of Ascorbic Acid from D-Glucose. Glucose is converted to D-glucuronate and L-gulonolactone through multiple reactions, L-gulonolactone is oxidized to produce ascorbate. Humans lack the last enzyme, gulonolactone oxidase, and are unable to synthesize ascorbate.

readily. The oxidized form of vitamin C is termed dehydroascorbic acid (**FIGURE 11.2**). Glutathione and dehydroascorbate reductase facilitate the production of the reduced form. Both forms of the vitamin are equally active, and this interconversion makes vitamin C a good antioxidant. This property also makes vitamin C useful for food preservation, especially in canned foods.

The vitamin has several centers of asymmetry. Both D and L isomer forms exist, but it is the L form that is active in humans. The reverse is true with regard to glucose, where the D form is the active form. If ascorbate is oxidized, it will form diketogulonic acid, which is inactive. Substitutions may also occur on carbon atoms of the molecular structure. The methoxyl group on carbon 6, for example, may be substituted by a methyl group. Also, a seven-carbon structure may exist in which an additional CH_2OH group may be added. In both situations, those forms are still active.

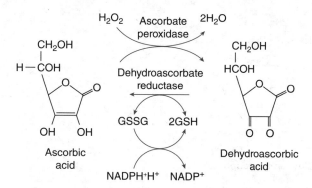

FIGURE 11.2 Chemical Structures of Ascorbic Acid and Dehydroascorbic Acid. Ascorbate can be reduced to dehydroascorbate by dehydroascorbate reductase and glutathione (GSH). The reduced ascorbate functions as an antioxidant.

Vitamin C is heat labile, readily dissolves in water, and is destroyed by alkali solutions but stabilized by acid solutions. Oxidation, as suggested previously, destroys the vitamin, whereas reduction stabilizes it. Vitamin C absorbs light, whereupon it is destroyed. Contact with iron and copper readily oxidizes ascorbate and destroys its activity.

Food Sources of Vitamin C

Vitamin C is available in many fruits and vegetables, with excellent sources being cantaloupe, kiwi, mango, honeydew, citrus fruits, papaya, strawberries, watermelon, asparagus, broccoli, brussels sprouts, cabbage, cauliflower, green and red peppers, and plantains. Vitamin C is susceptible to breakdown during certain cooking, processing, and storage procedures. For example, potatoes can lose almost half of their vitamin C by boiling, and spinach can lose nearly all its vitamin C if it is stored for 2 to 3 days at room temperature. Therefore, for practical purposes, citrus fruits and other vitamin C-containing fruits are better dietary sources of vitamin C because they are generally eaten fresh and raw. **TABLE 11.2** lists the vitamin C content of select foods.

Absorption of Vitamin C

Dehydroascorbic acid (DHA) and vitamin C can both be absorbed by passive diffusion, but the amount is small. DHA but not vitamin C can be absorbed by facilitated diffusion. DHA is rapidly converted to vitamin C when it enters the enterocyte, thereby maintaining a concentration gradient for DHA. Additionally, DHA binds to glucose transporters (GLUT 1-4) in the absorption process. However, the efficiency of vitamin C absorption appears to be high and occurs primarily

TABLE 11.2 Vitamin C Content of Select Foods

Food	Vitamin C (mg)
Fruits	
Orange juice, fresh (½ cup)	62
Kiwi (½ cup)	83
Grapefruit juice, fresh (½ cup)	47
Cranberry juice cocktail (½ cup)	54
Orange (½ cup)	74
Strawberries, fresh (1 cup)	89
Cantaloupe (½ cup)	33
Grapefruit (½ cup)	36
Raspberries, fresh (½ cup)	16
Watermelon (½ cup)	5
Vegetables	
Green peppers (½ cup)	60
Cauliflower, raw (½ cup)	23
Broccoli, raw (½ cup)	39
Brussels sprouts, cooked (½ cup)	48
Collard greens (½ cup)	17
Cauliflower, cooked (½ cup)	27
Potato, baked with skin (1 large)	29
Tomato (½ cup)	10

via a sodium-dependent and gradient-coupled carrier mechanism in the small intestine. Two transporters have been known to be involved with his mechanism: **sodium-ascorbate cotransporter 1 (SVCT1) and 2 (SVCT2).** DHA does not use this transport system. At an intake level of up to 180 milligrams per day, approximately 80% of vitamin C is absorbed. Above that level, saturable levels are achieved and much of the additional absorption is due to passive absorption. It is estimated that at doses approaching 5 grams, only about one-fourth of vitamin C is absorbed. However, this can still lead to significant levels of absorption, because 25% of 5 grams is 1.25 grams.

The brain has high levels of vitamin C compared with other organs. As such, the brain uses SVCT2. SVCT2 has a high affinity to vitamin C and there is a greater concentration of them in the brain. This likely explains the high level of vitamin C in the brain relative to other tissues and organs.

Functions of Vitamin C

Vitamin C is a cofactor in several important enzymatic reactions (**FIGURE 11.3**). It is an activator of a hydroxylase enzyme involved with collagen synthesis (see Figure 11.3a). Collagen is the most abundant protein in the human body and is found in tendons, bones, cartilage, skin, the cornea, and in interstitial spaces. Approximately 30% of its amino acids are glycine, with proline, hydroxyproline, and hydroxyserine each contributing approximately 20%. Collagen, as synthesized by fibroblasts, has a helical structure. Three collagen helices twisted together form a larger, left-handed helix called **tropocollagen**. Multiple tropocollagen helices are cross-linked together to form a strong collagen fiber. Hydroxylation of the proline to produce hydroxyproline in collagen chains allows for subsequent cross-linking via lysyl oxidase. This is significant because one-third of collagen is composed of proline. Prolyl and lysyl hydroxylases both require iron as a cofactor, and vitamin C functions as a reductant, maintaining iron in a reduced state. Lysyl oxidase requires copper for optimal activity.

Vitamin C is well known for aiding in the absorption of iron by promoting the **ferrous** (Fe^{2+}) iron state. Iron in this oxidation state is better absorbed, as opposed to the **ferric** (Fe^{3+}) state. Although this process may be extremely important in iron-deficient individuals, it is still not clear whether excessive vitamin C consumption increases the risk of iron overload. However, preliminary research indicates that it may not be a concern because consumption of 1 to 2 grams of vitamin C daily does not appear to increase iron status indicators, such as ferritin.

Vitamin C is probably necessary for two reactions in the formation of carnitine (see Figure 11.3b). The reactions involving vitamin C are hydroxylations and are very similar to those discussed for collagen synthesis. The two enzymes, trimethyllysine hydroxylase and 4-butyrobetaine hydroxylase, require iron as a cofactor, and vitamin C is the preferred reductant. Carnitine is needed to transport longer-chain fatty acids across the mitochondrial inner membrane so that they can engage in β-oxidation.

The hydroxylation reaction that converts the amino acid phenylalanine to tyrosine is catalyzed by phenylalanine hydroxylase, an iron-containing enzyme found in the liver and kidneys (see Figure 11.3c). A substrate for this reaction is tetrahydrobiopterin, which is converted to dihydrobiopterin. Vitamin C is needed to regenerate tetrahydrobiopterin from dihydrobiopterin. Vitamin C participates in another key reaction in the metabolism of tyrosine catalyzed by the copper-dependent enzyme p-hydroxyphenylpyruvate hydroxylase (reaction not shown).

Tyrosine is converted to DOPA by tyrosine monooxygenase, an iron-dependent enzyme. DOPA decarboxylase, a vitamin B_6-dependent enzyme, converts DOPA to dopamine. The dopamine β-hydroxylase (monoxygenase) reaction that produces norepinephrine from dopamine that was derived from tyrosine requires ascorbate to reduce copper at its active site. The adrenal glands are the primary site of this reaction, and this tissue has the highest concentration of vitamin C compared with other tissues or organs. Vitamin C appears to be needed to allow for a release of some of the adrenal hormones into the circulation. Vitamin C may, therefore, play a role in stress reactions. In another reaction related to neurotransmitters, vitamin C is needed for the conversion of the amino acid tryptophan to serotonin. The vitamin is needed to produce tetrahydrobiopterin from dihydrobiopterin in the reaction shown in Figure 11.3d.

Vitamin C is known for its antioxidant capacity, particularly in the aqueous portions of a cell. As an antioxidant, it seems to be very efficient in reducing superoxide (O_2^-) and hydroxyl radicals (OH^-) as well as hydrogen peroxide (H_2O_2). Recent investigative efforts have revealed that vitamin C promotes the reduced form of vitamin E, which itself can help protect LDL from oxidation. In this manner, vitamin C may indirectly decrease the development of atherosclerotic lesions.

Recommended Levels of Vitamin C Intake

The DRI for vitamin C is expressed as an RDA for those older than 1 year. Currently, the RDA for adults varies by sex. For adult women, it is set at 75 milligrams and for adult men, it is 90 milligrams per day. However, the actual requirements are probably much lower than the recommended amounts. During pregnancy, the RDA is 85 milligrams, and for the first 12 months of lactation, it is 120 milligrams.

Interestingly, smokers have lower serum levels of vitamin C than nonsmokers because the metabolism

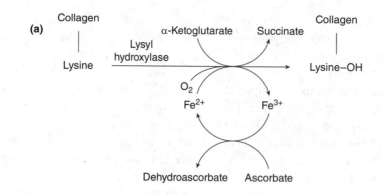

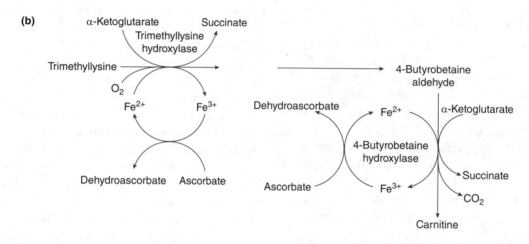

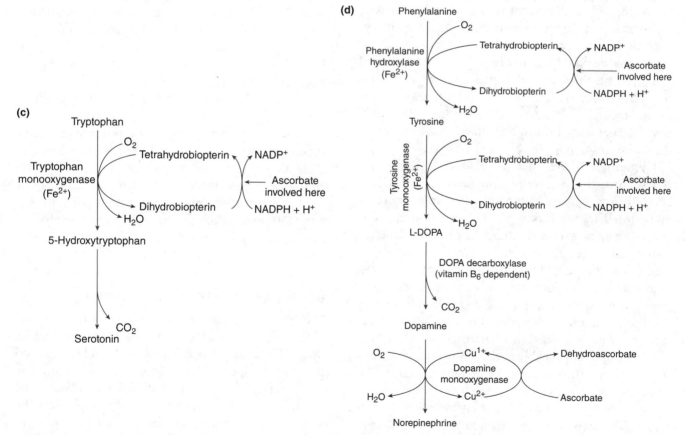

FIGURE 11.3 Different Metabolic Pathways in Which Vitamin C Plays a Critical Role. (a) collagen synthesis. (b) carnitine synthesis depends on vitamin C. (c) production of numerous neurotransmitters is facilitated by vitamin C. (d) production of serotonin from tryptophan depends on vitamin C.

of vitamin C is greatly enhanced. Thus, it takes about twice the amount of dietary vitamin C to achieve similar serum levels in smokers as in nonsmokers. As a general rule, it is recommended that male adult smokers consume 125 milligrams of vitamin C per day, and female adult smokers 110 milligrams per day.

Infants have an adequate intake (AI) of 40 milligrams per day from birth to 6 months of age, and 50 milligrams per day from 7 months until 12 months of age.

Vitamin C Deficiency

A deficiency of vitamin C is known to result in scurvy. This disease is characterized by abnormal bone growth, joint pains, bleeding gums, and tiny petechial hemorrhages beneath the skin. Normal blood clotting is hindered, and the capillaries become very weak because the underlying connective tissue is compromised due to impaired collagen synthesis. An abrasion to the surface of the skin may result in many petechial hemorrhages in individuals with scurvy. Hemorrhaging occurs around hair follicles and in the gums, muscles, bones, gastrointestinal tract, and kidneys. In severe cases, teeth may become loose and fall out. Susceptibility to infections due to wound exposure is a possibility. Edema occurs due to a shift in osmotic pressure, resulting from the loss of blood proteins during episodes of hemorrhaging. Infants develop a so-called scorbutic rosary in which the rib cage exhibits swollen bone joints. In milder cases, rheumatic-like pain is frequent. Signs and symptoms of mild deficiency include a yellowish complexion, listlessness, and some psychic disturbances (in both mild and severe deficiencies) as a result of imbalances in neurotransmitters.

As little as 10 milligrams of vitamin C may be enough to prevent signs of scurvy. The adult RDA of 90 milligrams for males and 75 milligrams for females allows for higher serum levels and will prevent the development of signs of scurvy for at least 1 month after vitamin C is removed from the diet. Scurvy is not a problem in the United States today, although individuals afflicted with poverty or alcohol addiction may show some of the symptoms.

Vitamin C Toxicity

Vitamin C is one of the most popular nutritional supplements. It has been purported to be a prophylactic or treatment for the common cold as well as for cancer. Vitamin C supplementation in quantities approaching gram doses has been advocated by several scientists, including Nobel Prize winner Linus Pauling. However, most of the scientific community does not support such aggressive supplementation suggestions.

Vitamin C toxicity can produce **rebound scurvy** among infants and pregnant women. Humans have developed an enzymatic mechanism to destroy excessive vitamin C. Vitamin C supplementation by individuals or pregnant women, therefore, results in higher levels of those enzymes in their tissue, including fetal tissue. Thus, an infant is at higher risk of vitamin C deficiency if he or she consumes only breast milk, which is a marginal vitamin C source at best. Children and adults supplementing with larger doses of vitamin C can also develop rebound scurvy once the supplementation is stopped. It is recommended that individuals taper their reduction of vitamin C supplementation.

Chronic excessive vitamin C ingestion can lead to inaccurate readings on blood glucose tests (due to pancreatic β-cell damage), intestinal bleeding and other anomalies of the digestive tract, adrenal failure, reduced fertility and bone growth, suppression of mitosis, hemolytic reactions, and kidney stone formation. Calcium oxalate crystals are the most prominent component of kidney stones. Oxalates are a primary metabolite of vitamin C and are voided in the urine.

Asians and individuals of African or Middle Eastern descent appear to be more sensitive to vitamin C toxicity. Hemolytic anemia is common among individuals in those groups who take supplemental vitamin C at well above normal doses. Supplementation of 100 to 300 milligrams per day is generally considered sufficient, and up to 1 gram per day is safe. Above that level, there may be increased risk associated with vitamin C supplementation.

● BEFORE YOU GO ON . . .

1. What happens to the content of vitamin C in food if the food is cooked in an iron skillet and why?

2. Why is vitamin C important for phenylalanine and tyrosine metabolism?

3. What role does vitamin C play in collagen formation from a biochemical perspective?

4. why does vitamin C improve the absorption of dietary iron?

5. How are ascorbate and dehydroascorbate absorbed by the small intestine?

Vitamin C and Disease Prevention and Treatment

The role of vitamin C in disease prevention is controversial. Claims that vitamin C can prevent the common cold, cancer, and other diseases have been widespread for years. Scientists, many of them notable, have advocated the intake of vitamin C supplements to prevent diseases. One such scientist was Nobel laureate Linus Pauling. Consumption of vitamin C supplements has been advocated to reduce the incidence of cancer, stroke, coronary heart disease, and cataracts. Many of the theoretical beneficial effects have been attributed to the role that vitamin C has as an antioxidant.

Scores of studies have examined whether vitamin C in large enough doses can prevent the common cold. Vitamin C does have an antihistamine effect, which has been hypothesized to lessen the symptoms of a cold. However, doses as large as 2 grams per day have not been shown to reduce the incidence or duration of symptoms of the common cold. The majority of studies suggest that vitamin C does not prevent or lessen a cold's symptoms.

Does vitamin C help in the treatment of cancer? Pauling advocated dosages of up to 10 grams per day to treat cancer and extend the life of cancer patients. Unfortunately, other researchers have not confirmed this hypothesis. There has been some concern and speculation that taking too large a dose of vitamin C may actually increase the progression of a tumor in cancer patients by increasing the growth of cancer cells. As an antioxidant, vitamin C could protect cancer cells against free radicals. Radiation and chemotherapy are used to create free radicals to kill cancer cells, and; therefore, vitamin C could also make cancer cells resistant to treatment.

The use of vitamin C in patients with coronary heart disease is a bit more promising. Vitamin C can cause blood vessels to widen or dilate and increase blood flow. Lipoprotein B oxidation is inhibited with vitamin C. Patients who consume 500 milligrams of vitamin C per day have fewer complications related to blood flow. High sensitivity C-reactive protein (hsCRP) is a predictor of coronary heart disease. A study on 200 heart failure patients revealed that those with a vitamin C deficiency had significantly elevated levels of hsCRP. Epidemiology studies suggest that the risk of mortality from heart disease is increased with vitamin C deficiency.

The studies just discussed focused on whether vitamin C could correct or cure a disease. Can vitamin C *prevent* a disease? The results here are a bit more promising. Five servings of fruits and vegetables per day provide a person with about 200 milligrams of vitamin C per day, almost three times the RDA. Increased intake of fruits and vegetables is associated with a decreased risk for various cancers, obesity, and other diseases. Is the level of vitamin C in those foods part of their protection against those diseases? Studies have suggested that taking vitamin C supplements at a level sufficient to saturate tissues and cells (400 milligrams per day) does have a cardioprotective effect.

Although taking large supplements of vitamin C cannot cure cancer, can vitamin C prevent cancer? Again, available studies show that people who consume more vitamin C have reduced cancer rates of various types. People who consume 80 to 110 milligrams of vitamin C daily have a reported decreased rate of incidence of cancers of the mouth, throat, esophagus, stomach, colon, rectum, and lung. Vitamin C may reduce the risk of esophageal and gastric cancers by preventing the formation of cancer-causing nitrosamines in the mouth. The results have been mixed for breast cancer, but some evidence suggests that those who consume more than 200 milligrams of vitamin C per day have a decreased risk compared with those who consume an average of 70 milligrams per day. Another study suggested that among those diagnosed with early-stage breast cancer, vitamin C supplementation decreased reccurrence. For more information about vitamin C and disease prevention, see http://lpi.oregonstate.edu/infocenter/vitamins/vitaminC/.

Thiamin, Riboflavin, Niacin, and Vitamin B$_6$

Thiamine, riboflavin, niacin, and vitamin B$_6$ are discussed separately from the other vitamins. The rationale is that these vitamins are linked in various ways to the TCA or Kreb's cycle. Thiamin, riboflavin, and niacin act as either co-factors or co-enzymes for many metabolic reactions, particularly those that impact energy utilization via the Kreb's cycle. Vitamin B$_6$ is involved in transamination of certain amino acids. The carbon skeleton for these reactions comprises amino acids or their derivatives that are intermediates of the Kreb's cycle. Vitamin B$_6$ also has a separate function: it is involved in enzymatic reactions that

may convert one type of amino acid into another, particularly non-essential amino acids.

Thiamin (Vitamin B$_1$)

Thiamin was first recognized as essential in 1896 by Christiaan Eijkman, a Dutch physician who traveled to the Dutch East Indies to help prisoners. He altered their food supply by removing brown rice and providing polished rice. The prisoners became sick, as did pigeons who normally fed from the rice. Some of the pigeons that had access to the hulls did not suffer or were found to be recovering from the disease. Eijkman shifted the diets of the prisoners back to the brown rice and noticed a reversal of symptoms. He

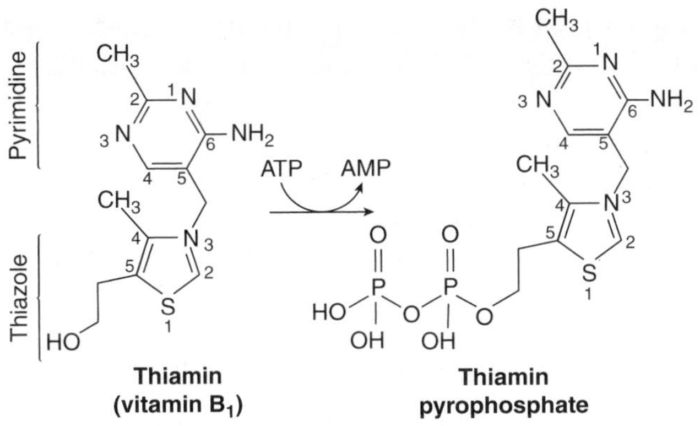

FIGURE 11.4 The Structure of Thiamin and the Metabolically Active Form, Thiamin Pyrophosphate. The methylene group bridges two components of thiamin: a pyrimidine group and a thiazole ring. Most thiamin in animals is phosphorylated with thiamin pyrophosphate being the predominant form participating in cell metabolism.

discovered that the process of polishing the rice left a water-soluble material behind. Later, Willem Donath and Barend Jansen, who worked in Eijkman's laboratory, isolated and crystallized the active factor. Then, in 1912, Casimir Funk determined that the active factor was an amide (nitrogen-containing structure) and referred to it as a vital amine, or *vitamine*. Robert Williams, at the University of Texas in 1936, discovered the structure and synthesized the vitamin.

Thiamin is composed of two chemical components: a pyrimidine group and a thiazole ring, as depicted in **FIGURE 11.4**. A methylene group bridges the two groups. The molecule may be split at this methylene group by sodium bisulfite or the enzyme thiaminase, the latter of which is found in fish or the bracken fern. At one time, mink breeders fed raw fish to the animals, and the minks died due to a thiamin deficiency caused by thiaminase activity. The methyl group at the 2 position of the thiamin pyrimidine group may be replaced with an ethyl or propyl group, but this results in a less-active vitamin. Replacement with a butyl group actually results in antithiamin activity.

When the amino group at position 6 is replaced by an OH group, the resulting compound is referred to as oxythiamin, which has antivitamin activity. Oxythiamin exacerbates thiamin deficiency symptoms related to nervous tissue. When the sulfur group at position 1 is replaced by an ethylene group, the compound is referred to as pyrithiamin, which is also an antivitamin and accentuates the fluid imbalance associated with thiamin deficiency. It should be pointed out that those derivatives are laboratory synthesized and do not occur in nature. Other compounds may interact with thiamin to cause it to become inactive, such as potassium phosphate, copper, and iron salts.

Dietary Sources of Thiamin

Good sources of thiamin in the diet are pork (probably the best source), whole grains, enriched or fortified cereals, liver, poultry, fish, eggs, potatoes, legumes, nuts, dark green vegetables, brewer's yeast, and wheat germ (**TABLE 11.3**). All of the thiamin available in plant sources is in the form of thiamin. In contrast, almost all of the thiamin in animal sources is phosphorylated, with 80% being thiamin pyrophosphate (TPP) [see Figure 11.4] and the remainder being thiamin monophosphate (TMP; sometimes referred to as thiamine diphosphate or TDP) and thiamin triphosphate (TTP). As mentioned earlier, certain foods, such as raw fish, contain thiaminases, which inactivate thiamin. Cooking (heat) inactivates thiaminases. Other antithiamin factors include tannic and caffeic acids. Those substances are heat stable and are found in foods such as coffee, tea, betel nuts, Brussels sprouts, and blueberries.

Digestion, Absorption, and Transport of Thiamin

Thiamin phosphates must be digested by intestinal phosphatases to yield free thiamin. Absorption is high and takes place rapidly, primarily in the jejunum and secondarily in the duodenum and ileum. The uptake actively occurs against a concentration gradient, with metabolic inhibitors reducing uptake. In vivo and in vitro findings have revealed that inhibitors of Na^+–K^+ ATPase and a lack of sodium could inhibit thiamin uptake. Two transport proteins have been identified: **THTR1 and THTR2**. They are saturable and pH dependent. In addition to the small intestine, these transports are found in a wide variety of tissues. In the small intestine, THTR2 is responsible for the absorption from the lumen to the enterocyte; whereas THTR1 is responsible for the transport of thiamin from the enterocyte to the blood. These carriers absorbed thiamin in the free form. Passive absorption does occur and may be significant when luminal thiamin content is high. Intake levels greater than 5 milligrams daily result in an increase in passive diffusion. Alcohol reduces thiamin absorption. However, it does not appear that mucosal uptake is inhibited; more likely, the transfer of thiamin to the serosal side is inhibited via an inhibition of Na^+–K^+ ATPase.

Thiamin can be phosphorylated within mucosal enterocytes to form thiamin pyrophosphate (TPP); sometimes also referred to as thiamin diphosphate (TDP). Thiamin that is in the TPP or TDP form can be converted to thiamin monophosphate (TMP). Thiamin triphosphate (TTP) is synthesized from TDP by a phosphoryl-transferase enzyme. This latter reaction is more common in the liver than enterocytes.

TABLE 11.3 Thiamin Content of Select Foods

Food	Thiamin (mg)
Meats	
Pork roast (3 oz)	0.49
Beef, ground cooked (3 oz)	0.055
Ham (3 oz)	0.27
Liver, pan fried, 1 slice	0.01
Nuts and seeds	
Sunflower seeds, roasted (¼ cup)	0.03
Peanuts, dry roasted (¼ cup)	0.16
Almonds (¼ cup)	0.06
Grains	
Bran flakes (1 cup)	0.50
Macaroni, cooked (½ cup)	0.19
Rice, white, cooked (½ cup)	0.17
Bread, wheat (1 slice)	0.08
Vegetables	
Peas, cooked (½ cup)	0.18
Lima beans (½ cup)	0.06
Corn (½ cup)	0.07
Broccoli, raw (½ cup)	0.03
Potato (1 large)	0.19
Fruits	
Orange juice (½ cup)	0.1
Orange (½ cup)	0.1
Avocado, raw, pureed (½ cup)	0.1

The TMP is the major form of thiamin that is absorbed and it is transported from the enterocyte to the blood by another carrier, reduced folate carrier (RFC). This is also thought to be an active sodium-dependent mechanism. Apparently, only TMP and thiamin are able to cross cellular plasma membranes, therefore, explaining the relative lack of the polyphosphorylated forms of thiamin in the blood.

Metabolism and Functions of Thiamin

An adult body may contain approximately 30 milligrams of thiamin. Approximately one-half of body thiamin can be found in skeletal muscle; other tissues with higher thiamin concentrations include those with high metabolic expenditure, such as the heart, liver, brain, and kidneys. Thiamin is necessary for biochemical reactions involving the metabolism and release of energy from carbohydrates. Thiamin is largely active as TPP, which is used by some tissues in glycolysis and the TCA cycle reaction series presented in **FIGURE 11.5**.

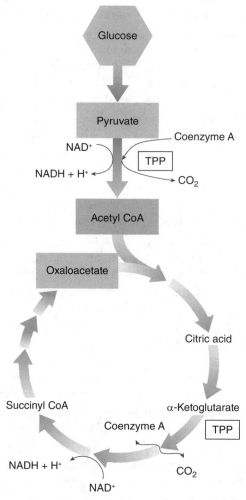

FIGURE 11.5 The Role of Thiamin via Thiamin Pyrophosphate in the Krebs Cycle. Thiamin functions in glycolysis and the Kreb's cycle in the form of thiamin pyrophosphate (TPP).

Most of this reaction occurs in the liver, but other tissues have the capability of producing TPP. Thiamin is phosphorylated using ATP in the presence of the enzyme thiamin pyrophosphokinase. Basically, this form of thiamin is a coenzyme needed for oxidative decarboxylation of α-ketoacids (pyruvate and α-ketoglutarate) and α-keto-sugars via a transketolase reaction, in which an aldehyde group is removed from the molecule (**FIGURE 11.6**).

The pyruvate dehydrogenase enzyme complex is necessary for the conversion of pyruvate to acetyl CoA. This reaction occurs within the mitochondrial matrix; the acetyl CoA created is then available to condense with oxaloacetate (OAA) to form citrate, the first molecule of the TCA or Krebs cycle. TPP is a critical component, along with lipoic acid, Mg^{2+}, NAD^+, and coenzyme A. Thiamin, as TPP, is also necessary for a key reaction of the Krebs cycle whereby α-ketoglutarate is converted to succinyl CoA. The necessary components of the α-ketoglutarate dehydrogenase enzyme complex, which catalyzes this reaction, are the same as for pyruvate dehydrogenase. In both of those thiamin-dependent reactions, NADH is produced, which delivers electrons to the electron transport chain for ATP generation.

Thiamin, as TPP, also functions at an important step in the cytosolic hexose monophosphate shunt or pentose phosphate pathway. Here, TPP functions as a coenzyme for a transketolase reaction. The metabolic significance of the pentose phosphate pathway is to generate NADPH for synthetic operations and

ribose for nucleic acid synthesis. Thiamin also appears to be important for impulse conduction in neuronal membranes. Although speculative at this time, it has been suggested that thiamine may be involved in active transport of chloride and promote nerve impulses by regulating sodium channels.

Branched-chain α-ketoacid dehydrogenase is another enzyme whose activity is dependent on thiamin. This enzyme is critical to the metabolism of the branched-chain amino acids leucine, isoleucine, and valine. A deficiency of this enzyme leads to maple syrup urine disease, a genetic disease in which the urine of infants smells like maple syrup, as described in Chapter 6. Acid metabolites accumulate in the blood, and mental retardation is a frequent outcome if it is not diagnosed in time. A medical food-based diet is needed for individuals with this disease to keep the branched-chain amino acid levels low.

Another function of thiamin is that it is thought to be anti-inflammatory and neuroprotective, although indirectly. Production of thiazole from thiamin is anti-inflammatory and thought to inhibit cyclooxygenase. Thiazole production is dependent on the production of thiazole synthase. The precursor to this enzyme is TPP. However, the conversion involves a unique mechanism involving a substance known as a **TPP-riboswitch**. Simply stated, a riboswitch is an mRNA that contains a regulatory portion. When TPP binds to this element or to the regulatory portion, thiazole synthase is produced, which results in increased thiazole production.

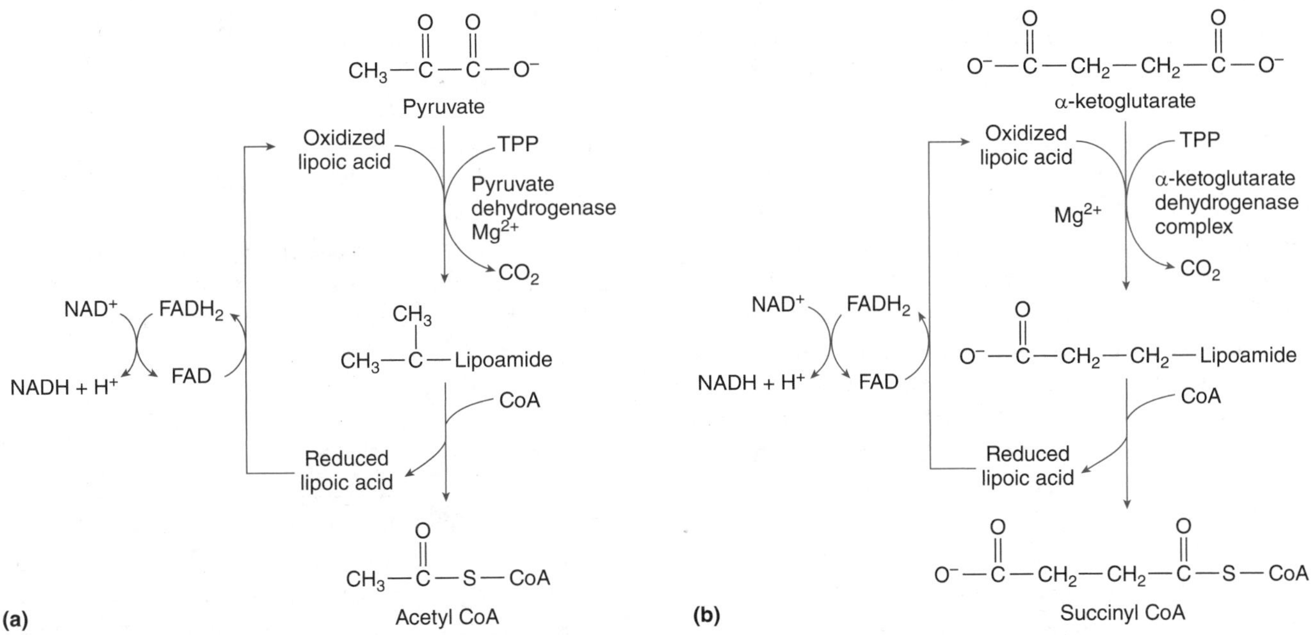

(a) Acetyl CoA

(b) Succinyl CoA

FIGURE 11.6 Role of Thiamine as a Coenzyme. Thiamine in the form of thiamine pyrophosphate (TPP) acts as a coenzyme to facilitate the conversion of (a) pyruvate to acetyl CoA and (b) α-ketoglutarate to succinyl CoA.

Recommended Levels for Thiamin Intake

Recommendations for thiamin intake are in milligram quantities. The AI is 0.2 milligram for infants younger than 6 months and 0.3 milligram for infants older than 6 months. An RDA is available for those older than 1 year and younger than 9 years: 0.5 to 0.6 milligram. For those 9 to 13 years old, the RDA is 0.9 milligram. For adolescent and adult males, it is 1.2 milligrams. For females aged 14 to 18 years, it is 1.0 milligram; the RDA rises to 1.1 milligrams thereafter. During pregnancy and lactation, the RDA increases to 1.4 milligrams.

Thiamin Deficiency

Severe thiamin deficiency produces mental confusion and muscular cramps, which are characteristic of the disease syndrome called **beriberi**. The polishing of rice, a staple food for many countries, leads to the development of beriberi by removing the thiamin in the rice hulls. The general refining (polishing, milling, refining) of grains, leaving only the endosperm, also results in the removal of most of the thiamin in grain. For instance, the endosperm only contains approximately 3% of the thiamin in a kernel of wheat. The remainder of thiamin is split between the germ (64%) and the bran layers (33%). Because of this, the U.S. government passed the Enrichment Act, which requires food manufacturers to resupply thiamin and other vitamins and minerals to products that use refined cereal products (e.g., flours).

One characteristic of beriberi is cardiac enlargement. The size of the heart can return to normal, however, if thiamin is returned to the diet in adequate amounts. In thiamin deficiency, there is inefficient utilization of carbohydrate, which can also lead to central nervous system–related problems, such as convulsions, head retractions, and spasms. Muscular anomalies can also occur, such as decreased tonus, improper peristalsis, and constipation. Anorexia is also a deficiency sign, as it is for many of the water-soluble vitamins, particularly the B vitamins.

In addition to cardiac enlargement, there appears to be a change in heart rate; however, this seems to vary among species. In humans, tachycardia is common; in rats, bradycardia results. Fluid imbalances are also frequent in beriberi. In humans, a marked loss of body fluids produces cachexia. An individual in this state appears to be a walking skeleton; this condition is frequently referred to as the "dry" type of beriberi. However, edema or fluid accumulation in tissue can occur, giving the affected individual a bloated appearance. When this occurs in thiamin-deficient individuals, it is referred to as "wet" beriberi.

Milder signs of thiamin deficiency that can be observed include fatigue, irregular heartbeat, a burning sensation in the feet, muscle cramps, and a loss of "tickle" in the fingers. A simple test used to diagnose thiamin deficiency is to have an individual sit on a table. Under normal conditions, the feet should be parallel to the floor. In deficiency, the feet point to the floor in what is referred to as foot drop syndrome.

There is another manner to obtain a thiamin deficiency that is of genetic origin. THTR1 mutations result in a thiamin-responsive megaloblastic anemia and many studies have focused on blood-related disorders. There is a variety of mutations in the gene that expresses THTR1. One consequence of the genetic defect appears to be aberrations within the mitochondria that mimic a mitochondrial disease. Some of the electron transport does not function normally. However, supplementation with thiamin appears to be beneficial in those patients with the defect. The other transporter, THTR2, also may have genetic mutations. In this deficiency, the brain appears to be impaired, particularly the basal ganglia. Patients develop what is termed a **Wernicke-like syndrome**, which affects the brain. Alcoholics often suffer from a thiamin deficiency and develop this disorder. In this genetic disease, patients respond to thiamin in combination with biotin. The role of biotin in modulating this disease with thiamin is not clear at the moment. Both of those diseases are rather rare with respect to the two genetic mutations.

Thiamin Toxicity

Thiamin ingestion in amounts exceeding 125 milligrams per kilogram body weight can cause physiologic problems. Edema, nervousness, sweating, tachycardia, tremors, an increased incidence of sores caused by the herpes virus, increased allergic reactions, fatty liver, and hypotension may occur. In rats, even sterility has been reported.

▶ Riboflavin (Vitamin B$_2$)

Riboflavin (**FIGURE 11.7**) was discovered shortly after the discovery of thiamin. It is synthesized by all plants and microorganisms, but not by higher organisms. This substance is fundamentally important in energy metabolism and occurs in foods and in the human body as either riboflavin or as flavin mononucleotide

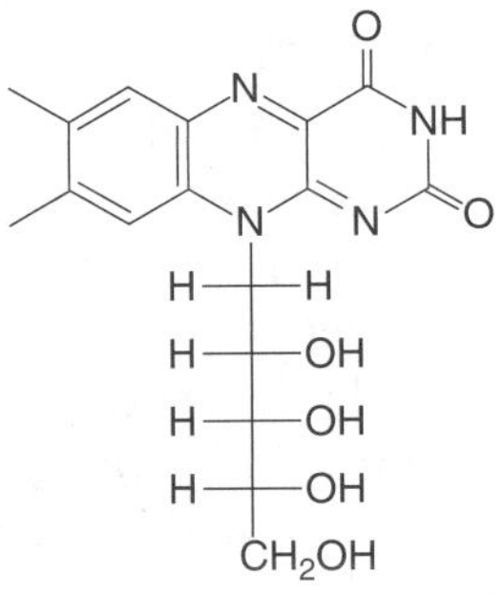

FIGURE 11.7 The Structure of Riboflavin. Riboflavin is synthesized by plants and microorganisms but not by higher organisms. It plays a key role in cell energy metabolism. Note that ribose is a component of riboflavin.

(FMN) or flavin adenine dinucleotide (FAD) bound to protein complexes (**FIGURE 11.8**). In 1917, riboflavin was shown to be a growth factor in yeast; it was also discovered that this substance was relatively heat stable yet was broken down to inactive structures with exposure to light. In solution, riboflavin produces a greenish-yellowish color that is readily obvious in urine. In 1935, the structure and synthesis of riboflavin were determined. The term *riboflavin* is derived from *ribose*, a component of this vitamin, and *flavus*, which is Latin for "yellow."

Dietary Sources of Riboflavin

Riboflavin is found in many foods, especially milk and dairy products (e.g., yogurt, cottage cheese), leafy green vegetables, beef liver, and beef and other meats (**TABLE 11.4**). Approximately one-half of the riboflavin provided in the American diet comes from milk and milk products. Meats are also a primary supplier of dietary riboflavin.

As mentioned previously, riboflavin appears to be relatively stable in heat—certainly more stable than vitamin C and thiamin. However, foods experience significant riboflavin losses when they are exposed to light. For instance, milk loses about one-third of its riboflavin activity when exposed to sunlight for about 1 hour. Fortunately, most milk producers no longer package their product in clear containers, such as glass bottles. This helps milk retain most of its riboflavin. Sun-drying and cooking foods in an open pot can lead to significant riboflavin losses as well. Like other water-soluble vitamins, riboflavin can also be washed away during boiling and thawing (thaw drip).

As is the case with so many other vitamins and minerals, the refining or milling of cereal grains removes most of the riboflavin. For instance, a kernel of wheat only has about 32% of its riboflavin in

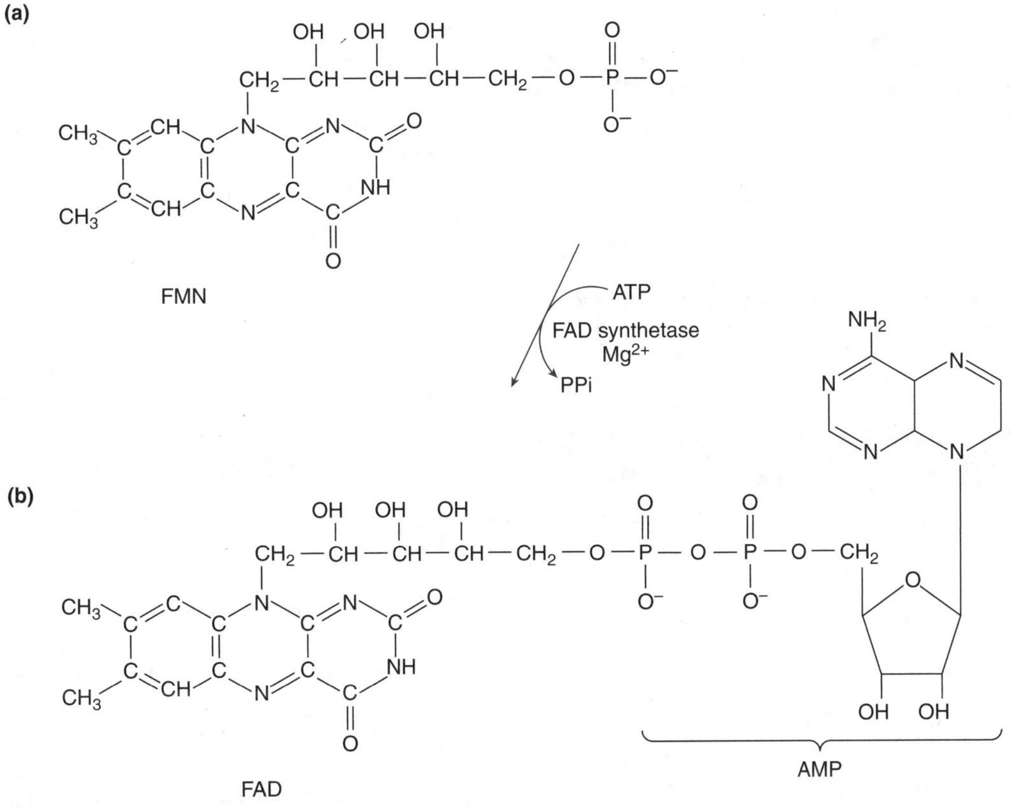

FIGURE 11.8 Structures of the Coenzyme Forms of Riboflavin. (a) flavin mononucleotide (FMN). (b) flavin adenine dinucleotide (FAD) are the two coenzyme forms. Both are involved in the transfer of electrons.

Food	Riboflavin (mg)
Milk and milk products	
Milk, whole (1 cup)	0.39
Milk, 2% (1 cup)	0.42
Yogurt, low fat (1 cup)	0.52
Milk, skim (1 cup)	0.45
Yogurt (1 cup)	0.35
Cheese, American (1 oz)	0.13
Cheese, cheddar (1 oz)	0.11
Meats	
Liver, pan fried (1 slice)	2.79
Pork chop, cooked (3 oz)	0.26
Beef, ground lean (3 oz)	0.13
Tuna, canned in water (3 oz)	0.04
Vegetables	
Collard greens (½ cup)	0.10
Broccoli, raw (½ cup)	0.05
Spinach, cooked (½ cup)	0.21
Eggs	
Egg (1 whole)	0.24
Grains	
Macaroni, cooked (½ cup)	0.10
Bread, wheat (1 slice)	0.08

TABLE 11.4 Riboflavin Content of Select Foods

the endosperm; the remaining riboflavin is distributed throughout the germ (26%) and bran layers (42%). Riboflavin is added to foods using refined cereal grain products in accordance with the Enrichment Act.

Absorption and Transport of Riboflavin

The coenzyme forms FAD and FMN represent most of the riboflavin in the diet. Pyrophosphatases and phosphatases in the upper portion of the small intestine act upon those coenzymes. The free riboflavin is absorbed by a saturable transport system that is rapid and dose proportional before reaching a plateau at approximately 25 milligrams per day. Riboflavin is absorbed by a transporter. Several riboflavin transporters in the absorption of riboflavin have been identified as described in a later section of this chapter. Three transporters are involved in the absorption of riboflavin: **RFVT1, RFVT2, and RFVT3**. RFVT2 may be involved in riboflavin transport by the small intestine but this transporter is found chiefly in the brain. RFVT3 is located on the brush border of the enterocyte and is responsible for riboflavin uptake from the lumen. RFVT1 and, perhaps RFVT2, are responsible for exporting riboflavin into the blood. Apparently, the presence of bile salts facilitates the uptake of riboflavin, and there is evidence to suggest that this uptake is also a sodium-dependent process. Once riboflavin is absorbed by the mucosal cells, it can be rephosphorylated to FMN. Riboflavin can dissolve into the plasma; about one-half is bound to proteins, primarily albumin and, secondarily, to globulins, fibrinogen, and other proteins. FMN is mostly found in the plasma bound to proteins, again, primarily albumin.

Metabolism and Roles of Riboflavin

Tissues and organs that have a greater riboflavin concentration include the heart, liver, and kidneys. Although the concentration of riboflavin in the brain is not as great as the tissues just mentioned, the brain seems more resistant to changes in riboflavin status than elsewhere in the human body. This suggests some form of regulation. It is estimated that the reserve of riboflavin in an adult is equivalent to metabolic demands for 2 to 6 weeks. Riboflavin is voided primarily in the urine.

In cells of all tissue, riboflavin can be interconverted to FMN and FAD. In the coenzyme forms (FAD and FMN), riboflavin facilitates the release of energy from carbohydrates, fat, and protein through the Krebs cycle, mitochondrial electron transport, and other electron transfer mechanisms. Both compounds play their basic roles in accepting electrons (and H$^+$) in biochemical reactions.

FMN is a cofactor for enzymes such as:

1. NADH dehydrogenase (transfers electrons from NADH to ubiquinone via the electron transport chain).

2.   L-amino acid oxidase and lactate dehydrogenase (used in the interconversion of pyruvate and lactic acid).

FAD is a coenzyme for enzymes such as:

1.   Cytochrome reductase (electron transport chain).
2.   Succinate dehydrogenase (Krebs cycle reaction).
3.   Acyl CoA dehydrogenase (β-oxidation of fatty acid).
4.   D-Amino acid oxidase (degradation of D-amino acids).
5.   Xanthine oxidase (oxidation of hypoxanthine and xanthine to uric acid).
6.   Monoamine oxidase (degradation of amine structures, such as tyramine).

Riboflavin is more than just a cofactor for enzyme activity. Riboflavin may be involved in protein stabilization and regulate apo-protein synthesis. Flavin homeostasis is a new and emerging field for this vitamin and involves some of the riboflavin transporters discussed above. There are a number of nervous and muscle disorders that are responsive to riboflavin supplementation. Mutations in the gene that encodes RFVT2 and RFVT3 lead to a neurodegenerative disorder sometimes referred to as **Brown-Vialetto-Van Laere syndrome** or multiple acylCoA dehydrogenase deficiencies, which are involved in fatty acid oxidations. The cranial nerves are most affected in infants, children, and young adults and can lead to deafness. Vision loss and weakness in the neck muscles may also occur. There can be significant mortality with this disease. However, it is now known that supplementation with large doses of riboflavin is used to successfully treat the disease. The range of supplementation used is rather large compared with the RDA and varies, ranging from 7 to 60 mg/kg body weight/day.

As suggested previously, the riboflavin transporters are distributed in various tissues. RFVT1 is found in placenta, intestine, and kidney; RFVT2 in almost all tissues but is especially high in brain and salivary glands; RFTV3 in prostate, testes, intestine, stomach, and pancreas. Thus, many tissues are susceptible to riboflavin transporter mutations. As much of the co-enzymes of riboflavin occur in the mitochondria, the impact upon cellular energetics can be profound.

Recommended Levels of Riboflavin Intake

The most recent RDAs for riboflavin are 1.3 milligrams for adolescent and adult males, and 1.0 milligram for adolescent females aged 14 to 18 years. The RDA increases to 1.1 milligrams for women older than age 18 years. During pregnancy, 1.4 milligrams is recommended. For lactation, the RDA is 1.6 milligrams. The requirements for riboflavin, like those of thiamin, are best described on an energy basis or, more specifically, on the basis of a 1,000-kilocalorie intake. In infancy, the DRI for riboflavin is expressed as an AI of 0.3 milligram per day from birth to 6 months of age and 0.4 milligram per day from 7 months until 12 months.

Riboflavin Deficiency and Toxicity

A decrease in energy release is the most obvious result of riboflavin deficiency because of riboflavin's critical role in the Krebs cycle and breakdown of fatty acids. The nervous system is typically the first region to develop problems due to its reliance on carbohydrate as an energy source. **Photophobia**, or sensitivity to light, can occur. There is increased vascularity around the eyeball, allowing for the appearance of bloodshot eyes. A riboflavin-deficient individual exhibits signs of dyscoordination. Overt signs of deficiency also include cracked skin around the mouth (cheilosis); inflamed lips; and a sore, inflamed tongue (glossitis) that develops a glossy appearance. The skin can oversecrete a waxy material (sebacea), resulting in seborrheic dermatitis, and anorexia is common. The enrichment of foods has made riboflavin deficiency rare in the United States. However, it is still prominent in countries where milled grains are a major component of the diet.

There does not appear to be great concern regarding riboflavin toxicity. Much of the excess riboflavin present in the human body is rapidly voided in the urine. Unlike the urinary loss of most other substances, riboflavin removal is visually obvious because urine turns a bright yellow. This effect is noticeable even with small doses of riboflavin. Riboflavin toxicity may result in gastrointestinal discomfort when intake levels exceed 1,000 milligrams per day.

▶ Niacin (Vitamin B₃)

Niacin has an interesting history and that history has been known since 1864. Niacin deficiency leads to **pellagra**, a disease that the southeastern portion of the United States experienced significant outbreaks of prior to 1935. In the mid-1920s, the U.S. Public Health Service sent a physician, Joseph Goldberger, to this area of the United States; at this time, pellagra was thought to be an infectious disease. Dr. Goldberger began to notice that if he changed the diets of those individuals who were afflicted, they appeared to experience less severe symptomatology. He realized that those with the disease consumed a monotonous diet of fatback, molasses, and grits (white corn). Adding milk, meat, or fresh vegetables either alone or in combination to the diet led to the resolution of symptoms. Dr. Goldberger was convinced that pellagra could be cured by dietary intervention. Later, in the 1930s, Conrad Elvehjem was able to show that niacin cured "black tongue" in dogs, which is the canine version of pellagra. Fatback and molasses are completely devoid of niacin, Grits are made from corn, and unless it is soaked in lime, niacin is unavailable for absorption. All three of those food items were common in the poor areas of southeastern United States.

Niacin is typically present as nicotinic acid (niacin) or nicotinamide, as shown in **FIGURE 11.9**. The pyrimidine ring with a carboxyl group at carbon number 3 is nicotinic acid. The presence of an amine group on this same carbon defines the structure as nicotinamide. Niacin is active in the human body in two coenzyme forms: nicotinamide adenine dinucleotide (NAD) and nicotinamide adenine dinucleotide phosphate (NADP) [**FIGURE 11.10**]. Both are involved in electron transfer operations.

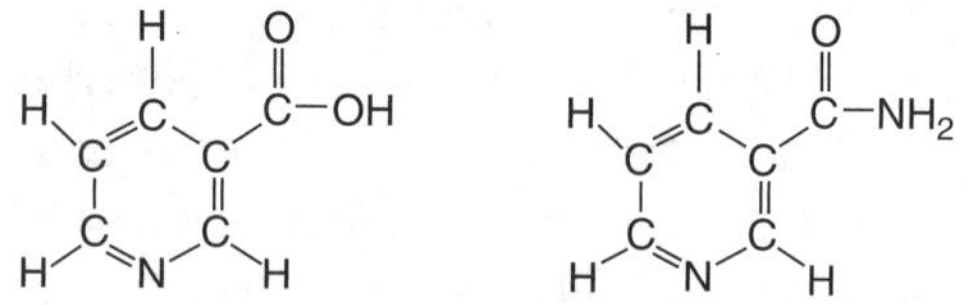

FIGURE 11.9 Chemical Structures of Niacin (Nicotinic Acid) and Nicotinamide. Nicotinic acid has a carboxyl group and nicotinamide an amine group. Nicotinamide is the form used in cell metabolism.

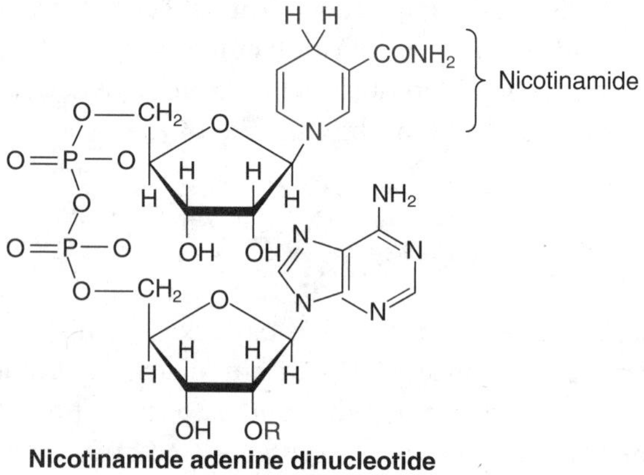

Nicotinamide adenine dinucleotide phosphate (NADPH)
R = PO(OH)$_2$
Nicotinamide adenine dinucleotide (NADH)
R = H

FIGURE 11.10 The Metabolically Active Forms of Niacin: Nicotinamide Adenine Dinucleotide (NAD) and Nicotinamide Adenine Dinucleotide Phosphate (NADP). NAD and NADP are coenzyme forms of nicotinamide and both are involved in the transfer of electrons.

Sources of Niacin

Nicotinic acid and nicotinamide are found well distributed throughout most foods. Brewer's yeast, most fish, pork, beef, poultry, mushrooms, and potatoes offer a higher niacin content than other foods (**TABLE 11.5**).

TABLE 11.5 Niacin Content of Select Foods

Food	Niacin (NE)
Meats and seafood	
Liver, pan fried (1 slice)	14.2
Tuna, canned in water (3 oz)	7.6
Turkey (3 oz)	5.8
Chicken (3 oz)	5.3
Salmon, cooked (3 oz)	6.3
Beef, round steak (3 oz)	4.5
Pork, cooked (3 oz)	4.0
Haddock, cooked (3 oz)	3.9
Scallops, steamed (1 oz)	1.9
Nuts and seeds	
Peanuts (1 oz)	3.8
Vegetables	
Asparagus, cooked (½ cup)	1.0
Grains	
Rice, brown (½ cup)	1.3
Noodles, egg, enriched (½ cup)	1.7
Rice, white, cooked, enriched (½ cup)	1.8
Bread, wheat (1 slice)	1.0
Milk and milk products	
Milk, whole (1 cup)	0.3
Cheese, cottage (½ cup)	0.2

1 niacin equivalent (NE) = 1 mg niacin and 60 mg tryptophan.

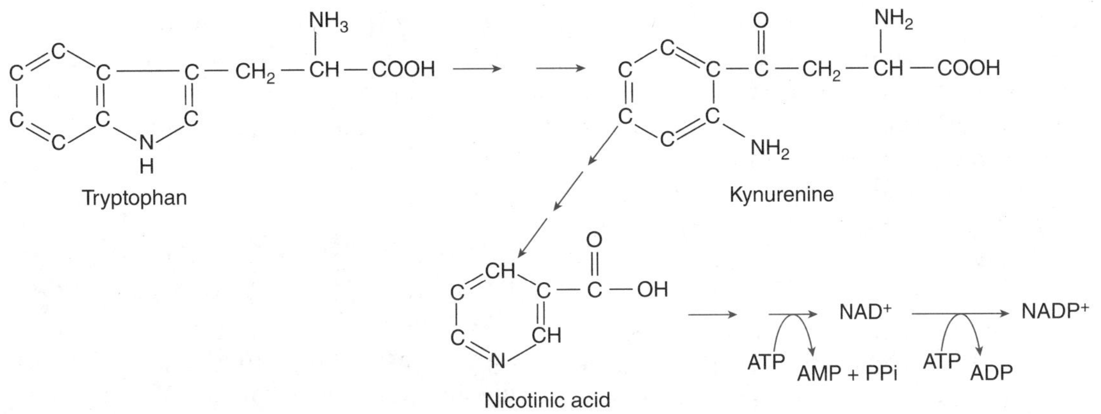

FIGURE 11.11 Biosynthesis of Niacin, NAD⁺, and NADP⁺ from Tryptophan. Not all sources of niacin are dietary. Three percent of the amino acid tryptophan may be converted to nicotinic acid, NAD⁺, and NADP⁺.

Plant foods contain nicotinic acid, whereas animal foods contain nicotinamide as well as the coenzyme forms NAD and NADP. Niacin forms in foods appear relatively stable during most methods of cooking and storage; some losses may be experienced when boiling foods and during thaw drip because the vitamin leaks out of a food.

Nicotinic acid can also be formed in human cells. The starting molecule is the essential amino acid tryptophan, as depicted in **FIGURE 11.11**. It is estimated that only about 3% of tryptophan is used in this manner. This process is considered inefficient for niacin production because it requires approximately 60 milligrams of tryptophan to create 1 milligram of niacin. This is largely due to the potential to irreversibly create intermediate molecules, such as kynurenic acid and xanthurenic acid. The process of niacin formation is also influenced by the levels of tryptophan and niacin ingested, protein and energy intake, and vitamin B$_6$ (involved in four reactions) and riboflavin nutriture. Finally, NAD⁺ and NADP⁺ are synthesized sequentially from niacin (nicotinic acid), which will be discussed in detail later.

Digestion and Absorption of Niacin

Niacin in its coenzyme forms must be digested to nicotinamide. This is accomplished by glycohydrolase in the small intestine. Although some absorption of nicotinic acid and nicotinamide can occur in the stomach, most absorption takes place in the small intestine. Nicotinamide and nicotinic acid appear to be taken up by mucosal enterocytes via a sodium-dependent, saturable, facilitated diffusion carrier mechanism at lower luminal concentrations. As the luminal concentration increases, more niacinamide and nicotinic acid are absorbed by simple passive diffusion.

Metabolism and Functions of Niacin

Nicotinic acid and niacinamide are both found in the plasma freely dissolved or bound to proteins (15 to 30%). In all human cells, nicotinamide is converted to NAD. Nicotinic acid can also be converted to NAD; however, this seems to occur mostly in the liver. NAD can be phosphorylated to form NADP (see Figure 11.11). NAD and NADP are involved in more than 200 enzymatic reactions, most of which are dehydrogenase reactions and many of which are reversible. Although most of the functions associated with NAD and NADP are attributable to their redox potential, more nonredox roles are becoming known.

With regard to carbohydrate utilization for ATP synthesis, NAD (NAD⁺) is reduced in one glycolytic reaction (the conversion of pyruvate to acetyl CoA in the mitochondria) and three reactions of the Krebs cycle. One NADH is created for each "turn" of β-oxidation of fatty acids, and the acetyl CoA created in this process can condense with oxaloacetate to form citrate. Two NADH molecules are generated per ethanol molecule metabolized by alcohol dehydrogenase. The NADH generated by those reactions can be transferred to the electron transport chain for ATP generation. Beyond energy metabolism, NAD is required for the conversion of pyridoxal (vitamin B$_6$) to its primary excretory metabolite, pyridoxic acid. Beyond redox operations, NAD probably serves as a donor of ADP ribose for post-translational modification of proteins associated with chromosomes (e.g., histone and nonhistone proteins). NAD is also speculated to be a possible component of glucose tolerance factor (GTF), but this is debatable.

NADP differs from NAD in that whereas most of the NADH generated is used to transfer electrons to the electron transport chain, most of the NADPH is used in synthetic processes. NADP is reduced to NADPH in two separate oxidative reactions of the pentose phosphate pathway. As mentioned previously, the pentose phosphate pathway is a means of generating NADPH for fatty acid synthesis. NADP is also reduced to NADPH by cytosolic malic enzyme; this NADPH can be used for fatty acid synthesis as well. NADPH is also needed for cholesterol synthesis. In the rate-limiting reaction involving HMG CoA reductase, two NADPH molecules are used. NADPH is also used in steroid hormone synthesis and the synthesis of deoxynucleotides for DNA. NADPH may also be used by cells to reduce dehydroascorbic acid to ascorbic acid.

Niacin in the form of $NAD^+/NADH^+$ or $NADP^+/NADPH^+$ functions more than just as cofactors in oxidative metabolism. It is known that NAD^+ and $NADP^+$ both have roles in mitochondrial health and age-related disorders.

The ratios of $NAD^+/NADH^+$ or $NADP^+/NADPH^+$ in essence can lead to mitochondrial biogenesis and better mitochondrial function. Those effects are modulated through a family of proteins called **sirtuins**. Sirtuins are sometimes referred to as silent information regulator 2 (Sir2), or **SIRT**. The function and activation of those proteins are dependent on the level of NAD^+ present in the cells. In mammals, there are seven sirtuins (1–7) and the different forms are located in various parts of the cell. In the nucleus, there is SIRT 1, 6, and 7; cytosol has SIRT 2; and the mitochondria SIRT 3, 4, and 5. SIRTs can have a variety of enzymatic activities. An example of a major function is the removal of acetyl groups from lysine or proteins and removal of succinate from enzymes as well. SIRTs may affect insulin secretion, gluconeogenesis, mitochondrial biogenesis, endothelial function, lipid metabolism, cell cycling, and apoptosis. This indicates clearly that the link between NAD^+ levels and SIRTs have profound effects.

In Chapter 1, we discussed PGC-1α as the master regulator of mitochondrial biogenesis. PGC-1α can be activated by deacetylation, demonstrating a molecular role for niacin. Another transcriptional factor is **forkhead box protein O1 (FOXO1)**, which controls mitochondria fatty acid metabolism and promotes protection from oxidative stress. SIRT 3 is a mitochondria deacetylase that affects proteins involved with fatty acid metabolism, ketogenesis, and antioxidant protection.

Taken together, increased NAD^+ levels are sensors to optimize mitochondria function. Decreased levels of $NAD^+/NADH^+$ ratios are observed in a number of mitochondria disorders (eg., diabetes, cancer, obesity, neurodegenerative disease) and aging. Experimental studies reveal that increasing the levels of NAD^+ can reduce mitochondria dysfunction and attenuate those diseases.

Recommended Levels for Niacin Intake

Recommended intakes of niacin are expressed as niacin equivalents, or milligrams NE. Sixty milligrams of tryptophan is equal to 1 milligram of niacin, and this factor is taken into consideration when determining the recommendations. The AI recommended for infants ranges from 2 to 4 milligrams NE per day. For adolescents and adults, the RDA ranges from 12 to 16 milligrams NE per day. During pregnancy and lactation, 18 milligrams NE per day and 17 milligrams NE per day are recommended, respectively.

Niacin Deficiency

As mentioned earlier, niacin deficiency can result in a syndrome called pellagra. Severe pellagra is characterized by the four Ds: dermatitis, diarrhea, dementia, and death. Gastrointestinal disturbances are common, including glossitis, stomatitis, abdominal discomfort, and severe diarrhea. The skin tends to become affected in areas exposed to light and in contact with heat. Lesions on the skin develop, with loss of cells and desquamation. Dementia can occur, characterized by disorientation and confusion. A manic type of behavior may also be observed. Many victims of pellagra in the past ended up in mental institutions because the dementia is irreversible.

The use of isoniazid, an antituberculosis drug and an antivitamin, can produce niacin deficiency symptoms relatively quickly, especially if the diet was previously marginal in niacin. An encephalopathy syndrome can develop. Uncontrollable sucking reflexes, stupor, delirium, and agitated depression are common mental symptoms.

Pharmacologic Use of Niacin and Toxicity

Nicotinic acid (niacin) is often prescribed in gram doses as a drug to lower total blood cholesterol, LDL-cholesterol, and triglyceride levels in individuals with hypercholesterolemia and hypertriglyceridemia. Usually, the dose required varies depending on the activity level, age, and sex of the individual. It is believed that nicotinic acid decreases mobilization of fatty acids from adipocytes, thereby decreasing circulation and uptake by the liver and incorporation into VLDL.

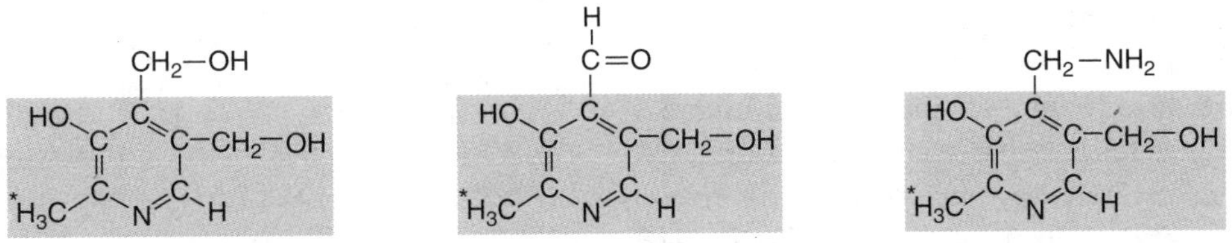

Pyridoxine (alcohol) Pyridoxal (aldehyde) Pyridoxamine (amine)

FIGURE 11.12 Structures of Naturally Occurring Vitamin B_6. Three forms of vitamin B_6. The asterisk (*) is the site of the PO_4 group to form pyridoxine phosphate, pyridoxal phosphate, and pyridoxamine phosphate, respectively.

Large doses of niacin in this form may produce toxic side effects, such as heart abnormalities, gastrointestinal problems, abnormal blood tests, hot flashes, skin irritations, liver damage, elevated blood glucose levels, and peptic ulcers.

Vitamin B_6

In 1935, Paul György demonstrated that dermatitis in rats was due to a new B complex factor. In 1939, Harris and Folks synthesized vitamin B_6. A few years later, compounds were identified that had similar properties to the synthesized vitamin. In 1945, pyridoxal phosphate was discovered as an active coenzyme.

Vitamin B_6 appears in the human body in six chemical forms. Three basic forms are pyridoxamine (the amine form), pyridoxal (the aldehyde form), and pyridoxine or pyridoxol (the alcohol form). The other three forms are 5′-phosphate derivatives of each of the basic forms. (**FIGURE 11.12**). Chemically, pyridoxine is stable to light and heat in acid solutions, but not at neutral or alkaline pH. Pyridoxal is probably the least stable form.

Food Sources of Vitamin B_6

All six forms of vitamin B_6 are found in foods. Pyridoxine is mostly found in plant foods, with good sources being bananas, navy beans, and walnuts (**TABLE 11.6**).

TABLE 11.6 Vitamin B_6 Content of Select Foods

Food	Vitamin B_6 (mg)	Food	Vitamin B_6 (mg)
Meat and seafood		*Fruits*	
Liver, pan fried (1 slice)	0.84	Banana (1)	0.43
Salmon, cooked (3 oz)	0.48	Avocado, pureed (½ cup)	0.33
Chicken, cooked (3 oz)	0.55	Cantaloupe (½ cup)	0.06
Ham (3 oz)	0.26	*Vegetables*	
Hamburger, lean cooked (3 oz)	0.34	Brussels sprouts, cooked (½ cup)	0.14
Pork, cooked (3 oz)	0.35	Potato, baked (1 large)	0.93
Eggs		Sweet potato, baked (½ cup)	0.29
Egg (1 whole)	0.07	Carrots, raw (½ cup)	0.09
Legumes		Peas, cooked (½ cup)	0.12
Kidney beans, cooked (½ cup)	0.18	*Nuts*	
Lentils, cooked (½ cup)	0.15	Walnuts (¼ cup)	0.16

Pyridoxal and pyridoxamine and their 5'-phosphorylated derivatives are almost exclusively found in animal products, with good sources being meats, fish, and poultry. Vitamin B$_6$ is fairly stable in cooking processes; however, some losses are experienced with prolonged exposure to heat, light, or alkaline conditions, as mentioned earlier. Also, the milling or refining of cereal grains removes vitamin B$_6$. For instance, the endosperm of a kernel of wheat contains only 6% of the wheat's pyridoxine, whereas the remainder is located in the germ (21%) and bran layers (73%).

Absorption of Vitamin B$_6$

Pyridoxal phosphate in the gut reacts with an intraluminal intestinal alkaline phosphatase or other phosphatases to remove the phosphate group. Absorption of the three nonphosphorylated forms of vitamin B$_6$ may occur by diffusion, primarily in the jejunum. There is also evidence that there is a pH-dependent, carrier-mediated mechanism of uptake that is sodium independent.

If the luminal concentration of the phosphorylated forms of vitamin B$_6$ is high, some will be absorbed as well. Vitamin B$_6$ absorption is relatively efficient and ranges roughly between 70 and 85% at physiologic doses. However, the efficiency of absorption decreases as intake increases. Within enterocytes, some of the pyridoxine can be phosphorylated to pyridoxine phosphate via pyruvate kinase. Also, pyridoxal can be converted to pyridoxal phosphate (PLP) via the kinase. In essence, this is a method of trapping the vitamin within the mucosal cell and preventing movement back into the lumen.

Metabolism and Function of Vitamin B$_6$

Approximately 60% of the circulating vitamin B$_6$ is in the form of PLP and is transported either within cells, such as erythrocytes, or is bound to albumin. Circulating pyridoxal is also found in red blood cells as well as bound to albumin. Some pyridoxamine is also found in the blood. The liver is a primary organ involved in the metabolism of vitamin B$_6$. Pyridoxal enters hepatocytes and is phosphorylated with ATP to produce pyridoxal phosphate in the presence of pyridoxal kinase, which requires magnesium. Pyridoxine and pyridoxamine can be oxidized to pyridoxal phosphate by FMN oxidase. Pyridoxal is also catabolized in the liver with 4-pyridoxic acid and pyridoxal lactone produced from pyridoxal. Those two compounds are excreted from the liver and other tissues and then excreted in the urine (**FIGURE 11.13**). The former compound represents as much as one-half of the vitamin B$_6$ found in the urine. There are also two anti-vitamin B$_6$ compounds: desoxypyridoxamine and a methyl ester of pyridoxamine. Those are thought to be produced by bacterial synthesis of the vitamin in the gut, but the general consensus is that they are insignificant to overall human vitamin B$_6$ status.

The functions of PLP are numerous, because they are involved in several metabolic pathways. The main function of PLP is to convert one type of amino acid to another type by transferring the amino group of one amino acid to a carbon skeleton in a Schiff base mechanism, a process called transamination

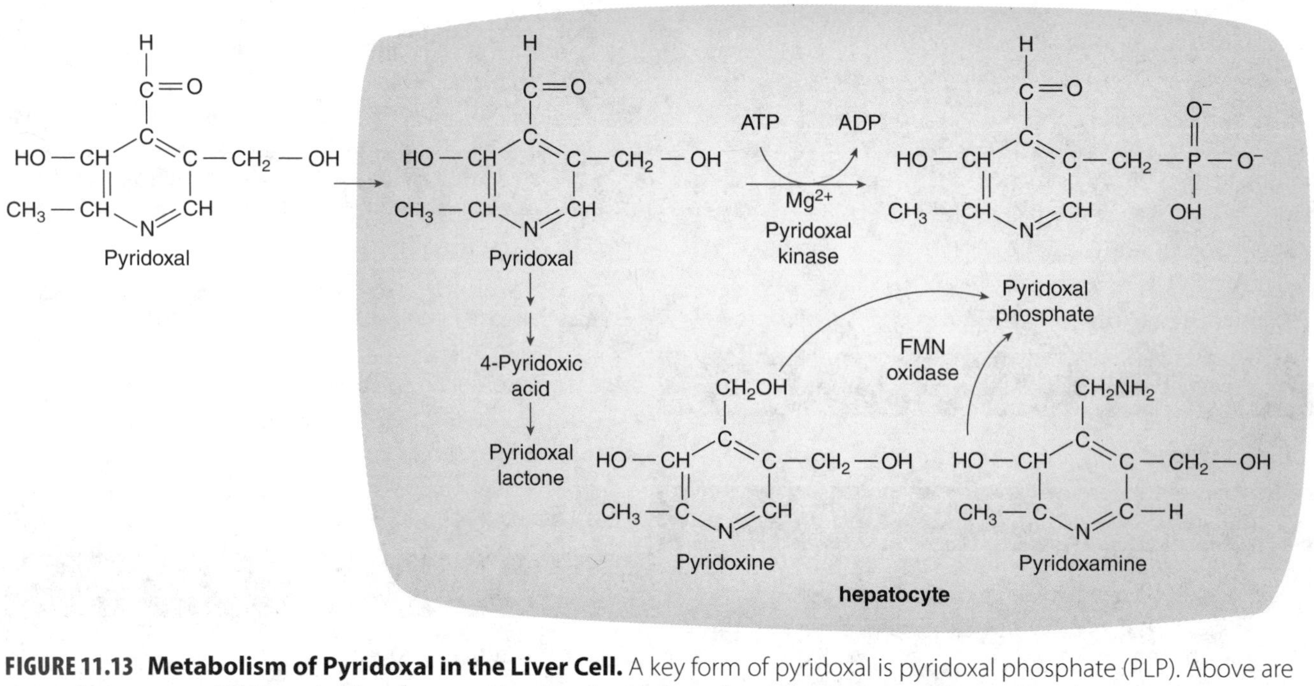

FIGURE 11.13 Metabolism of Pyridoxal in the Liver Cell. A key form of pyridoxal is pyridoxal phosphate (PLP). Above are the various routes of PLP production: from pyridoxal and oxidation of pyridoxine and pyridoxamine in hepatocytes.

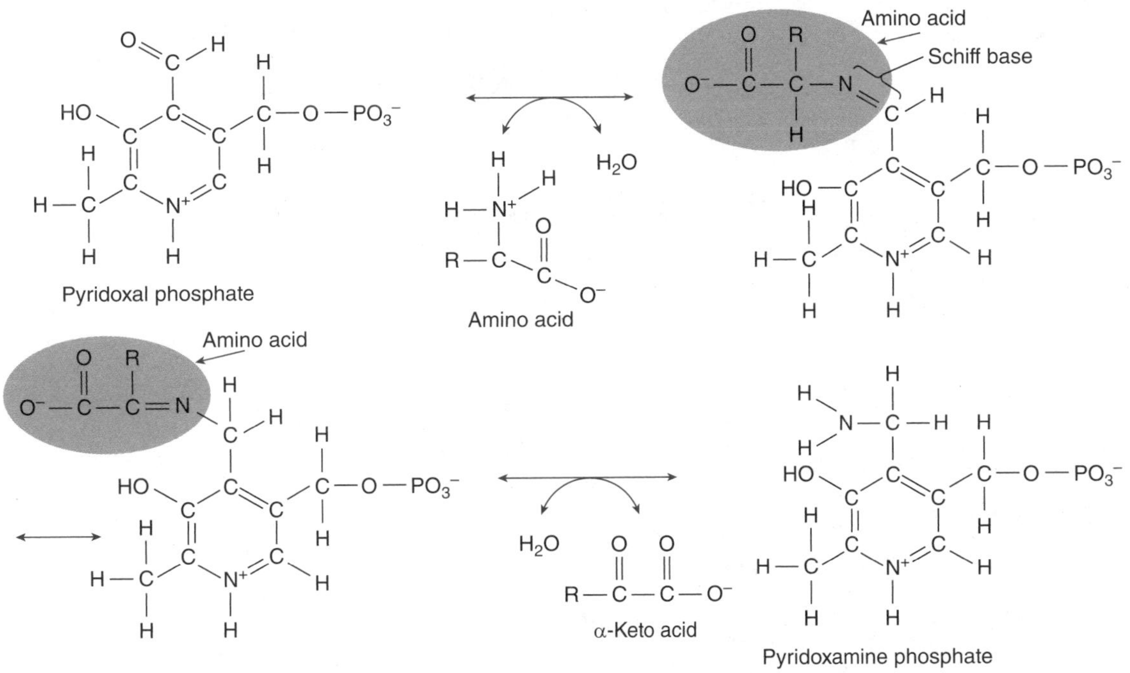

FIGURE 11.14 Schiff Base Mechanism for Pyridoxal Phosphate in Amino Acid Transamination Reactions.
R represents the carbon side chain of an amino acid.

(**FIGURE 11.14**). A Schiff base is a compound with a C=N group. The nitrogen is bonded to a hydrocarbon group. Transamination reactions reversibly pass an amino group from a donor amino acid to an α-ketoacid, such as pyruvate and α-ketoglutarate. For instance, alanine amino transferase (ALT) passesthe amino group from alanine to an α-keto acid to form pyruvate and an α-amino acid. More likely than not, α-ketoglutarate accepts the amino group to form glutamic acid (glutamate). In another reaction, aspartate amino transferase (AST) catalyzes the transfer of an amino group from aspartate to an α-ketoacid to form an α-amino acid and oxaloacetate.

During fasting and starvation or prolonged aerobic exercise, muscle cell α-ketoglutarate receives an amino group from branched-chain amino acids (leucine, isoleucine, valine) and aspartate to form glutamate. Subsequently, the amino group of glutamate can be transferred to pyruvate to form alanine via ALT. Alanine can then be released from skeletal muscle and circulate to the liver for conversion back to pyruvate and gluconeogenesis. PLP is also critical for the deamination of certain amino acids via deaminase enzymes. Transamination and deaminase reactions are important for several reasons. First, they may enable the generation of carbon skeletons of amino acids for energy and other metabolic pathways. Second, transamination reactions allow for the creation of certain nonessential amino acids. PLP is also involved in decarboxylation reactions as well as transulfhydration and desulfhydration reactions. For instance, the formation of γ-aminobutyric

acid (GABA) from glutamate (**FIGURE 11.15a**) and the synthesis of serotonin from 5-hydroxytryptophan (Figure 11.15b) require PLP. PLP is pivotal in the formation of several other neurotransmitters, such as histamine, dopamine, and norepinephrine (Figure 11.15c). PLP is involved in the creation of the nonessential amino acid cysteine from methionine, the conversion of tryptophan to niacin, and the breakdown of glycogen because it may positively influence glycogen phosphorylase activity.

PLP is important to the production of aminolevulinic acid (ALA), which is necessary in heme production (**FIGURE 11.16**). Succinyl CoA condenses with glycine to form an intermediate molecule that is subsequently decarboxylated by ALA synthetase (involving PLP), forming aminolevulinic acid. This compound is, in turn, dehydrated to form protoporphyrin and heme. PLP also appears to be required for the incorporation of iron into the heme molecule. The role of vitamin B$_6$ in hemoglobin formation is very important, as is demonstrated during a deficient state in which hypochromic microcytic anemia occurs.

Interestingly, vitamin B$_6$ is probably involved in sphingolipid and other phospholipid synthetic processes. Studies conducted as early as the 1930s involving rodents demonstrated that a vitamin B$_6$ deficiency resulted in decreased body fat, decreased liver lipids, and an impairment in lysosomal lipid degradation. The conversion of the ω-6 polyunsaturated fatty acid linoleic acid to arachidonic acid is also dependent on PLP. Vitamin B$_6$ status also influences the immune system; deficient animals demonstrate a hindered cell-mediated immune response.

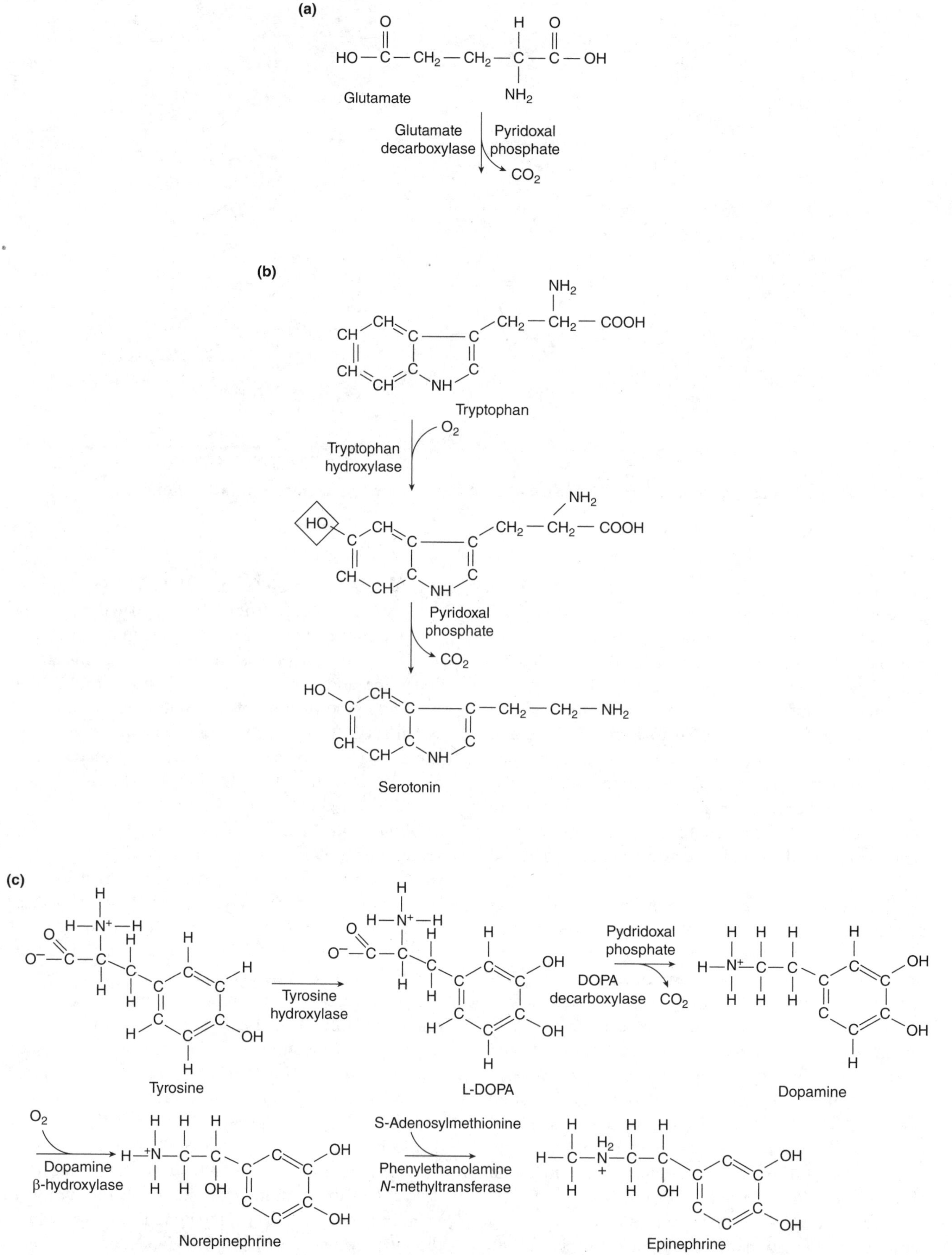

(a)

Glutamate

Glutamate decarboxylase | Pyridoxal phosphate

CO_2

(b)

Tryptophan

O_2

Tryptophan hydroxylase

Pyridoxal phosphate

CO_2

Serotonin

(c)

Tyrosine

Tyrosine hydroxylase

L-DOPA

Pyridoxal phosphate

DOPA decarboxylase CO_2

Dopamine

O_2

Dopamine β-hydroxylase

Norepinephrine

S-Adenosylmethionine

Phenylethanolamine N-methyltransferase

Epinephrine

FIGURE 11.15 Formation of Key Neurotransmitters Involving Vitamin B$_6$. (a) γ-aminobutyric acid (GABA), (b) serotonin, (c) DOPA, dopamine, norepinephrine, and epinephrine.

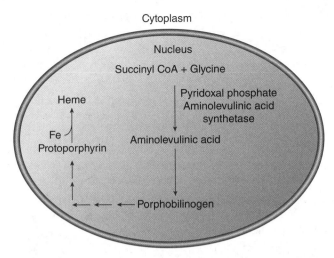

FIGURE 11.16 Role of Pyridoxal Phosphate in Heme Biosynthesis. Pyridoxal phosphate is a cofactor for aminolevulinic acid synthetase, the rate-limiting enzyme in heme biosynthesis.

Several tests can be performed to evaluate vitamin B$_6$ status. The most direct and perhaps most commonly applied measure is plasma PLP levels. However, it is important to note that other physiologic factors, such as increased protein intake, smoking, and age, can also influence PLP levels. In addition to plasma PLP levels, vitamin B$_6$ status can be evaluated by measuring urinary metabolites of tryptophan and methionine pathways as well as erythrocyte transaminase activity. However, the use of oral contraceptives is known to increase the activity of those transaminases but decrease vitamin B$_6$ pools, particularly in the blood.

Recommended Levels of Vitamin B$_6$ Intake

The DRI for infants is expressed as an AI; for those older than 12 months, it is expressed as an RDA. The RDA for vitamin B$_6$ ranges from 1.0 to 1.3 milligrams for adolescents and adults. For those over 50 years old, the RDA increases to 1.5 milligrams for females and 1.7 for males. During pregnancy, the RDA is 1.9 milligrams; and for lactation, it is 2.0 milligrams.

Vitamin B$_6$ Deficiency and Toxicity

Cases of vitamin B$_6$ deficiency, although rare, have been reported. Infants fed formula in which vitamin B$_6$ was accidentally destroyed by high-heat autoclaving developed vitamin B$_6$ deficiency. Individuals being treated for tuberculosis are at increased risk of vitamin B$_6$ deficiency because the isoniazid commonly prescribed for treatment is an antagonist to vitamin B$_6$. Drugs, such as penicillamine, corticosteroids, and anticonvulsants, can also inhibit vitamin B$_6$ activity. The production of acetaldehyde formed by alcohol (ethanol) metabolism may, in turn, destroy some vitamin B$_6$–associated structures.

Vitamin B$_6$ deficiency affects the central nervous system and can cause convulsions, particularly in infants and children, as well as other behavioral abnormalities. Depressive symptoms and peripheral neuritis are often observed. Poor growth, decreased antibody formation, and some vague symptoms such as weakness, irritability, and insomnia have also been reported. Dermatitis with lesions around the mouth, eyes, and nose is common. Niacin levels may also be depleted or lowered, which may confound the deficiency signs. Some inborn errors of metabolism have an impact on vitamin B$_6$ metabolism. An example is cystathionurea, in which cystathione lyase is deficient; supplementation with vitamin B$_6$ may be used to help treat the disease. The immune response in humans may be compromised by poor vitamin B$_6$ status, increasing the risk of infection and illness.

At one time, vitamin B$_6$ was advocated by health food stores as a treatment for premenstrual syndrome. Some women who were taking 2 grams per day developed toxic symptoms, such as pins and needles in the feet caused by irreversible nerve damage. Numbness of the mouth can also occur. With regard to pregnancy, a drug once used for morning sickness called Bendectin, a derivative of vitamin B$_6$, was commonly prescribed. This drug was banned by the FDA because of evidence that women who consumed it had a higher incidence of stillbirths, infants born with birth defects, and infants who suffered sudden infant death syndrom.

● BEFORE YOU GO ON . . .

1. How are thiamin, riboflavin, and niacin involved in the energy-yielding biochemical pathways?

2. Explain how thiamin and riboflavin are absorbed?

3. If dietary sources of niacin are deficient, how can the body adapt to maintain some levels of tissue niacin?

4. Of the four water-soluble vitamins just discussed, which ones will lead to dementia and other central nervous system disorders in deficiency states?

5. What are SIRTS, including which vitamin they interact with and what their function(s) is (are)?

6. What is the main biochemical function of pyridoxal phosphate?

7. Which of the four water-soluble vitamins that were discussed can lower blood lipid levels when used in large doses?

▸ Folate, Vitamin B₁₂, Biotin, and Pantothenic Acid

Folate, Vitamin B_{12}, biotin, and pantothenic acid are discussed here under a separate category as they are different from the other water-soluble vitamins discussed earlier. Folate and vitamin B_{12} overlap each other in that a deficiency of either results in a megoblastic anemia that is characterized by immature red blood cells. Often, people with this type of anemia were misdiagnosed as to whether folate or vitamin B_{12} was deficient. Folate, as explained in this section, is part of a pathway known as the methyl folate trap in which Vitamin B_{12} plays a critical role if folate is deficient in the diet.

Biotin and pantothenic acid are different. Biotin is critical to the metabolism of carbohydrates, fatty acids, and leucine as it is a co-enzyme for enzymes that play key roles in their metabolism. Pantothenic acid is a part of acetyl CoA, which has a multitude of functions in metabolism, particularly energy metabolism, as discussed throughout this text.

▸ Folic Acid (Folate)

In 1930, folic acid was identified by Lucy Wills and became known as the Wills factor. For a while, it was confused with vitamin B_{12} because a deficiency in either led to a similar type of anemia. In 1938, the name vitamin M was given to the folate in food because it was recognized as an essential growth factor in monkeys. In 1939, folate was also called factor U, and by 1940, the term *Lactobacillus casei* growth factor had been coined.

The structure of folic acid is best described as a complex of individual compounds, as depicted in **FIGURE 11.17**. A pterin nucleus is bound to para-aminobenzoic acid (PABA) to form pteroic acid. Glutamic acid is linked to the PABA portion of pteroic acid, forming folate or pteroylmonoglutamic acid or pteroylmonoglutamate. Although all three components of folate can be synthesized in the human body, humans lack the conjugase enzyme that condenses those components to form folate. Therefore, folate is nutritionally essential.

Dietary Sources of Folate

Folate is available in a wide variety of foods derived from both animal and plant sources (**TABLE 11.7**). Good sources include vegetables such as asparagus, spinach, mushrooms, Brussels sprouts, broccoli,

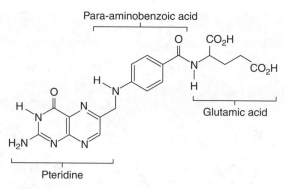

FIGURE 11.17 Structure of Folic Acid. Folic acid is composed of 3 compounds bonded together: a pteridine nucleus, para-aminobenzoic acid, and glutamic acid. These three compounds can be synthesized in humans, but the conjugase enzyme that binds these components together is absent in humans. Thus folate is required in the diet.

turnip greens, and legumes, such as lima beans and peas; nuts; some fruits, such as citrus fruits and their juices; organ meats; and whole grain products. The word *folate* is derived from **folium** (Latin for "leaf") in reference to some of the better providers of this vitamin in the diet. Nonorgan meats are not a good source of folate. Furthermore, the limited availability of folate in meats is drastically reduced during cooking because folate is generally unstable in heat. That also means that foods consumed raw retain more of their folate content. It is estimated that as much as 50 to 80% of the folate in foods may be lost during processing and preparation.

Folate is different from folic acid. Folate is the natural compound found in foods, and folic acid is the synthetic form used in supplements and enriched foods. Folic acid is more potent than folate because more folic acid is absorbed by the small intestine.

Absorption of Folate

As naturally found in foods, folate may have as many as nine or more glutamate residues attached to PABA. However, only the monoglutamate form is found in human plasma. Thus, polyglutamates must be digested to the absorbable monoglutamate form. This process is performed by intestinal conjugases or γ-glutamylcarboxypeptidases that are primarily active in the jejunum. Those enzymes are both soluble and membrane-bound proteins. The folate produced by bacteria in the colon is normally in the monoglutamate form. Most of the folate absorption is believed to occur via a sodium-independent, saturable,

TABLE 11.7 Folate Content of Select Foods	
Food	**Folate (µg)**
Vegetables	
Asparagus, cooked (½ cup)	134
Brussels sprouts, cooked (½ cup)	47
Peas, cooked (½ cup)	37
Spinach, cooked (½ cup)	131
Lettuce, romaine (½ cup)	32
Lima beans (½ cup)	18
Sweet potato, cooked (½ cup)	6
Broccoli, raw (½ cup)	28
Fruits	
Cantaloupe (½ cup)	19
Orange juice (½ cup)	23
Orange (½ cup)	42
Grains	
Rice, white, enriched, cooked (½ cup)	107

carrier-mediated mechanism on the brush border or more simply, facilitative diffusion. Two types of folate transporters have been identified: 1) **reduced folate carrier (RFC)** and 2) **proton-coupled folate transporter (PCFT)**. RFC operates in both the small and large intestine, whereas little PCFT is found in the large intestine. RFC functions in a neutral pH environment and PCFT in an acidic environment. Folates do not diffuse across membranes efficiently. Those transporters are found in many other tissues outside of the gastrointestinal system, but RFC appears to be the major transporter of folate in other tissues. Hereditary folate malabsorption, while rare, is due to a mutation in the gene that expresses PCFT. Because the defect results in severe folate deficiency, PCFT is thought to be the major transporter of folate for intestinal absorption.

Because at least one of the conjugases is zinc dependent, zinc deficiency can decrease folate absorption. Excessive alcohol consumption and drugs, such as sulfin-pyrazone, phenylbutazone, ethacrynic acid, and furosemide (Lasix) also decrease folate absorption by inhibiting digestion or competing for absorptive mechanisms. Once inside the mucosal enterocyte, folic acid may be reduced to dihydrofolate, tetrahydrofolate (THF), and methylated primarily at the N^5 position to form 5-methyl THF.

Metabolism and Functions of Folate

Folate may be transported in portal and systemic blood will either be freely dissolved or bound to blood proteins. Although some of the folate is bound to albumin, albumin has a relatively low affinity for folate. Folate circulates as a monoglutamate. Folate-binding proteins (FBPs) have also been identified within blood cells and have a higher binding affinity. Folate is taken into cells in a carrier-mediated fashion, which may require energy. Those human cells that turn over, such as red blood cells, hepatocytes, and epithelial cells, have higher folate content.

Within cells, the folate molecular structure can be metabolized in three ways. First, glutamic acid residues can be added to form polyglutamate forms of folic acid. This probably serves to trap folate within a particular cell. Second, folate is reduced on the pterin nucleus, at N^5 and N^8 and at C^6 and C^7, giving rise to tetrahydrofolate, as depicted in **FIGURE 11.18**. $NADPH_2$ is required for this reduction, which is catalyzed by dihydrofolate reductase. Third, once in the THF form, which is sometimes referred to as the active form, the structure can accept single-carbon moieties (**FIGURE 11.19**).

Carbon moieties or units can attach at the N^5 or N^{10} position or form a bridge between those positions. The carbon units can be in the form of a methyl group (as in 5-methyl THF), an aldehyde group (as in 10-formyl THF), an imino group (as in N^5-formimino THF), a methylene bridge (as in 5,10-methylene THF), or a methylidyne bridge (as in 5,10-methylidyne/methyl THF).

Once carbon moieties are attached to THF, folate can become involved in a variety of synthetic and other metabolic processes. For instance, the single-carbon unit from folate is used to make the amino acid methionine from homocysteine and the amino acid glycine from serine as well as to synthesize nucleic acid precursor molecules (e.g., dTMP and purines) [see Figure 11.19]. Because of this function and the need for replicating cells to copy their DNA prior to cell

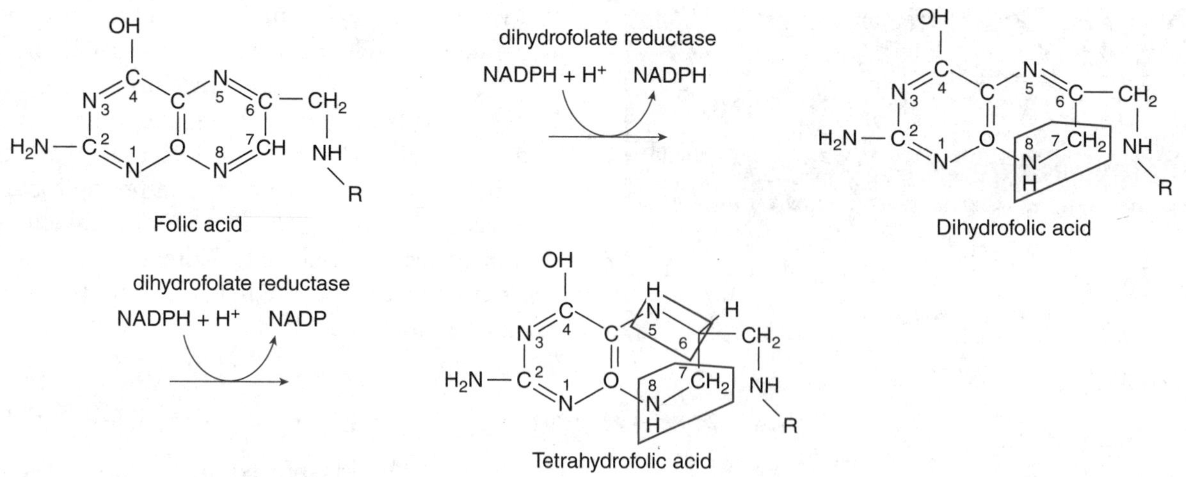

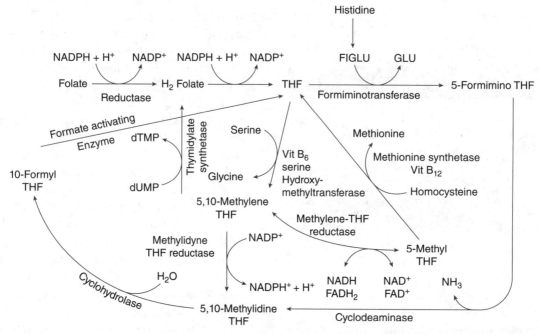

FIGURE 11.18 Activation of Folic Acid. Tetrahydrofolic acid (THF) is produced from folic acid. THF is the active form of folate. Boxes show where changes are occurring.

FIGURE 11.19 The Interconversion of One-Carbon Moieties Attached to Tetrahydrofolate (THF). Once tetrahydrofolate is formed, folate becomes involved in a variety of reactions involving one-carbon moieties. For example, glycine and methionine may be produced. dTMP and purines are also synthesized, which are precursors to nucleic acid molecules for DNA.

division, folate is recognized as one of the most important vitamins with regard to tissue turnover. Folate is also necessary in the complete catabolism of histidine to glutamate. One of the metabolites involved in the conversion of histidine to glutamic acid is *N*-formiminoglutamic acid (FIGLU), which requires THF as a cofactor to remove a formimino group. The concentration of FIGLU increases in tissues and the blood and FIGLU appears in the urine if folate stores are compromised.

Beyond the acquisition of single-carbon units by THF, other molecular derivatives that have physiologic significance are possible. An aldehyde group at N^5 or N^{10} is possible, as is an imino group at the N^5 position. Aminopterin, which has an amino group at N^4, is an antineoplastic drug and has antifolate activity. Other antivitamin forms are possible and are useful as chemotherapeutic agents because folate is required for cell division. Methotrexate is one such chemotherapeutic agent that inhibits folate metabolism because it hinders dihydrofolate reductase activity. The net result of methotrexate inhibition is to decrease the conversion of folate to THF.

The Methyl–Folate Trap

Once THF is formed, it can become involved in several reactions in which a single-carbon unit is attached. The major reaction, however, results in the formation of 5,10-methylene THF. This reaction is bidirectional. 5,10-Methylene THF can be converted irreversibly to 5-methyl THF via catalysis by methylene-THF reductase. 5-Methyl THF can then be converted back to THF via the transfer of the methyl group to homocysteine to form methionine (see Figure 11.19). This reaction is catalyzed by methionine synthase, which requires vitamin B_{12} as a coenzyme. If vitamin B_{12} is deficient within a cell, folate can become trapped as 5-methyl folate. As more and more THF follows the pathway just described, a cell becomes void of THF. Thus, a vitamin B_{12} deficiency can create a conditional folate deficiency, thereby explaining why many of the manifestations associated with deficiencies in those vitamins are the same. In fact, the macrocytic anemia that results from the conditional folate deficiency is used as a diagnostic indicator of a vitamin B_{12} deficiency.

If folate is provided by dietary means in large doses, as with supplements, it decreases the need for THF recycling within cells via the reaction that requires vitamin B_{12}. Therefore, the macrocytic anemia will not result and a vitamin B_{12} deficiency can go undetected. Because folic acid supplementation can mask a vitamin B_{12} deficiency, folate levels in supplemental form are federally limited. One of the manifestations of a protracted and severe vitamin B_{12} deficiency is irreversible neurologic alterations, and the most critical manifestation is death.

Recommended Levels for Folate Intake

The DRI for folate has an AI for infants and an RDA for those older than 12 months. In 1989, the RDA for folate ranged from 150 to 200 micrograms for adolescents and adults. Given the concern over folate status and birth defects and perhaps other disorders, the DRI was increased to 400 micrograms for adolescents and adults of both sexes. During pregnancy, the RDA is 600 micrograms, declining to 500 micrograms during lactation.

The actual recommended levels are based on folic acid, not folate. A **dietary folate equivalent** is a unit of measure used to indicate the conversion of folic acid to folate. If 200 micrograms of folic acid in supplemental form is consumed along with 150 micrograms of folate from food, a correction factor is needed. The 200 micrograms of folic acid are multiplied by the factor 1.7 and are equal to 340 micrograms of folate activity. Add to this number the 150 micrograms from the diet, and a total of 490 micrograms of dietary folate equivalents is obtained.

Folate Deficiency and Toxicity

Folate deficiency leads to a **megaloblastic macrocytic anemia**, as just discussed. In this type of anemia, red blood cells are large and immature and their numbers are reduced, which results in a reduced oxygen-carrying capacity of the blood. Pathologic changes to the digestive tract mucosa also result from a folate deficiency. Mucosal villi shorten and the digestive tract wall thins. Much of this change is due to a reduced ability of the mucosal lining to replace enterocytes that are being sloughed off into the lumen of the intestinal tract. Leukopenia, or decreased white blood cell count, is another sign of folate deficiency.

Because folate is fundamentally important in rapidly dividing cells, good folate status is paramount during pregnancy, and the requirement increases accordingly. Individuals at greater risk of folate deficiency include those with chronically poor folate intake; women who have experienced multiple births; those enduring malabsorption situations (e.g., celiac disease), leukemia, Hodgkin disease, cancer, or burns; and alcoholics. Cancer increases folate requirements because of the high proliferation rate of cancerous tissue.

Psychosis and mental deterioration is associated with folate deficiency. In pregnancy, neural tube defects have been associated with elevated plasma homocysteine levels and low levels of folate. In a multinational study spanning nearly a decade, the risk of neural tube defect was reduced by 72% with periconceptual (4 weeks before and 8 weeks after conception) folate supplementation of 4 milligrams daily.

Folate supplements greater than 400 micrograms daily are considered a pharmacologic dose. Although intakes of 15,000 micrograms resulted in insomnia, malaise, irritability, gastrointestinal problems, and decreased zinc status, other reports of folate supplementation stated that there were no significant effects from taking 10,000 micrograms daily for months to years. However, as mentioned earlier, folate supplementation potentially can mask a vitamin B_{12} deficiency.

▶ Vitamin B₁₂

Vitamin B_{12} was the last of the water-soluble vitamins to be isolated and have its structure identified. This is partly due to this vitamin's relatively small requirement compared with other water-soluble vitamins. However, as far back as 1822, cases of anemia were described that were at that time believed to be due to a disorder of the gastrointestinal tract. Because that particular type of anemia was associated with a potentially fatal prognosis, it became known as **pernicious anemia** (*pernicious* means "leading to death"). In 1860, Flint noted that many of the individuals with this particular type of anemia exhibited degeneration of the stomach and that the glandular structures of the stomach appeared abnormal. In 1929, Castle demonstrated that normal gastric secretions contained a peptide that he called intrinsic factor (IF). Furthermore, it was hypothesized that this IF combined with an extrinsic factor, and that the combination of the two factors alleviated pernicious anemia. In 1948, Rickes, Smith, and Packer isolated vitamin B_{12}; in that same year, Beck demonstrated that vitamin B_{12} was the extrinsic factor or antipernicious anemia factor.

Vitamin B_{12} is composed of four pyrrole rings that form a porphyrin structure, as shown in **FIGURE 11.20**. This central part of the compound is called a corrin ring. The central core of the molecule contains cobalt; thus, the chemical name for this vitamin is cobalamin. A number of related compounds have cobalamin-like activity. One such compound is cyanocobalamin,

in which a cyanide (CN) group is attached to the cobalt atom and exists above the ring complex. The CN group must be removed before the molecule can be used as an active vitamin. Other substances can be attached to cobalt, such as OH (hydroxocobalamin), CH_3 (methylcobalamin), H_2O (hydrocobalamin), NO_2 (nitrocobalamin), and 5'-deoxyadenosyl (5'-deoxyadenosylcobalamin), in addition to others. Below the ring a heterocyclic nitrogen side chain may be present, or nothing may be attached. Often, a 5,6-dimethylbenzimidazole moiety is present as part of the attachment below the ring. Cobalt is in the Co^{3+} oxidation state and may form six bonds: four with the pyrrole nitrogen atoms, one with an attachment structure below the ring, and one with the substances mentioned previously (e.g., CN, CH_3) above the ring.

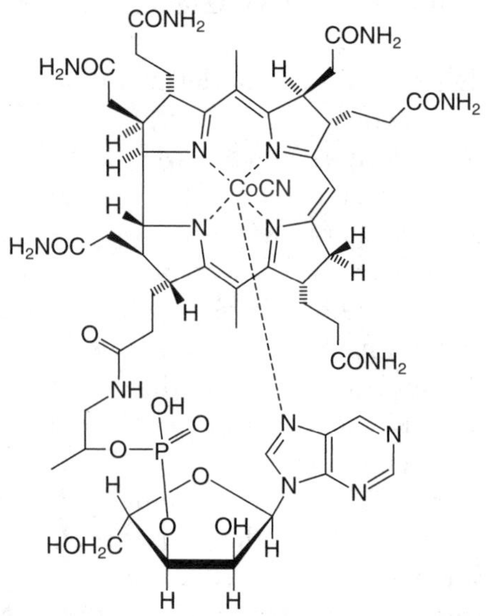

Vitamin B_{12} is a rather stable compound. Subjecting it to extreme heat (100–120°C) does not destroy the vitamin; however, intense ultraviolet light and visible light will result in significant destruction. Vitamin B_{12} is water soluble, especially in acid-type solutions; however, acids reduce its activity. The presence of other metals, such as iron and copper, which are strong oxidizing elements, can also destroy the vitamin. It is insoluble in chloroform and other fat solvents. Vitamin B_{12} is synthesized by micro-organisms and may also be synthesized in a laboratory, although the latter is a difficult procedure.

FIGURE 11.20 The Vitamin B₁₂ Form Cyanocobalamin.
Cobalt at the center of the ring (corrin ring) may have different compounds bound to it and maintain vitamin B_{12} activity once the compounds are removed from cobalt.

Food Sources, Digestion, and Absorption of Vitamin B₁₂

Vitamin B_{12} is only available from animal sources. Animals derive their vitamin B_{12} from microbes inhabiting their digestive tract. The best sources of vitamin B_{12} are meats, fish, poultry, shellfish, eggs, and milk and milk products (**TABLE 11.8**). The vitamin B_{12} content in those foods is modest, but compatible with human needs.

For vitamin B_{12} to be absorbed, it must bind to intrinsic factor (IF), which is produced by the parietal cells of the stomach mucosa. IF is a glycoprotein with a molecular weight of approximately 50,000. That protein essentially protects vitamin B_{12} from degradation as it moves through the intestinal tract to the ileum, the site of absorption. Although the large intestine can also absorb some vitamin B_{12}, the mechanism is generally undefined. That absorption is more significant for vitamin B_{12} of bacterial origin.

Vitamin B_{12} in foods is generally bound to proteins. Cooking food will release some of the vitamin, and pepsin in stomach juice will free the remaining

TABLE 11.8 Vitamin B$_{12}$ Content of Select Foods

Food	Vitamin B$_{12}$ (µg)
Meats/Fish	
Liver, pan fried (1 slice)	67.8
Salmon, cooked (3 oz)	2.8
Beef, hamburger, lean (3 oz)	2.2
Oysters (3 oz)	23.6
Crab (3 oz)	6.2
Lamb, cooked (3 oz)	2.1
Tuna, canned in water (2 oz)	1.7
Eggs	
Egg, fried (1)	0.6
Milk and milk products	
Milk, skim (1 cup)	1.0
Milk, whole (1 cup)	1.1
Yogurt (1 cup)	0.9
Cottage cheese (½ cup)	0.8
Cheese, American (1 oz)	0.4
Cheese, cheddar (1 oz)	0.2

protein-bound vitamin B$_{12}$ (**FIGURE 11.21**) The free vitamin then attaches to R proteins that are present in the saliva and gastric juices. R proteins are simply those proteins that bind to vitamin B$_{12}$. Vitamin B$_{12}$ bound to R proteins will eventually be picked up by IF even though the vitamin has a greater affinity for the R proteins. This is due to the digestion of R proteins by gastric proteases. Vitamin B$_{12}$ is released to IF to create a B$_{12}$-IF complex. Next, the B$_{12}$-IF complex binds to specific receptors on the brush border and crosses the intestinal mucosa via pinocytosis, where B$_{12}$ is released from IF and transferred to transcobalamin II. For the B$_{12}$-IF complex to attach to the receptor site, ionic

calcium and a pH greater than 6.0 are needed. Vitamin B$_{12}$ is transported into the mucosal enterocytes against a concentration gradient, so it is an active process and saturable as well. Once inside the cell, it binds to transcobalamin II. With pharmacologic doses of vitamin B$_{12}$, an increasing percentage of absorption is attributable to passive diffusion. At lower levels of ingestion (e.g., 0.1 microgram), absorption is approximately 80% efficient; however, as the dose increases, the percentage of absorption decreases.

Vitamin B$_{12}$ is released on the serosal side to the portal blood supply, most likely by means of exocytosis. Transcobalamin II is the major plasma transport protein for this vitamin. Transcobalamin I is another protein that can transport vitamin B$_{12}$ in the plasma; it is also involved in vitamin B$_{12}$ storage in the liver. Transcobalamin II is the major form in which the vitamin is delivered to the tissues. Methylcobalamin is the primary vitamin B$_{12}$ form found in the blood, accounting for as much as 80%; 5′-deoxyadenosylcobalamin makes up most of the remaining vitamin B$_{12}$ in the blood.

Metabolism and Function of Vitamin B$_{12}$

Vitamin B$_{12}$ is somewhat different from the other water-soluble vitamins in that it has significant storage and retention in the human body. The liver possesses the greatest concentration of vitamin B$_{12}$, and the total content in the liver may be 1.5 milligrams. Other tissues, such as the brain, kidneys, bone, spleen, and muscle, also present relatively higher concentrations. In the liver, the major form of the vitamin is 5′-deoxyadeno-sylcobalamin; as mentioned earlier, this contrasts with the situation in the blood, in which the major form is methylcobalamin. In hepatocytes, vitamin B$_{12}$ is added to bile that flows to the small intestine. As mentioned earlier, vitamin B$_{12}$ complexes with IF and is subsequently reabsorbed in the ileum and returned to the liver in the portal blood. Therefore, vitamin B$_{12}$ experiences enterohepatic circulation. The vitamin B$_{12}$ that is not absorbed from biliary secretions is excreted in the feces, thus making bile the primary means of ridding the body of excessive vitamin B$_{12}$. About 40 micrograms enters biliary secretions daily; however, almost all is reabsorbed. Some urinary losses occur as well; a typical urinary loss might be 0.025 microgram per day.

Vitamin B$_{12}$ appears to be involved in perhaps as few as three chemical reactions. One of the reactions involves the conversion of homocysteine to methionine (see Figure 11.19). Here, methylcobalamin is the coenzyme form and N^5-methyl THF is the methyl

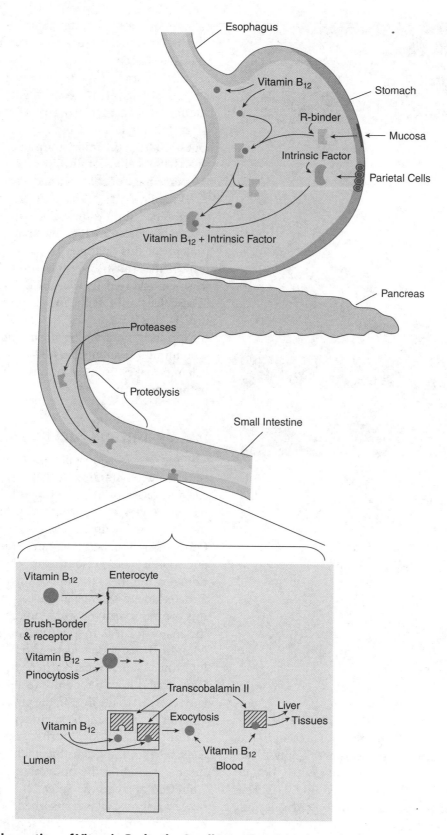

FIGURE 11.21 The Absorption of Vitamin B$_{12}$ by the Small Intestine. R-binder and Intrinsic Factor proteins protect vitamin B$_{12}$ in the stomach until they enter the small intestine. Vitamin B$_{12}$ binds to a receptor on the brush border of the enterocyte and is absorbed by pinocytosis into the enterocyte. It subsequently transverses the lumen bound to transcobalamin II and through exocytosis released into the blood where it is picked up by blood transcobalamin II. Here, the vitamin can be delivered to the liver or others tissues.

source. In this reaction, homocysteine methyltransferase (methionine synthetase) binds to vitamin B_{12}, and N^5-methyl THF transfers the methyl moiety to the cobalt of vitamin B_{12}. At this point, the methyl group, now bound to vitamin B_{12}, is transferred to homocysteine to produce methionine. As mentioned in the discussion of folate, if there is a lack of vitamin B_{12}, an accumulation of N^5-methyl THF occurs (the methyl–folate trap). That creates a lack of the folate or THF that is needed for nucleic acid metabolism. Such a block is responsible for the megaloblastic anemia characteristic of both vitamin B_{12} and folate deficiency.

Another reaction in which vitamin B_{12} plays a critical role is the conversion of L-proprionyl CoA to succinyl CoA (**FIGURE 11.22**). D-methylmalonyl CoA is produced from the catabolism of propionyl CoA, which itself is produced from the β-oxidation of odd-chain-length fatty acids as well as the amino acids methionine, threonine, and isoleucine. D-methylmalonyl CoA in the presence of an isomerase is converted to L-methylmalonyl CoA. L-methylmalonyl CoA is converted to succinyl CoA by methylmalonyl CoA mutase and vitamin B_{12}. In vitamin B_{12} deficiency, methylmalonyl CoA and methylmalonic acid accumulate in the blood. The latter compound is formed when methylmalonyl CoA is split. Because neural tissue uses propionic acid, that may explain the peripheral neuritis that accompanies vitamin B_{12} deficiency.

In another chemical reaction using vitamin B_{12} as a coenzyme, L-leucine is isomerized to β-leucine and vice versa. β-Leucine is created by intestinal bacteria and can be converted to L-leucine in a limited manner. Conversely, L-leucine can be converted to β-leucine, which can undergo subsequent transamination. The latter mechanism requires PLP and is believed to be an alternative means of leucine catabolism.

Recommended Levels of Vitamin B_{12} Intake

The DRI has an AI for infants until 12 months of age and an RDA for those older than 12 months. The RDA for vitamin B_{12} is 2.4 micrograms for both adults and adolescents aged 14 years and older. For pregnancy, the RDA is 2.6 micrograms; the RDA increases to 2.8 micrograms during lactation. As mentioned earlier, the recommendations for vitamin B_{12} are small relative to other water-soluble vitamins. For instance, the next lowest recommendation for a water-soluble vitamin is that for folate, which is still 100 times greater than the recommendation for vitamin B_{12} for adult males.

Vitamin B_{12} Deficiency

Individuals with limited amounts of vitamin B_{12} in their diets or who lack intrinsic factor can develop pernicious anemia. The whole-body turnover of vitamin B_{12} in an otherwise healthy adult is only about 0.1% daily. Therefore, it takes many months to years to develop a deficiency in an adult who previously was well nourished. Infants, however, have limited vitamin B_{12} stores, so infants being weaned to a vegetarian-based diet are at greater risk. Adult vegans

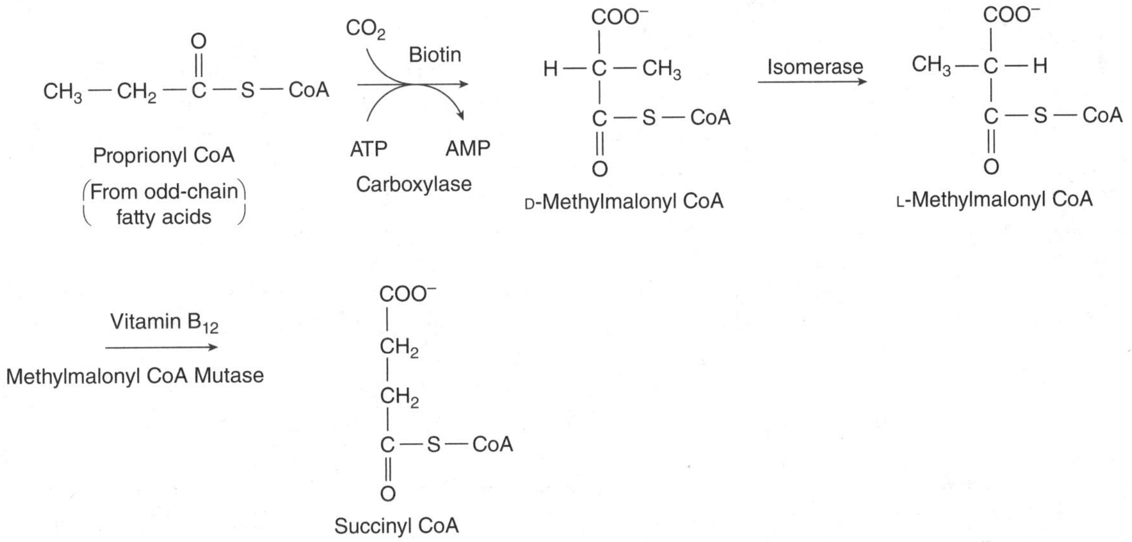

FIGURE 11.22 Overall Reaction Sequence in the Conversion of Propionate to Succinyl CoA. Note the involvement of biotin and vitamin B_{12} as coenzymes.

are a more common risk group. Individuals with gastric anomalies, such as gastric bypass and stapling or excessive pathology of the gastric mucosa, are at increased risk as well. Those individuals have a decreased ability to reabsorb the biliary vitamin B_{12} due to a reduced presence of IF and R proteins. In fact, as many as 95% of the cases of vitamin B_{12} deficiency in America are explained by malabsorption, not low dietary intake.

Vitamin B_{12} deficiency is characterized by abnormally large, immature red blood cells (macrocytic megaloblastic anemia). Accompanying symptoms include weakness, indigestion, abdominal pain, constipation alternating with diarrhea, sore and glossy tongue, and damaged nerve fibers via demyelination and degeneration. An individual can also exhibit psychosis. The state of the red blood cells is identical to that developed in a folate deficiency, leading to some confusion regarding treatment. As mentioned previously, treating an individual with macrocytic megaloblastic anemia with folate supplements may reverse the anemia while worsening the vitamin B_{12} deficiency.

SPECIAL FEATURE 11.2

The Role of Vitamin B_{12}, Folate, and Homocysteine in Mental Disorders and Alzheimer's Disease

In the previous chapter, vitamin E and other fat-soluble vitamins and their possible role in dementia and Alzheimer's disease was discussed. Some water-soluble vitamins may also have a role in the development of similar disorders. The possible role of vitamin B_{12} in preventing dementia and Alzheimer's disease has received scientific scrutiny. Some even suggest that this vitamin may improve overall cognitive function. A number of studies have demonstrated reduced blood levels of vitamin B_{12} in patients with Alzheimer's disease. Low levels of both vitamin B_{12} and folate were found to double the risk of developing Alzheimer's disease in one study of 370 older men and women. However, this study did not find a similar relationship for individuals with non-Alzheimer types of dementia. Another study followed more than 1,000 people for 10 years; those who had high levels of blood homocysteine at the beginning of the study had twice the risk of developing not only Alzheimer's disease but other types of dementia as well.

Psychological testing for short- and long-term memory and overall cognition in one study revealed poorer outcomes in Alzheimer's patients with elevated homocysteine levels. However, similar outcomes were not observed in those with only mild cognitive impairment and elevated homocysteine levels. In nondemented subjects, poorer language function scores were linked with higher blood homocysteine levels; however, there was no link with memory scores.

It is difficult to conclude whether the mental defects are due to the effect of elevated blood homocysteine levels or if they are caused by decreased vitamin B_{12} or folate status. One possible reason for this is that people with Alzheimer's disease have higher levels of homocysteine independent of vitamin B_{12} or folate status. The elevated homocysteine levels could disrupt the integrity of the blood vessels that serve the brain, much as with heart disease.

In other studies, lower levels of folate or vitamin B_{12} have been linked to both dementia and Alzheimer's disease.

In a key study, blood levels of homocysteine and folate were measured in dementia-free subjects in their mid-60s to mid-70s. A follow-up, 7 years later, revealed that those who had higher blood homocysteine levels earlier had lower scores for a wide variety of cognitive tests, such as those testing for memory, executive function, and verbal expression, among other measures. Furthermore, those who had higher folate levels earlier achieved higher global cognition scores and performed better on tests of verbal expression. Those studies suggest that folate may be a significant nutrient in relation to cognitive function, particularly in older adults; however, other studies suggest that vitamin B_{12} may be the major factor Survey studies of older women found that those who were vitamin B_{12} deficient were highly likely to suffer from depression. In one study, blood levels of both folate and vitamin B_{12} were determined, along with levels of cognitive functioning. Aptitudes such as response speed, sustained attention, visual spatial skills, associative learning, and memory were evaluated. Those subjects with normal folate but low vitamin B_{12} levels performed the worst, and those with normal levels of folate and vitamin B_{12} performed the best. That suggests that vitamin B_{12}, not folate, played the role of key nutrient. It should also be noted that people hospitalized with depression were found to have lower levels of Vitamin B_{12}.

In addition to the psychological measures discussed above, elevated homocysteine levels have been linked to changes in brain structure, in particular, reduced white matter of the cerebrum. Also, cerebral atrophy, decreased cerebral tissue volume, cerebral infarction, and other brain and nervous system defects, have been linked to higher blood homocysteine levels. Vitamin B_{12} deficiency can lead to the disruption in the myelin sheath, the fatty coating surrounding nerve fibers that causes nerve conduction to move faster. Whether there is a direct link with folate or vitamin B_{12} or if supplementation can prevent or delay, those changes remain largely unknown.

▶ Biotin

In 1916, Bateman observed that feeding raw egg whites to animals resulted in symptoms of dermatitis. In 1927, Boas further demonstrated that feeding particular food items could prevent this dermatitis. In 1936, Kögl and Tönnis isolated biotin from the liver and, at the same time, proposed its structure. It was not until 1942, however, that the definite structure of biotin was proven by du Vigneaud. Biotin is sometimes referred to as vitamin H.

Biotin is composed of two rings and a carbon chain that ends with a carboxyl group, as shown in **FIGURE 11.23**. Its scientific name is *cis*-hexahydro-2-oxo-1H-thieno-[3,4-d]-imidazole-4-pentanoic acid. One of its two rings contains sulfur at the number 1 position. Biotin is stable in heat and light, both ultraviolet and visible, as well as air when in its dry state. It is relatively soluble in both ethanol and water, with a relatively greater solubility in the former medium. When biotin is dissolved in an aqueous or solution environment, its properties change and it is susceptible to destruction by ultraviolet light or oxidation in either strong acid or alkali conditions. Humans are unable to synthesize biotin; however, microorganisms in the gut do so and use cysteine as the source of sulfur. This allows gut microbial synthesis to be a source of biotin to humans. There are as many as eight isomeric forms of biotin, but what is termed the D-biotin form has the greatest vitamin activity in humans. Biotinol and biocytin are two derivatives that have some biotin activity.

Sources of Biotin

Biotin in foods is fairly widespread because it is found in every living cell. Good sources include organ meats, egg yolks, brewer's yeast, legumes, nuts, soy flour and soybeans, whole grains, and certain ocean fish. Although egg yolks are a concentrated source of biotin, egg whites contain a protein called **avidin**, which has an extremely high affinity for biotin and substantially decreases its availability for absorption. Avidin is not stable in heat and is inactivated by cooking. In

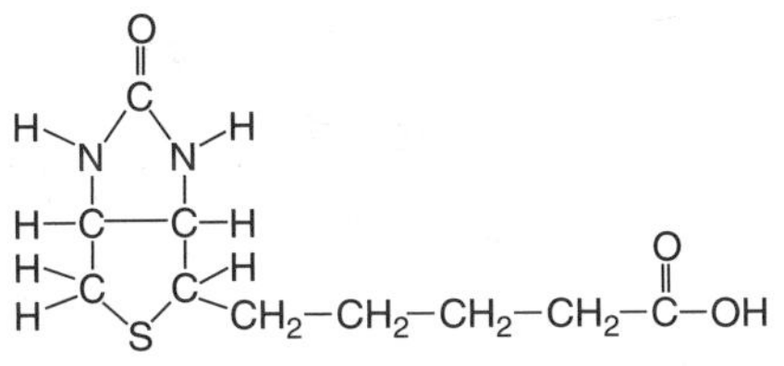

FIGURE 11.23 Biotin. Biotin has two rings and a carbon side chain. One of the rings contains sulfur.

addition to its presence in food, biotin is produced by microbes in the human colon. Some of this biotin is believed to be absorbed. Biotin may also be produced by intestinal microflora and absorbed.

Digestion and Absorption of Biotin

In food, biotin is found either free or bound to proteins. The protein-bound form can be liberated via proteases, yielding free biotin forms, predominantly biotin and secondarily biocytin. Biocytin is essentially biotin bound to the amino acid lysine. An intestinal enzyme, biotinidase, which also appears to be in the blood, can cleave the lysine portion bound to biocytin to release biotin. In some instances, there may be a mutation for the gene that encodes biotinidase. This can lead to a biotin deficiency. At one time, it was thought that biotin was absorbed by facilitative diffusion. There is a sodium-dependent, carrier-mediated update mechanism and a transporter for biotin on the surface of enterocytes. The protein is referred to as sodium-dependent multivitamin transporter or **SMVT**. This transporter is also present in the large intestine for biotin uptake. SMVT is also important for renal reabsorption and the transport of biotin in liver and other tissues. This carrier also is responsible for the absorption of pantothenic acid. Biotin deficiency is rare. Chronic alcohol intake can impair the transporter, leading to low blood biotin levels. The presence of avidin, as provided by raw egg whites, significantly decreases biotin absorption efficiency. Cooking eggs denatures the avidin and eliminates this potential problem.

Metabolism and Function of Biotin

Biotin is transported primarily as free biotin and bound to plasma proteins such as albumin, α- and β-globulins, and a biotin-binding protein. It is excreted largely by urinary filtration as biotin and, to a minor degree, as biotin metabolites, such as bisnorbiotin, biotin sulfone, and biotin sulfoxide. Biotin appears to be stored, at least to a minor degree, in muscle, brain, and the liver. As noted above, SMVT is responsible for renal reabsorption of biotin and transport across the cell membranes of other tissues.

Biotin is critical because it is needed to metabolize carbohydrates, fatty acids, and the amino acid leucine. The carboxylase enzymes that require biotin as a coenzyme are acetyl CoA carboxylase, β-methylcrotonyl CoA carboxylase, pyruvate carboxylase, and propionyl CoA carboxylase. Essentially, those enzymes attach to biotin, as does carbon dioxide, where the carbon dioxide (via HCO_3^-) is added to a substrate. Biotin is activated in cells to biotinyl 5′-adenylate before it becomes involved in those complex processes. The activation process requires ATP and magnesium.

Acetyl CoA carboxylase catalyzes the addition of carbon dioxide to acetyl CoA to form malonyl CoA in the cytosol of cells, such as hepatocytes and adipocytes. This energy-requiring reaction is the first step in fatty acid synthesis. Propionyl carboxylase catalyzes another biotin-dependent reaction. Here, the addition of carbon dioxide to propionyl CoA, again via HCO_3^-, results in D-methylmalonyl CoA, which is subsequently converted to succinyl CoA and enters the Krebs cycle (see Figure 11.22).

In a third biotin-dependent reaction, pyruvate carboxylase converts pyruvate in the mitochondria to oxaloacetate. Depending on the metabolic state of the cell, oxaloacetate can be used for gluconeogenesis or can condense with acetyl CoA to form citrate, the first molecule of the Krebs cycle.

The last carboxylase reaction is involved in the catabolism of leucine. Here β-methylcrotonyl CoA carboxylase catalyzes the conversion of β-methylcrotonyl CoA to β-methylglutaconyl CoA, which is subsequently split to acetoacetate and acetyl CoA. There may be other, not-well-defined reaction pathways in which biotin has a role, including deamination of some amino acids, tryptophan metabolism, purine synthesis, oxidative phosphorylation, and synthesis of tRNA.

Recommended Levels for Biotin Intake

At this time, there is no RDA for biotin; however, there is an AI. For adolescents and adults, the range is from 20 to 30 micrograms. The AI for infants is 5 micrograms per day for the first 6 months and 6 micrograms for the second 6 months. Recommendations for children between 1 and 8 years of age range from 8 to 12 micrograms.

Biotin Deficiency and Toxicity

Biotin deficiency rarely occurs naturally. A marginal biotin status or limited tissue/organ levels are possible if there is chronic consumption of raw egg whites. Most of the cases of known biotin deficiency are the result of individuals with an inborn error of metabolism in which there is insufficient biotinidase activity to free the lysine from the biotin. In documented animal studies, as in cases of human biotin deficiency, dermatitis is the most striking deficiency symptom. The skin presents patches of dried-out tissue and has a scaly nature. In those areas, the loss of cells results in a grayish hue.

Biotin deficiency results in a loss of epithelial cells; the tongue papillae are compromised, as is the mucosal lining of the gastrointestinal tract. Anorexia and nausea have also been documented. Alopecia, growth retardation, auditory and visual loss, metabolic acidosis, and elevated blood ammonia levels are also some of the symptoms of biotin deficiency. Biotin toxicity has yet to be documented.

▶ Pantothenic Acid

Pantothenic acid first gained notice around 1931 when a pellagra-like dermatitis was described by Ringrose. In 1933, Williams gave the name pantothenic acid to a compound that was a growth factor for yeast. In 1939, the compound was identified as an antidermatitis factor in chicks. Then, in 1940, Williams synthesized pantothenic acid. That was followed by the characterization of coenzyme A as the active form of pantothenic acid by Kaplan and Lipmann in 1948.

Although pantothenic acid (**FIGURE 11.24**) is active as a structural component of coenzyme A (**FIGURE 11.25**), pantothenic acid itself is composed of two principal parts: β-alanine and pantoic acid (see Figure 11.24). Its

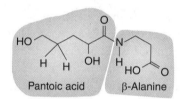

FIGURE 11.24 Pantothenic Acid. Pantothenic acid is composed of two molecules: pantoic acid and the amino acid alanine.

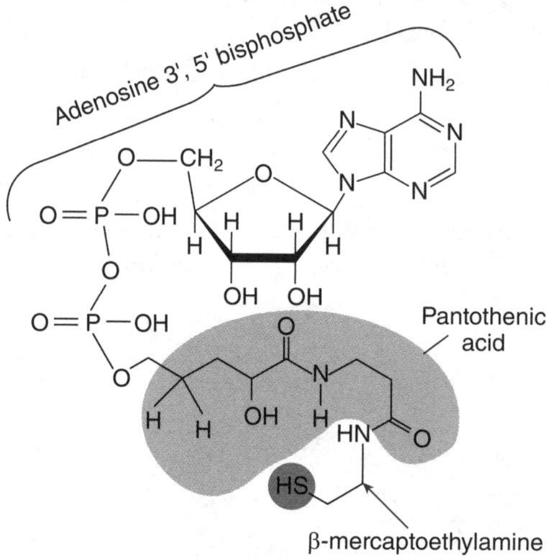

FIGURE 11.25 Coenzyme A. Pantothenic acid is a component of coenzyme A.

scientific name is dihydroxy-β,β-dimethylbutyryl-β-alanine. Pantothenic acid is stable in air and light when in the dry state. It is soluble in both water and acetic acid. At neutral pH in solution, it is stable, but it is readily destroyed by heat and at alkali or acid pH. It may also decompose when heated.

Food Sources of Pantothenic Acid

Pantothenic acid is widespread in foods, both animal and plant sources. In fact, its name is derived from the Greek word *pantos*, which means "from every side" or "from everywhere." Rich sources include certain organ meats, egg yolk, meats, fish, whole grain cereals, legumes, mushrooms, broccoli, avocados, and royal jelly from bees. Pantothenic acid can be made in plants and by intestinal bacteria.

Digestion and Absorption of Pantothenic Acid

Almost all (85%) of the pantothenic acid in foods is provided as part of coenzyme A. During digestion, pantothenic acid is liberated first to pantotheine, which is then converted to pantothenic acid. Absorption, occurring principally in the jejunum, is via SMVT as discussed under biotin absorption. The large intestine can also absorb biotin via SMVT. Some absorption may be by passive diffusion. The efficiency of absorption is approximately 50% with physiologic doses and decreases as the dose increases. Pantothenol and salts of pantothenate (e.g., calcium pantothenate) are typically used in supplements.

Metabolism and Function of Pantothenic Acid

Absorbed pantothenic acid is transported in the portal vein. In the blood, pantothenic acid is found largely in the form of coenzyme A in red blood cells. Free coenzyme A is also found in red blood cells, as well as dissolved in the plasma, but to a lesser extent. Pantothenic acid excretion is mainly by renal filtration; typical urinary pantothenic acid levels are 1 to 4 milligrams daily. The mechanism for uptake of pantothenic acid by various tissues includes both active and passive processes. For instance, in the liver and cardiac and skeletal muscle, pantothenic acid is transported into cells in a sodium-dependent, active process. Conversely, in the central nervous system, as well as in adipose and renal tissue, uptake appears to be passive.

Once in cells, pantothenic acid is largely used to make coenzyme A. Because of the general involvement of coenzyme A in energy metabolism, its concentration is higher in more metabolically active organs, such as the heart, liver, kidneys, adrenal gland, and brain. The structure of coenzyme A is shown in Figure 11.24. Briefly, pantothenic acid is phosphorylated to 4′-phosphopantothenate in an ATP-requiring step catalyzed by the enzyme pantothenate kinase (**FIGURE 11.26**). Then, cysteine is attached to 4′-phosphopantothenate to form 4′-phosphopantothenyl cysteine in another ATP-requiring reaction. The addition of cysteine provides the final coenzyme A structure with a fairly exposed sulfur region. Subsequently, CO_2 is removed from 4′-phosphopantothenyl cysteine, producing 4′-phosphopantotheine, which, in turn, is converted to dephosphocoenzyme A and then to coenzyme A in two ATP-requiring reactions. The first of those last two reactions uses ATP as a source of AMP. AMP is added to the molecule, and the last step involves phosphorylation of a hydroxyl group of dephosphocoenzyme A.

Coenzyme A, and thus pantothenic acid, is fundamentally involved in the metabolism of the energy-providing nutrients, carbohydrates, protein, and fat, as well as alcohol (ethanol). Coenzyme A bonds to the carboxylic acid portion of molecules as its sulfur forms a **thio-ester** covalent link. That is said to activate the molecules, thereby allowing them to proceed in subsequent reactions of energy pathways. One of the most common molecules that coenzyme A activates is acetic acid (acetyl CoA), which is the product of a fatty acid and certain amino acid oxidation as well as the product of pyruvate and ethanol oxidation. Propionic acid is also activated by coenzyme A to form propionyl CoA. Propionic acid can either be found in foods such as fish or be derived from the oxidation of odd-chain-length fatty acids and certain amino acids (methionine, leucine, and isoleucine). Methylmalonic acid (methylmalonyl CoA) is formed as an intermediate in the conversion of propionyl CoA to succinyl CoA. Succinic acid is also activated to succinyl CoA, which is a Krebs cycle intermediate, as well as other key intermediate acids.

Acetyl CoA can condense with oxaloacetate to form citrate, the first molecule of the Krebs cycle. Acetyl CoA can also be used to make ketone bodies in the liver and is the building block for fatty acid and cholesterol synthesis. Furthermore, if fatty acids are to become involved in processes such as β-oxidation or attachment in phospholipids, they must first be activated by the binding of coenzyme A.

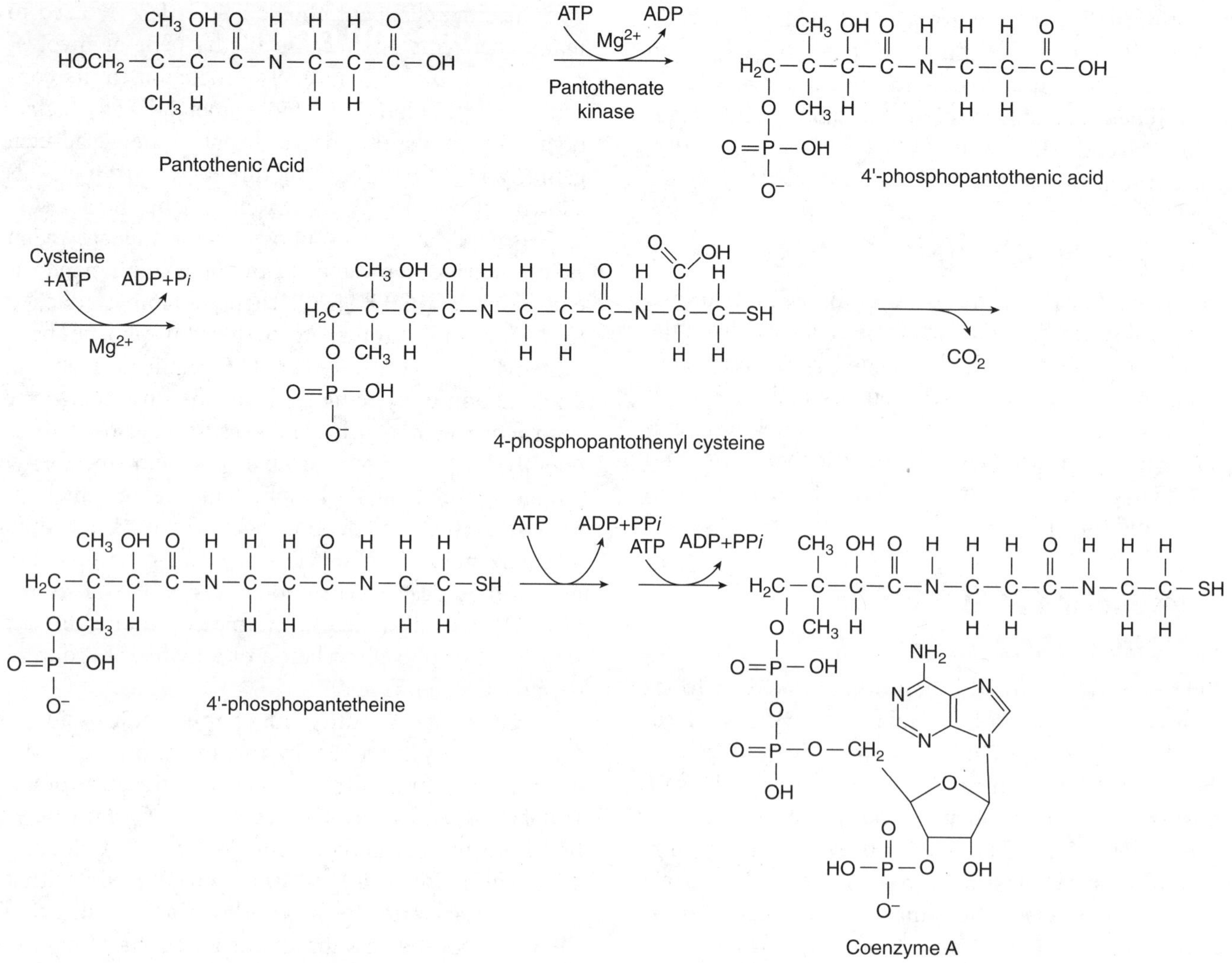

FIGURE 11.26 Synthesis of Coenzyme A from Pantothenic Acid. Indirectly, pantothenic acid has a role in energy metabolism via Coenzyme A synthesis. Coenzyme A is fundamental in energy-providing reactions of carbohydrates, proteins, fat, and alcohol.

A second function of pantothenic acid is to serve as a component of acyl carrier protein (ACP). ACP is a component of the large fatty acid synthase (FAS) enzyme complex. ACP, as a component of FAS, binds to nascent fatty acids during the synthetic process. Other functions of pantothenic acid are somewhat more vague. As coenzyme A, pantothenic acid may be involved in the post-translational acetylation of key cellular proteins, such as histones and cytoskeletal proteins, thereby increasing their stability against proteases such as ubiquitin.

Recently, pantothenic acid has been receiving greater interest because of its ability to protect against free radicals. Evidence exists for pantothenate protecting against free radical-induced apoptosis or programmed cell death. Pantothenate is believed to also play a role in preventing the decay of mitochondria.

Recommended Levels of Pantothenic Acid Intake

Currently, there is no RDA for pantothenic acid. An AI of 5 milligrams for adults has been established. For infants, 1.7 milligrams in the first 6 months and 1.8 milligrams after the first 6 months are recommended. Children have an AI of 2 to 3 milligrams from 1 to 8 years of age, and adolescents aged 9 to 13 years old have an AI of 4 milligrams. Thereafter, the AI reaches the adult level of 5 milligrams. It is 6 milligrams during pregnancy and 7 milligrams during lactation.

Deficiency and Toxicity of Pantothenic Acid

Deficiency of pantothenic acid is rare and takes several weeks to develop. In experimental studies, a pantothenic acid deficiency can be produced by feeding subjects l isomers of pantothenic acid. Other antagonists of pantothenic acid include methyl-pantothenic acid, pantoylaminoethanethiol, and pantoyl taurine. Symptoms of a pantothenic acid deficiency include burning feet syndrome, which is a feeling of tingling and tenderness in the feet; headache; fatigue; impaired motor function; muscle cramps; disturbances of the digestive tract; and vomiting. More extreme manifestations can result, such as ulcerations, cardiac tachycardia, hypotension, reduced eosinophil output, hypochromic anemia, and hypoglycemia. Pantothenic acid is not stored well in the human body, and urinary levels reflect dietary intake. There have been no reports of pantothenic acid toxicity at present.

⬡ BEFORE YOU GO ON . . .

1. What is meant by the term *methyl–folate trap*?
2. How are folate and biotin absorbed by the small intestine?
3. Although symptoms of folate and vitamin B_{12} deficiency appear similar, a misdiagnosis can lead to serious problems. Which of those two vitamins, when deficient, can result in a deficiency sign in one and not the other, resulting in serious consequences?
4. List the three major biochemical reactions in which vitamin B_{12} is involved.
5. How can a biotin deficiency occur?
6. What is the major biochemical role of pantothenic acid?

🩺 CLINICAL INSIGHT

Elevated Blood Homocysteine and Heart Disease: the Link with Vitamin B_6, Folate, and Vitamin B_{12}

For some time, it has been known that elevated homocysteine levels are a risk factor for heart disease. Research suggests that higher blood homocysteine levels are linked to atherosclerosis, primarily due to enhanced plaque development. A deficiency of folate, vitamin B_6, or vitamin B_{12} can interfere with the enzymatic conversion of homocysteine to methionine. Even moderate elevations in blood homocysteine levels are associated with an increased risk of heart disease. For example, an increase of 5 micromoles per liter in plasma homocysteine levels is estimated to increase heart disease risk by 70%. This is equivalent to the increase in risk when serum cholesterol levels increase by 0.5 micromoles per liter. An increased intake of folic acid by 200 micrograms per day reduces homocysteine levels by about 4 micromoles per liter.

Homocysteine levels can be regulated by both genetic and environmental (nutritional) factors. Genetic defects in the enzymes cystathione β-synthase, methionine synthase, and methylenetetrahydrofolate reductase can all lead to an augmentation of homocysteine levels. Research has shown that folic acid, riboflavin, methionine, choline, and vitamins B_6 and B_{12} may all affect homocysteine metabolism. Elevated serum homocysteine has been suggested to cause oxidative damage, in particular that of LDL. It may also interfere with the blood coagulation process, in particular, those events associated with dissolution of the fibrin clot. However, many studies have shown that folic acid and vitamin B_{12} supplementation can lower blood homocysteine levels without reducing cardiovascular risk. That suggests that routine supplementation of those vitamins to reduce heart disease may not be effective or useful in reducing heart disease even though homocysteine levels may be normalized.

▶ Here's What You Have Learned

1. Ascorbate, or vitamin C, is water soluble and derived from glucose. Its prime function is as an antioxidant, but it also has other functions. Collagen formation is dependent on vitamin C metabolism. Vitamin C can reduce iron to the ferrous form, which is more available for intestinal absorption. It is central in two reactions in the formation of carnitine to allow for longer-chain fatty acids to cross the inner membrane of mitochondria for β-oxidation. Dehydroascorbic acid and vitamin C have different modes of intestinal absorption.

2. Thiamin, riboflavin, and niacin are all involved in energy-yielding pathways. Thiamin is a component of thiamin pyrophosphate (TPP) that works with the enzyme pyruvate dehydrogenase, which is necessary for the conversion of pyruvate to acetyl CoA. TPP is also critical for

the hexose monophosphate shunt. Riboflavin and niacin have roles as coenzymes. Riboflavin plays a role as FAD and FMN, which facilitate the release of energy from macronutrients via the Krebs cycle. Specific transport proteins have been identified for thiamin and riboflavin absorption. Niacin is functional as NAD or the phosphorylated form, NADP. Both forms are reduced in glycolysis and the Krebs cycle and transfer electrons to the electron transport chain for ATP formation. Niacin may protect mitochondria by interacting with a family of proteins referred to as SIRTs.

3. The metabolically active form of vitamin B_6 is pyridoxal phosphate (PLP). The major function of vitamin B_6 is to facilitate the conversion of one amino acid into another, or transamination, in a Schiff base mechanism. It is also involved in decarboxylation, transulfhydration, and desulfhydration reactions. It is pivotal in the synthesis of neurotransmitters, such as GABA and serotonin. Finally, it is important for the production of aminolevulinic acid in the biosynthesis of heme.

4. Folate and vitamin B_{12} deficiency signs may appear similar in some instances, and yet, both are distinct in terms of their chemistry and some unique deficiency signs. Folate may be absorbed by two transporter proteins: 1) reduced folate carrier (RFC) and 2) proton-coupled folate transporter (PCFT). Folic acid's main function is to carry a carbon unit in biochemical reactions. The active form of folate is tetrahydrofolate (THF), in which two nitrogens and two carbons are reduced. It is this active form that accepts carbon moieties. Methionine can be made from homocysteine, and serine from glycine, by the THF form. The methyl–folate trap refers to the fact that when THF becomes methylated, it can be converted back to the THF form via the transfer of the methyl group to homocysteine to form methionine. This requires vitamin B_{12}; if vitamin B_{12} is deficient in a cell, folate is trapped in the methylated form.

5. Vitamin B_{12} needs to be bound to the protein intrinsic factor in order to be absorbed without destruction. Vitamin B_{12} is needed in (1) the conversion of homocysteine to methionine, (2) the conversion of L-methylmalonyl CoA to succinyl CoA in the oxidation of odd-chain-length fatty acids, and (3) the isomerization of L-leucine to D-leucine.

6. Biotin deficiency is rare. A deficiency can be produced experimentally in animals by feeding them raw egg whites, which contain avidin. Deficiency may also occur in a genetic mutation in the gene that encodes biotinase, which hydrolyzes biotin complexes in the gut to a free form for absorption. SMVT is a transport protein for biotin in the intestine and other tissues. Biotin is needed to metabolize the macronutrients and the amino acid leucine in a variety of carboxylation reactions. The carboxylase enzymes that require biotin are acetyl CoA carboxylase, β-methylcrotonyl CoA carboxylase, pyruvate carboxylase, and propionyl CoA carboxylase.

7. Pantothenic acid is a vitamin that is incorporated into another compound used in intermediary metabolism, namely, coenzyme A. Pantothenic acid is consumed as a nutrient and absorbed in the portal vein. Various tissues take up pantothenic acid, either by a sodium-dependent, active process or by passive diffusion, depending on the tissue. Pantothenic acid is made into coenzyme A once inside the cells. Another function of pantothenic acid is to serve as a component of acyl carrier protein, which is a component of the large fatty acid synthase (FAS) enzyme complex.

8. Vitamin C, thiamin, riboflavin, folate, biotin, and pantothenic acid are absorbed by specific transport proteins. Those proteins may be nonfunctional in cases of gene mutations that can lead to impaired status of each vitamin.

▶ Suggested Reading

Alsulaimani S, Gardner H, Elkind MS, Cheung K, Sacco RL, Rundek T. Elevated homocysteine and carotid plaque area and densitometry in the Northern Manhattan Study. *Stroke.* 2013;44(2):457–461.

Ames BN. Delaying the mitochondrial decay of aging. *Ann N Y Acad Sci.* 2004;1019:406–411.

Barile M, Giancaspero TA, Leone P, Galluccio M, Indiveri C. Riboflavin transport and metabolism in humans. *J Inherit Metab Dis.* 2016; 39(4):545–557.

Bender DA. Optimum nutrition: thiamin, biotin and pantothenate. *Proc Nutr Soc.* 1999;58(2):427–433.

Bogan KL, Brenner C. Nicotinic acid, nicotinamide, and nicotinamide riboside: a molecular evaluation of NAD⁺ precursor vitamins in human nutrition. *Annu Rev Nutr.* 2008;28:115–130.

Boushey CJ, Beresford SA, Omenn GS, Motulsky AG. A quantitative assessment of plasma homocysteine as a risk factor for vascular disease. Probable benefits of increasing folic acid intakes. *JAMA.* 1995;274(13):1049–1057.

Brown G. Defects of thiamine transport and metabolism. *J Inherit Metab Dis.* 2014;37(4):577–585.

Brownsey RW, Boone AN, Elliott JE, Kulpa JE, Lee WM. Regulation of acetyl-CoA carboxylase. *Biochem Soc Trans.* 2006;34(pt 2):223–227.

Butterworth RF. Thiamine deficiency-related brain dysfunction in chronic liver failure. *Metab Brain Dis.* 2009;24(1):189–196.

Cacciapuoti F. Lowering homocysteine levels with folic acid and B-vitamins do not reduce early atherosclerosis, but could interfere with cognitive decline and Alzheimer's disease. *J Thromb Thrombolysis.* 2013;36(3):258–262.

Ciaccio M, Bellia C. Hyperhomocysteinemia and cardiovascular risk: effect of vitamin supplementation in risk reduction. *Curr Clin Pharmacol.* 2010;5(1):30–36.

Combs GF. *The Vitamins.* San Diego, CA: Academic Press; 1992.

Eichholzer M, Tönz O, Zimmermann R. Folic acid: a public-health challenge. *Lancet.* 2006;367(9519):1352–1361.

Farmer JA. Nicotinic acid: a new look at an old drug. *Curr Atheroscler Rep.* 2009;11(2):87–92.

Faux NG, Ellis KA, Porter L, et al. Homocysteine, vitamin B12, and folic acid levels in Alzheimer's disease, mild cognitive impairment, and health elderly: baseline characteristics in subjects of the Australian Imaging Biomarker Lifestyle study. *J Alzheimers Dis.* 2011;27(4):909–922.

Feng L, Isaac V, Sim S, Ng TP, Krishnan KR, Chee MW. Associations between elevated homocysteine, cognitive impairment, and reduced white volume matter in healthy old adults. *Am J Geriatr Psychiatry.* 2013;21(2):164–172.

Fischer M, Bacher A. Biosynthesis of vitamin B_2: structure and mechanism of riboflavin synthase. *Arch Biochem Biophys.* 2008;474(2):252–265.

Graham IM, Daly LE, Refsum HM, et al. Plasma homocysteine as a risk factor for vascular disease: The European Concerted Action Project. *JAMA.* 1997;277(22):1775–1781.

Green R. Is it time for vitamin B-12 fortification? What are the questions? *Am J Clin Nutr.* 2009;89(2):712S–716S.

Greenlee H, Kwan ML, Kushi L, et al. Antioxidant supplement use after diagnosis and breast cancer outcomes. *Cancer.* 2012;118(8):2048–2058.

Gropper SS, Smith JL, Groff JL. *Advanced Nutrition and Human Metabolism.* Belmont, CA: Wadsworth; 2005.

Hooshmand B, Solomon A, Kåreholt I, et al. Associations between serum homocysteine, holotranscobalamin, folate and cognition in the elderly: a longitudinal study. *J Int Med.* 2012;271(2):204–212.

Hou Z, Matherly LH. Biology of the major facilitative folate transporters SLC19A1 and SLC46A1. *Curr Top Membr.* 2014;73:175–204.

Jaeger B, Bosch AM. Clinical presentation and outcome of riboflavin transporter deficiency: mini review after five years of experience. *J Inherit Metab Dis.* 2016;39(4):559–564.

Jurgenson CT, Begley TP, Ealick SE. The structural and biochemical foundations of thiamin biosynthesis. *Annu Rev Biochem.* 2009;78:569–603.

Lai EC. RNA sensors and riboswitches: self-regulating messages. *Curr Biol.* 2003;13(7):R285–R291.

Leonardi R, Zhang YM, Rock CO, Jackowski S. Coenzyme A: back in action. *Prog Lipid Res.* 2005;44(2):125–153.

Lindblad M, Tveden-Nyborg P, Lykkesfeldt J. Regulation of vitamin C homeostasis during deficiency. *Nutrients.* 2013;5(8):2860–2879.

Magni G, Orsomando G, Raffelli N, Ruggieri S. Enzymology of mammalian NAD metabolism in health and disease. *Front Biosci.* 2008;13:6135–6154.

Mandl J, Szarka A, Bánhegyi G. Vitamin C: update on physiology and pharmacology. *Br J Pharmacol.* 2009;157(7):1097–1110.

McMahon RJ. Biotin in metabolism and molecular biology. *Annu Rev Nutr.* 2002;22:221–239.

McNulty H, Pentieva K, Hoey L, Ward M. Homocysteine, B-vitamins and CVD. *Proc Nutr Soc.* 2008;67(2):232–237.

McNulty H, Scott JM. Intake and status of folate and related B-vitamins: considerations and challenges in achieving optimal status. *Br J Nutr.* 2008;99(suppl 3):48S–54S.

Morris MS, Jacques PF, Rosenberg IH, Selhub J. Folate and vitamin B-12 status in relation to anemia, macrocytosis, and cognitive impairment in older Americans in the age of folic acid fortification. *Am J Clin Nutr.* 2007;85(1):193–200.

Moser MA, Chun OK. Vitamin C and heart health: a review based on findings from epidemiologic studies. *Int J Mol Sci.* 2016;17(8):E1328.

Myllyharju J. Prolyl 4-hydroxylases, key enzymes in the synthesis of collagens and regulation of the response to hypoxia, and their roles as treatment targets. *Ann Med.* 2008;40(6):402–417.

Ohno S, Ohno Y, Suzuki N, Soma G, Inoue M. High-dose vitamin C (ascorbic acid) therapy in the treatment of patients with advanced cancer. *Anticancer Res.* 2009;29(3):809–815.

Pitkin RM. Folate and neural tube defects. *Am J Clin Nutr.* 2007;85(1):285S–288S.

Ragsdale SW. Catalysis of methyl group transfers involving tetrahydrofolate and B(12). *Vitam Horm.* 2008;79:293–324.

Said HM. Cellular uptake of biotin: mechanisms and regulation. *J Nutr.* 1999;129(2 suppl):490S–493S.

Said HM. Intestinal absorption of water-soluble vitamins in health and disease. *Biochem J.* 2011;437(3):357–372.

Said HM. Recent advances in carrier-mediated intestinal absorption of water-soluble vitamins. *Annu Rev Physiol.* 2004;66:419–446.

Sánchez-Moreno C, Jiménez-Escrig A, Martín A. Stroke: roles of B vitamins, homocysteine and antioxidants. *Nutr Res Rev.* 2009;22(1):49–67.

Shane B. Folate and vitamin B12 metabolism: overview and interaction with riboflavin, vitamin B6, and polymorphisms. *Food Nutr Bull.* 2008;29(2 suppl):5S–16S.

Srivastava S. Emerging therapeutic roles for NAD^+ metabolism in mitochondrial and age-related disorders. *Clin Trans Med.* 2016;5(1):25.

Varela-Moreiras G, Murphy MM, Scott JM. Cobalamin, folic acid, and homocysteine. *Nutr Rev.* 2009;67(suppl 1):69S–72S.

Vosper H. Niacin: a re-emerging pharmaceutical for the treatment of dyslipidaemia. *Br J Pharmacol.* 2009;158(2):429–441.

West RK, Beeri MS, Schmeidler J, et al. Homocysteine and cognitive function in very elderly nondemented subjects. *Am J Geriatr Psychiatry.* 2011;19(7):673–677.

Winkler W, Nahvi A, Breaker RR: Thiamine derivatives bind messenger RNAs directly to regulate bacterial gene expression. *Nature.* 2002;419(6910):952–956.

Wojtczak L, Slyshenkov VS. Protection by pantothenic acid against apoptosis and cell damage by oxygen free radicals—the role of glutathione. *Biofactors.* 2003;17(1–4):61–73.

Wolff T, Witkop CT, Miller T, Syed SB; U.S. Preventive Services Task Force. Folic acid supplementation for the prevention of neural tube defects: an update of the evidence for the U.S. Preventive Services Task Force. *Ann Intern Med.* 2009;150(9):632–639.

Zempleni J. Uptake, localization, and noncarboxylase roles of biotin. *Annu Rev Nutr.* 2005;25:175–196.

Zempleni J, Hassan YI, Wijeratne SS. Biotin and biotinidase deficiency. *Expert Rev Endocrinol Metab.* 2008;3(6):715–724.

Zempleni J, Wijeratne SS, Hassan YI. Biotin. *Biofactors.* 2009;35(1):36–46.

Ziegler EE, Filer LJ, eds. *Present Knowledge in Nutrition.* Washington, DC: ILSI Press; 1996.

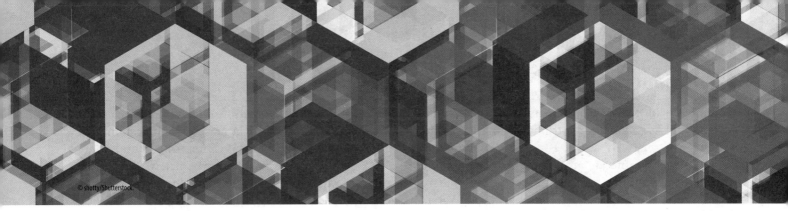

© shotty/Shutterstock.

CHAPTER 12

Major Minerals

← HERE'S WHERE YOU HAVE BEEN

1. Our understanding of the functions of water- and fat-soluble vitamins continues to evolve as new research provides insights into the mechanisms by which they optimize human health.
2. Vitamins A, D, E, and B_{12} and folic acid are examples of vitamins that may play a role at the gene level.
3. Fat- and water-soluble vitamins play a central role in many biochemical reactions, with many of the water-soluble vitamins acting as cofactors for enzymes.
4. Exercise requires special nutrition considerations related to energy and micronutrients.
5. Vitamins are supplied by a wide variety of food sources, and some can be synthesized by gut bacteria.

HERE'S WHERE YOU ARE GOING →

1. Sodium, potassium, and chloride are referred to as electrolytes and play an important role in water balance, electric activity, and biochemical reactions.
2. Although calcium and phosphorus have major roles in bone metabolism, their functions go far beyond that role.
3. The blood concentrations of the major minerals are tightly regulated by hormonal, absorption, and renal mechanisms.
4. A key aspect of determining the nutrition status of the major minerals is their relative bioavailability in a diet.
5. Calcium, magnesium, and potassium provide cardioprotection.

▶ Introduction

Compared with the macronutrients, the requirements for minerals—and their contribution to total body weight—are relatively small. For instance, although some 20 to 25 minerals are known to have human physiological significance, collectively, they constitute less than 5 to 6% of total human mass. Water, protein, fat, and carbohydrates make up the majority of the remaining human mass.

Minerals are typically divided into two general categories: major minerals and trace minerals (**TABLE 12.1**). Minerals whose estimated average daily dietary need is 100 milligrams or more and that represent more than 0.01% of total human mass are considered **major minerals**. For a 70-kilogram individual, for example, a particular major mineral would contribute at least 7 grams to his or her total body mass. However, many nutritionists prefer to classify the minerals based solely on dietary need. The major minerals include calcium (Ca), phosphorus (P), sodium (Na), potassium (K), chloride (Cl), and magnesium (Mg). Sulfur (S) is often included in this category because of its contribution to human mass; however, its dietary need remains questionable. The major minerals are discussed in detail in this chapter.

TABLE 12.1 Minerals of the Human Body

Major Minerals	Trace Minerals	
Calcium	Arsenic	Lithium[a]
Chloride	Boron	Manganese
Magnesium	Cadmium[a]	Molybdenum
Phosphorus	Chromium	Nickel
Potassium	Cobalt[a]	Selenium
Sodium	Copper	Silicon[a]
Sulfur	Fluoride	Tin[a]
	Iodine	Vanadium
	Iron	Zinc

[a]Dietary essentiality is questionable despite presence in the body.

▶ Calcium

Calcium is a divalent cation (Ca^{2+}) and is the most abundant mineral in the human body. It accounts for approximately 40% of total mineral mass and about 1.5% of total body mass. Approximately 99% of the calcium within the human body is located within the bones and teeth, where it provides a structural service. The remaining 1% of body calcium is found within intracellular and extracellular fluids. Thus, calcium plays many functional roles. Calcium nutrition has become a concern for many individuals because of the increased incidence of osteoporosis as human life expectancy continues to increase. Research findings have suggested the potential involvement of calcium in cancer prevention and hypertension. More recently, its role in weight control has been highlighted in research literature.

Dietary Calcium Sources

Dairy products tend to be the greatest contributors of calcium to the human diet. As much as 55% of calcium in the American diet is derived from dairy products. For instance, a glass of milk supplies approximately 300 milligrams of calcium. Beyond dairy products, good sources of calcium include sardines, oysters, clams, tofu, molasses, almonds, calcium-fortified foods, and dark green, leafy vegetables, such as broccoli, kale, collards, and mustard and turnip greens (**TABLE 12.2**). Other vegetables such as spinach, rhubarb, chard, and beet greens contain respectable amounts of calcium. However, oxalates and phytate found in those foods can bind to calcium in the digestive tract and decrease its absorption. For example, as little as 5% of the calcium in spinach is actually absorbed.

Calcium-containing complexes rank among the most popular individual nutrient supplements. For the most part, those supplements are used with the hope of increasing bone density or minimizing the rate of bone calcium loss. Amino acid chelates of calcium, calcium carbonate, calcium acetate, and calcium citrate, as well as calcium gluconates, phosphates, lactates, and oyster shells, are the most common forms of calcium supplements. In those substances, the associated molecule is ionically complexed to calcium. Approximately 36 to 42% of the calcium in calcium carbonate, perhaps the most widely used calcium supplemental form, is absorbed. About 24 to 36% of the calcium in calcium citrate, calcium acetate, calcium lactate, and calcium gluconate is absorbed. Calcium citrate malate (CCM) has been used by some food manufacturers (e.g., manufacturers of orange

TABLE 12.2 Calcium Content of Select Foods

Food Source	Calcium (mg)
Milk and milk products	
Yogurt, low fat (1 cup)	419
Milk, skim (1 cup)	299
Cheese, Swiss (1 oz)	224
Cheese, cheddar (1 oz)	204
Ice cream (1 cup)	226
Ice milk (1 cup)	470
Custard (½ cup)	151
Cottage cheese (1 cup)	156
Vegetables	
Collard greens (1 cup)	266
Spinach, cooked (1 cup)	245
Broccoli, cooked (1 cup)	42
Legumes and legume products	
Tofu, soft (1 cup)	275
Snap beans (1 cup)	58
Lima beans (1 cup)	54

juice) because researchers have reported very efficient absorption. Calcium supplements should be taken with a snack or meal; it is not advisable to take single large doses because calcium supplements are better absorbed when distributed throughout the day. One final note is that oyster shell calcium supplements pose a risk of lead contamination and generally are not recommended.

Calcium Absorption

Calcium, derived either from foods or supplements, is in the form of insoluble salts. Therefore, in order for calcium to be absorbed, it must be liberated to its ionized form. However, calcium in its ionized form may also form chelates with certain dietary factors, such as other minerals and fiber-associated substances. Those ionic chelations can potentially decrease calcium absorption, especially in more neutral pH environments, such as the small intestine.

Several factors that may decrease the absorption of calcium include the presence of oxalate, phytate, and fibers in foods; rapid movement of food through the intestine, as with higher fiber intake; a very high-fat diet or decreased fat digestion; excess vitamin A intake; and excessive dietary phosphorus and magnesium. A calcium-to-phosphorus ratio of 1:1 to 3:1 is considered optimal. Magnesium is also a divalent cation, and it is believed that magnesium can compete with calcium for absorptive mechanisms. Interestingly, decreased physical activity may also be associated with decreased calcium absorption efficiency. **TABLE 12.3** lists many of the factors that influence calcium absorption.

Phytate (inositol hexaphosphate) is found in fibrous plant sources, such as legumes, nuts, and cereals (**FIGURE 12.1**). A molar ratio of phytate to calcium greater than 0.2 has been suggested to increase the risk of calcium deficiency. Oxalate can also bind ionized calcium in the digestive tract and decrease its

TABLE 12.3 Factors Influencing Calcium Absorption

Increased Calcium Absorption	Decreased Calcium Absorption
Increased vitamin D and PTH[a]	Decreased vitamin D and PTH
Consuming lactose during same meal	Consuming phytate, fiber and oxalates during same meal
Increased need (growth, pregnancy, lactation)	Decreased need
Distribution of intake throughout the day	Increased diet zinc or magnesium
Acidic pH in digestive tract	High-fat diets or decreased-fat digestion
	Excess diet phosphorus, magnesium, and vitamin A

[a]PTH, parathyroid hormone.

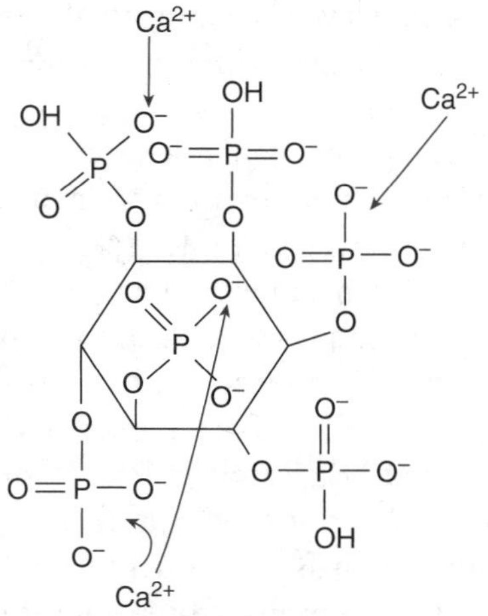

FIGURE 12.1 Structure of Phytate or Phytic Acid with Potential Calcium-Binding Sites. The phosphate groups allows ions to bind to it. Phytate is present in plant sources, such as legumes, nuts, and cereals. Too much dietary phytate may cause a calcium deficiency and it is also known to cause a zinc deficiency.

absorption (**FIGURE 12.2**). Oxalate is found in various vegetables (spinach, eggplants, beets, celery, greens, okra), fruits (berries), nuts (peanuts and pecans), and beverages (tea, Ovaltine, cocoa).

High-fat diets, or decreased fat digestion, may decrease calcium absorption by allowing for the formation of calcium soaps (saponification). Those soaps are ionically formed between the acid portion of a fatty acid and calcium.

Calcium absorption is enhanced by several factors. Those factors include healthy vitamin D status; acid conditions in the digestive tract (prevents precipitation); the presence of lactose in the digestive tract; lack of physical stress on bone; distribution of calcium intake throughout the day rather than at one time; and

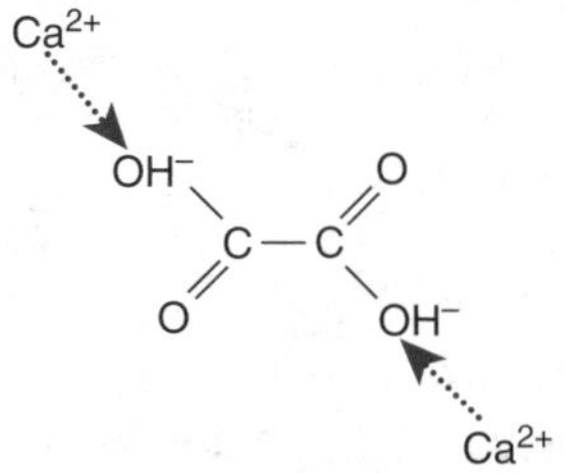

FIGURE 12.2 Structure of Oxalate or Oxalic Acid with Potential Calcium-Binding Sites. The negative hydroxyl groups are binding sites for minerals. Oxalate is present in vegetables, such as spinach, eggplant, beets, celery, and okra; in fruits, such as berries; nuts; and in beverages such as tea. As with phytate, excess consumption of oxalate can bind to calcium and zinc and lead to deficiency.

increased physiologic need (e.g., growth, pregnancy, lactation, decreased calcium status).

The positive effect of a more acidic pH in the digestive tract is most likely related to a reduction in the formation of calcium chelations. Lactose can facilitate the absorption of calcium. Lactose's constituent monosaccharides may be more responsible for the positive influence on calcium absorption, as opposed to its influence on intestinal pH. That effect is probably more significant in infants than adults because infants rely more on milk for nourishment. Also, although some fermentable fibers, such as pectin, can bind calcium in the digestive tract; microbes in the colon can liberate calcium as they ferment those fibers, thereby increasing calcium availability and the potential for absorption. It has been suggested that as much as 4% of dietary calcium is absorbed in the colon. The presence of normal bile acid may assist in calcium absorption by promoting proper fat digestion and decreasing the formation of calcium-fatty acid soaps.

The absorption of calcium (**FIGURE 12.3**) occurs along the length of the small intestine. Two transport processes appear to be responsible for the absorption

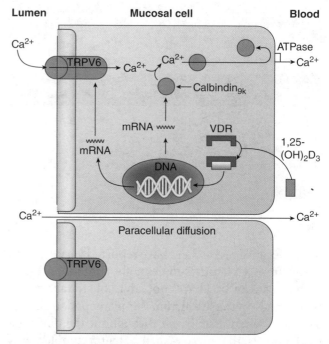

FIGURE 12.3 The Absorption of Calcium by Enterocytes. Calcium is absorbed by two mechanisms. One mechanism is dependent on vitamin D and its nuclear receptor that enhances synthesis of a membrane calcium channel, such as TRPV6; a calcium-binding protein, calbindin$_{9k}$; and export to the blood via a vitamin D-regulated Ca^{++}-Mg^{++} ATPase. This mechanism is both saturable and energy dependent. The second mechanism of calcium absorption is paracellular diffusion between the enterocytes.

of calcium. The first process is a saturable, active mechanism that involves a calcium-binding protein (CBP) known as **calbindin**. Calbindin is located all along the small intestine but is more abundant in the duodenum and proximal jejunum. Different isoforms of this protein exist, designated calbindin$_{9K}$ and calbindin$_{28K}$. Calbindin$_{9K}$ occurs in mammalian species, whereas calbindin$_{28K}$ occurs in avian species. In the upper portion of the small intestine, the efficiency of calcium absorption is greater, but because the chyme stays in contact with the remainder of the small intestine for a greater period of time, the total amount absorbed is greater in the distal portion of the small intestine.

The absorption of calcium is a three-step process (see Figure 12.3). First, calcium is transferred through the microvilli membrane. Next, calcium is transported or escorted through the cell to decrease its interaction with intracellular molecules. Finally, calcium exits from the cell across the basolateral membrane into the extracellular fluid and subsequently into the blood.

Vitamin D (1,25-$(OH)_2D_3$) regulates all three steps. Vitamin D enters intestinal mucosal cells and binds to a receptor. The vitamin D-receptor complex translocates to the nucleus and binds to promoter regions of DNA to stimulate the transcription of CBP as well as an intracellular membrane calcium-binding protein (IMCBP). The proteins produced in response to the vitamin D receptor mediate calcium metabolism—for example, an apical membrane calcium channel; the transient receptor potential cation channel, subfamily V, member 6 (TRPV6); and calcium-binding protein D$_{9K}$ (calbindin D$_{9K}$). TRPV6s are channels for calcium absorption. The calbindin protein binds to the calcium that enters the mucosal cells. This may keep the free calcium levels minimized, thereby decreasing any potential interference with other intracellular metabolic processes. Organelles, such as the mitochondria and Golgi apparatus, may also bind calcium and facilitate its absorption by movement toward the basolateral membrane. In any event, the calcium bound to those proteins or organelles is released into the extracellular fluid. Release into the extracellular fluid requires ATP and a vitamin D-regulated Ca^{++}-Mg^{++} ATPase. Sodium may also be exchanged for calcium during membrane transport.

Aging appears to decrease the efficiency of calcium absorption. Vitamin D-regulated absorption of calcium becomes impaired as less 1,25-$(OH)_2D_3$ is made in response to parathyroid hormone. Reduction in estrogen in menopausal and postmenopausal women is also associated with a reduction in vitamin D-mediated calcium absorption.

The second mechanism for calcium absorption also occurs throughout the small intestine and appears to be a nonsaturable, paracellular process. Here, calcium moves between enterocytes instead of moving through them. This route of calcium absorption becomes more significant as calcium intake increases. Also, it should be mentioned that larger intakes of calcium appear to hinder iron absorption.

Blood Calcium Levels and Homeostasis

The total amount of calcium in the blood ranges from 8.8 to 10.8 milligrams per 100 milliliters. Calcium is found in the blood mainly bound to protein (approximately 40%) or free (approximately 50%). Albumin is the primary transport protein. The remaining 10% of circulating calcium is complexed with sulfate, phosphate, or citrate.

Blood calcium is very tightly regulated by several endocrine factors. Contrary to popular belief, dietary calcium levels do not significantly influence blood calcium levels. Alterations in blood calcium levels occur as a result of endocrine balance. As blood calcium levels fluctuate toward the lower end of the normal range, parathyroid hormone (PTH) levels in the blood increase. Parathyroid hormone supports the reestablishment of normal serum calcium levels by increasing calcium absorption from the intestine, mobilizing calcium from bone via stimulating osteoclasts, and reducing kidney excretion of calcium and increasing tubular reabsorption (**FIGURE 12.4**). Vitamin D also helps to regulate the level of calcium in the blood by interacting with PTH, which is how PTH exerts its major function in the intestine. Vitamin D stimulates the production of CBP and IMCBP in the small intestinal mucosa, as discussed earlier, thereby facilitating calcium absorption. In contrast, calcitonin is secreted by the thyroid glands when blood calcium levels increase. Calcitonin increases calcium deposition into bones, thereby removing it from the blood. That effect, along with a decreased influence of PTH and vitamin D, results in a lowering of the serum calcium level.

Physiologic Roles of Calcium

As stated previously, calcium has both structural and functional significance. Because most body calcium is found as part of mineral complexes in hard tissue, such as bone and teeth, that has become its most recognized role. However, calcium is involved in several functional aspects of human physiology as well, such as transmission of nerve impulses, regulation of

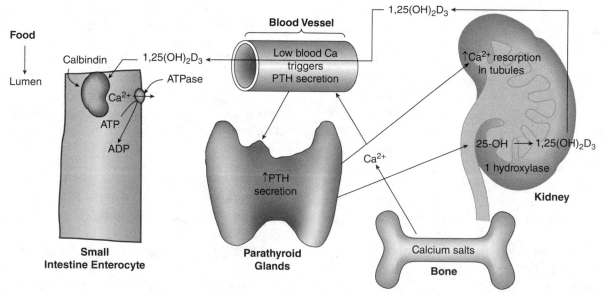

FIGURE 12.4 Calcium Balance as Mediated by Parathyroid Hormone (PTH), Calcitonin, and Vitamin D (25-OH). Low blood calcium increases secretion of PTH. PTH stimulates 1) calcium release from bone; 2) 1 α-hydroxylase to produce 1,25 $(OH)_2D$, and 3) the reabsorption of calcium by the kidney tubules. 1,25 $(OH)_2$ will enhance calcium absorption by stimulating small intestinal cells to produce the calcium uptake protein, calbindin, the TRPV6 calcium channel, and a vitamin D-regulated $Ca^{++}-Mg^{++}$ ATPase. These series of reactions maintain calcium levels within a normal range.

muscle contraction, maintenance of acid–base (pH) balance, regulation of biochemical reactions, and coagulation of blood.

Calcium is part of structurally important components of bones and teeth. Bones and teeth are about two-thirds mineral by weight, with the remaining one-third being mostly water, protein, and small amounts of lipid and other organic substances. Two complexes containing mostly calcium and phosphate provide strength and rigidity to bones and teeth: calcium phosphate $(Ca_3(PO_4)_2)$ and hydroxyapatite $(Ca_{10}(PO_4)_6OH_2)$. Hydroxyapatite is a complex molecule (**FIGURE 12.5**) and is responsible for a "hardening" effect on bone. Those mineral complexes also serve as a storage area for calcium and phosphorus. It is this portion of bone that is depleted during bone demineralization diseases, such as osteomalacia and osteoporosis.

Calcium is also associated with proteins in bone, cartilage, and dentin; ionic calcium binds with proteins, such as bone Gla protein (BGP, or osteocalcin) and matrix Gla protein (MGP). Both of those proteins are believed to promote mobilization of bone calcium. That notion is supported by reports that their expression is stimulated by 1,25-$(OH)_2D_3$.

Beyond bone, the remaining 1% of calcium in our body is found distributed in the blood and other tissue, such as muscle, nerves, and glands. As mentioned previously, it is this portion of body calcium that is crucial to human function and survival on a

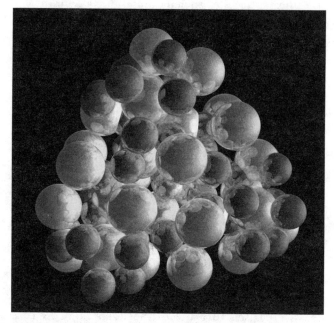

FIGURE 12.5 Structure of Hydroxyapatite. This is one of the primary crystalline forms of calcium in bone.
© Scott Camazine/Science Source.

millisecond-to-millisecond, second-to-second, minute-to-minute basis. The level of ionized calcium in the intracellular fluid is about 1/10,000 of that of extracellular levels. The concentration of calcium in the intracellular fluid is maintained at 100 nanomoles per liter. Maintaining such low intracellular levels of calcium prevents activation events, as described below, as well as precipitation with phosphates and other anions.

When cytosolic calcium levels are at their lowest levels, calcium is sequestered within organelles such as mitochondria, nuclei, and the endoplasmic reticulum (or sarcoplasmic reticulum in muscle tissue). Low calcium levels in the intracellular fluid are maintained by Ca^{2+} pumps located on the plasma or organelle membranes. Cell calcium levels can be regulated partly by the release of calcium from the endoplasmic reticulum. The mechanism responsible for that is rather complex and is initiated by a ligand (hormone or neurotransmitter) that binds to a G protein receptor on the cell membrane surface. Through a series of reactions, inositol triphosphate (IP_3) is produced and targets the endoplasmic reticulum to release calcium into the cell cytoplasm. Calcium ATPase pumps can cause cytoplasmic calcium to be pumped back into the endoplasmic reticulum. The cell, therefore, has several mechanisms to tightly control intracellular calcium levels.

Calcium is involved in the function of excitable cells, namely muscle fibers and neurons. Via so-called slow calcium–sodium channels in the sinoatrial node of the heart, calcium initiates the electric signal or action potential that stimulates cardiac muscle to contract. The influx of calcium via voltage-gated membrane channels on the plasma membrane and sarcoplasmic reticulum initiates cardiac muscle contraction (**FIGURE 12.6**). In skeletal muscle, an increase in the intracellular calcium concentration evokes fiber

contraction as well (**FIGURE 12.7**). Calcium binds with troponin C, which evokes a conformational change in this protein that ultimately uncovers binding sites on actin. This allows myosin to form cross bridges and perform a power stroke that results in sarcomere shortening and fiber contraction. After the stimulus for contraction is removed, calcium is pumped back into the sarcoplasmic reticulum and across the plasma membrane to reestablish the extremely low ionized calcium concentration in the intracellular fluid. The sarcoplasmic reticulum contains a calcium-binding protein called calsequestrin, which allows for a 10,000-fold greater calcium concentration during an unstimulated state.

Smooth muscle contraction differs somewhat from skeletal and cardiac muscle contraction. First, smooth muscle contains relatively fewer voltage-gated sodium channels and many more voltage-gated calcium channels. Therefore, calcium, not sodium, is responsible for the initiation and propagation of the action potential. Second, the source of calcium to initiate contraction is derived primarily from the extracellular fluid because the sarcoplasmic reticulum system is not developed in smooth muscle. Thus, whereas most of the calcium influx in stimulated skeletal muscle is derived from the sarcoplasmic reticulum, nearly all of the calcium influx in smooth muscle is across the plasma membrane. Finally, smooth muscle does not contain troponin.

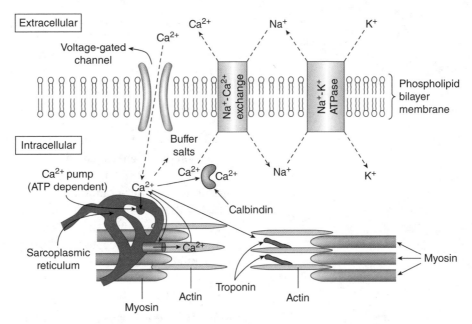

FIGURE 12.6 Calcium Channels and Pumps in Muscle Cells That Control Various Functions. Intracellular calcium levels are tightly controlled. Calcium may be sequestered by organelles (mitochondria, nuclei, and sarcoplasmic reticulum). Calcium ATP-dependent pumps cause cytoplasmic calcium to be pumped back into the sarcoplasmic reticulum. This returns intracellular levels of calcium to low levels once a calcium-dependent reaction has occurred. One such reaction would be the calcium-troponin reaction for muscle contraction, as illustrated here by forming cross-bridges with myosin. Extracellular calcium levels are controlled through voltage-gated channels and Na-Ca and Na-K ATPase pumps. This is important so that Ca levels remain high in the extracellular fluids but low within the cell.

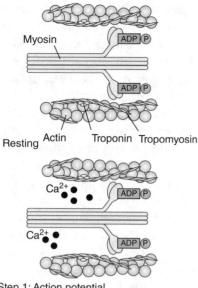

Myosin

ADP P

ADP P

Resting   Actin   Troponin   Tropomyosin

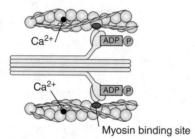

Ca²⁺

ADP P

Ca²⁺

ADP P

Step 1: Action potential

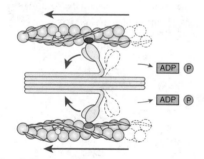

Ca²⁺

ADP P

Ca²⁺

ADP P

Myosin binding site

Step 2: Myosin-actin binding

ADP P

ADP P

Step 3: Power stroke

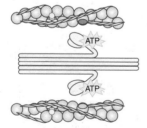

ATP

ATP

Step 4: ATP binding and actin-myosin release

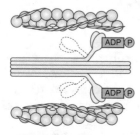

ADP P

ADP P

Step 5: ATP cleavage

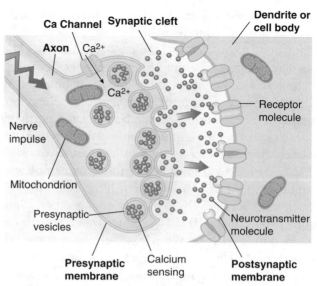

FIGURE 12.8 Role of Calcium in Synaptic Junctions and Neurotransmission. Calcium enters the axon from the synaptic cleft through calcium channels when an action potential occurs. The calcium causes the presynaptic vesicles that contain the neurotransmitter to fuse with the presynaptic membrane. The neurotransmitter is released into the synaptic cleft. The neurotransmitter binds to the receptor molecule on the postsynaptic membrane of the dendrite where an action potential is initiated to continue the impulse. The vesicles that contained the neurotransmitter are recycled by the axon for subsequent reactions.

Therefore, calcium has the capability to evoke smooth muscle contraction by a mechanism that is different from other muscle tissue.

Whereas the initiation and propagation of neuron action potentials is largely attributable to other ions, namely sodium and potassium, the release of neurotransmitters at synaptic junctions is reliant on calcium (**FIGURE 12.8**). As an action potential reaches a nerve terminal, voltage-gated calcium channels open and calcium enters the intracellular fluid of the axon from the synaptic cleft via calcium channels. It is believed that the increase in intracellular calcium allows for neurotransmitter-containing vesicles to migrate to and fuse with the plasma membrane. Neurotransmitters are thereby released into the synaptic gap. The neurotransmitters bind to a receptor on the dendrite and an action potential is initiated to continue the neural impulse.

FIGURE 12.7 Role of Calcium in Muscle Contraction. This scheme demonstrates the role of calcium binding to muscle troponin C to exposed binding sites on actin to allow myosin cross-bridges to form. These bridges are essential to allow for a power stroke to occur and cause a shortening of the microfibrils that compose the sarcomere. ATP is used in this process. After contraction, calcium is released from troponin and pumped back into the sarcoplasmic reticulum.

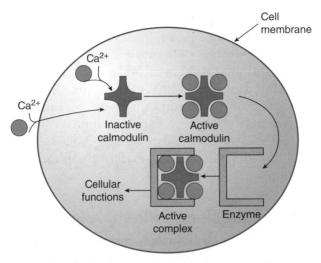

FIGURE 12.9 Calcium as a Second Messenger with Calmodulin Protein to Activate Enzymes. Calmodulin is a protein with four calcium-binding sites. When calcium binds to calmodulin, a conformational change occurs that allows the complex to interact with a variety of cellular enzymes that control cell functions.

Calcium functions as a second messenger. The binding of certain hormones to plasma membrane receptors results in the opening of calcium channels and an increase in the intracellular calcium concentration (**FIGURE 12.9**). Calcium is then able to bind with calmodulin, a protein with four calcium-binding sites. The binding of calcium to calmodulin evokes a conformational change in the protein structure. The presence of calmodulin–calcium complexes results in several intracellular events, including the regulation of the activity of key enzymes. For example, myosin light-chain kinase, which is involved in smooth muscle cell contraction, is dependent on calmodulin. Phosphorylase kinase is also calmodulin dependent. Phosphorylase kinase activates phosphorylase, which is a key enzyme involved in glycogen degradation. Calcium can also influence the activity of other enzymes, such as phospholipase A_2, protein kinase C, and phosphodiesterase. When intracellular levels of calcium increase, phospholipase A_2 becomes activated and will hydrolyze fatty acids. A good example of this is with the fatty acid arachidonic acid. Arachidonic acid may be hydrolyzed from membrane phospholipids, which allows it to feed into the production of thromboxanes and prostaglandins. When protein kinase C is activated, that enzyme can phosphorylate a number of proteins, including enzymes. Depending on the enzyme that is phosphorylated, the enzyme can either be activated or inactivated, thereby modulating metabolic pathways. When phosphodiesterase is activated, cAMP, a second messenger, is hydrolyzed and is thus inactivated.

Calcium is pivotal for blood clotting. Calcium is necessary for the conversion of factors VII, IX, and X to their active forms, as well as for the conversion of prothrombin to thrombin during the clotting cascade. Finally, calcium appears to be involved in sperm motility and in enzyme release upon penetration of the granulosa cell mass surrounding the ovum.

Recommended Levels for Calcium Intake

The DRI for calcium is expressed as an RDA. The RDA quantities for calcium are the highest among the non-energy-providing nutrients. For adolescents aged 11 to 18 years, the RDA for calcium is 1,300 milligrams per day. For those aged 18 to 50 years, it is 1,000 milligrams per day. The RDA increases to 1,200 milligrams per day for females older than 50 years but remains at 1,000 milligrams per day for males. It increases to 1,200 milligrams per day after 70 years of age for both sexes. For pregnant and lactating females, the RDA is 1,300 milligrams per day for those younger than 18 years of age and 1,000 milligrams per day for older women. On a per-weight basis, children have a higher calcium requirement than adults. Some organizations, such as the World Health Organization (WHO), suggest lower calcium intakes (400 to 500 milligrams per day) for adults.

Calcium Deficiency

A deficiency of calcium, whether from decreased provision, decreased absorption, or increased excretion, can result in numerous disease situations, especially pertaining to bone. If the deficiency occurs during the growing years, poor bone mineralization occurs. Bones become soft and pliable as a result of a lack of mineralization, which can result in a bowing of the legs.

In adults, two forms of bone disease may develop related to calcium deficiency. Osteomalacia is a demineralization of bone, primarily peripheral bones, due to a loss of calcium and phosphorus crystals that renders the remaining bone soft. That bone disease can result from a diet that is chronically poor in calcium or from poor vitamin D status. Osteoporosis, which mostly affects older women, is characterized by loss in the total amount of bone. Osteoporosis has a complex etiology that extends beyond insufficient dietary calcium intake over time and includes genetic and ethnic backgrounds, decreased estrogen, and lack of exercise. The bones affected in osteoporosis are more likely to be central bones, such as the hip and spine.

Blood pressure is thought to be regulated, in part, by dietary calcium. The connection between dietary calcium and blood pressure was first observed in pregnancy. The disorder preeclampsia, a toxic condition accompanied by hypertension, can occur in some pregnant women. Increased intake of calcium, primarily through dairy products, has been demonstrated to lower hypertension in preeclampsia. Follow-up studies on nonpregnant subjects revealed that hypertensive individuals who increased their calcium intake via dairy products or dietary supplements had lower blood pressure. Decreased calcium has been linked with greater adiposity: animal studies and some human studies suggest a link between calcium intake and body weight, although that remains controversial.

Situations, such as excessive urinary calcium losses in the urine or a vitamin D deficiency, may also result in a reduction in blood calcium. Whatever the cause of reduced blood calcium, it also affects the calcium concentrations in tissues such as nerve, muscle, and glands. Low blood calcium levels are associated with irritability of nervous tissue, including the central nervous system (CNS), and skeletal muscle cramping.

Calcium Toxicity

It is not uncommon today to find people ingesting large supplemental amounts of calcium. Sometimes, their intake can climb above several times their RDA. Although the efficiency of calcium absorption decreases as its dietary content increases and with optimal physiologic status, passive paracellular absorption can still lead to increased absorption. Other factors, such as gram doses of vitamin C and increased vitamin D ingestion or hyperparathyroidism, may also increase calcium status. Although fairly uncommon, excessive body calcium, over time, can lead to increased calcium deposition in tissue, such as muscle (including the heart), blood vessels, and lungs. That affects the activity of those tissues by making them more rigid. Renal filtration is the primary route of calcium excretion, and increased calcium in the ultrafiltrate may render an individual more prone to calcium-containing renal stones (i.e., calcium oxalates).

⬢ BEFORE YOU GO ON . . .

1. List the factors that both decrease and increase calcium absorption by the small intestine.

2. List the steps involved in the active uptake of calcium, including the proteins involved and how they are regulated in the absorptive cell.

3. How does the body best maintain calcium levels in the blood within a narrow range?

4. How does calcium play a role in muscle contraction and in neuroexcitation?

5. Describe the role that the protein calmodulin plays in calcium function.

▶ Phosphorus

Phosphorus is the sixth most abundant element (by weight) in the human body and the second most abundant mineral behind calcium. Like calcium, most of the phosphorus in the human body (approximately 85%) is found in bone. Whether one is discussing the phosphorus in food or in the body, this mineral is almost exclusively in the form of phosphate (PO_4^-).

Dietary Phosphorus Sources

Food sources with a higher content of phosphorus include meat, poultry, eggs, fish, milk and milk products, cereals, legumes, grains, and chocolate (**TABLE 12.4**). Many soft drinks contain phosphorus in the form of phosphoric acid. Coffee and tea also provide some phosphorus. Phosphorus occurs in foods in both an inorganic form as well as a component of organic molecules, such as phospholipids, phosphoproteins, and phosphorylated sugars. The type of food determines the relative amount of either inorganic or organic sources. For instance, most phosphorus in meats and more than half of the phosphorus in milk is complexed in organic molecules. As much as 80% of the phosphorus in grains (e.g., wheat, oats, corn, rice) is part of phytate (inositol hexaphosphate). Phytate is composed of the carbohydrate inositol with up to six phosphate groups esterified to the carbon atoms in the ring (see Figure 12.1). Phytate is the plant storage form of phosphorus.

Digestion and Absorption of Phosphorus

Most phosphorus is absorbed in its inorganic form. Therefore, phosphate that is part of organic molecules must be liberated by digestive enzymes. A notable exception is the phosphate from phytate, which has very limited absorption due to the lack of the **phytase** enzyme in humans. However, yeast preparations used in the production of breads contain phytase. The phytase can liberate as much as one-half of the phosphate available from the grain's phytate.

A meal containing a considerable quantity of magnesium or calcium or both can decrease phosphorus absorption. Magnesium and phosphates may form chelates in the intestinal lumen, thereby decreasing the absorption efficiency for both substances. In contrast, a meal low in magnesium enhances phosphate absorption. Aluminum-containing substances ingested with a meal can also decrease phosphate absorption. For instance, 3 grams of aluminum hydroxide can reduce phosphorus absorption by one-half. Aluminum

TABLE 12.4 Phosphorus Content of Select Foods

Food	Phosphorus (mg)	Food	Phosphorus (mg)
Milk and milk products		*Grains*	
Yogurt (cup)	331	Bran flakes (1 serving, ¾ cup)	105
Milk (1 cup)	205	Bread, whole wheat (1 slice)	57
Cheese, American (1 oz)	211	Noodles, cooked (1 cup)	122
Meat and alternatives		Rice, cooked (1 cup)	68
Pork (3 oz)	178	Bread, white (1 slice)	25
Hamburger (3 oz)	174	*Vegetables*	
Tuna (3 oz)	264	Potato, large (1)	209
Lobster (3 oz)	157	Corn (1 cup)	107
Chicken (3 oz)	192	Peas (1 cup)	88
Nuts and seeds		Broccoli, raw, chopped (1 cup)	60
Sunflower seeds (1 oz)	209	*Other*	
Peanuts (1 oz)	101	Cola (12 oz)	37
Peanut butter (1 Tbsp)	179	Diet cola (12 oz)	32

hydroxide and magnesium hydroxide are common ingredients in antacids.

Phosphorus absorption is believed to take place throughout the small intestine. The efficiency of absorption is about 50 to 70% with a typical intake and as high as 90% when phosphorus intake is low. The efficiency of absorption is not impaired by physiologic phosphorus status; thus, hyperphosphatemia is possible with higher intakes over time.

The absorption of phosphorus probably involves two mechanisms: first, an active, saturable, carrier-mediated process; and second, a diffusion system that demonstrates a linear nature. Vitamin D stimulates the absorption of phosphorus via the active transport mechanism. Active transport predominates when luminal phosphorus is low. However, when luminal phosphorus is high, diffusion predominates. For active transport of phosphorus, sodium cotransport with phosphate occurs and is ATPase dependent.

Serum Phosphorus Levels and Homeostasis

Approximately 70% of the phosphorus in the blood circulates as part of phospholipids, primarily in lipoproteins, cells, and platelets. The remaining 30% is largely dissolved inorganic phosphates (HPO_4^{2-} and $H_2PO_4^-$). To a lesser degree, phosphate is also bound to proteins or complexed to calcium or magnesium. The range for inorganic phosphate levels in adult blood is approximately 2.5 to 4.5 milligrams per 100 milliliters. Because a large portion of dietary phosphorus is absorbed, proper renal excretion is paramount. As much as two-thirds of dietary phosphorus is excreted in the urine.

Serum phosphorus levels are under tight homeostatic control, similar to that of calcium. Parathyroid hormone and 1,25 $(OH)_2$ cholcalciferol control phosphorus homeostasis, similar to that of calcium.

Specific proteins have been identified that function to control phosphorus absorption by the small intestine and the amount of phosphorus either reabsorbed or eliminated through the urine. Those proteins are under genetic control. Studies have revealed that mutations in the genes that encode those proteins can lead to serious health consequences. If serum phosphorus becomes elevated, that will increase calcification of the vascular tissue, arteriosclerosis, cardiovascular disease, and increased mortality, especially for those already afflicted with kidney disease.

The two specific proteins that regulate serum phosphorus levels are: 1) **Fibroblast Growth Factor 23 (FGF 23)**, and 2) **Klotho**. FGF 23 is synthesized in bone osteocytes. When serum phosphorus becomes elevated (hyperphosphatemia), FGF 23 will be released and lower serum phosphorus levels by three mechanisms: 1) the protein will reduce the synthesis of 1,25 $(OH)_2$ cholcalciferol by inhibiting the 1-α hydroxylase enzyme in the small intestine enterocytes. It will stimulate the production of 24, 25 $(OH)_2$ cholcalciferol; 2) FGF 23 decreases renal phosphorus reabsorption by the proximal tubules. Klotho binds to FGF 23 and collectively this complex binds to the receptor in the proximal tubule. The overall effect is that sodium-phosphorus transporter (NaPi) 2a and 2c has reduced gene expression and protein produced. That decreases the reabsorption of phosphorus, resulting in increased phosphorus elimination through the urine; 3) FGF 23 will suppress PTH gene expression. Taken together, those events tend to normalize serum phosphorus levels.

There are genetic mutations that can lead to abnormal serum phosphorus levels. Genetic defects in the genes that encode FGF 23 and/or Klotho results in hyperphosphatemia. That results in calcification of soft tissues and can be problematic around hips, shoulders, and knee joints and could accelerate the development of chronic kidney failure and onset of cardiovascular disease.

Physiologic Roles of Phosphorus

There are many significant roles of phosphorus. Phosphorus as phosphate is the form of much of its physiologic/biochemical effects. Phosphorus is important in energy metabolism in that the phosphate bond in ATP, GTP, and creatine phosphate drives most of the energy requiring reactions (**FIGURES 12.10** and **12.11**). Absorption of nutrients via active transport pumps, maintenance of the balance of cellular ions, and muscle contraction are dependent on these nucleoside triphosphates. Another nucleoside phosphate derivative, UTP, is important in the production of glycogen.

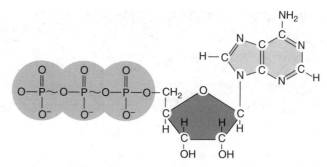

FIGURE 12.10 ATP Molecule. The energy of ATP is contained within the high energy bonds of the three phosphate groups. Other nucleotides (e.g., GTP) have the same function.

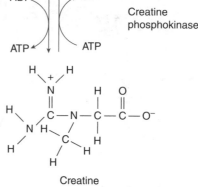

FIGURE 12.11 Production of ATP from Creatine Phosphate with the Enzyme Creatine Phosphokinase. Another source of energy is creatine phosphate, in which the energy from the phosphate group can be liberated by creatine phosphokinase. Note that this reaction is reversible.

Phosphate is part of cAMP, a critical component of cell signaling. ATP is the precursor to cAMP and is referred to as a second messenger. Hormones may bind to cell receptors and activate adenyl cyclase to convert ATP to cAMP. The cAMP can influence enzyme activity by activating kinases. cGMP is another nucleoside form that may activate other kinases. Finally, inositol phosphate (iP_3) can cause the release of calcium from specific organelles in cells via activating protein kinases.

DNA and RNA are dependent on phosphate (See Figure 1.8). A phosphodiester bond links the ribose components together. Phosphorus is also required for vitamin B_6 and thiamin to function. Examples of this are pyridoxal phosphate and thiamin pyrophosphate.

Phospholipids are a component of various lipoproteins and cell membranes. The polar nature of phosphate allows lipids to be miscible in aqueous environments, such as plasma.

It is essential that phosphorus play a role in teeth and bone structure as a component of hydroxyapatite. Phosphorus is a part of the calcium-phosphate crystals, which are a part of calcium hydroxyapatite. This is important as calcium hydroxyapatite increases the mechanical hardness and strength of both bone and teeth.

Finally, phosphate is involved in the regulation of the pH of extracellular fluid. Phosphates in the ultrafiltrate, largely as sodium phosphate, can react with hydrogen ions and keep them from being reabsorbed:

$$Na_2HPO_4 + H^+ \rightarrow NaH_2PO_4 + Na^+$$

Recommended Levels of Phosphorus Intake

The current RDAs for phosphorus are different from those for calcium (previous recommendations had the levels the same). The RDA for phosphorus in those aged 9 to 18 years is 1,250 milligrams per day. This decreases to 700 milligrams per day for people who are older than 18 years. Pregnant and lactating females have an RDA of 1,250 milligrams per day for people who are younger than 18 years; that RDA decreases to 700 milligrams per day for pregnant and lactating females older than 18 years.

Phosphorus Deficiency and Toxicity

Because most foods contain phosphorus, a deficiency is somewhat rare under normal circumstances. Toxicity is also rare, with the exception of infants who receive a formula that is high in phosphorus. However, most commercially available infant formulas are not a threat with regard to their phosphorus content.

● BEFORE YOU GO ON . . .

1. In what form is phosphorus found in the blood?
2. List the physiologic roles that phosphorus plays in the body.
3. List some good sources of dietary phosphorus.
4. How is serum phosphorus homeostasis maintained?
5. What are FGF 23 and Klothos?

▶ Magnesium

Like calcium, magnesium is a divalent cation. Typically an adult body contains 20 to 28 grams of magnesium. More than one-half and up to two-thirds of this mineral is associated with bone tissue. On a mass basis, magnesium is the twelfth most abundant element in the human body, contributing about 1% of human mass. It is the fourth most abundant cation in the human body; however, it is the second most abundant intracellular cation, after potassium.

Dietary Magnesium Sources

Magnesium is the third largest consumed element in the human diet, following calcium and phosphorus. Unfortunately, magnesium intake has been lowered over the past century, possibly due to increased intake of refined foods. However, there has been an increase in intake in the last couple of decades, but the intake is well below recommended levels. This low intake is thought to be related to a number of chronic diseases, as discussed later. Magnesium is found in a variety of foods, with good sources, including whole grain cereals, nuts, legumes, spices, seafood, coffee, tea, and cocoa (**TABLE 12.5**). Chlorophyll contains magnesium. Therefore, plant components rich in chlorophyll, such as green leaves, are a source of magnesium. Certain processing techniques, such as the refining of grains and polishing of rice, may result in significant losses of magnesium. Some magnesium can also dissolve into cooking water during boiling, resulting in some losses as well.

There has been much work published pertaining to the correct dietary ratio of calcium to magnesium intake. Studies have revealed that Ca:Mg ratios greater than 2.7 is detrimental to human health. Colorectal adenomas are increased in ratios greater than 2.7. On the other hand, Ca:Mg intake less than 1.7 leads to a greater risk of ischemic heart disease. It seems as though a safe ratio of Ca:Mg is 1.7 to 2.7.

Magnesium Absorption

The absorption of magnesium occurs along the length of the small intestine, as well as, to a limited degree, in the colon. However, if small-intestinal absorption of magnesium is impaired, the absorption in the colon can play a major role in maintaining magnesium balance in the body. Absorption in the ileum may be a saturable process, whereas absorption in the more proximal small intestine is not. The saturable mechanism involves the protein transient receptor potential melastatin divalent cation-permeable channel protein,

TABLE 12.5 Magnesium Content of Select Foods

Food	Magnesium (mg)	Food	Magnesium (mg)
Legumes		*Vegetables*	
Lentils, cooked (1 cup)	71	Bean sprouts (1 cup)	17
Split peas, cooked (1 cup)	71	Peas (1 cup)	36
Tofu (1 cup)	146	Spinach, cooked (1 cup)	157
Nuts		Lima beans (1 cup)	100
Peanuts (1 oz)	50	*Milk and milk products*	
Cashews (1 oz)	73	Milk (1 cup)	24
Almonds (1 oz)	81	Cheese, cheddar (1 oz)	8
Grains		Cheese, American (1 oz)	9
Bran Buds (1 serving, ⅓ cup)	62	*Meats*	
Rice, wild, cooked (1 cup)	52	Chicken (3 oz)	23
Wheat germ (2 Tbsp)	45	Beef (3 oz)	16
		Pork (3 oz)	20

which is more simply designated as **TRPV6**. That is not an energy-dependent absorption process, but it is more significant when luminal magnesium concentrations are low. The paracellular diffusion route is more significant with high luminal magnesium concentration. In contrast, export of magnesium from the enterocyte to the blood is an energy-dependent process where sodium is exchanged for magnesium via an ATPase-dependent mechanism (**FIGURE 12.12**).

Magnesium absorption from the human digestive tract is fair (25 to 60%), although certain factors can influence this efficiency. For example, a low body magnesium status results in a higher percentage of absorption. Vitamin D also appears to increase magnesium absorption to a limited, yet significant, degree. In contrast, a high-magnesium diet and excessive dietary calcium, phosphate, phytate, and fatty acids decrease the efficiency of magnesium absorption. The unabsorbed fatty acids can form magnesium–fatty acid soaps in a manner similar to the formation of calcium–fatty acid soaps. As mentioned earlier, calcium and magnesium may compete for similar absorptive mechanisms.

Tissue Magnesium Content and Excretion

An adult contains about 0.5 gram of magnesium per kilogram of fat-free body weight. About 60% of the magnesium in humans is located in bones; the remaining portion is found in the extracellular fluid (approximately 1%) and in soft tissue (approximately 39%). Approximately 50 to 55% of plasma magnesium is dissolved as an independent ion. About 32% of circulating magnesium is bound to plasma proteins, such as albumin, and the remaining magnesium is complexed to negatively charged substances, such as citrate, phosphate, or other anions. While **TRPM6** is the transport protein for magnesium absorption in the small intestine, another transporter for tissues has been identified as **TRPM7**. That transport protein is ubiquitously expressed.

Whereas unabsorbed magnesium is removed from the digestive tract in feces, magnesium is excreted from within the body, primarily through urinary loss. Circulating magnesium becomes part of the ultrafiltrate, with the exception of that associated with plasma proteins. As much as 95 to 97% of the magnesium in the ultrafiltrate is reabsorbed. However,

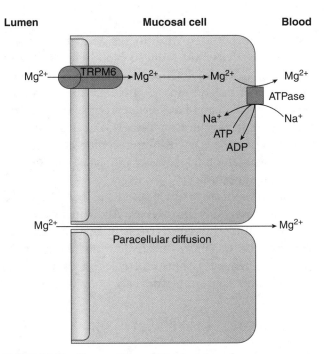

FIGURE 12.12 Absorption of Magnesium by Enterocytes. Similar to calcium absorption, there are two mechanisms of magnesium absorption by the enterocytes. One mechanism is saturable and energy dependent. Magnesium enters the cell through TRPM6, a channel protein, and exits the cell to the blood via an ATPase-dependent mechanism. The second mechanism is paracellular diffusion between the enterocytes.

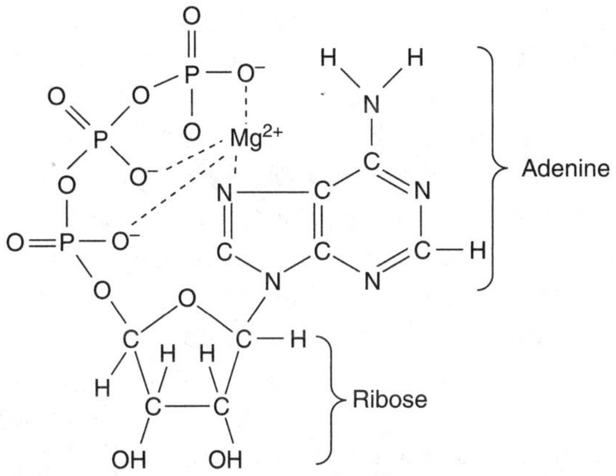

as circulating levels of magnesium increase, so does renal excretion.

Physiologic Roles of Magnesium

Bone magnesium should be separated into (1) the magnesium associated with the crystal lattice, which may have been laid down during development; and (2) magnesium associated with the surface of bone, which represents a magnesium pool. Most of the nonbone magnesium is found in soft tissue, especially skeletal muscle. In those tissues, it is ionically associated with membrane phospholipids, proteins, nucleic acids, and ATP.

Magnesium forms an electric union with the negatively charged oxygen atoms of the phosphate tail of ATP (**FIGURE 12.13**). This interaction appears to add stability to the molecule and to assist ATP-dependent reactions, especially kinase reactions that transfer an ATP phosphate group to another molecule.

Magnesium is believed to be necessary, or at least important, in over 300 enzyme-catalyzed reactions. Therefore, magnesium is a key factor for most metabolic pathways. For instance, hexokinase, glucokinase, and phosphofructokinase (PFK), key enzymes in glycolysis, depend on magnesium (**FIGURE 12.14**). Other

FIGURE 12.13 Magnesium's Role in Stabilizing Chemical Compounds, such as ATP. Magnesium binds to the phosphate groups of ATP to stabilize the structure. This structure stability is especially important for kinase reactions.

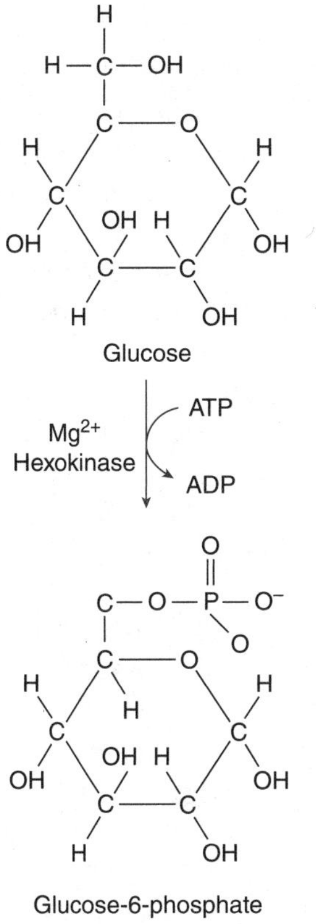

Glucose

Mg^{2+}
Hexokinase

ATP

ADP

Glucose-6-phosphate

FIGURE 12.14 Magnesium's Involvement in Hexokinase Activity. Magnesium is a key factor in most metabolic pathways. Magnesium is especially important in many kinase reactions, including several key kinases in glycolysis. The above reaction with hexokinase adding a phosphate group to glucose to produce glucose-6-phosphate is only one example of many such reactions.

magnesium-dependent enzymes include mevalonate kinase, phosphomevalonate kinase, and squalene synthetase, which are involved in cholesterol synthesis. Creatine kinase, which synthesizes creatine phosphate, and acyl CoA synthetase, a key enzyme in β-oxidation, are also magnesium dependent, as are alkaline phosphatase and pyrophosphatase. Some general operations that require magnesium include amino acid activation, DNA replication and RNA transcription, nucleic acid synthesis, protein synthesis, and cAMP formation from adenylate cyclase.

Magnesium is also thought to have an anti-inflammatory role. Low magnesium levels exacerbate or stimulate hypoxia, which produces free radicals and stimulates interleukin 1 (IL-1), IL-17, and interferon λ production. Those chemicals target NFκB, which, in turn, stimulates the expression of TNF-α, which also leads to an inflammatory response. An inflammatory response under low magnesium levels can lead to asthma, arthritis, atherosclerosis, and neuroinflammation, among other similar diseases.

Magnesium is vital for the proper activity and metabolism of other nutrients. For instance, magnesium is needed for parathyroid hormone secretion as well as its hormonal effects on bone, the kidney, and intestines. Magnesium is also necessary for the hydroxylation of vitamin D (cholecalciferol) in hepatocytes. This reaction is the preliminary step in converting vitamin D to its most active form. Specifically, magnesium is required for the activity of 25-hydroxylase, 24-hydroxylase, and 1α-hydroxylase. Magnesium deficiency can consequently lead to decreased parathyroid function and reduced levels of 1, 25 $(OH)_2$ cholcalciferol. This can impact bone integrity.

A large number of studies have revealed that a lack of magnesium in the diet has been linked to a wide variety of diseases. There appears to be a link between low magnesium status with Type II diabetes, metabolic syndrome, some cancers, and ischemic heart disease. Magnesium has been linked to blood pressure, but the data remain inconclusive. Intakes of 500 to 1,000 mg/day appeared to reduce blood pressure in several studies. Other studies suggest that the possible blood pressure-lowering effect of magnesium is more significant when there is a low-sodium and high-potassium diet. Taurine supplementation, in combination with magnesium supplementation, has also been reported as being more effective in lowering blood pressure than with magnesium supplementation alone. That combination has been reported to enhance insulin sensitivity. Reduced vascular tone and cardiac hypertrophy have been reported with increased dietary magnesium.

The role of magnesium as it relates to Type II diabetes has been studied extensively. Type II diabetics supplemented with 300 mg magnesium per day for 3 months increased serum magnesium levels and resulted in a significant improvement in insulin sensitivity. In addition, overweight subjects, who were not diabetic but were insulin resistant, had greater insulin sensitivity and reduced blood glucose levels. That latter aspect is related to metabolic syndrome and the ability of magnesium to attenuate the condition. Several mechanisms have been proposed to explain the role of magnesium on Type II diabetes. Tyrosine kinase activity of the insulin receptor and GLUT4 (which facilitates glucose entry into a cell) are dependent on magnesium.

Magnesium supplementation has been reported to reduce migraine headaches, Alzheimer's disease, and dementia. The effectiveness of magnesium supplementation was more effective in modulating those diseases when potassium and calcium supplements were administered simultaneously.

Recommended Levels for Magnesium Intake

The RDA is 30 and 75 milligrams per day for infants during their first 6 months and second 6 months of life, respectively. The dietary levels of magnesium recommended (RDA) are systematically raised during childhood, from 80 milligrams for those 1 to 3 years old to 130 milligrams per day for children between 4 and 8 years old. Males and females between the ages of 9 and 13 years have an RDA of 240 milligrams per day. During adolescence and adulthood, recommendations range from 410 to 420 milligrams per day for males and from 310 to 360 milligrams per day for nonpregnant females. Pregnancy increases the recommendation to 400 milligrams per day for those younger than 18 years of age, whereas it decreases the RDA to 350 per day for those aged 19 to 30 years and to 260 milligrams for those aged 31 to 50 years. During lactation, the RDA is 360 milligrams per day for those younger than 18 years, 310 milligrams per day for those aged 19 to 30 years, and 320 milligrams per day for those aged 31 to 50 years.

Deficiency and Toxicity of Magnesium

Although magnesium is found in a variety of foods and deficiency is somewhat rare, excessive vomiting and diarrhea, alcohol abuse, renal and endocrine disease, and protein malnutrition may lead to a deficient status. Excess use of diuretics may result in deficiency of magnesium as well as other nutrients. Subtle reductions in blood magnesium content can affect the release and activity of the parathyroid hormone. Furthermore, a magnesium deficiency can alter the ability of protein pumps to maintain optimal sodium and potassium concentration differences across cell membranes. That largely reflects magnesium's ability to stabilize ATP, which is the power source for pumping ions across cell membranes. Thus, the proper function of excitable and other cells is jeopardized during magnesium deficiency. Clinical signs of a magnesium deficiency can be nonspecific, such as anorexia and nausea and vomiting. Specific symptoms, such as muscle spasms and tremors; and abnormal CNS function, which would include seizures, paresthesias (pins and needles), and rapid heartbeat or tachycardia may be present. Decreased blood levels of PTH, serum calcium, and potassium are also present.

Toxicity induced by a high dietary intake of magnesium can be thwarted by appropriately functioning kidneys. However, magnesium, in excess, may pose physiologic problems in that it may enhance the excretion of calcium, phosphorus, and potassium. It has been suggested that a chronic excess of magnesium can result in renal damage or renal insufficiency.

● BEFORE YOU GO ON . . .

1. Why are green plants a good source of magnesium?

2. List some factors than can decrease magnesium absorption.

3. What is the role of magnesium with respect to ATP chemistry?

4. Do you believe that magnesium can play a role in glycolysis, and why?

5. What can lead to a magnesium deficiency, and what are some of the clinical signs?

6. Discuss the various diseases linked to low magnesium intake.

▶ Sodium, Chloride, and Potassium

Sodium, potassium, and chloride (chlorine) can be discussed in tandem because their metabolic and biochemical functions are so interrelated. Furthermore, the heavy use of sodium chloride (table salt) as a flavoring agent and food preservative allows for many foods to be significant providers of both sodium and chloride.

Sodium is the primary cation found in the extracellular fluid, whereas potassium is the primary intracellular cation. The chloride anion is usually associated with sodium and, therefore, is more concentrated in the extracellular fluid. Those elements are heavily involved in the proper maintenance of water balance across cellular membranes as well as in establishing the electric potential across plasma membranes. Often, those elements, as well as other ions, are referred to as **electrolytes** because of their ability to conduct an electric charge when dissolved in water.

Dietary Sources of Sodium, Potassium, and Chloride

The typical American diet includes approximately 3 to 7 grams of sodium daily; however, the natural sodium content of most foods is very low. As much as 50 to 75% of the sodium in the American diet is actually added to foods by food manufacturers for taste or preservation. Another 15% is added by individuals during cooking and by salting foods at the table. The sodium occurring naturally in foods, such as eggs, milk, meats, and vegetables, may only account for about 10 to 15% of the total sodium intake by Americans. Drinking water may contribute to sodium intake, along with certain medicines, mouthwashes, and toothpastes (sodium fluoride). Foods with the greatest contribution of sodium to the American diet include luncheon meats, snack chips, French fries, hot dogs, cheeses, soups, and gravies. **TABLE 12.6** provides a list of select foods and their sodium content. Food labels in the United States require manufacturers to list the sodium content of a food on a per-serving basis. Any claims made by the manufacturer regarding the sodium content must follow the criteria listed in **TABLE 12.7**.

Like sodium, the natural chloride content of most foods is very low. However, some fruits and vegetables do contain respectable amounts of chloride. Sodium chloride (NaCl) provides nearly all of the chloride in the diet. NaCl is approximately 60% chloride and 40% sodium by weight. Thus, a food containing 1 gram of NaCl contains approximately 400 milligrams of sodium and 600 milligrams of chloride.

Unlike sodium and chloride, potassium is not routinely added to foods. Potassium is naturally found in most foods in the diet. Rich sources of potassium are typically fresh, unprocessed foods. Fresh fruits and vegetables rank among the best potassium sources. Tomatoes, carrots, potatoes, beans, peaches, pears, squash, oranges, and bananas are all notable for their high potassium content (**TABLE 12.8**). Milk, meats, whole grains, coffee, and tea are also among the significant contributors to our daily potassium intake. Many athletes refer to bananas as "potassium sticks" in reference to their potassium content, although their potassium content is not necessarily outstanding compared with many other fruits or vegetables.

TABLE 12.6 Sodium Content of Select Foods

Food	Sodium (mg)	Food	Sodium (mg)
Meat and alternatives		*Other*	
Corned beef (3 oz)	964	Salt (1 tsp)	2,325
Ham (3 oz)	936	Pickle, dill (1 large)	1,181
Fish, canned (3 oz)	185	Broth, chicken (1 cup)	763
Sausage (3 oz)	629	Ravioli, canned (1 cup)	1,091
Hot dog (1)	1, 140	Broth, beef (1 cup)	893
Bologna (1 oz)	1,302	Gravy (1 cup)	1,080
Milk and milk products		Italian dressing (1 tbsp)	150
Cream of potato soup (1 cup)	645	Pretzels (10)	814
Cottage cheese (1 cup)	819	Olives, green (5)	210
Cheese, American (1 oz)	452	Pizza, cheese (1 slice)	890
Cheese, Parmesan (1 oz)	433	Soy sauce (1 tsp)	341
Milk, skim (1 cup)	103	Bacon (3 slices)	534
Milk, whole (1 cup)	105	French dressing (2 tbsp)	268
Grains		Potato chips (1 oz)	149
Bran flakes (1 serving, ¾ cup)	220	Ketchup (1 tbsp)	167
Corn flakes (1 cup)	220		
Bagel (1)	530		
English muffin (1)	206		
Bread, white (1 slice)	128		
Bread, whole wheat (1 slice)	130		
Crackers, saltines (5 squares)	167		

Absorption of Sodium, Potassium, and Chloride

The absorption efficiencies of sodium, potassium, and chloride rank among the highest of the nutrients. As much as 90 to 95% of those minerals are absorbed, because less than 10% of dietary sodium, potassium, or chloride appears in the feces. Thus, renal excretion becomes the primary route of regulating physiologic levels of those minerals.

TABLE 12.7 Labeling Guidelines for Sodium Claims

Label Claim	Sodium Content
Sodium free	Must contain < 5 mg sodium per serving
Very low sodium	Must contain ≤ 35 mg sodium per serving
Low sodium	Must contain ≤145 mg sodium per serving
Reduced sodium	25% reduction in sodium content
Unsalted	No salt added to recipe
No added salt	No salt added to recipe

throughout the small intestine and in the proximal colon; and (3) an electrogenic Na^+ transport mechanism occurring in the colon (**FIGURE 12.15**). Sodium is also involved in the transport of certain amino acids, dipeptides, tripeptides, and some of the water-soluble vitamins across the apical membrane of enterocytes in a mechanism similar to the Na^+-glucose co-transporter.

Unlike sodium, the mechanisms for potassium absorption are not entirely clear. Absorption appears to take place along the length of the intestines, with the colon perhaps being a major site of absorption. Some research has suggested that potassium enters enterocytes via a K^+-H^+ antiport ATPase pump. Potassium also appears to diffuse across the apical membrane and across the basolateral membrane into the extracellular fluid via potassium channels. Extracellular potassium is necessary for the movement of sodium across the basolateral membrane as well because it is used in a Na^+-K^+ ATPase antiport system.

Chloride is absorbed along the length of the small intestine, and its absorption is often associated with sodium absorption in efforts to maintain electric neutrality. With the exception of the Na^+-Cl^-

Sodium appears to be absorbed by three primary mechanisms: (1) a Na^+-glucose co-transport system occurring along the length of the small intestine; (2) a Na^+-Cl^- co-transport system occurring

TABLE 12.8 Potassium Content of Select Foods

Food	Potassium (mg)	Food	Potassium (mg)
Vegetables		*Milk and milk products*	
Potato, large (1)	1,627	Yogurt, low fat (1 cup)	573
Squash, winter (1 cup)	896	Milk, skim (1 cup)	382
Tomato (1)	235	*Meats/Fish*	
Celery (1 stalk)	104	Fish, trout (3 oz)	394
Carrots (1)	195	Hamburger (3 oz)	258
Broccoli (½ cup)	139	Lamb (3 oz)	263
Fruit		Pork (3 oz)	280
Avocado (1)	975	Chicken (3 oz)	207
Orange juice (1 cup)	443	*Grains*	
Banana (1)	422	Bran buds (1 serving, ⅓ cup)	300
Raisins (1 cup)	1,236	Bran flakes (1 serving, ¾ cup)	185
Prunes (1 cup)	774	Raisin bran (1 cup)	335
Watermelon (1 cup)	172	Wheat flakes (1 serving, ¾ cup)	171

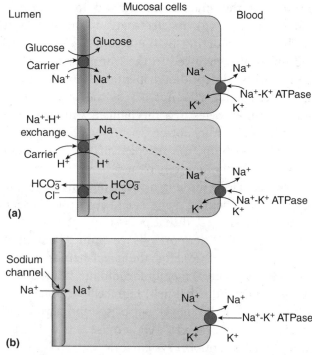

FIGURE 12.15 Various Absorption Routes of Sodium.
(a) Two absorption routes are shown here: sodium–glucose co-transport and sodium–hydrogen exchange. (b) Another route is via a sodium channel that is often termed electrogenic and is more common in the colon.

co-transporter mentioned previously, most chloride absorption occurs in a paracellular manner because chloride appears to be able to navigate the tight junctions between enterocytes.

Tissue, Urinary, and Sweat Content of Sodium, Potassium, and Chloride

Humans have approximately 1.8 grams of sodium per kilogram of fat-free body weight. For example, an average 70-kilogram adult male body would contain about 83 to 97 grams of sodium. The serum concentration averages in the range of 300 to 355 milligrams of sodium per 100 milliliters. Approximately 30 to 35% of total body sodium is located in bone associated with the surface of mineral crystals. That probably serves as a reservoir of blood sodium to avoid potential hyponatremia. The remainder of body sodium is primarily found dissolved within extracellular fluid, and sodium accounts for more than 90% of the blood cation content. Meanwhile, about 88% of chloride is found in the extracellular fluid, and the remainder is located intracellularly. Chloride's negative charge serves to neutralize the positive charge of sodium. The

sodium and chloride content of sweat increases with the rate of sweating.

In contrast to sodium and chloride, about 97 to 98% of body potassium is located within intracellular fluid. It is the predominant intracellular cation. Approximately 2.6 grams of potassium per kilogram fat-free body weight can be expected. The concentration of potassium in serum is 14 to 22 milligrams per 100 milliliters.

The regulation of those elements in the body is primarily accomplished by the adrenal corticoids deoxycorticosterone and aldosterone, and the pituitary peptides antidiuretic hormone (ADH, or vasopressin) and oxytocin. Those hormones all act on the kidney tubules to increase sodium retention. For instance, increased aldosterone output increases sodium retention and blood calcium. The kidney filters sodium out, and the element is reabsorbed by the proximal tubule. The distal tubules are also active in secreting potassium promoted by those hormones.

Physiologic Functions of Sodium, Potassium, and Chloride

Sodium, potassium, and chloride are the primary electrolytes in human fluids. Other important electrolytes include bicarbonate (HCO_3^-), magnesium, calcium, sulfate (SO_4^{2-}), and phosphates (PO_4^{2-}). All are dispersed throughout the extracellular and intracellular fluids; **TABLE 12.9** lists their concentrations. Although all electrolytes contribute at least to some degree to the establishment of the electric potential across plasma membranes, in general, sodium, potassium, and chloride contribute the most. Although an electric potential exists across the plasma membrane of essentially all cells, without a doubt, it is most important in the so-called excitable cells (muscle cells and neurons). In excitable cells, ion flux through gated channels allows for rapid and transient changes in the membrane potential. This, of course, is the action potential, the hallmark of excitable cells. During nerve transmission and muscle contraction, sodium diffuses intracellularly and potassium diffuses extracellularly, serving as the basis of the action potential. The cell quickly reestablishes the concentration gradients after an impulse or contraction has occurred by using a Na^+-K^+ ATPase pump.

Chloride is a component of hydrochloric acid, which is responsible for the acidic nature of the stomach. Hydrochloric acid is secreted by parietal cells in the oxyntic glands of the stomach mucosa.

TABLE 12.9 Electrolyte Composition in the Extracellular and Intracellular Fluid

	Extracellular Fluid (mEq/L)	Intracellular Fluid (mEq/L)
Sodium (Na$^+$)	142	10
Potassium (K$^+$)	4	140
Chloride (Cl$^-$)	103	4
Calcium (Ca^{2+})	2.4	0.0001
Magnesium (Mg^{2+})	1.2	58
Bicarbonate (HCO$_3^-$)	28	10
Phosphates (PO$_4^{2-}$)	4	75
Sulfates (SO$_4^{2-}$)	1	2

Chloride is also secreted along the digestive tract as a means of maintaining electric neutrality. Chloride may be the only ion actively secreted by the digestive tract mucosa.

In red blood cells, the cellular waste product CO_2 reacts with water in the presence of carbonic anhydrase to produce HCO_3^-. When the HCO_3^- content increases in the cell, it diffuses out of the cell. Chloride is brought into the cell to maintain electric neutrality. The transport of chloride and HCO_3^- occurs simultaneously via a transmembrane transport protein. This process allows for more carbon dioxide to circulate to the lungs. In the lungs, the reverse occurs. Because the reversible carbonic anhydrase catalyzes an equilibrium reaction, more and more HCO_3^- is converted to CO_2 and water. The equilibrium reaction proceeds in this direction in the lungs as CO_2 diffuses into the alveoli and is expired. Those reactions are collectively referred to as the **chloride shift**.

Recommended Levels of Intake for Sodium, Potassium, and Chloride

In contrast to the typical American sodium intake of several grams per day, the adult AI for adolescents and adults ranges from only 1.2 to 1.5 grams per day. The AI for chloride of adults is about 1.8 to 2.3 grams per day. As with sodium, the average American dietary intake of chloride is in tremendous excess of requirements. As mentioned previously, the major provider of sodium and chloride is NaCl used as a food manufacturing or consumer additive. The average American consumes 10 to 15 grams of NaCl per day. The adult AI for potassium is 4.7 grams daily. Although this level should be achievable by consuming a variety of foods, many Americans do not consume adequate potassium.

Deficiency, Toxicity, and Health Concerns for Sodium, Potassium, and Chloride

As noted earlier with regard to the extremely efficient absorption of sodium, potassium, and chloride, renal excretion is the primary mechanism of body content regulation of those minerals. Given normal renal filtration and urinary excretion, removal of those ions can easily occur.

The sodium-to-potassium ratio in the human diet is believed to have changed for many cultures in comparison with the hypothesized Paleolithic diet. The sodium-to-potassium ratio has been estimated at about 0.1:1 for Paleolithic humans and at between 1.5:1 and 2:1 for many developed societies today. Many researchers have suggested that this seemingly lifelong reversal of the sodium-to-potassium ratio has affected humans from a pathophysiologic perspective.

There is some evidence to suggest that diets high in sodium increase the renal excretion of calcium. In contrast, diets rich in potassium seem to decrease the excretion of calcium. This may be significant with regard to lifelong diets and the risk of osteoporosis. The excess consumption of sodium, or the reversed sodium-to-potassium ratio, has also been implicated as a possible risk factor in the development of hypertension. Some evidence suggests that potassium can lower blood pressure in some individuals and, therefore, has potential therapeutic value. Excess sodium in the blood is called **hypernatremia**, whereas high blood potassium is called **hyperkalemia**.

Excessive loss of sodium by the body normally results in a concomitant loss of water from the extracellular compartments. This can lead to a shock-like syndrome as blood volume falls, perfusion of tissue becomes insufficient, and veins collapse. Loss of sodium via sweat followed by replacement of only water may lead to water intoxication as the sodium concentration in the extracellular fluids becomes further depressed. Also, the concentration of sodium in the extracellular fluids becomes diluted.

SPECIAL FEATURE 12.1

Hypertension and Diet

Approximately one-fourth of Americans have high blood pressure, or hypertension, a confirmed risk factor for coronary heart disease and stroke. Millions of Americans are afflicted with those diseases. Fortunately, most hypertension is treatable with lifestyle modifications (diet and exercise), medications, or both. The cause of 85% of hypertension cases is unknown. High blood pressure from an unknown cause is called **essential hypertension**. The remaining 15% of cases have a known cause, such as kidney disease.

Much debate has centered on what constitutes high blood pressure. Because blood pressure increases with age, what may be normal for an adult may be considered high for a child or teenager. Blood pressure readings consist of two components. When the heart contracts and forces blood to move due to an increase in pressure from the pumping action, the peak pressure generated is termed the **systolic blood pressure**. When the heart relaxes and blood pressure falls, the lowest blood pressure reading during cardiac relaxation is called the **diastolic blood pressure**. High blood pressure is generally defined as a systolic reading of 140 mm Hg or a diastolic reading of 90 mm Hg or greater, or both. **TABLE 1** outlines normal and high blood pressure readings for adults (≥ 18 years old). People with stage 1 high blood pressure are at risk for a heart attack or kidney disease. Normalization of blood pressure, either through lifestyle change, medication, or a combination of both, is critical to prevent the onset of those diseases.

Regardless of the classification scheme used, the role of diet in the control of hypertension has been studied and debated for years. In many cases, hypertension is associated with obesity; losing weight can result in a significant drop in blood pressure. Sodium has long been linked with an increased incidence of hypertension. For many years, health professionals advocated for reduced salt intake to decrease the incidence of hypertension. Not all individuals with a high sodium intake develop hypertension, however. Some studies show that individuals who have a difficult time excreting the sodium they consume experience higher blood pressure. Other studies suggest that the greater the reduction of sodium in the diet, the greater the reduction in blood pressure. However, there are many other factors involved with high blood pressure, such as consumption of other nutrients and physical activity. Potassium appears to exert an antihypertensive effect by relaxing blood vessels and lowering blood pressure. Nutritionists often refer to the sodium–potassium consumption ratio as a critical determinant of hypertension. Reports also suggest that lack of dietary calcium may be as much of a factor in hypertension as excessive sodium. Sodium excretion may increase with increased calcium intake because calcium may block reabsorption of sodium in the kidneys.

One of the most effective campaigns against hypertension is the **DASH (Dietary Approaches to Stop Hypertension) eating plan** (**TABLE 2**), which is rich in fruits, vegetables, and low-fat dairy products, which are low in fat and saturated fat. When used in combination with moderate salt intake, the DASH plan has a significant lowering effect on blood pressure. Given those findings and those outlined earlier, it would seem that a moderately restricted sodium diet, rich in low-fat dairy products, fruits, and vegetables and restricted in fat, can go a long way toward reducing high blood pressure. The DASH plan also calls for ample calcium and potassium—two nutrients that can help reduce blood pressure.

TABLE 1   Normal and High Blood Pressure Measurements for Adults 18 Years Old or Older

Category	Blood Pressure (mm Hg)		
	Systolic		Diastolic
Normal	<130	and	< 85
Best	<120	and	< 80
High-normal	130–139	or	85–89
High blood pressure (three categories)			
Stage 1	140–159	or	90–99
Stage 2	160–179	or	100–109
Stage 3	≥ 180	or	≥ 110

TABLE 2   The DASH Eating Plan

Food Group	Daily Servings	Serving Sizes	Examples and Notes	Significance of Each Food Group to the DASH Eating Pattern
Grains[a]	6–8	1 slice bread 1 oz dry cereal[b] ½ cup cooked rice, pasta, or cereal	Whole wheat bread and rolls, whole wheat pasta, English muffin, pita bread, bagel, cereals, grits, oatmeal, brown rice, unsalted pretzels, and popcorn	Major sources of energy and fiber
Vegetables	4–5	1 cup raw leafy vegetable ½ cup cut-up raw or cooked vegetable ½ cup vegetable juice	Broccoli, carrots, collards, green beans, green peas, kale, lima beans, potatoes, spinach, squash, sweet potatoes, tomatoes	Rich sources of potassium, magnesium, and fiber
Fruits	4–5	1 medium fruit ¼ cup dried fruit ½ cup fresh, frozen, or canned fruit ½ cup fruit juice	Apples, apricots, bananas, dates, grapes, oranges, grapefruit, grapefruit juice, mangoes, melons, peaches, pineapple, raisins, strawberries, tangerines	Important sources of potassium, magnesium, and fiber
Fat-free or low-fat milk and milk products	2–3	1 cup milk or yogurt 1½ oz cheese	Fat-free (skim) or low-fat (1%) milk or buttermilk; fat-free, low-fat, or reduced-fat cheese; fat-free or low-fat regular or frozen yogurt	Major sources of calcium and protein
Lean meats, poultry, and fish	6 or fewer	1 oz cooked meats, poultry, or fish 1 egg[c]	Select only lean portions; trim away visible fats; broil, roast, or poach; remove skin from poultry	Rich sources of protein and magnesium
Nuts, seeds, and legumes	4–5 per week	⅓ cup or 1½ oz nuts 2 tbsp peanut butter 2 tbsp or ½ oz seeds ½ cup cooked legumes (dry beans and peas)	Almonds, hazelnuts, mixed nuts, peanuts, walnuts, sunflower seeds, peanut butter, kidney beans, lentils, split peas	Rich sources of energy, magnesium, protein, and fiber
Fats and oils[d]	2–3	1 tsp soft margarine 1 tsp vegetable oil 1 tbsp mayonnaise 2 tbsp salad dressing	Soft margarine, vegetable oil (such as canola, corn, olive, or safflower), low-fat mayonnaise, light salad dressing	The DASH study had 27% of calories as fat, including fat in or added to foods
Sweets and added sugars	5 or fewer per week	1 tbsp sugar 1 tbsp jelly or jam ½ cup sorbet or gelatin 1 cup lemonade	Fruit-flavored gelatin, fruit punch, hard candy, jelly, maple syrup, sorbet and ices, sugar	Sweets should be low in fat

[a]Whole grains are recommended for most grain servings as a good source of fiber and nutrients.

[b]Serving sizes vary between ½ cup and 1 ¼ cup, depending on cereal type. Check the product's Nutrition Facts label.

[c]Because eggs are high in cholesterol, limit egg yolk intake to no more than four per week; two egg whites have the same protein content as 1 oz of meat.

[d]Fat content changes the serving amount for fats and oils. For example, 1 tbsp of regular salad dressing equals one serving; 1 tbsp of a low-fat dressing equals one-half serving; 1 tbsp of a fat-free dressing equals zero servings.

Reproduced from: National Heart, Lung and Blood Institute. *Your Guide to Lowering Your Blood Pressure with DASH*. April 2006. NIH Publication No. 06-4082: http://www.nhlbi.nih.gov/health/public/heart/hbp/dash/how_make_dash.html

This condition is called **hyponatremia**. Symptoms, such as loss of appetite, weakness, mental apathy, and uncontrolled muscle twitching are common. Death can result if the condition is severe.

Although the dietary potassium intake is by and large adequate to meet human needs, certain situations can place an individual at risk for potassium deficiency. Persistent use of laxatives can result in a lowering of body potassium levels by decreasing the amount absorbed from the digestive tract. Chronic use of certain diuretics used to control blood pressure may also result in increased urinary loss of potassium and decreased concentration of potassium intracellularly. The latter state is termed **hypokalemia**. Physicians routinely monitor the potassium levels of patients who are following either of those prescribed protocols. Frequent vomiting after a meal, either involuntarily or voluntarily, also ultimately reduces potassium absorption.

Renal disease may result in excess excretion of potassium. However, as the disease continues to end-stage renal disease, potassium excretion decreases and serum potassium levels increase. Diabetic acidosis and the use of certain diuretics (e.g., furosemide) may lead to those conditions. Diarrhea and vomiting over a period of a few days can lead to a potassium loss that manifests as muscle weakness, complete paralysis, and failure of the gastrointestinal tract musculature. Tachycardia and hypotension may occur.

▶ Sulfur

Sulfur is not really an essential nutrient but rather is a vital component of essential nutrients, such as the amino acid methionine and the vitamins biotin and thiamin. Therefore, sulfur's physiologic significance is really as a reflection of the metabolism of those substances rather than as an independent nutrient. Sulfur is also part of several food additives.

● BEFORE YOU GO ON . . .

1. Approximately what percentage of sodium, potassium, and chloride are absorbed by the small intestine and how does that compare with the absorption of the other minerals discussed thus far?

2. Discuss the three mechanisms by which sodium can be absorbed by the cells of the small intestine.

3. What effect does increased aldosterone secretion have on sodium levels in the blood?

4. What is the chloride shift?

5. How can a potassium deficiency occur?

🩺 CLINICAL INSIGHT

Should Magnesium Supplementation Be Encouraged?

Studies suggest that dietary magnesium intake is lower than recommended. While severe magnesium deficiency is rare, concern on "marginal" cases of deficiency has received attention as it relates to specific health issues. Historically, magnesium supplementation has not been advocated by nutritionists. Often, when supplementation is advocated, it is for micronutrients, such as iron, calcium, and vitamin D.

In the last 10 to 15 years, scientists have learned more about possible health conditions linked to low dietary magnesium intake. Historically, magnesium deficiency has been known to negatively affect bones and also enzyme activities due to its cofactor roles in about 300 enzymes. As reported earlier in this chapter, low dietary magnesium intake and low serum magnesium levels have been linked to hypertension and blood pressure, heart disease, cognition, bone health, metabolic syndrome, and, most significantly, Type II diabetes.

Dietary intake of magnesium ranges from 175 to 225 mg/d according to national surveys. This is well below recommended levels. Diet consumption of processed foods that are high in fat and sugar and include refined grains is correlated with the low magnesium status. Prior to the era of food processing, dietary magnesium intake was estimated at 500 mg/d. It is estimated that half of the population have diet magnesium intakes well below the RDA.

A critical factor that also should be considered with magnesium status is diet calcium intake, including the increasing use of calcium supplements. The balance of calcium and magnesium is significant since both minerals interact with each other. Calcium intakes either from dietary or supplemental sources at 1,200 mg/d or above result in increased urinary excretion of magnesium. While diet intake of magnesium is lower than recommended, there has been an increase in both males and females, but have not reached recommended levels. However, there has been an increase in calcium consumption that has been double the level of magnesium, further increasing the Ca:Mg intake. As indicated earlier in this chapter, a calcium to magnesium intake of 1.7 to 2.7 is thought to be ideal in terms of health maintenance.

On the other hand, excess magnesium coupled with low calcium intake can lower calcium status. It would appear that consideration of calcium intake, especially low intake, be considered as a factor prior to advocating magnesium supplementation. Increased magnesium to calcium at the cellular level can be beneficial in that intracellular levels of calcium and sodium are lowered, which reduces blood pressure.

There are studies that suggest that combining magnesium supplements with potassium and vitamin D supplements will enhance magnesium absorption. Therefore, another question that should be addressed is whether multiple supplements of nutrients should be advocated for magnesium to have its full health effects.

Studies that reported health benefits from magnesium supplementation have used 500 to 1,000 mg/d levels. How does one know when magnesium supplements are warranted? Serum magnesium levels are often used as a guide in making a decision. However, serum magnesium levels do have their limitations as, like calcium and other minerals in blood, they are often tightly regulated. Approximately 0.3% of the total body magnesium is in the serum. A normal range of serum magnesium levels range from 0.76 to 1.15 nmol/l; but some clinicians suggest that 0.85 nmol/l be used as the lower limit of "normal." The cutoff levels were determined when clinical symptoms of magnesium deficiency appear and corresponded with blood magnesium levels. Such symptoms, as discussed earlier, include muscle tremors and spasms, rapid heartbeat, ataxia, and even blood levels of PTH, calcium, and potassium.

If magnesium supplements are advised, consideration as to whether other micronutrients, such as potassium, calcium, and vitamin D, may need to be considered. This is especially important with blood pressure where all of those nutrients may act synergistically to lower blood pressure. A major question facing scientists and clinicians is whether routine magnesium supplementation should be advocated as a preventative measure for the diseases outlined in this chapter. Magnesium supplementation may only be warranted when clinical deficiency signs are apparent; but the public at large should be encouraged to consume more magnesium-rich foods.

▶ Here's What You Have Learned

1. Dairy products are the major source of calcium in U.S. diets. For those who do not consume dairy products, some calcium supplements have good bioavailability.

2. Several factors can decrease calcium absorption: the presence of oxalate, phytate, and fibers in foods; the rapid movement of food through the intestine; a very high-fat diet or decreased fat digestion; excess vitamin A intake; and excessive dietary phosphorus and magnesium.

3. Blood calcium levels are tightly regulated through the actions of parathyroid hormone, calcitonin, and vitamin D.

4. Although bone integrity is a major function of calcium, that mineral has many other functions. Calcium is important in muscle contraction, neuroexcitation, blood clotting, and cell signaling via its role as a second messenger.

5. Good sources of dietary phosphorus include meat, poultry, eggs, fish, milk and milk products, cereals, legumes, grains, and chocolate. Grains are a good source, but the phosphorus in grains is found in the form of phytate (the plant storage form of phosphorus). Because of the negative charges of the phosphorus groups in phytate, it can bind with other positively charged minerals and make them unavailable for absorption.

6. A major role of phosphorus is as an energy source via bonding to various compounds such as ATP and GTP. Because of its polarity, it is found as a component in phospholipids to allow better miscibility in aqueous environments for cell membranes and lipoproteins. It is also the backbone of DNA and RNA.

7. Magnesium is found in whole grain cereals, nuts, legumes, spices, seafood, coffee, tea, and cocoa. Chlorophyll contains magnesium; therefore, plant components rich in chlorophyll, such as green leaves, are a good source of magnesium.

8. Magnesium is important for bone integrity, stabilizing high-energy phosphate molecules such as ATP, and as a cofactor for more than 300 enzymes.

9. Dietary magnesium deficiency is rare. However, a loss of magnesium may occur that leads to a deficiency of stores. Excessive vomiting, diarrhea, alcohol abuse, renal and endocrine disease, and protein malnutrition may lead to a deficient status. Excess use of diuretics may

also result in magnesium deficiency. However, many westerners consume less than the recommended levels of magnesium. Those low levels have been linked to metabolic syndrome, Type II diabetes, hypertension, heart disease, Alzheimer's disease, dementia, and migraine headaches.

10. Sodium, potassium, and chloride are sometimes called electrolytes because they take on a charge when dissolved in water. Sodium is found extracellularly, whereas potassium is an intracellular mineral. A sodium–potassium pump that requires ATP keeps the two minerals separated across cell membranes. Chloride is normally associated with sodium and hence is found mostly outside of cells.

11. The current U.S. diet is high in sodium but low in potassium. Sodium chloride added through food processing is the major source of sodium in our diets. The lack of potassium in our diets is due to the low consumption of potassium-rich foods, such as fruits.

12. A major role of sodium, potassium, and chloride is water balance. Other roles include electric stimulation of nerve cells or action potentials as well as a role in neuromuscular junctions to initiate muscle contraction.

13. Sodium is absorbed by three mechanisms: (1) a Na^+-glucose co-transport system along the length of the small intestine; (2) a Na^+–Cl^- co-transport system throughout the small intestine and in the proximal colon; and (3) an electrogenic Na^+ transport mechanism in the colon. The mechanism for potassium absorption is not certain. Absorption appears to take place along the length of the intestines, with the colon perhaps being a major site of absorption. Some research suggests that potassium enters enterocytes via a K^+–H^+ antiport ATPase pump. Chloride is absorbed along the length of the small intestine; its absorption is often associated with sodium absorption in efforts to maintain electric neutrality.

14. Sulfur can be found in the amino acid methionine and the vitamins biotin and thiamin.

▶ Suggested Reading

Bronner F. Calcium and osteoporosis. *Am J Clin Nutr.* 1994;60(6):831–836.

Bronner F. Recent developments in intestinal calcium absorption. *Nutr Rev.* 2009;67(2):109–113.

Centeno V, de Barboza GD, Marchionatti A, Rodríguez V, Tolosa de Talamoni N. Molecular mechanisms triggered by low-calcium diets. *Nutr Res Rev.* 2009;22(2):163–174.

Chandrasekaran NC, Weir C, Alfraji S, Grice J, Roberts MS, Barnard RT. Effects of magnesium deficiency–more than skin deep. *Exp Biol Med.* 2014;239(10):1280-1291.

Chow M, Hinderliter AL, Kris-Etherton PM. Effects of dairy products on intracellular calcium and blood pressure in adults with essential hypertension. *J Am Coll Nutr.* 2009;28(2):142–149.

Craddick SR, Elmer PJ, Obarzanek E, Vollmer WM, Svetkey LP, Swain MC. The DASH diet and blood pressure. *Curr Atheroscler Rep.* 2003;5(6):484–491.

Crowe MJ, Weatherson JN, Bowden BF. Effects of dietary leucine supplementation on exercise performance. *Eur J Appl Physiol.* 2006;97(6):664–672.

Desroches S, Chouinard PY, Galibois I, et al. Lack of effect of dietary conjugated linoleic acids naturally incorporated into butter on the lipid profile and body composition of overweight and obese men. *Am J Clin Nutr.* 2005;82(2):309–325.

Freis ED. The role of salt in hypertension. *Blood Press.* 1992;1(4):196–200.

French SA, Story M, Jeffery RW. Environmental influences on eating and physical activity. *Annu Rev Public Health.* 2001;22:309–335.

Gröber U, Schmidt J, Kisters K. Magnesium in prevention and therapy. *Nutrients.* 2015;7(9):8199–8226.

Gropper SS, Smith JL, Groff JL. *Advanced Nutrition and Human Metabolism.* Belmont, CA: Wadsworth; 2005.

Hilpert KF, West SG, Bagshaw DM, et al. Calciotropic and magnesiotropic TRP channels. *Physiology (Bethesda).* 2008;23:32–40.

Houston M. The role of magnesium in hypertension and cardiovascular disease. *J Clin Hypertens.* 2011;13(11): 843–847.

Huth PJ, DiRienzo DB, Miller GD. Major advances with dairy foods in nutrition and health. *J Dairy Sci.* 2006;89(4): 1207–1221.

Hyppönen E, Power C. Vitamin D status and glucose homeostasis in the 1958 British birth cohort: the role of obesity. *Diabetes Care.* 2006;29(10):2244–2246.

Institute of Medicine, Food and Nutrition Board. *Dietary Reference Intakes for Calcium, Phosphorus, Magnesium, Vitamin D, and Fluoride.* Washington, DC: National Academies Press; 1997.

Ito S, Ishida H, Uenishi K. Fibroblast growth factor-23 and phosphorus related factors in young Japanese women: a cross-sectional study. *Asia Pac J Nutr.* 2016; 25(3):549–555.

Jurutka PW, Bartik L, Whitfield GK, et al. Vitamin D receptor: key roles in bone mineral pathophysiology, molecular mechanism of action, and novel nutritional ligands. *J Bone Miner Res.* 2007;22(suppl 2):V2–V10.

Larson TM, Toubro S, Gudmundsen O, Astrup A. Conjugated linoleic acid supplementation for 1 y does not prevent weight or body fat regain. *Am J Clin Nutr.* 2006;83(3):606–612.

Layman DK, Baum JI. Dietary protein impact on glycemic control during weight loss. *J Nutr.* 2004;134(4):968S–973S.

Lee R, Weber TJ. Disorders of phosphorus homeostasis. *Curr Opin Endocrinol Diabetes Obes.* 2010;17(6):561-567.

Lin PH, Aickin M, Champagne C, et al. Food group sources of nutrients in the dietary patterns of the DASH-Sodium trial. *J Am Diet Assoc.* 2003;103(4):488–496.

McCarron DA, Morris CD, Henry HJ, Stanton JL. Blood pressure and nutrients in the United States. *Science.* 1984;224(4656):1392–1398.

Musso CG. Magnesium metabolism in health and disease. *Int Urol Nephrol.* 2009;41(2):357–362.

Nowson CA, Morgan TO, Gibbons C. Decreasing dietary sodium while following a self-selected potassium-rich diet reduces blood pressure. *J Nutr.* 2003;133(12):4118–4123.

Obarzanek E, Proschan MA, Vollmer WM, et al. Individual blood pressure responses to changes in salt intake: results from the DASH-Sodium trial. *Hypertension.* 2003;42(4):459–467.

Ogden CL, Carroll MD, Curtin LR, McDowell MA, Tabak CJ, Flegal KM. Prevalence of overweight and obesity in the United States, 1999–2004. *JAMA.* 2006;295(13):1549–1555.

Ogden CL, Flegal KM, Carroll MD, Johnson CL. Prevalence and trends in overweight among US children and adolescents, 1999–2000. *JAMA.* 2002;288(14):1728–1732.

Ohta H, Sakuma M, Suzuki A, Morimoto Y, Ishikawa M, Umeda M, Arai H. Effects of gender and body weight on fibroblast growth factor 23 responsiveness to estimated dietary phosphorus. *J Med Invest.* 2016; 63(12):58–62.

Papakonstantinou E, Flatt WP, Huth PJ, Harris RB. High dietary calcium reduces body fat content, digestibility of fat, and serum vitamin D in rats. *Obes Res.* 2003;11(3):387–394.

Pérez AV, Picotto G, Carpentieri AR, Rivoira MA, Peralta López ME, Tolosa de Talamoni NG. Minireview on regulation of intestinal calcium absorption. Emphasis on molecular mechanisms of transcellular pathway. *Digestion.* 2008;77(1):22–34.

Ramos JG, Brietzke E, Martins-Costa SH, Vettorazzi-Stuczynski J, Barros E, Carvalho C. Reported calcium intake is reduced in women with preeclampsia. *Hypertens Pregnancy.* 2006;25(3):229–239.

Renkema KY, Alexander RT, Bindels RJ, Hoenderop JG. Calcium and phosphate homeostasis: concerted interplay of new regulators. *Ann Med.* 2008;40(2):82–91.

Rosanoff A, Dai Q, Shapses SA. Essential nutrient interactions: does low or suboptimal magnesium status interact with vitamin D and/or calcium status? *Adv Nutr.* 2016;7(1):25–43.

Rude RK, Singer FR, Gruber HE. Skeletal and hormonal effects of magnesium deficiency. *J Am Coll Nutr.* 2009;28(2):131–141.

Song Y, Fleet JC. Intestinal resistance to 1,25 dihydroxyvitamin D in mice heterozygous for the vitamin D receptor knockout allele. *Endocrinology.* 2007;148(3):1396–1402.

Suzuki Y, Landowski CP, Hediger MA. Mechanisms and regulation of epithelial Ca^{2+} absorption in health and disease. *Annu Rev Physiol.* 2008;70:257–271.

Tricon S, Burdge GC, Williams CM, Calder PC, Yaqoobb P. The effects of conjugated linoleic acid on human health-related outcomes. *Proc Nutr Soc.* 2005;64(2):171–182.

Volpe SL. Magnesium in disease prevention and overall health. *Adv Nutr.* 2013;4:378S-383S.

Xue Y, Fleet JC. Intestinal vitamin D receptor is required for normal calcium and bone metabolism in mice. *Gastroenterology.* 2009; 136(4):1317–1327.

Yang CY. Calcium and magnesium in drinking water and risk of death from cerebrovascular disease. *Stroke.* 1998;29(2):411–414.

Ziegler EE, Filer LJ, eds. *Present Knowledge in Nutrition.* Washington, DC: ILSI Press; 1996.

Zimmerman E, Wylie-Rosett J. Nutrition therapy for hypertension. *Curr Diab Rep.* 2003;3(5):404–411.

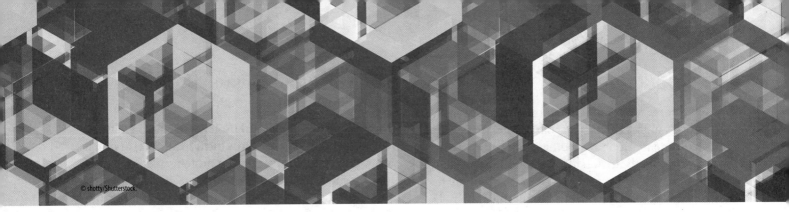

CHAPTER 13

Minor Minerals

← HERE'S WHERE YOU HAVE BEEN

1. Major minerals have structural and functional roles.
2. Calcium is the most prevalent mineral in the body, largely due to the body's large skeletal mass.
3. A major role of phosphorus is as an energy source contained in the chemical bonds in such compounds as ATP and GTP.
4. Magnesium is important for bone integrity, for stabilizing high-energy phosphate molecules such as ATP, and as a cofactor for more than 300 enzymes.
5. Sodium is an extracellular mineral and potassium an intracellular mineral; the separation of those two minerals across a cell membrane requires energy in the form of ATP.

HERE'S WHERE YOU ARE GOING →

1. Many of the minor minerals are bound to specific proteins for transport across membranes and for cell function.
2. Many trace elements can function at the gene level or have a molecular mechanism of action in metabolism.
3. Iron regulatory proteins are able to help control the amount of iron stored and absorbed, depending on iron status.
4. Copper and zinc may interact with one another at the intestinal level due to the ability of dietary zinc to control the synthesis of a metal binding protein that can bind both zinc and copper.
5. Selenium can be incorporated into proteins through the process of translation. This mechanism is different from that of other minerals, which are often added to proteins post-translationally.

▶ Introduction

Minor minerals, or trace elements, are present in the human body at less than 0.01% of the total mass. Current recommendations regarding intakes for each of the minor minerals are less than 100 milligrams daily. Minor minerals may act as cofactors in human tissues or may be part of various compounds, or both. A growing body of evidence suggests that certain minor minerals function at the genetic level. Even though they are present in relatively small amounts, certain minor minerals can be fatal if omitted from the diet or if taken in excess of needs. Deficiencies of trace elements may result from either lack in the diet or malabsorption over a period of time. Furthermore, the amount of a minor mineral in a plant or animal source can vary based on the soil and water content of the area in which the plant was grown or the animal grazed.

Minor minerals are often called *trace elements* or *trace metals*. It is important to recognize that although all the trace minerals that are important to human nutrition are indeed elements, they are not all metals. For instance, selenium is not a metal and neither are the halogens—fluorine and iodine. In contrast, manganese, iron, copper, molybdenum, vanadium, zinc, and nickel are indeed metals. Metals are generally solid and tend to have shiny surfaces. Furthermore, they can be pounded into sheets and drawn into wires. They are also very good conductors of electricity. Nonmetals typically lack luster and are poor conductors of electricity in their elemental form. Nonmetals exist as gases, liquids, and solids. With some exceptions, metals tend to have one, two, or three valence electrons, whereas nonmetals tend to have anywhere from four to eight valence electrons.

▶ Iron

Iron occurs in the human body, as well as in food, in either the ferrous (Fe^{2+}) or ferric (Fe^{3+}) state. (Iron has a broader range of oxidation states in nature.) Iron is among the top three most recognizable minerals of all types, along with calcium and sodium. From a disease perspective, iron deficiency is second only to obesity as the most prevalent nutritional problem in the United States today, and iron deficiency affects millions of individuals worldwide. Whereas much of the attention regarding iron imbalance has focused on iron deficiency, recently, more attention has been afforded to iron overload.

Dietary Sources of Iron and Iron Absorption

There are many factors and proteins that are involved in iron absorption. These factors include the level of iron in food, the form of iron, and the proteins that are bound to iron which are critical for both iron absorption by the small intestine and transport to the liver. Other dietary components will influence the absorption of iron.

Dietary Iron and Availability

Iron is present in both animal and plant foods in the form of either **heme iron** or **nonheme iron**. Animal foods contain both heme and nonheme iron, whereas plants and plant-derived products contain only nonheme iron. About 50 to 60% of the iron in meat, fish, and poultry is in the heme form. Heme iron is complexed in heme structures, such as myoglobin and cytochromes (**FIGURE 13.1**). Nonheme iron is found in foods, such as cereal grains, legumes, and milk and dairy products. **TABLE 13.1** presents the iron content of select foods. Cooking in nonenamel pots increases the iron content of food.

Nonheme iron is less efficiently absorbed (2 to 20%) than heme iron (25 to 35%). Because the absorption efficiency of both forms of iron is relatively low, it seems likely that the iron content of the human body is primarily regulated at the point of absorption. This hypothesis is reinforced by the fact that the efficiency of iron absorption increases significantly during times of greater iron need, such as when iron stores are low, or during periods of growth, menstruation, and pregnancy.

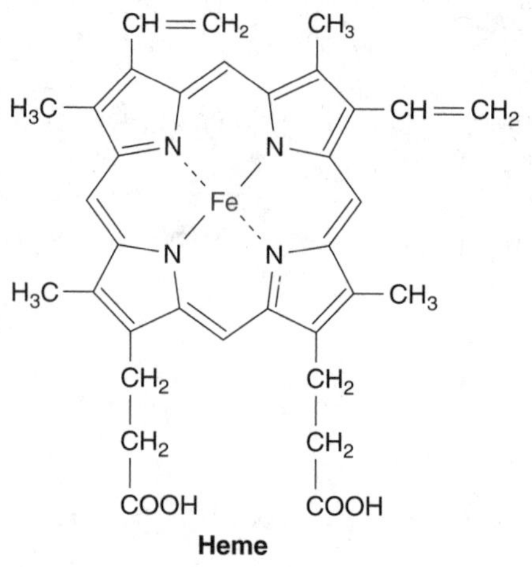

FIGURE 13.1 The Structure of Heme, Showing the Centralized Atom of Iron. Heme iron is present in meat, poultry, and fish and its absorption is greater than nonheme iron. In addition to hemoglobin, heme is found in myoglobin and the cytochromes.

TABLE 13.1 Iron Content of Select Foods

Food	Iron (mg)	Food	Iron (mg)
Meat and alternatives		*Grains*	
Liver (3 oz)	5.2	Breakfast cereal, fortified (1 cup)	4–18
Round steak (3 oz)	1.9	Oatmeal, fortified (1 cup)	14.0
Hamburger, lean (3 oz)	2.4	Bagel (1)	0.9
Baked beans (1 cup)	0.7	English muffin (1)	2.3
Pork (3 oz)	1.0	Bread, rye (1 slice)	0.9
White beans (1 cup)	5.1	Bread, wheat (1 slice)	0.9
Soybeans (1 cup)	8.8	Bread, white (1 slice)	0.9
Fish (3 oz)	1.2	*Fruits*	
Chicken (3 oz)	1.0	Prune juice (1 cup)	2.0
Vegetables		Apricots, dried (1 cup)	4.1
Spinach, cooked (1 cup)	6.4	Prunes (1 cup)	4.6
Lima beans (1 cup)	4.5	Raisins (1 cup)	4.3
Peas (1 cup)	1.6	Plums (3 medium)	0.5
Asparagus (1 cup)	1.6		

Dietary Components That Effect Absorption

Beyond iron status and need, many factors within the digestive tract appear to affect iron absorption into the human body (**TABLE 13.2**). This is the primary reason why the ranges of absorption for both forms of dietary iron are so broad.

Vitamin C intake plays a significant role in iron absorption. Quite simply, as vitamin C intake increases in conjunction with iron-containing sources, iron absorption is enhanced. It is likely that vitamin C promotes the formation and stabilization of ferrous iron, which, as mentioned earlier, is much better absorbed than the ferric form. Living at a high altitude appears to create a greater need for iron. Therefore, greater iron absorption is needed to synthesize more red blood cells under the control of erythropoietin.

Consumption of meat, fish, or poultry (MFP) enhances iron absorption. In fact, 75 units of MFP (1 unit is equal to 1.3 grams of raw or 1 gram of cooked meat, fish, or poultry) can enhance the absorption of nonheme iron from about 2 to 3% to about 7 to 8%. Similarly, 75 units of ascorbic acid, where 1 unit is equal to 1 milligram of vitamin C, enhances nonheme absorption tremendously.

Several factors decrease iron absorption (see Table 13.2). A high phytic acid intake decreases absorption. Polyphenolic substances, such as tannins in tea; oxalates in spinach, chard, berries, chocolate, teas, and other foods; phytate in whole grains; and the preservative EDTA can decrease iron absorption

TABLE 13.2 Factors Influencing Iron Absorption

Increased Iron Absorption	Decreased Iron Absorption
Vitamin C	Phytate
Gastric acidity	Oxalates
Meat, fish, poultry	Tannins (in tea)
Increased need	Decreased need
Pregnancy	Use of antacids
Menstruation	
Growth	

by chelation. Interestingly, supplemental doses of calcium may also decrease iron absorption. Supplemental calcium at 600 milligrams taken in conjunction with 18 milligrams of either a ferrous or ferric iron salt decreases iron absorption by about 50 to 60%. Beyond supplements, the calcium in milk has also been suggested to reduce iron absorption. Those findings suggest that an iron supplement may be most beneficial when taken in the absence of a significant source of calcium. Zinc may also compete with ferrous iron for absorption via a common transporter, and thus, decrease its absorption.

Iron Absorption Proteins and Mechanisms

Iron that is part of heme structures requires two stages of digestion (**FIGURE 13.2**). First, iron-containing heme must be liberated from associated

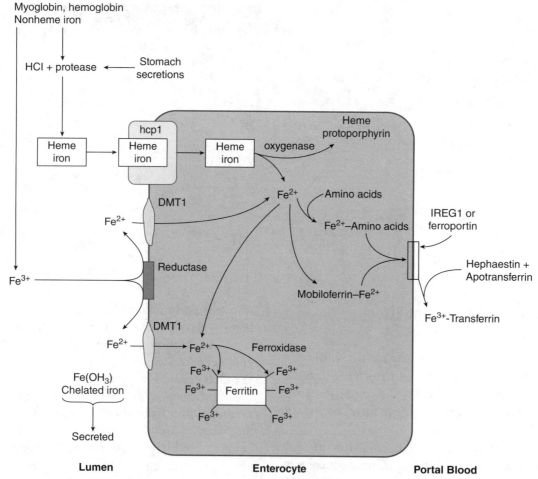

FIGURE 13.2 The Absorption of Heme and Nonheme Iron by the Gastrointestinal System. Note the various carriers involved with nonheme iron uptake and the fates of the iron that are absorbed. Heme carrier protein (hcp1) binds heme iron on the luminal side of the enterocyte. Heme iron enters the cell and the enzyme, heme oxygenase, liberates the iron in the ferrous form. Inorganic iron is transported into the enterocyte by divalent metal transporter (DMT1). Ferroportin (IREG1) will absorb the ferrous iron from the enterocyte to the blood, where iron will be converted to the ferric form by hephaestin and subsequently picked up by transferrin for delivery to the liver. Only a small portion of iron is absorbed, depending on total body status. Iron bound to ferritin in the ferric acid form will be eliminated as enterocytes are replaced.

protein structures. That occurs in the stomach and small intestine via the activity of proteases in digestive secretions. Heme, endowed with iron, then crosses the luminal membrane of small-intestinal enterocytes intact. It does this by binding to a carrier on the intestinal membrane called **heme carrier protein 1 (hcp1)**. Once inside the cell, iron is liberated from the protoporphyrin ring by the action of **heme oxygenase**.

Nonheme iron includes the iron complexed into the iron storage proteins ferritin and hemosiderin and iron-containing enzymes and salts. Nonheme iron is released from food components by digestive secretions. If the iron is associated with a protein, proteases and hydrochloric acid are necessary for its liberation. Hydrochloric acid also assists in maintaining the stability of ionic iron by inhibiting its precipitation to anionic entities. Other acids, such as lactic acid, citric acid, and tartaric acid, also seem to enhance iron absorption, probably by stabilizing ionic iron.

Ionic iron appears to be more efficiently absorbed in the ferrous state than the ferric state. The duodenum appears to be the site of most nonheme iron absorption, with several transporters likely involved. The protein **divalent metal transporter 1 (DMT1)** can bind nonheme iron and then deliver it either to **ferritin** or **mobiloferrin** (see Figure 13.2). DMT1 transports ferrous iron only. Ferric iron must be converted to ferrous iron before it can be absorbed. A number of reductases on the intestinal cell membrane can reduce the ferric iron to the ferrous form prior to binding to DMT1 for absorption. If iron binds to mobiloferrin, the iron is delivered to the basolateral side of the enterocyte and given to the membrane protein **IREG1**, which is sometimes called **ferroportin**. Another protein involved in this process is **hephaestin**, a copper-containing enzyme. This enzyme oxidizes the ferrous to the ferric form of iron so that it can be picked up by serum transferrin, because the ferrous form cannot bind to transferrin.

Iron Homeostasis

There are several proteins that influence iron homeostasis. One protein involved with iron absorption is **HFE**, which is often referred to as an overall iron absorption regulator. It is produced in both liver and small intestinal cells. HFE may regulate the ability of transferrin to bind to the transferrin receptor. It is thought that the HFE protein blocks iron absorption, but whether this entails decreased transferrin binding to transferrin receptors is currently

speculation. The exact mechanism by which HFE regulates iron absorption is poorly understood. As mentioned earlier, iron absorption is directly related to physiologic need. Absorption may be regulated systemically by the level of plasma transferrin receptors and the rate of erythropoiesis. Some evidence exists for local regulatory factors in mucosal tissue as well. Iron is transported in the plasma to various tissue bound to the glycoprotein **transferrin**, which has a molecular weight of 79,550. Transferrin can accommodate two atoms of iron; however, only about 30% of the iron-binding sites are occupied with iron under normal conditions. In liver hepatocytes, transferrin bound to transferrin receptors is engulfed by endocytosis (**FIGURE 13.3**). In the endosome, the ferric form of iron is removed from the transferrin receptor and converted to the ferrous form by the metalloreductase enzyme **Steap3**. The ferrous iron is transported out of the endosome by DMT1. Once the ferrous iron is in the liver cytoplasm, it is then reconverted to the ferric form to be stored as ferritin. The apotransferrin is recycled to the cell surface to bind to other iron-containing transferrin molecules.

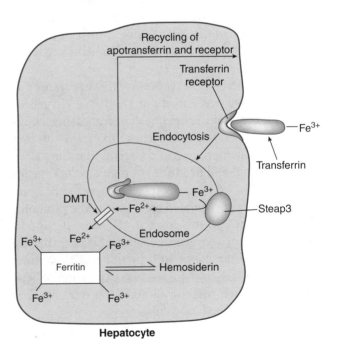

FIGURE 13.3 Regulation of Iron Uptake by Hepatocytes Through the Transferrin Receptor. The transferrin receptor with bound transferrin is engulfed by the cell, and iron is reduced from the ferric to the ferrous form so that it can be subsequently delivered to ferritin. In ferritin, iron is in the ferric form. Hemosiderin is a breakdown product of ferritin.

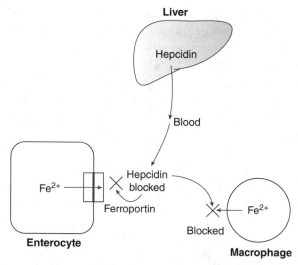

FIGURE 13.4 Role of the Liver Hormone Hepcidin in Iron Absorption. Hepcidin blocks iron absorption when iron stores are sufficient.

Another regulator in iron absorption is **hepcidin** (**FIGURE 13.4**), a liver hormone that regulates iron homeostasis. When liver iron stores are high, this hormone is released into the bloodstream and binds to the iron transporter ferroportin in the small intestine as well as to macrophage ferroportin protein. In the small intestine, it blocks the uptake of iron by binding to ferroportin and causes the complex to be internalized by the enterocyte or macrophage; that degrades the ferroportin so that iron is not absorbed. Instead, it is eliminated when the intestinal mucosal cells are sloughed off.

Hypoxia inducible factors (HIF) are transcription factors that are sensors of low tissue oxygen or hypoxic states that may exist when iron deficiency is present. As such, when low-tissue oxygen is present in such as the enterocyte of the small intestine, HIFs are upregulated and produced to regulate those genes involved with iron homeostasis. In particular, one HIF, HIF-2α is upregulated and binds to the promoter of specific genes. In this context, HIF-2α will bind to the promoter of the gene encoding DMT1, thereby increasing the uptake of iron by the small intestine. Furthermore, HIF-2α will decrease expression of hepcidin by the liver, thereby allowing a greater absorption of iron into the blood supply.

Metabolism and Function of Iron

An adult human has about 2 to 5 grams of iron distributed throughout his or her body, depending on diet, gender, size, and menstrual status. Iron is engaged in operations in all human cells and is distributed among metabolic, structural, and transport compartments.

Approximately two-thirds of the iron in the human body is found within red blood cells as part of the oxygen-binding pigment hemoglobin, which transports oxygen to the tissues. Each hemoglobin molecule can carry four atoms of iron, and a healthy red blood cell can contain 250 million molecules of hemoglobin. Thus, each red blood cell can carry 1 billion oxygen molecules. Muscle myoglobin accounts for 10% of body iron, and heme and nonheme enzymes account for 2 to 4%.

Hemoglobin

Heme synthesis begins in the mitochondria of liver and bone marrow cells, where the Krebs cycle intermediate succinyl CoA reacts with the amino acid glycine to form α-aminolevulinic acid (ALA), which is catalyzed by the enzyme ALA synthase (**FIGURE 13.5**). After ALA is formed, it enters the cytoplasm, and two molecules of ALA condense where ALA dehydratase removes a water molecule to form porphobilinogen. After a series of additional reactions, the compound reenters the mitochondria as coproporphyrinogen III. That compound is oxidized to protoporphyrinogen. That step is followed by another oxidation step. Finally, the addition of iron occurs to form heme.

Iron Storage Proteins

Ferritin is the primary iron storage protein and is found in many tissues, especially the liver, bone marrow, intestine, and spleen. Augmented synthesis of ferritin occurs in those tissues because they are sites of iron absorption, storage, or red blood cell catabolism. Ferritin is synthesized as apoferritin, a large protein with 24 subunits and a molecular weight of 440,000. Apoferritin has a three-dimensional design believed to be similar to a cornucopia or hollow horn. When apoferritin is associated with iron, it is called ferritin. Each ferritin structure can store as many as 4,300 atoms of iron. There are two types of ferritin: H ferritin and L ferritin. H ferritin has ferroxidase activity. Ferrous iron is oxidized by the ferroxidase activity in H ferritin found in its porous shell; the resultant product, ferric oxyhydroxide (FeOOH), is stored. The H ferritin form promotes more rapid incorporation of iron into its shell and is more likely found in the heart muscle and red blood cells. L ferritin takes up iron more slowly but holds onto it longer than the H form. Liver and spleen are rich sources of the L ferritin. Regardless of the form, ferritin molecules are constantly being synthesized and catabolized, allowing for a controlled intracellular iron pool. Ferritin found in the serum is used as a sensitive indicator of tissue

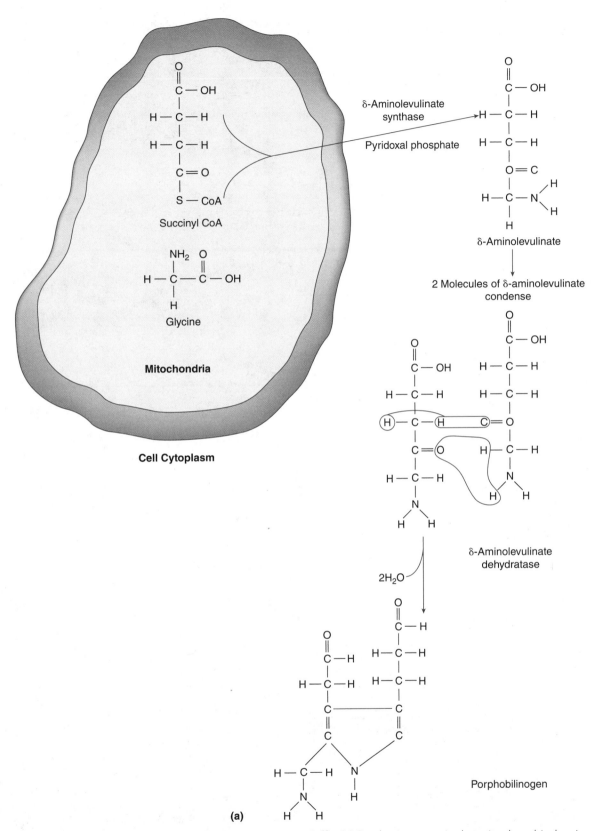

FIGURE 13.5 Synthesis of Heme in Liver and Bone Marrow Cells. (a) Synthesis occurs in the mitochondria, beginning with condensation of the amino acid glycine and the Krebs cycle intermediate succinyl CoA in the mitochondria and partly in the cell cytoplasm. (*continues*)

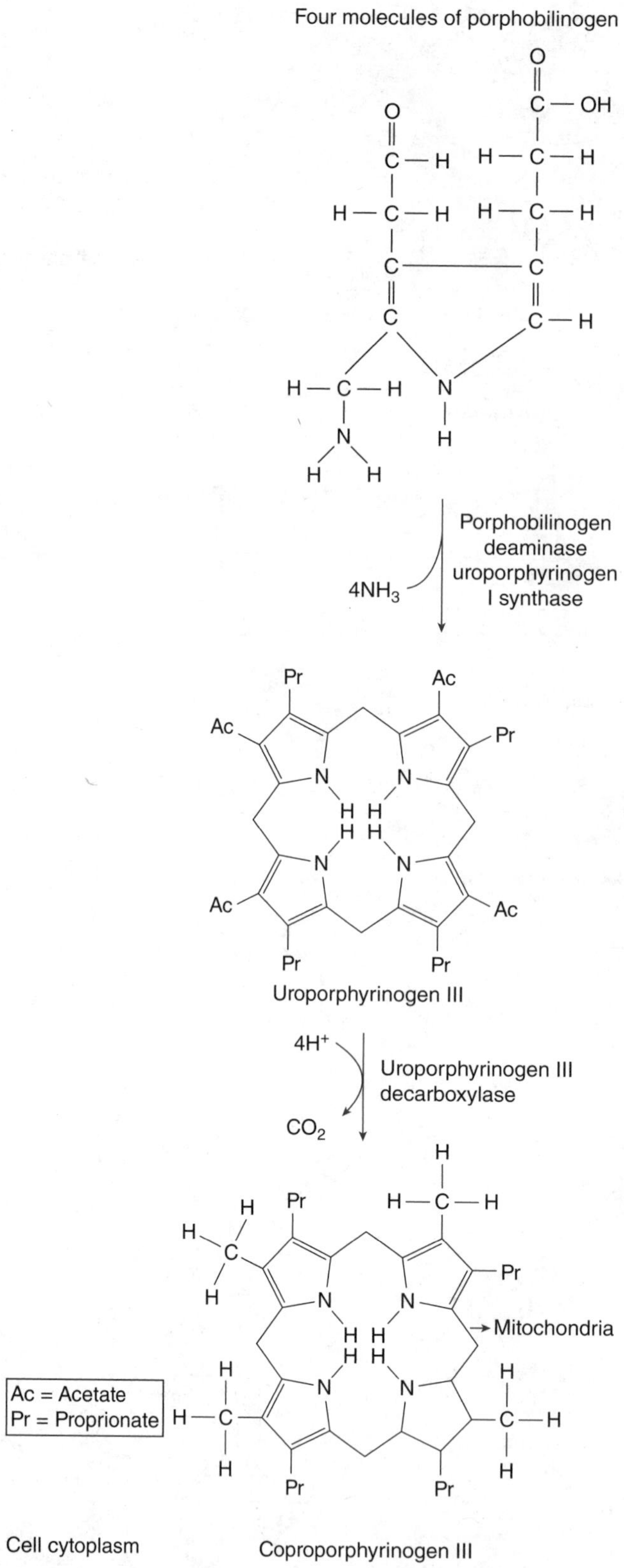

Four molecules of porphobilinogen

Porphobilinogen
deaminase
uroporphyrinogen
I synthase

$4NH_3$

Uroporphyrinogen III

$4H^+$

Uroporphyrinogen III
decarboxylase

CO_2

→ Mitochondria

Ac = Acetate
Pr = Proprionate

(b)   Cell cytoplasm   Coproporphyrinogen III

FIGURE 13.5 (*continued*) (b) In the cytoplasm, porphobilinogen is formed from the glycine and succinyl CoA reaction and, subsequently, a series of reactions forms the ring structure, coproporphyrinogen III. (*continues*)

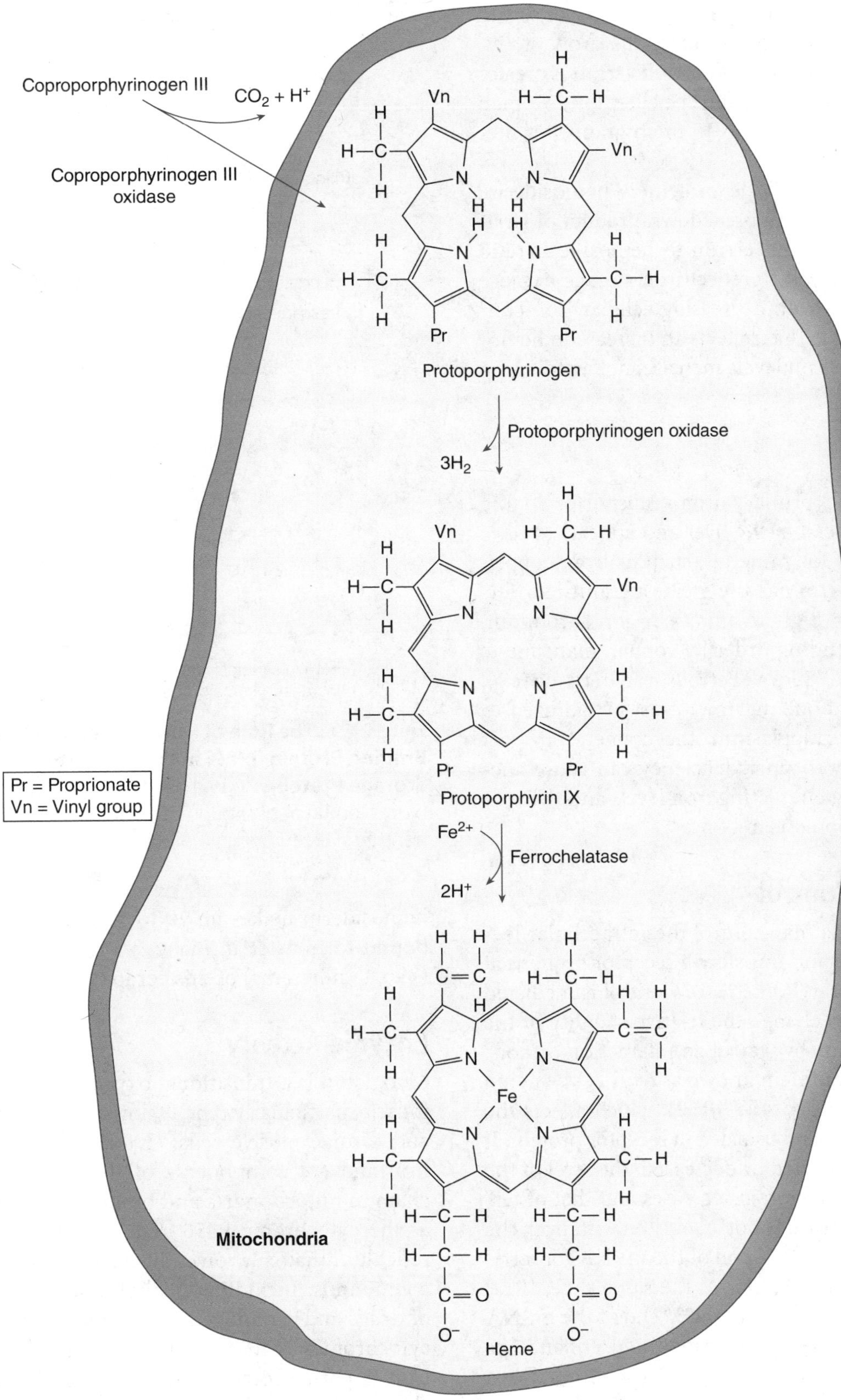

FIGURE 13.5 (*continued*) (c) This compound is subsequently oxidized to protoporphyrinogen IX in the mitochondria, and eventually, iron is added to form heme.

(c)

iron status: 1 microgram of ferritin per liter of serum approximates 10 milligrams of tissue iron stores. Typically, the ferritin content of adult serum is greater than or equal to 12 micrograms per liter for a woman and greater than or equal to 15 micrograms per liter for a man.

The other iron storage protein is hemosiderin, which is believed to be a breakdown product of ferritin (see Figure 13.3). The ferritin-to-hemosiderin ratio in the liver is believed to reflect iron storage because the ratio increases with decreasing cellular iron content, and vice versa. That reflects an increase in hemosiderin as cellular iron levels increase, not a reduction in ferritin content.

Transferrin

Transferrin is the primary iron transporter in the blood. It is produced in the liver and appears to have two binding sites for minerals, such as iron, copper, and zinc. Transferrin has the greatest affinity for ferric iron. Its next highest affinity is for chromium, followed in descending order by copper, manganese, cadmium, zinc, and nickel. Ferrous iron in tissue (e.g., liver, spleen, and bone marrow) must be oxidized to ferric iron via ceruloplasmin, the copper transport protein. Therefore, copper deficiency can cause anemia by decreasing circulating iron levels and delivery to sites of erythropoiesis in bone.

Cellular Iron Control

Cellular iron levels may control the intracellular levels of both ferritin and transferrin receptor proteins at the molecular level (**FIGURE 13.6**). Control is mediated via iron's ability to change the relative stability of the mRNA. That occurs by way of an interaction or noninteraction with a protein known as **iron-responsive element-binding protein (IREP)**, which affects the synthesis of ferritin and transferrin receptor protein. If iron in the cell is limited or decreased, the level of the transferrin receptor protein increases and that of ferritin decreases. If IREP is not associated with iron, the protein will bind to the 5′ end of the mRNA for ferritin and block its translation. At the same time, IREP without iron will also bind to the 3′ end of the mRNA for the transferrin receptor protein and enhance its stability to prevent degradation. That allows for a greater synthesis of the receptor protein and, consequently, a greater iron uptake by cells. Conversely, when intracellular iron is high, iron binds to the IREP, thereby preventing it from binding to the mRNA for either protein. Collectively, the iron that is transported as transferrin and stored in the form of ferritin and

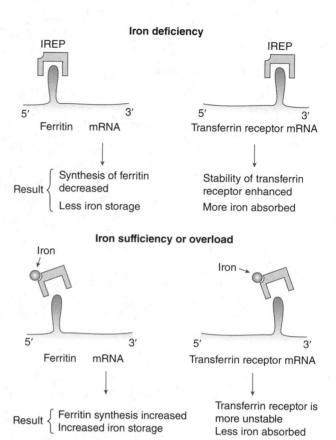

FIGURE 13.6 The Role of Iron-Responsive Element-Binding Protein (IREP) in the Regulation of Iron Storage Proteins. In iron deficiency, IREP is active and blocks ferritin transcription but stabilizes the mRNA of the transferrin receptors.

hemosiderin makes up 20 to 30% of body iron. Iron bound to transferrin makes up a very small portion (3 to 4 milligrams) of this compartment.

Enzyme Activity

Myoglobin is a transitional oxygen storage protein in muscle, particularly type I (slow-twitch) muscle fibers and cardiac muscle cells. Cytochromes also contain iron and are components of the electron transport chain in mitochondria and other redox systems, such as the cytochrome P450 system in the endoplasmic reticulum that is involved in the oxidation of organic compounds, including alcohol, and the metabolism of drugs and carcinogens. The iron in myoglobin and cytochromes is found within the heme component. Iron is part of other complexes associated with the electron transport system, namely NADH dehydrogenase, succinate dehydrogenase, and ubiquinone-cytochrome c reductase. Here, iron is present, but not as a component of heme.

Outside of electron transport systems, iron is a component of several heme-containing enzymes, namely, in certain peroxidases, myeloperoxidase, and catalase. Peroxidases are found in leukocytes, platelets, and other tissue involving eicosanoid metabolism. They catalyze the reduction of hydrogen peroxide (H_2O_2) to two water molecules in a reaction that proceeds as follows:

$$H_2O_2 + XH_2 \xrightarrow{\text{peroxidase}} 2\ H_2O + X$$

In this equation, X represents several substances that are willing to act as electron acceptors, namely ascorbate, quinones, and cytochrome c. It is important to note that not all peroxidases contain iron. For instance, glutathione peroxidase contains selenium at its prosthetic site.

Myeloperoxidase, in contrast, does contain iron at its prosthetic site and is found in relatively large amounts in neutrophil granules. Here, H_2O_2 is used to form a hypohalous acid (an acid that contains a halide element, such as Cl^-, Br^-, or I^-). However, because of the relative abundance of H_2O_2, the hypohalous acid formed is hypochlorous acid (HOCl). Hypochlorous acid is the active ingredient in household bleach and is a powerful oxidant and antimicrobial agent. In humans, hypochlorous acid can react with primary and secondary amines in neutrophils and form chloramines, which are also oxidants, only less potent. Those are released at sites of trauma that allow microbial infection.

Finally, catalase is an antioxidant that converts H_2O_2 to molecular oxygen and water in the following reaction:

$$2\ H_2O_2 \xrightarrow{\text{catalase}} 2\ H_2O + O_2$$

Recommended Levels of Intake for Iron

For adult women (19 years or older) of childbearing years, the RDA is 18 milligrams per day; for adult men, it is 8 milligrams per day. For males aged 14 to 18 years, the RDA is 11 milligrams per day; for females in this same age range, it is 15 milligrams per day. The RDA drops to 8 milligrams per day for women older than 50 years. During pregnancy, a total of 27 milligrams of iron per day is recommended. The RDA decreases to 9 milligrams per day during lactation for those aged 19 years or older, and to 10 milligrams per day for those younger than 18 years.

Iron Deficiency

When iron stores, which are estimated at about 300 milligrams in adults, become exhausted, an individual is said to be iron deficient. About 20% of American females of all ages have minimal iron stores and are iron deficient, compared with 3% of males.

Inadequate iron intake or excessive loss, or both, results in a reduction of blood hemoglobin levels. The anemia that results is a **hypochromic microcytic anemia**, in which the red blood cells are small and pale. **Iron deficiency anemia** is defined as occurring when hemoglobin levels fall well below normal, to a level less than 7 grams per 100 milliliters of blood.

There are various forms of inherited anemia—homozygous 8-thalassemia, 8-thalassemia/hemoglobin E, and hemoglobin H disease—all result in ineffectual erythropoiesis in bone marrow. Although the mechanisms are unclear, the ineffective erythropoiesis ultimately leads to augmented iron absorption. The treatment of these diseases involves multiple blood transfusions, which contribute even more iron to these individuals. Initially, the overloading of iron results in deposits in the liver; however, with time, iron accumulates in other organs, such as the heart and pancreas.

Other forms of anemia associated with ineffective erythropoiesis can increase iron absorption and potentially lead to overload. Those anemias include congenital dyserythropoietic anemias (subdivided into type 1, type 2, and type 3, based on genetic disease causes), a number of sideroblastic anemias (a defect in inserting iron into the heme molecule), and many anemias associated with poor iron incorporation into hemoglobin.

Normal hemoglobin levels for men and women are 14 and 12 milligrams or more per 100 milliliters of blood, respectively. Borderline anemia is defined as blood hemoglobin levels that are lower than normal yet still greater than 7 grams per 100 milliliters of blood. When hemoglobin levels are reduced, there is a reduction in the oxygen-carrying ability of the blood. Ultimately, less oxygen delivery to cells can result in lethargy and in early fatigue when a person is active. Iron deficiency also decreases the ability of cells to make ATP by aerobic mechanisms. The activity of all other iron-containing enzymes is likely reduced as well.

Iron Toxicity (Overload)
Conditions Under Which Iron Toxicity Occurs

Iron toxicity has been reported in both humans and animals. HLA-linked hemochromatosis appears to be one of the most common inborn errors in metabolism among white people of European descent. The hemochromatosis locus is linked to the HLA region on the short arm of chromosome 6 and is an autosomal recessive trait. This genetic abnormality may be as prevalent as 12 per 1,000 individuals of

European descent and is characterized by excessive iron absorption, elevated plasma iron concentration and transferrin saturation, and high iron content in liver parenchymal cells. In contrast, macrophage iron content is relatively low. One specific gene on the HLA region of chromosome 6 involved in iron absorption is HFE. Mutations in the HFE gene lead to increased iron absorption.

Congenital atransferrinemia is an extremely rare disorder characterized by a nearly complete lack of transferrin. That disorder is probably an autosomal recessive anomaly and is accompanied by hypochromic anemia and iron overload involving the liver, heart, and pancreas and an almost complete lack of iron in bone marrow. That disorder, along with a mouse model of hypotransferrin, suggests that plasma transferrin is not necessary for the transport of absorbed iron.

More isolated examples of human genetic disposition for iron overload have also been described. One-third of the members of a large Melanesian family have been reported to develop an iron overload disorder. Although many characteristics of this disorder are similar to HLA-linked hemochromatosis, the mode of inheritance appears to be autosomal dominant. Another instance of inherited iron overload was reported in two siblings in a Yemenite Jewish family. This inherited trait is also believed to be different from HLA-linked hemochromatosis.

Iron overload has been reported in at least 15 sub-Saharan African countries as a result of drinking locally brewed beer with a high iron content. The histologic alterations to the liver are distinct from alcohol-related insult, and iron accumulates in both hepatic parenchymal cells and macrophages. Necropsy evaluation estimated the incidence of iron overload-induced liver cirrhosis to be greater than 10% in those geographic regions. Further investigation suggested that there is likely an underlying genetic factor concomitant with the high dietary iron consumption.

Iron overload may also be induced clinically by frequent blood transfusions in patients with aplastic anemia, pure red blood cell anemia, Blackfan-Diamond syndrome, myelodysplasia, and sickle cell disease. The iron is derived primarily from erythrocytic hemoglobin, and excessive iron initially accumulates in macrophages and then in the liver parenchyma. In this list of blood diseases, the causes vary from genetic to environmental to unknown.

Neonatal iron overload has been described as being associated with certain perinatal metabolic disorders, such as hypermethioninemia and severe fatal liver disease. Animal models have been developed to study iron overload and its related pathology. Rats fed a diet enriched with 2 to 3% elemental (carbonyl) iron over a period of 2 to 4 months develop hepatic nonheme iron concentrations 50 to 100 times normal. Excessive iron deposition in cardiac and pancreatic tissue is modest, and nonhepatic organ toxicity is not evident.

Mechanism of Iron Toxicity

The exact mechanisms of toxicity from iron overload are not completely established. However, many investigators agree that the pathologic alterations associated with iron overload are probably the result of increased free radical activity initiated by excessive iron. Under normal conditions, iron is found almost entirely bound to proteins. However, unbound iron in the reduced ferrous form is believed to contribute to free radical activity by participating in the Fenton reaction, which results in the production of the highly reactive hydroxyl radical (OH^-):

$$Fe^{2+} + H_2O_2 \rightarrow Fe^{3+} + OH^- + HO^\bullet$$

Many investigators have reported the products of lipid peroxidation in various tissue, including liver, plasma, kidney, spleen, muscle, and skin. Increased iron absorption results in hepatic iron overload, which ultimately leads to organelle dysfunction and injury, lipocyte collagen synthesis that leads to fibrosis, and, possibly, alterations in hepatic DNA that initiate tumor formation.

Although iron is deposited in many organ tissues during overload; such as the heart, lung, kidney, and brain; the liver has received the most investigative attention, most likely because of its prominent involvement in iron storage and because cirrhosis is recognized as one of the most common causes of death from genetically based hemochromatosis in humans. Rats fed a diet enriched with 2 to 3% carbonyl for 2 to 4 months develop hepatic iron concentrations of 3,000 to 6,000 micrograms of iron per gram of liver. The iron preferentially deposits in periportal hepatocytes, similar to the early stages of HLA-linked hemochromatosis and African iron overload. The iron-overloaded rats present direct evidence of mitochondrial and microsomal lipid peroxidation along with an increase in the low-molecular-weight pool of catalytically active iron. Furthermore, at a hepatic iron concentration at which lipid peroxidation is observed, specific mitochondrial membrane-associated activities, such as oxidative metabolism and calcium sequestering, are decreased. Similarly, microsomal membranes demonstrate decreased cytochrome concentrations, enzyme activities, and calcium sequestration.

Iron overload results in excessive accumulation of iron in hepatocellular lysosomes and appears to increase their fragility. This increase in fragility results in the release of hydrolytic enzymes into the cytosol of hepatocytes and the initiation of cellular damage. In one study, experimental iron-overloaded rat hepatocytes demonstrated lysosomes that were more fragile. Those membranes also demonstrated decreased fluidity and increased lipid peroxidation.

At liver iron concentrations similar to those observed in HLA-linked hemochromatosis (3,000 to 6,000 micrograms of iron per gram liver), experimental iron-overloaded rat mitochondria show increased lipid peroxidation. Furthermore, at modest increases in hepatic liver iron concentration, there was a significant impediment of mitochondrial electron transport, as exemplified by a 70% reduction in cytochrome c oxidase activity and a 48% decrease in cellular oxygen consumption.

Iron Toxicity and Diseases

Iron overload also results in hepatic fibrosis. The mechanisms of fibrogenesis in this condition are poorly understood. Hepatic levels of type I procollagen mRNA are augmented and nonparenchymal cells are predominantly involved, most likely activated lipocytes.

Iron overload is also associated with a greater incidence of cancer. Humans with HLA-linked hemochromatosis have about a 200 times greater risk of hepatocellular carcinoma. Experimental iron-overloaded rats have shown evidence of an increase in DNA strand breaks with a liver iron concentration of 3,130 micrograms per gram of tissue, but not at lower liver iron concentrations (approximately 600 micrograms per gram). Furthermore, a synergistic carcinogenic effect was reported with the combination of iron in conjunction with polychlorinated biphenyls.

Concern has been expressed over the reported association of serum ferritin levels with increased myocardial infarction. In a study of over 1,900 Finnish men aged 40 to 64 years, those with serum ferritin levels greater than 200 micrograms per liter had a 2.2 times greater risk of myocardial infarct compared with men with lower levels. This risk level was after adjustment for other known risk factors, such as cigarette smoking, higher systolic blood pressure, lipoprotein cholesterol levels, and so on. In fact, those men with a serum LDL-cholesterol level greater than 193 milligrams per 100 milliliters plus high serum ferritin levels had a greater risk compared with those men with only high serum ferritin levels. The mechanism for this effect may be related to the role of iron in free-radical generation, as discussed previously. Oxidation of LDL-cholesterol is known to result in greater cholesterol uptake by macrophages, which is a key mechanism in foam cell production and subsequent plaque formation.

Finally, iron overload has been associated with neurodegenerative diseases (**SPECIAL FEATURE 13.1**). Alzheimer's disease, Parkinson's disease, and amyotrophic lateral sclerosis (ALS) have a high association with increased iron levels, in particular, nerve cells related to those pathologies.

● BEFORE YOU GO ON . . .

1. List the factors that increase the uptake of nonheme iron.

2. How do iron-responsive, element-binding proteins affect ferritin and transferrin receptors in terms of intracellular iron levels and mechanisms?

3. Explain the mechanism by which the liver may affect small intestine iron absorption?

4. What is HLA-linked hemochromatosis?

5. What are the various types of iron toxicity?

SPECIAL FEATURE 13.1

Iron and Neurodegenerative Disorders

Brain iron metabolism may have a significant role in the pathogenesis of several neurodegenerative disorders. Alzheimer's disease, Parkinson's disease, and amyotrophic lateral sclerosis (ALS) are some of the neurologic diseases in which iron has been implicated. Iron is taken up by the brain via transferrin receptors. In all of those brain disorders, the common thread is iron overload or accumulation as a potential underlying factor. Accumulation of iron by different cell types may lead to oxidative stress, which could result in cell damage and the onset of disease. That theory is, in part, supported by the observation that treatment with certain iron chelators appears to improve some of the symptoms of the diseases, or at a minimum, improves the quality of life of patients.

(continues)

SPECIAL FEATURE 13.1 (*continued*)

The link with oxidative stress has been suggested for those patients with ALS who have a genetic basis for this disease. Mutations in the antioxidant enzyme Cu/Zn-SOD are common in some types of ALS. Often, there is a point mutation of Cu/Zn-SOD in those patients, and approximately 25 missense mutations have been identified for Cu/Zn-SOD thus far. Decreased Cu/Zn-SOD activity increases oxidative stress. The role of iron in ALS is less certain with respect to a mechanism compared with the mutations related to Cu/Zn-SOD. Iron is implicated in ALS due to the fact that there is altered expression of transferrin receptors, DMT1, ferroportin, and ferritin, to name a few proteins involved with iron metabolism. Iron accumulation in the central nervous system of ALS patients occurs, which can lead to greater oxidative stress. How all of the iron regulator proteins interact to result in increased iron accumulation in ALS is speculative.

In Alzheimer's disease, the key pathologies include the accumulation of insoluble amyloid β-protein and neurofibrillary tangles, which are the primary marker of the disease. The neurofibrillary tangles have hyperphosphorylated proteins in which ferric iron (Fe^{3+}) binds and then is reduced to ferrous (Fe^{+2}) iron. This reduction leads to the production of neurofibrillary tangles. However, a key protein in the disease is APP, which is a precursor to amyloid β-protein. This protein is found in neurons and glial cells of the brain and is believed to be regulated in part by iron, but it also functions in iron export from cells to extracellular fluid. Iron accumulation may cause oxidative damage to APP and further misregulate iron export.

Parkinson disease is characterized by damaged dopaminergic neuronal cells in the substantia nigra. Iron deposits have been found in those cells from Parkinson's patients. The substantia nigra is the site of the pigment neuromelanin, which complexes with iron. This neuromelanin protects nerve cells from oxidative stress. However, with aging, the level of neuromelanin produced declines, and thus, the capacity to bind excess iron also decreases. The extra nonbound iron leads to cellular dysfunction. In addition, DMT1 has also been reported to increase in neuronal cells of the substantia nigra of Parkinson's patients, which results in greater levels of iron in those cells, as well as greater oxidative stress.

The role of iron in those neurodegenerative brain diseases has resulted in increased research on the efficacy of iron chelators as a treatment option. However, the role of dietary iron in those diseases is largely unknown at this time.

▶ Zinc

The major metabolic function of zinc in the human body is as a cofactor for more than 200 enzymes affecting probably every general function in the human body. That makes zinc one of the most ubiquitous micronutrients. Special attention was paid to zinc after it was determined that zinc works directly at the level of gene expression. Zinc is commonly found as a divalent cation (Zn^{2+}).

Dietary Zinc and Absorption
Food Sources

Because zinc is mostly associated with proteins and nucleic acids in organisms, good protein sources are also better zinc sources. For example, some of the best zinc sources in the diet include herring, oysters, clams, poultry, meats, eggs, and legumes (**TABLE 13.3**). Although whole cereal grains are also a good source of zinc, the refining or milling process removes most of that mineral. Fruits are relatively poor sources.

Dietary Factors That Affect Zinc Absorption

Zinc in the intestinal lumen is derived not only from dietary sources but also from biliary and pancreatic digestive secretions. Zinc associated with proteins and nucleic acids is liberated from those structures via digestive secretions. Although the exact mechanisms are not completely resolved, zinc absorption appears to occur along the length of the small intestine, with the jejunum being responsible for most of the absorption. Several factors influence the efficiency of zinc absorption and contribute to its relatively wide range of absorption (12 to 60%). As with several of the transition elements, the absorption of zinc increases as its physiologic status decreases, and vice versa. Several dietary factors can also influence zinc absorption. For instance, zinc availability from soy and wheat may be improved by the addition of casein, cysteine, or histidine, to which zinc binds preferentially (a beneficial chelation). In contrast, phytate present in grains and legumes can bind zinc and decrease its absorption. However, phytate seems to only have a negative effect in the presence of increased intraluminal calcium.

TABLE 13.3 Zinc Content of Select Foods

Food	Zinc (mg)	Food	Zinc (mg)
Meat and alternatives		*Legumes*	
Liver (3 oz)	4.4	Baked beans, cooked (1 cup)	3.5
Hamburger (3 oz)	5.4	Peas, cooked (1 cup)	1.8
Crab (1 cup)	3.2	*Nuts and seeds*	
Lamb (3 oz)	3.5	Pecans (1 cup)	4.9
Pork (3 oz)	2.4	Cashews (1 cup)	7.7
Chicken leg (3 oz)	2.2	Sunflower seeds (1 cup)	6.8
Grains		Peanut butter (2 tbsp)	0.9
Oatmeal, cooked (1 cup)	1.5	*Milk and milk products*	
Bran flakes (1 serving, ¾ cup)	1.5	Cheese, cheddar (1 oz)	0.9
Rice, brown (1 cup)	1.2	Milk, whole (1 cup)	0.9
Rice, white (1 cup)	0.7	Cheese, American (1 oz)	0.9

Zinc absorption is also decreased by substances such as oxalic acid (found in teas, chocolate, berries, and spinach) and polyphenols, such as the tannins present in tea. High dietary fiber intake may also decrease zinc absorption.

Zinc and iron may compete for absorption, because an iron-to-zinc intake ratio of 2:1 or higher substantially reduces zinc absorption in humans. Zinc is more bioavailable as amino acid chelates (e.g., zinc alanine, zinc glycine) and as zinc gluconate. It appears to be less available as zinc sulfate and zinc carbonate. Zinc absorption appears to be somewhat positively influenced by the presence of meat. A pancreatic substance, such as citrate or picolinic acid may enhance the absorption of zinc.

Zinc Absorption Proteins and Mechanism

At physiologic levels of intestinal zinc, the predominant mechanism of absorption appears to be a carrier-mediated system (**FIGURE 13.7**). Zinc is absorbed against a concentration gradient, which is certainly suggestive of an active transport mechanism. Interestingly, metabolic inhibitors do not appear to influence zinc uptake, nor does zinc uptake display saturation kinetics. Therefore, zinc absorption is still somewhat enigmatic and likely does not require an energy source such as ATP. DMT1 (the same protein that was involved in nonheme iron absorption) binds zinc and transfers it across the brush border membrane. However, this mechanism may only be responsible for minor amounts of zinc absorbed. The current thinking is that there is a specific zinc transporter, referred to as **transporter ZIP4**. The level of this protein is dependent on zinc status in that during zinc deficiency, the production of this protein is upregulated. This effect is at the transcriptional level where increased mRNA is expressed. This protein is also important in an inherited disease called **acrodermatitis enteropathica**.

Individuals with that disorder have a mutation in the gene that encodes ZIP4 and thus results in a zinc deficiency. Another protein that can transport zinc from the lumen into the enterocyte is ZIP14, but it appears that its role is more limited and may be more upregulated in the small intestine in response to infection. At higher dietary intake levels, some paracellular absorption is thought to contribute to the overall

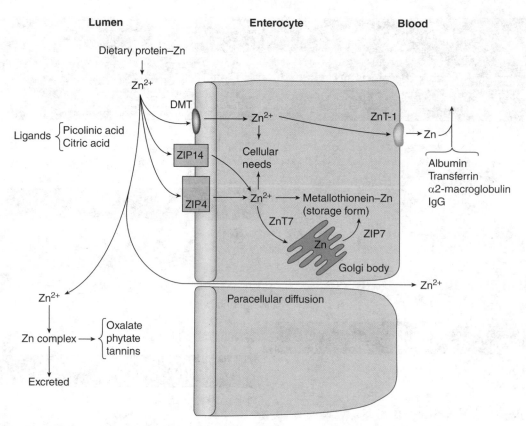

FIGURE 13.7 Absorption Routes and Mechanisms of Zinc in the Enterocytes of the Small Intestine. Zinc is liberated to the free form from dietary protein. Several transport proteins (ZIP 4, ZIP14, and DMT) are responsible for the uptake of zinc by enterocytes. If there is a physiologic need for zinc, it is exported to the blood by the ZnT-1 transport protein and picked up by blood proteins. The protein metallothionein will bind excess zinc and will be eliminated along with enterocytes as they are sloughed off. Paracellular diffusion also contributes to zinc absorption.

absorption. Using this mechanism, high dosages of zinc supplements can be used to help overcome the lack of zinc absorption via the ZIP4 protein in acrodermatitis enteropathica.

When zinc enters the mucosal cell, it is destined for one or more of the following fates: (1) it may perform functions within the mucosal cell, (2) it may move into the blood, or (3) it may bind to the small-molecular-weight protein **metallothionein**. High intramucosal zinc levels induce the transcription of mRNA for metallothionein, a protein with a molecular weight of between 6,000 and 8,000. This compound has a high number of sulfhydryl groups capable of generally chelating divalent cations. The excessive zinc, bound to metallothionein, can then be excreted as mucosal cells are sloughed off (see Figure 13.7). Zinc that is to be absorbed can transverse the enterocyte and exit via the **zinc transporter 1 (ZnT-1)** on the basolateral side of the enterocyte. When zinc exits the enterocyte, it can be picked up in the portal blood by binding to albumin, transferrin, α2-macroglobulin, or immunoglobin G

(IgG). At one time, it was thought that the protein cysteine-rich intestinal polypeptide, or CRIP, was responsible for binding zinc in the enterocyte and transferring it to ZnT-1, but this proposed mechanism has fallen out of favor.

Within the enterocyte, zinc is stored in various organelles and vesicles. The manner in which zinc is partitioned within the cell is regulated by a variety of zinc-binding proteins. Note the following nomenclature for the zinc-transporting proteins: ZnT protein function in zinc efflux from the cytoplasm, and ZIP protein function to move zinc into the cytoplasm. Thus, ZIP4 moves zinc into the cytoplasm of the enterocyte; ZnT-1 moves zinc out of the cytoplasm of the enterocyte. Within the enterocyte, transporters are available that import zinc into the Golgi apparatus and other vesicles. Conversely, there are zinc transporters that will function to export zinc from those cell structures. For instance, ZnT-7 will result in zinc import into the Golgi apparatus; ZIP7 will export zinc from that organelle to the cytoplasm. ZnT-2 will import zinc into cell vesicles, and ZIP proteins will export zinc from those structures. In this fashion, zinc is bound to protein as opposed to being in its ionic form. Approximately 20 zinc-transporting proteins have been identified, and each tissue may have different ones.

One potential consequence of excessive zinc ingestion and the resultant increase in the synthesis of metallothionein is a sequestering of copper and its subsequent loss in sloughed-off cells. Metallothionein has a greater affinity for copper than zinc, and it has become known that ingesting as little as 18.5 milligrams of zinc for a couple of weeks significantly decreases copper absorption.

Metabolism and Function of Zinc

Overall Metabolism

Zinc is found in every human cell. Its average content in the body ranges from 1.5 to 2.5 grams, depending on an individual's size. Tissues demonstrating a higher concentration of zinc include bone, liver, muscle, kidneys, and the skin. Zinc is a cofactor for more than 200 enzymes, many of which deal with various aspects of protein synthesis or hormone function of some type. Whereas the physiologic consequences of an absolute or marginal deficiency of dietary zinc often relate to the effect that zinc has on those enzymes, zinc excess may not have a direct influence on those target enzymes, and in fact, some of the associated physiologic consequences of excess may be related to resulting imbalances of other nutrients. This is well documented in the case of copper and zinc antagonism, mentioned previously. Excess dietary zinc may lead to a copper deficiency, which has different symptoms. Therefore, it becomes a challenge to separate the direct effects of zinc toxicity from the indirect or secondary effects that it may have in perturbing the balance of another essential element.

Although zinc is found in all tissue, most of this mineral is actually located in skeletal muscle (approximately 60%) and bone (approximately 30%). The skin, liver, brain, kidneys, and heart also have higher concentrations of zinc; however, these concentrations are still small relative to bone and skeletal muscle. The level of zinc in the liver of a newborn infant is greater than that found in an adult. For instance, 25% of the zinc in newborns is found in the liver. More zinc is probably also found in the bones of newborns compared with adults.

Zinc is primarily found within cells because its concentration in extracellular fluids is relatively low. A zinc-selective transport system allows for the uptake of zinc into tissue. It is possible that zinc carriers, or at least one zinc carrier, is positively influenced by amino acid metabolism within that tissue. Hormonal balance may influence the distribution of zinc between extracellular and intracellular fluids. Insulin, glucagon, and glucocorticoids appear to influence liver zinc levels. Glucocorticoids are known to stimulate zinc uptake in hepatic cultured cells. Glucagon may also stimulate zinc uptake by liver cells.

Zinc largely functions as a necessary component of various enzymes. In fact, the number of enzymes whose optimal function rely on zinc is probably greater than the total number of enzymes that rely on all of the other minor minerals combined. In general, zinc is involved with enzymes that affect pH regulation, ethanol (alcohol) metabolism, bone mineralization, protein digestion, heme manufacturing, antioxidation, immunity, and protein and nucleic acid metabolism. **TABLE 13.4** lists several zinc-dependent enzymes and their functions. It is important to note that zinc may have a structural role instead of a catalytic role in enzymes. An example is with copper-zinc, superoxide dismutase (SOD), where copper has a catalytic role and zinc a structural role.

Function of Zinc-Containing Proteins

Zinc also functions directly at the genetic level, where it is associated with specialized proteins to form **zinc finger proteins (FIGURE 13.8)**. Here, zinc binds to histidine and cysteine amino acids in proteins that are known to bind to DNA in the cell nucleus. These proteins are referred to as **transcription factors** and control gene expression or repression primarily by targeting the promoter

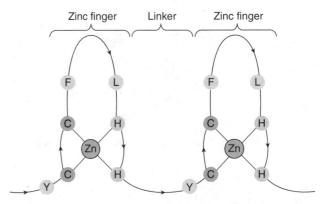

FIGURE 13.8 Zinc Finger Proteins Interact with DNA.
Cysteine and histidine residues form tetrahedral complexes to result in the fingerlike projections of certain proteins that act as transcription factors to allow proteins to bind to DNA.

Data from Stryer L. *Biochemistry*, 4th ed. New York: W. H. Freeman and Company, 1995.

TABLE 13.4 Zinc-Dependent Enzymes and Function	
Enzyme	**General Function**
Alcohol dehydrogenase	Oxidation of ethanol in the cytosol, primarily in hepatocytes
Lactate dehydrogenase	Reversible oxidation/reduction interconversion of pyruvate and lactic acid
Alkaline phosphatase	Primarily involved in mineralization of bone matrix
Angiotensin-converting enzyme	Converts angiotensin I to angiotensin II
Carbonic anhydrase	Interconverts CO_2 and H_2O to carbonic acid to assist in the regulation of CO_2 content of blood as well as pH
Pyruvate dehydrogenase	Converts pyruvate to acetyl CoA within mitochondria
DNA and RNA polymerases	DNA replication and transcription
Superoxide dismutase	Cytosolic antioxidant
Aspartate transcarbamylase	Pyrimidine synthesis
Carboxypeptidases A and B	Protein digestion
Phosphodiesterase	Cleaves phosphodiester bonds (i.e., nucleic acids)
Fructose 1,6-bisphosphatase	Gluconeogenesis
Leukotriene hydrolase	Eicosanoid metabolism
Elastase	Digestion of connective tissue elastin
Reverse transcriptase	DNA replication
Gustin	Taste acuity

regions of genes. Proteins, such as ZIP4, ZnT-1, and metallothionein appear to be regulated by the level of dietary zinc. With respect to ZIP4, the gene promoter encoding this zinc transport protein has a binding site for a transcription factor called **Kruppel-like factor 4 (KLF4)**, which upregulates the mRNA transcript for ZIP4 in zinc restriction. Apparently, in zinc restriction, the KLF4 transcription factor becomes "active" and enhanced binding to the promoter of the gene encoding ZIP4 occurs. Zn-T1 and metallothionein are under the control of **metal transcription factor-1 (MTF-1)**, which is a zinc finger protein. The gene promoters for these two proteins have binding sites for MTF-1. However, here, when zinc becomes abundant, the binding of MTF-1 to the gene promoters is enhanced. Apparently, zinc will induce a conformational change in shape of MTF-1 and will allow it to bind to the promoters to upregulate the mRNA transcripts for both ZnT-1 and metallothionein.

Zinc Excretion

Zinc excretion from the human body occurs by several routes. Zinc is primarily lost from the body via fecal excretion. Fecal zinc represents unabsorbed dietary zinc and zinc secreted into the digestive tract via digestion juices (e.g., zinc-containing enzymes, biliary fluids). Sloughed-off mucosal enterocytes containing metallothionein-bound zinc also contribute significantly to fecal zinc content. Exfoliation of skin and sweating allow for about 1 milligram of zinc loss daily. Urinary zinc is typically less than 600 micrograms daily, thus representing a minor route of excretion. A relatively small amount of zinc loss occurs from the loss of body hair (0.1 to 0.2 milligrams of zinc per gram).

Recommended Levels of Intake of Zinc

Zinc RDAs are influenced by age, gender, health status, condition (e.g., pregnancy, lactation), physical activity, and other dietary components. Males have a higher zinc requirement than females after 13 years of age, primarily because of their increased muscle mass. For males older than 13 years, 11 milligrams per day of zinc is recommended, compared with 8 milligrams per day for females.

During pregnancy, the RDA for females is increased to 12 milligrams per day for those aged 18 years or younger, but is 11 milligrams per day for those aged 19 years or older. This recommendation is followed by a further increase to 13 milligrams per day during lactation for those younger than 18 years, and 12 milligrams per day for those aged 19 years and older.

Zinc Deficiency

Zinc deficiency is characterized by dwarfism, poor sexual performance, deformed bones, poor wound healing, abnormal hair and nails, loss of taste (hypogeusia), gastrointestinal disturbances, poor chylomicron formation, central nervous system anomalies, and impaired folate and vitamin A absorption. Zinc deficiency has been commonly observed among Middle Eastern children, especially males, and also in the Hispanic population of Denver, Colorado. In the Middle East, unleavened bread is frequently consumed, which is high in phytate. Yeast contains phytase, which can digest some of the phytate. However, the recipe for the dough of unleavened bread does not include yeast. The high fiber content of the Middle Eastern diet and low meat intake contribute to the problem. In Denver, Colorado, the diets were low in zinc and plant based, which led to decreased zinc stores over time. As already mentioned, a defect in ZIP4 results in the genetic zinc deficiency of acrodermatitis enteropathica.

Zinc Toxicity

Acute human zinc toxicity rarely occurs. Much of the current knowledge regarding zinc toxicity comes from animal studies and through supplementation with mineral preparations. Animals provided a high dietary level of zinc generally manifest dysphagia. This could be the result of a reduction in the palatability of food. Growth rate declines and even weight loss can occur as a result of decreased food intake. Zinc toxicity has been reported to result in rough hair, achromotrichia, emphysema, diarrhea, arthritis-like symptoms, abortive fetuses, and stillbirths. A microcytic anemia develops. However, this may be partly explained by a decreased uptake of either copper or iron, or both. Hemolytic anemia is not uncommon, and renal fibrosis, fatty liver, and liver necrosis have been reported by some scientists. Hypercholesterolemia sometimes occurs with excess zinc intake, which again may be at least partially explained by a secondary copper deficiency. However, large doses of zinc have been known to lower HDL-cholesterol. Excess zinc normally would produce symptoms that mimic deficiencies of copper, iron, manganese, or calcium. When the level of one or more of these elements is increased in the diet, the signs of zinc toxicity are markedly reduced.

● BEFORE YOU GO ON . . .

1. How can excess dietary zinc lead to a copper deficiency?
2. Describe the roles the following proteins play in intestinal zinc metabolism: ZIP4, ZnT-1, and metallothionein. What are zinc finger proteins?
3. What are the major roles of zinc in tissues?
4. List some of the common signs of a zinc deficiency.
5. How is zinc absorbed by the small intestine?

▶ Iodine

The role of iodine in human and animal nutrition has been recognized for a long time. At one time, deficiency of iodine was widespread globally, including the United States. Today, it is still rather problematic in certain areas of the world, such as parts of Africa, where an estimated 200 million people are affected. Deficiency of iodine results in hypertrophy of the thyroid gland, termed **goiter**. Historically, goiter has been documented in the records of the early Greeks. The ancient Greeks used burnt sponges to treat goiter, but this information was lost for a long period of time. It was not until 1850 that the French physician Chatin measured the iodine content of water and various foods of France and noted that the iodine content of the soil correlated with the incidence of goiter. This information was published but forgotten as well. By the early part of the 20th century, iodine became known as a treatment for goiter.

Iodine, as an element, is a halogen. Like other halogens, iodine tends to accept an electron and exists in nature as a negatively charged ion. Therefore, the anion name *iodide* is used interchangeably with *iodine*, as is *fluoride* with *fluorine*, *chloride* with *chlorine*, and *bromide* with *bromine*. *Iodide* will be used in this text because it is the natural state for this element.

Dietary Sources of Iodide

The amount of iodide in food varies widely, and intake typically ranges between 100 to 200 micrograms per day in the United States. **TABLE 13.5** lists the iodide content of select foods. The iodide content of a plant is mostly related to the soil content in which the plant was grown, including the iodide content of any fertilizers used to cultivate the soil. The iodide content in drinking water usually reflects

TABLE 13.5 Iodide Content of Select Foods	
Food	**Iodide (µg)**
Salt, iodized (1 tsp)	400
Haddock (3 oz)	104–145
Cottage cheese (2 cups)	26–71
Shrimp (3 oz)	21–37
Egg (1)	18–26
Cheese, cheddar (1 oz)	5–23
Ground beef (3 oz)	8

the iodide content of the rocks and soils through which the water flows or is maintained. The content of iodide in animals depends on the plants they consumed or the feed they were provided. For carnivores, it depends on the plant consumption of their prey. Animal iodide content is also influenced by the content in their water source.

Marine seafood (shrimp, oysters, ocean fish, mollusks) is typically a better source of iodide than freshwater fish. Dairy foods may be a fair source of iodide. Again, the iodide content of cow's milk reflects the iodide content of the cow's feed or the soil of its grazing region. Iodide deficiency has been eradicated for the most part from many regions of the world, including the United States, where iodide is added to salt (iodized salt). Iodized salt contains one part sodium iodide for every 1,000 parts sodium chloride.

Today, concern is developing about the overconsumption of iodide in countries that use iodized salt. For instance, in the United States, excessive use of iodized salt in food manufacturing, preparation, and seasoning results in the ingestion of iodide well in excess of recommendations.

Absorption of Iodide

Along with dietary iodide, some iodide enters the small intestine via biliary secretions. The amount of iodide in biliary secretions is influenced by iodide status. The absorption of iodine occurs efficiently along the length of the intestinal tract, including the stomach. This results in nearly complete absorption of iodide, similar to several other monovalent

ions, such as sodium, potassium, and chloride. Very efficient absorption results in very low fecal iodide content. Iodide appears to dissolve freely into the blood, and excessive iodide is primarily excreted by the kidneys.

Metabolism and Function of Iodide

An adult human contains roughly 15 to 20 milligrams of iodide. For the most part, iodide is concentrated in the thyroid gland as well as the salivary and gastric glands. The thyroid gland contains roughly 75 to 80% of body iodide. In thyroid gland parenchyma, the concentration of intracellular iodide may be 30-fold higher than the extracellular fluid. These cells must use aggressive active transport systems to acquire such a large concentration of iodide. The thyroid gland uses iodide to synthesize thyroid hormone. At least 60 micrograms of iodide must be taken up by the thyroid gland daily to produce adequate thyroid hormone. Salivary glands also use an active transport mechanism to accrue iodide.

The iodine in the thyroid gland is incorporated into a globulin protein and termed **thyroglobin**, which is the storage form of iodine. It can be removed from storage and react with the amino acid tyrosine. Iodination may occur on the 3, 5, 3′, and 5′ carbon positions of the six-member rings of the thyronine structure. When iodide is bound to all four positions, the compound is called **thyroxin (T4)** [**FIGURE 13.9**].

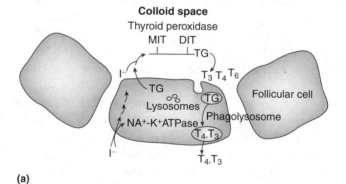

FIGURE13.9 Thyroid Hormones. (a) Synthesis of thyroxin and related hormones in the cells of the thyroid glands. MIT, monoiodotyrosine; DIT, di-iodotyrosine; TG, thyroglobulin. (b) Two key hormones: thyroxin (T$_4$) and the more metabolically active tri-iodothyronine (T$_3$).

Iodination at the 3, 5, and 3' ring positions results in a molecule called **triiodothyronine (T3)**. Collectively, T_3 and T_4 are referred to as *thyroid hormone*. Roughly 90% of the thyroid hormone released daily is T_4, and the remaining 10% is T_3, with T_4 predominating in the blood. However, T_3 is about 5 to 10 times more potent than T_4. In the blood, approximately 80% of thyroid hormone binds to thyroxine-binding protein (TBP), about 10 to 15% to thyroxine-binding prealbumin, and the remainder to albumin.

A unique control mechanism regulates the production of these compounds. The hypothalamus releases the peptide thyrotropin-releasing hormone (TRH), which, in turn, stimulates the pituitary to produce thyroid-stimulating hormone (TSH), which is also called thyrotropin. TSH circulates to the thyroid gland and initiates the production of thyroid hormone, which then enters the blood and circulates to peripheral tissue. Thyroid hormone output thus increases and exerts a negative feedback on the release of TRH. TSH may do the same, but to a lesser extent. Almost all of the thyroxine in the circulation may become converted (deiodinated) to T_3 after entering peripheral tissue. Thyroid hormone has its receptors in the nucleus of the cells; thus, its activity is largely attributed to influence on gene expression. Thyroid hormone also undergoes some low-affinity binding in the cytoplasm; however, the binding is not to the same protein receptor found in the nucleus.

How does thyroxin work at the gene level? Target cells for thyroxin have a thyroid receptor. The thyroid receptor binds to thyroid response elements, or DNA base pairs of DNA promoter regions of target proteins (**FIGURE 13.10**). The thyroid receptor can form homodimers with itself, but heterodimers with retinoid X receptors (RXR) are more common. RXR and the thyroid receptor bind to the promoter with a corepressor that blocks transcription. However, with T_3 present, the repressor dissociates and co-activators are recruited, which turns transcription on.

Thyroid hormone affects virtually every cell in the human body, perhaps with the exception of the adult brain, testes, spleen, uterus, and the thyroid gland itself. Thyroid hormone promotes the activities associated with glucose breakdown and thereby increases metabolism and heat production. Thyroid hormone generally acts by inducing or suppressing the expression of certain genes. One outstanding function of thyroid hormone is the induction of expression of the gene for growth hormone. This explains why earlier studies demonstrated that animals deficient in thyroid hormone had lower amounts of growth hormone in

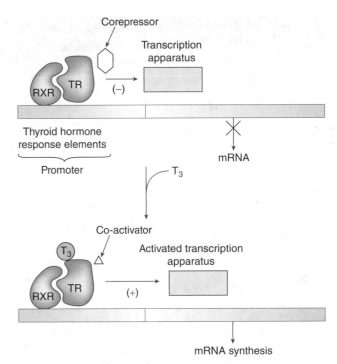

FIGURE 13.10 Mechanism by which T$_3$ Interacts with the Thyroid Receptor and Targets Certain Genes to Turn on the Gene Promoter. The thyroid receptor (TR) and retinoic acid receptor (RXR) both bind to the gene promoter. In the absence of the hormone, a corepressor remains activated. However, once T$_3$ binds to the thyroid receptor, a coactivator is recruited and the transcription process is turned on.

their pituitary gland. It also helps explain some of the general anabolic effects of thyroid hormone. **TABLE 13.6** lists more specific effects of thyroid hormone.

Because a higher blood thyroid hormone concentration increases metabolic rate, synthetic thyroid hormone was once prescribed to treat morbidly obese people. However, the effects of thyroid hormone are not limited to increasing cell metabolism, and potentially deleterious side effects limited its use for this purpose. Therapeutic thyroid hormone therapy affects blood pressure and heart activity, as well as producing nausea, sweating, diarrhea, anxiety, headaches, and insomnia. Today, thyroid hormone is prescribed mostly to treat hypothyroidism, a condition in which the thyroid gland fails to produce adequate thyroid hormone. During the growing years, thyroid hormone is very important because it promotes growth and maturation of the skeleton, central nervous system, and reproductive organs.

Recommended Levels for Iodide Intake

The RDA is 150 micrograms per day for adults. During pregnancy, the RDA is 220 micrograms per

TABLE 13.6 Effects of Thyroid Hormone on Specific Human Mechanisms

Tissue or Mechanism	Effect of Thyroid Hormone
Carbohydrate metabolism	Stimulates glucose absorption as well as uptake by cells; enhances carbohydrate metabolism, especially glycolysis and gluconeogenesis; enhances insulin release
Fat metabolism	Enhances fat mobilization from adipocytes; increases free fatty acid content of plasma and increases fatty acid oxidation in cells; decreases plasma cholesterol and triglycerides, probably by increasing bile cholesterol content and subsequent fecal loss
Protein synthesis	Increases general protein synthesis; however, excessive amounts result in protein catabolism
Basal metabolism	Increases general metabolism of most cells; lack of thyroid hormone results in a 50% reduction in basal metabolic rate
Cardiovascular system	Increases heart rate and stroke strength; increases blood volume slightly; blood pressure is generally unchanged, although systolic pressure can be elevated and diastolic pressure relatively decreased
Respiration	Increased respiration associated with increased cellular metabolism
Feeding/digestion	Increased appetite and food intake; increased rate of digestive juice secretion and motility of digestive tract; lack of thyroid hormone results in constipation
Skeletal muscle	Increases vigor of contraction
Central nervous system	Increases rapidity of elation; excessive amounts result in nervousness and anxiety
Endocrine glands	Increases rate of most endocrine secretions

day, followed by an increase to 290 micrograms per day during lactation. Most individuals in developed countries receive at least the recommended amounts of iodide via consumption of iodized salt. However, as mentioned earlier, iodide deficiency is still one of the most prevalent nutrition-based problems globally. The Upper Limit (UL) is 1,000 micrograms per day.

Iodide Deficiency

A deficiency of iodide limits thyroid hormone synthesis in the thyroid gland. Thus, most of the signs and symptoms of iodide deficiency result from hypothyroidism. An iodide deficiency in childhood can result in poor growth, poor organ maturation, delayed sexual maturity, and mental deficits. Over 30% of the world's population may have insufficient dietary iodine intake. Children are most susceptible to having iodine deficiency. The consequence of iodine deficiency on

the brain is significant in that early treatment with iodine is one of the most easily treatable brain diseases in the world. A striking characteristic of iodide deficiency is an enlargement of the thyroid gland (goiter). Treatment of goiter usually begins with iodide-rich foods, including iodized salt, which will shrink the goiter with time but will not necessarily correct any of the developmental problems (growth and mental aptitude) in children. Before the widespread use of iodized salt, various regions of the American Midwest were referred to as the "goiter belt" because of their low soil iodide content and decreased availability of iodide-rich fish. If goiter or thyroid enlargement is sufficiently significant, health issues with the trachea, esophagus, and laryngeal nerves are possible.

There are several methods to determine if iodine deficiency is present. The first method is urine iodine concentration. Approximately 90% of iodine is excreted in the urine within one or two days.

Insufficient iodine status is dependent on age and in women, pregnancy or breastfeeding. Low urine iodine status are levels below 100 µg/l. For pregnant and breastfeeding mothers, low urine iodine status are levels below 150 µg/l and 100 µg/l, respectively. A second method is the size of the thyroid gland which can be measured but may require an ultrasound to enhance sensitivity. A third method is TSH level. A TSH level above 5 µU/l indicates low iodine status. A fourth method is the measurement of serum thyroglobulin . Individuals with readings greater than 10 µg/l is considered low iodine status.

Infants born to mothers with low dietary iodine consumption, particularly during the third trimester of pregnancy, may suffer from a condition called **cretinism**, in which they often demonstrate stunted growth and present deficits in mental development. These individuals exhibit large heads relative to the body, are deaf, and have coarse features. This condition is permanent once the child is born. Cretinism is high in areas of the world that have endemic goiter regions: the Himalayas, central Africa, and Central America.

Pre-eclampsia, low-birth-weight infants, miscarriages, and stillbirths are possible consequences of iodine deficiency during pregnancy. The impact of iodine deficiency during pregnancy upon the developing fetal brain most likely involves decreased transfer of thyroxin from the mother to the fetus before the fetus has been able to develop adequate thyroid function on its own. Thyroid function in the fetus is active in the second trimester, thus iodine deficiency in the mother during the first trimester is likely to have the most significant effect. Thyroid hormones are important for the developing fetal brain because they are key in dendrite and axon formation, nerve myelination, neurogenesis, neuronal migration, and the development of synapses and the ability for neurotransmission. Some reports suggest that even mild iodine deficiency can lead to these brain disorders.

It is surprising that when it comes to determining inadequate iodine nutrition in the absence of goiter, the prevalence is about 60% in Europe compared with 10% in North and South America. A large number of affected individuals are children. Almost 2 billion people worldwide suffer from inadequate iodine nutrition, with slightly less than 300 million being children.

Certain foods contain substances called **goitrogens**, which appear to block iodide entry into the thyroid gland. Foods containing goitrogens include broccoli, kale, cauliflower, rutabaga, turnips, Brussels sprouts, and mustard greens. However, most individuals do not eat enough of these vegetables to pose a threat to normal iodide metabolism and thyroid gland activity.

Routine blood tests include T_3 and T_4 concentrations, thus providing a screening tool for thyroid deficiency or other diseases that affect the thyroid hormone.

⬡ BEFORE YOU GO ON . . .

1. List some good sources of iodine in the diet.
2. Explain what happens to iodine in terms of metabolism when it is in the thyroid gland.
3. What hormones control iodine metabolism?

▶ Copper

Copper in the human body shifts between two oxidation states: the **cuprous** (Cu^{1+}) and **cupric** (Cu^{2+}) states. By and large, the cupric state predominates. Copper exerts much of its action by being a cofactor for several enzymes, which are often referred to as cuproenzymes. Copper is fundamentally involved in iron metabolism. If a copper deficiency occurs, the signs and symptoms are similar to those of iron deficiency anemia. Copper is required for the proper synthesis of collagen and is needed to maintain the integrity of connective tissue.

Dietary Copper and Absorption
Food Sources

Dietary sources of copper include a wide variety of foods with very little in common (**TABLE 13.7**). Copper is found in foods such as nuts, shellfish, organ meats, dried fruits, seeds, and legumes. Grains and grain products, as well as chocolate, have appreciable levels of copper. Although these food items are good to excellent sources of copper, the absolute amount of copper absorbed may be influenced by other dietary components. Furthermore, the origin of a food or its processing and handling can greatly change the copper content. As with iodide and certain other minerals, the soil content in which plants were grown and the feed content and water sources of livestock influence the copper content of the final food product. Surveys reveal that copper consumption in the United States ranges between 0.7 and 7.5 milligrams daily.

Dietary Factors That Affect Copper Absorption

Several minerals influence copper absorption. Excess dietary iron can decrease copper absorption, whereas too much copper may cause an iron deficiency. Excessive

TABLE 13.7 Copper Content of Select Foods

Food	Copper (mg)
Liver, beef (3 oz)	12.3
Cashews, dry roasted (1 cup)	3.0
Peas (1 cup)	0.2
Molasses, blackstrap (2 tbsp)	0.2
Sunflower seeds (1 cup)	2.6
V-8 juice (1 cup)	0.02
Tofu, firm (½ cup)	0.5
Beans, refried (1 cup)	0.4
Cocoa powder (3 heaping tsp)	0.08
Prunes, dried (1 cup)	0.5
Salmon, baked (3 oz)	0.3
Pizza, cheese (1 slice)	0.3
Bread, whole wheat (1 slice)	0.04
Milk chocolate (1 oz)	0.02
Milk, 2% (1 cup)	0.02

zinc consumption also decreases copper absorption. The mechanism by which dietary zinc inhibits the uptake of copper involves the intestinal protein metallothionein, which was mentioned earlier. As dietary zinc levels increase, metallothionein synthesis in mucosal enterocytes increases. This results in the binding and trapping of zinc within the mucosal cell. Zinc is not easily dissociated from metallothionein; consequently, when enterocytes are sloughed off in normal mucosal turnover, zinc is lost through the fecal compartment. However, metallothionein has a greater affinity for copper. Thus, when excess zinc is consumed, the increased metallothionein production causes copper to be sequestered within enterocytes and eventually excreted in the feces. As little as 18.5 milligrams of zinc daily can decrease copper absorption, and even higher intakes (25 milligrams)

for several weeks can reduce the activity of key cuproenzymes such as superoxide dismutase.

The presence of certain amino acids, histidine and cysteine in particular, can enhance copper absorption. In addition, binding ligands, such as gluconate and citrate, can assist in copper absorption. The type of carbohydrate consumed may also influence copper absorption efficiency, although more information is needed in this area. One interesting aspect of copper absorption is that it is not as strongly affected by the presence of phytate as are zinc and iron absorption.

Copper may be absorbed by both the stomach and small intestinal mucosa; however, most of the absorption is attributed to the latter (**FIGURE 13.11**). The percentage of copper absorption is decreased as the luminal content of copper increases. For instance, with intakes approximating 7.5 milligrams, about 10 to 20% of the copper is absorbed. A much lower copper intake, meanwhile, such as approximately 1.0 milligram, results in as much as 50 to 75% absorption.

Most copper in the diet is in the cupric form (Cu^{2+}). For most of the copper to be absorbed, it must be converted to the cuprous form (Cu^{1+}). A group of reductases, or Steap proteins, are found along the cell membrane of the enterocyte that will convert the cupric form to the cuprous form. Once in the cuprous form, copper transport along the brush border may involve a couple of protein carriers. One of the copper carriers is **Ctr1**, and the cuprous form is required for this transport protein. Another possible, but less likely, candidate is divalent mineral transporter 1 (DMT1), as mentioned in the discussion regarding iron and zinc absorption. Ctr1 is more likely the prime player in copper absorption. However, uptake of the cupric form cannot be ruled out. It is unclear whether copper diffuses across the enterocyte. Young mice lacking Ctr1 have high tissue copper, suggesting that diffusion or other transport systems may be involved in copper absorption. Once copper is in a cell, it must be bound to a protein; otherwise, it will act as a pro-oxidant. One such group of proteins is termed **chaperone proteins** (**FIGURE 13.12**). In cells, copper may be incorporated into various enzymes or proteins, such as the antioxidant enzyme copper-zinc superoxide dismutase (Cu/Zn-SOD), cytochrome c oxidase in the electron transport system, or an enzyme called ATP7A, which is responsible for exporting copper from the enterocyte. The chaperone protein responsible for ferrying copper to Cu/Zn-SOD is CCS; for cytochrome c oxidase, it is Cox17; and for ATP7A, it is Atox1. Cox17 will deliver copper to other mitochondria chaperone proteins (e.g., Cox11, Sco1, Sco2).

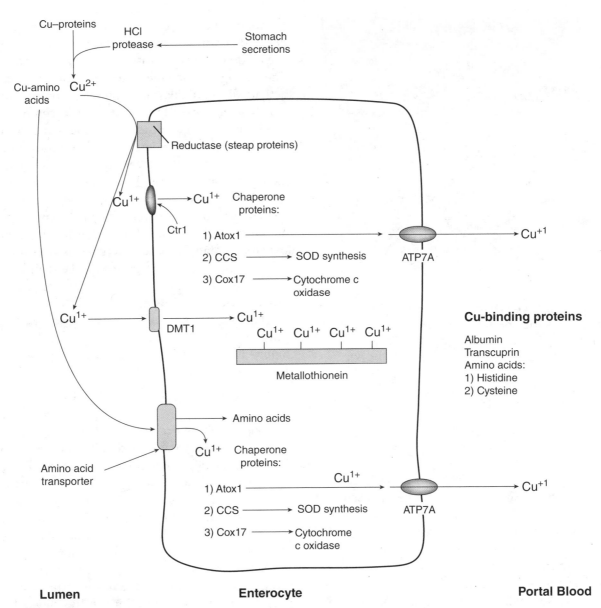

FIGURE 13.11 Absorption Routes and Mechanisms for Copper. Copper is converted from the cupric to the cuprous form by a reductase in order to be absorbed. The transport proteins Ctr1 and DMT1 and certain amino acid transporters are responsible for copper uptake by the enterocytes. Once in the enterocyte, copper may bind to various chaperone proteins (Atox1, CCS, and Cox17). Copper bound to Atox1 will be absorbed into the blood via ATP7A. Copper bound to CCS will be incorporated into super-oxide dismutase (SOD) and copper bound to Cox17 will be incorporated into cytochrome c oxidase (CCO). Excess copper may bind to metallothionein and be excreted when enterocytes are sloughed off. Excess zinc will stimulate metallothionein synthesis. Copper will bind to this protein and be eliminated. This mechanism is why excess zinc decreases copper absorption.

Metabolism and Function of Copper

Copper, once absorbed, is transported bound primarily to albumin and transcuprin. The half-life of the copper-albumin interaction is brief (10 minutes). Copper that is delivered to the liver may reenter circulation, however, this time, in association with the α-macroglobulin ceruloplasmin. This compound transports copper to other tissues and assists with the transport of iron aboard transferrin because it functions as a **ferroxidase**, converting iron to the appropriate oxidation state (ferric) for transport aboard transferrin.

Ceruloplasmin, which can carry up to six atoms of copper, has a molecular weight of approximately 160,000 and contains as much as 60 to 90% of the copper found in plasma. The remainder of copper in the systemic circulation is loosely bound to plasma albumin. A normal level of plasma copper is 0.9 microgram per milliliter; the ceruloplasmin level varies between 15 and 60 milligrams per 100 milliliters.

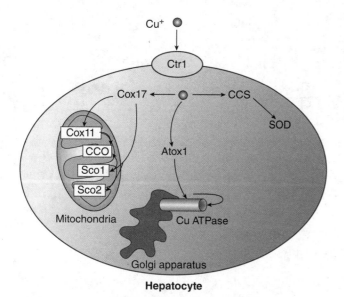

FIGURE 13.12 Liver Cell Demonstrating Copper Absorption via the Copper Transporter Ctr1. Note that there are several chaperone proteins that will bind and transport copper to other proteins once inside the cell. CCS, chaperone protein for Cu/Zn-superoxide dismutase (SOD); Atox1, chaperone protein for copper ATPase; Cox17, chaperone protein for mitochondria; Cox11, Sco1, and Sco2, chaperone proteins to bring copper to cytochrome c oxidase (CCO).

An adult body may contain 50 to 120 milligrams of copper, with the tissue having the highest concentration in the liver. The heart, brain, kidneys, and spleen are also concentrated with copper relative to other tissue. Interestingly, on a body weight basis, infants and younger children have a higher copper content than adults. For adults, bile represents the primary route of excretion. Approximately 2 milligrams of copper is excreted via bile daily. Copper is also excreted from the human body in the urine (10 to 50 micrograms per day) and through the loss of hair and skin.

Excess copper binds to liver metallothionein, thereby decreasing the potential for copper toxicity. It seems that copper, iron, and zinc are all involved in regulating the synthesis of metallothionein. Each of these minerals has specific metal-responsive elements that influence metallothionein expression.

Most of the functions of copper are mediated through its role as a component of key enzymes. Copper-containing **amine oxidases** are present in the plasma and catabolize some physiologically active amines, such as tyramine, histidine, and polyamines. Monoamine oxidases break down catecholamines (norepinephrine, tyramine, dopamine, and serotonin). Diamine oxidase inactivates histamine, particularly in the small intestine, where activity of the enzyme is high, as well as in the kidney. **Lysyl oxidase** is a cuproenzyme that facilitates bonding of lysine and

hydroxylysine or hydroxyproline side chains of collagen and elastin. In particular, lysine is deaminated by lysyl oxidase so that cross-links may be synthesized. The strength of connective tissue depends on the activity of lysyl oxidase and, therefore, on copper.

Copper is used by most cells as a component of the enzyme **cytochrome c oxidase**, which is at the terminal end of the mitochondrial electron transport chain. This enzyme is involved with the reduction of oxygen to form water and is the rate-limiting enzyme in electron transport. Its activity is dependent on tissue copper content. Levels of cytochrome c oxidase are very high in tissue such as the heart, where the oxidation of fatty acids and pyruvate is greater than in other tissue. **Dopamine hydroxylase** is another significant enzyme in that it catalyzes the conversion of dopamine to norepinephrine.

Cytosolic **superoxide dismutase**, which not only contains copper but zinc as well (Cu/Zn-SOD), is a powerful antioxidant that squelches superoxide radicals, as depicted in the following reaction:

$$2\ O_2^- + 2\ H^+ \xrightarrow{Cu/Zn\text{-}SOD} H_2O_2 + O_2$$

Superoxide radicals can be destructive to cellular structures by causing peroxidative damage, primarily to phospholipid components of membranes. The hydrogen peroxide formed by Cu/Zn-SOD can then be metabolized by peroxidases such as glutathione peroxidase, a selenium-containing enzyme. Higher levels of cytosolic superoxide dismutase are present in the brain, thyroid, liver, pituitary, erythrocytes, and kidneys. Cu/Zn-SOD has two atoms of copper per molecule. There is also an extracellular superoxide dismutase that is found in higher concentrations in the lungs, thyroid, and uterus and in small amounts in blood plasma. This antioxidant does not contain copper.

Tyrosine metabolism involves copper in three reactions. First, **tyrosine** can be metabolized further, serving as a precursor for dopamine or melanin synthetic processes. Dopamine can then be converted to norepinephrine, which is catalyzed by dopamine hydroxylase, a cuproenzyme. Dopamine hydroxylase requires at least eight atoms of copper and requires the redux potential of vitamin C. Metabolism of l-DOPA to melanin occurs in pigment cells called melanocytes. The color of skin, hair, and eyes is dependent on the enzyme. In copper deficiency, tyrosinase activity is low and leads to decreased pigmentation. This is especially obvious in animals, because dark fur can begin to lighten or turn gray. Finally, a copper-containing hydroxylase enzyme is involved in tyrosine catabolism.

Copper is also a part of other proteins, such as **transcuprin**, a plasma protein that may involve copper transport. Blood clotting factor V, although nonenzymatic, contains copper. Interestingly, however, copper deficiency is not known to impair blood clotting. Copper is also required for proper myelination of the central nervous system. Phospholipid synthesis depends on cytochrome c oxidase, which may be a reason why copper deficiency leads to decreased myelination, necrosis of nerve tissue, and neonatal ataxia in copper-deficient animals.

Copper Transport Proteins and Cell Distribution

Copper transport in hepatocytes and neurons is similar to absorption by the small intestine. Copper is transported into cells by the transport protein, Ctr1. Next, copper is transferred to one of 3 proteins: 1) CCS, 2) Atox1, and Cox17. CCS will ferry copper to the antioxidant enzyme, superoxide dismutase (SOD). Atox1 will ferry copper to ATPB in the golgi bodies. This will 1) facilitate the excretion of excess copper; or 2) allow copper to be available to be inserted to holoceruloplasmin to produce active ceruloplasmin. Cox17 will ferry copper to the mitochondria, where copper is delivered to Cox11 and/or Sco1 and 2 within the mitochondria. At this point, copper from Cox11 is transferred to cytochrome c oxidase. Sco1 and 2 are involved in this transfer. Thus, Cox17, Cox11, Sco1, and Sco2 are all essential for the delivery of copper to cytochrome c oxidase. Excess copper in a cell may be stored by binding to metallothionein, as it is important to bind ionic copper to a protein to prevent its pro-oxidant effects within cells.

Recommended Levels of Intake for Copper

The results of nutrition surveys suggest that most Americans consume 1 milligram or fewer of copper per day, a less than adequate amount. Some researchers speculate that over a lifetime, a marginal dietary intake of copper may be a contributing factor in the development of heart disease (**SPECIAL FEATURE 13.2**). The RDA for copper is 900 micrograms per day for adult men and women. The AI increases to 1,000 micrograms per day in pregnancy and to 1,300 micrograms per day during lactation. The UL of copper is 10 milligrams per day.

Copper Deficiency

Copper deficiency has been observed in premature infants and in infants suffering from malnutrition. Infants who are afflicted with short gut syndrome and are on enteral nutrition have demonstrated symptoms of copper deficiency. Many such infants present with the bone disease, *osteogenesis imperfecta* or brittle bones, which are subject to fracture. Individuals with celiac sprue may also demonstrate deficiency.

A more recent concern has been the observation of a decrease in copper status of patients who have had bariatric surgery. While copper may be absorbed by the stomach and, therefore, have less absorptive area, it is likely that bypassing a portion of the proximal small intestine is responsible for decrease in most of the copper absorption. Overt symptoms of copper deficiency may not present themselves, with the exception of low serum copper; however, long-term effects are unknown.

Overt symptoms in adults are rare but may occur with long-term patients or those who consume zinc supplements for a period of time. Animals that are fed diets deficient in copper often exhibit cardiac abnormalities such as cardiac hypertrophy, blood vessel and heart rupture, and abnormal electrocardiograms and have elevated levels of serum cholesterol, triglycerides, and glucose.

Genetic Anomalies Influencing Copper Status

Two well-known genetic diseases affect copper metabolism. Menkes disease (also known as kinky-hair disease), which was first characterized and reported in the early 1960s, is an X-linked chromosomal disorder that manifests abnormalities in copper absorption. This results in a copper deficiency-like syndrome despite what may be adequate dietary copper consumption. The mutation occurs in the enzyme ATP7A, discussed earlier, which is involved in copper export from the enterocyte. In contrast, Wilson disease, first described in the early part of the 1900s, is characterized by increased liver copper content, leading to severe hepatic damage, followed by increased brain copper levels and neurologic aberrations. Thus, Wilson disease results in a copper toxicity syndrome. Copper is unable to be exported from the Golgi bodies of the liver, the liver storage site for copper, because the copper transport enzyme ATP7B is defective.

In Menkes syndrome, individuals experience depigmentation of the skin, kinky hair, central nervous system damage, and muscle and connective tissue abnormalities. Interestingly, anemia is not common, nor is neutropenia. The problem lies in the transport of copper from intestinal mucosal enterocytes. Although parenteral copper administration is able to correct plasma levels, there remains a deficit in neurologic tissue. Infants with Menkes syndrome experience cerebral degeneration and generally do not survive beyond infancy.

Wilson disease is an autosomal recessive disorder that is associated with excessive copper accumulation. Individuals with Wilson disease typically experience premature death. The major flaw in this disorder is a decreased ability to incorporate copper into ceruloplasmin as well as a decreased ability to excrete copper in the bile. This appears to be a manifestation of a defective gene for P-type ATPase cation transporters and results in excess copper accumulation in the liver and brain tissue. The defect occurs on chromosome 13 for humans. Preliminary signs of Wilson disease include liver dysfunction, neurologic disorders, and copper deposits in the cornea of the eye that result in a halo-like appearance around the pupil that is referred to as a Kayser-Fleischer ring. Kidney stones and acidic urine can also occur. Wilson disease is managed with copper chelators such as D-penicillamine as well as zinc supplements, which decrease copper absorption by promoting the synthesis of metallothionein in enterocytes.

● BEFORE YOU GO ON . . .

1. List some good food sources of copper.
2. Explain the role of the following copper-containing enzymes: (a) ceruloplasmin, (b) amine oxidases, (c) lysyl oxidase, (d) super-oxide dismutase, (e) dopamine hydroxylase, (f) tyrosine hydroxylase, and (g) transcuprin.
3. Discuss the differences between Menkes disease and Wilson disease.
4. What are the key transporters in copper absorption?
5. What are the major chaperone proteins in hepatocytes and their function?

SPECIAL FEATURE 13.2

Can a Lack of Dietary Copper Lead to Heart Disease?

For a number of years, nutritionists have expressed concern that Americans may not be obtaining sufficient levels of copper in their diets. Only recently has there been sufficient evidence to make a recommendation for adequate copper intake. The AI for copper is 900 micrograms per day for adults. Prior to the issuing of this AI, copper did not have a specific recommended intake; rather, a range of 1,500 to 2,000 micrograms per day was recommended. Using the latter values as a basis, survey studies suggested that many Americans were not coming close to this level. With the new DRI, many more meet the requirement, but there are concerns that a significant segment of the public consumes less than 900 micrograms of copper per day.

It is difficult to determine whether people are getting enough copper per day. First, food composition tables have only recently become more complete for copper. Second, water is a good source of copper but is not often considered in intake studies. Third, a sensitive biochemical test is not available to determine whether an individual is mildly deficient in copper. Ceruloplasmin, while a marker for copper status in deficiency states, may not be as sensitive in detecting marginal copper status.

Animals fed a copper-deficient diet rapidly develop heart disease that is characterized by enlargement. The animals have abnormal electrocardiograms (a measure of electrical heart activity) and have elevated levels of blood cholesterol, triglycerides, and glucose. The deficiency sets in rapidly (within 4 to 5 weeks), and almost all of the experimental animals die from heart-related deaths. A unique feature is the increased number of mitochondria in the heart, resulting from copper deficiency. The increase may be an attempt to maintain normal levels of ATP. The copper-containing enzymes, cytochrome c oxidase, on which ATP formation is dependent, is dramatically decreased. The molecular set of signals to initiate mitochondria to multiply are increased accordingly.

Might this also be the case in humans? To date, no convincing studies have linked copper deficiency to heart disease in humans. There is some evidence that those individuals with a genetic inability to handle copper do have heart disease, but these individuals are rare. This does not mean that people with some copper in the diet, but below the AI, will eventually have heart problems. Although researchers have been able to show cause and effect with animals in the laboratory, a definite real-world link has not been made with regard to copper deficiency and heart disease in humans. Does this mean that copper may not have a role in heart disease? Some studies report that the addition of extra copper in the diet that are above adequate may block the development of cardiac hypertrophy. This has only been demonstrated in mice and not humans.

While this section focused on copper deficiency and heart disease, there is evidence that elevated copper may lead to heart disease. Copper is a pro-oxidant and can oxidize LDL-cholesterol, making it more atherogenic. However, such studies have been *in vitro* and studies in humans and animal models are lacking, with respect to elevated copper and atherosclerosis.

▸ Selenium

Selenium has achieved worldwide attention as the nutrient whose deficiency is responsible for Keshan disease. Lately, interest in selenium and disease prevention has focused on its possible role in the chemoprevention of cancers (**SPECIAL FEATURE 13.3**). Selenium primarily functions as part of the antioxidant complex glutathione peroxidase, although other functions are being revealed.

Dietary Selenium

Like other minor minerals, the amount of selenium in a food is highly dependent on the level found in the soil where crops were grown and animals grazed and drank. Therefore, deficiency or toxicity could be a concern if regional inhabitants subsist solely on crops and livestock from a deficient or superabundant area. However, in countries such as the United States, the varying level of selenium in the soil is not that great a concern because the inhabitants of most regions consume foods grown throughout the country as well as internationally. Good dietary sources of selenium are seafood, including tuna; meat; and cereals, especially wheat-based cereals (**TABLE 13.8**). In areas where the soil is high in selenium, cow's milk may be a more concentrated source.

Absorption of Selenium

Selenium is efficiently absorbed in the gastrointestinal tract in several forms (**FIGURE 13.13**). However, the absorption of two distinct selenium forms (seleno-methionine and selenite) has been studied the most in humans, using stable isotopes. Selenomethionine is a selenium analogue of a sulfur-containing amino acid. Selenium and sulfur are exchanged in methionine because of their chemical similarities. The major site of absorption is the duodenum, although some selenium is absorbed in the ileum and jejunum. Selenium absorption does not occur in the stomach. There is no known regulatory mechanism for selenium absorption. An absorption range of from 50 to 100% has been demonstrated for these two forms.

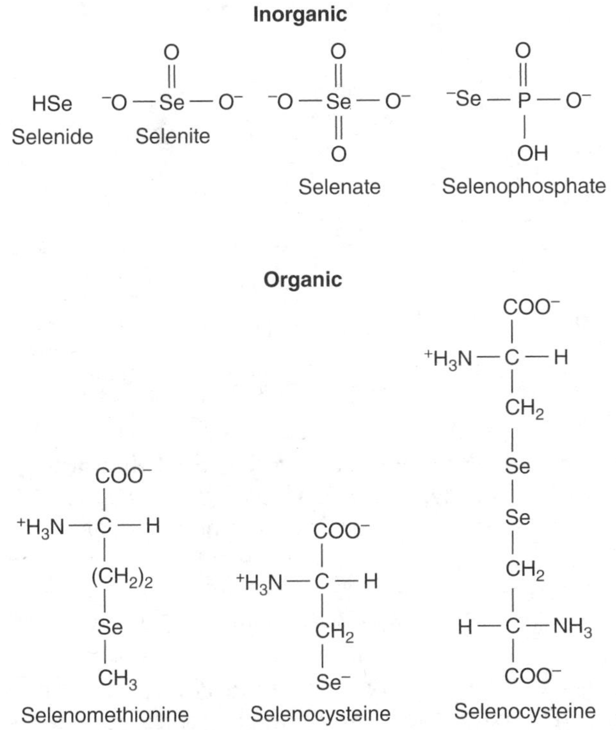

Metabolism and Function of Selenium

When selenium is absorbed as selenomethionine, it is incorporated into a plasma protein called **selenoprotein P**. It may also be synthesized in the liver and released into the plasma. This protein

TABLE 13.8 Selenium Content of Select Foods

Food	Selenium (μg)
Snapper, baked (3 oz)	42
Halibut, baked (3 oz)	47
Salmon, baked (3 oz)	32
Scallops, steamed (3 oz)	18
Clams, steamed (20 small)	121
Oysters, raw (3 oz)	54
Molasses, blackstrap (2 tbsp)	7
Sunflower seeds (1 cup)	102
Ground beef (3 oz)	18
Chicken, baked (3 oz)	20
Bread, whole wheat (1 slice)	11
Egg (1)	16
Milk, 2% (1 cup)	6

FIGURE 13.13 Different Selenium Forms. Dietary selenium may be present in either inorganic or organic forms. 50 to 100% of selenium may be absorbed. There is no known regulatory mechanism for selenium absorption.

transports and stores selenium and is thought to function as an antioxidant. It appears to be involved in selenium homeostasis in both brain and testes.

As selenite, selenium becomes incorporated into the metalloenzyme glutathione peroxidase. About 50 to 60% of selenium excreted is lost through urine and 40 to 50% through feces. Body stores of selenium greatly influence renal clearance of this mineral. Therefore, the kidneys appear to be the principal regulatory mechanism for selenium homeostasis. Endogenous selenium is also lost through the feces. This was demonstrated by showing that fecal selenium excretion remains the same regardless of dietary intake. At toxic intakes of dietary selenium, volatile selenium compounds such as dimethylselenide are exhaled and can escape through the skin.

Selenium exerts some of its physiologic effects as a coenzyme for **glutathione peroxidase**, which is often abbreviated as GPX. Glutathione peroxidase functions to reduce organic and hydrogen peroxides (**FIGURE 13.14a**). This is especially important for phagocytic cells, such as leukocytes and macrophages. In these cells, peroxides are the by-products of the oxidative destruction of foreign matter; therefore, glutathione peroxidase protects these cells from autodestruction.

Another site of glutathione peroxidase activity is platelets. Here, GPX acts in an antiaggregative capacity. This metalloenzyme reduces fatty acid peroxide

formation and increases the ratio of prostacyclin (an antiaggregating factor) to thromboxane (a pro-aggregant). Through this mechanism, selenium is prophylactically linked to cardiovascular disease by decreasing platelet aggregation, which reduces the incidence of clots and atherosclerosis.

In general, glutathione peroxidase stabilizes cell membranes, because they are composed of unsaturated fatty acids that may be susceptible to oxidation. Free radical production has been implicated in the aging process and as an initiating event in tumor development. Adequate levels of selenium ensure that sufficient glutathione peroxidase is available and protect against tumor development and the aging process. Glutathione peroxidase is important for the stability of red blood cells because oxygen is certainly abundant. The lack of mitochondria in red blood cells further depletes these cells of antioxidants, making glutathione peroxidase much more important. There are several isoforms of glutathione peroxidase, which are indicated by the numerals 1 through 4. The tissue distribution of these isoforms varies. For instance, whereas GPX1 and GPX4 are expressed in most tissue, red blood cells contain more GPX1, liver more GPX2 and GPX3, kidneys more GPX1 and GPX3, and the testes more GPX4.

A group of enzymes that is not often discussed in nutrition texts is thioredoxin reductases. **Thioredoxin reductases** have selenocysteine in their composition. There are three isoenzymes: cytoplasmic TrxR1, mitochondrial TrxR3, and one that is found in the testes, TGR. These enzymes contain FAD and NADPH binding sites. TrxRs are catalysts for the reduction of substrates for the regeneration of antioxidants (Figure 13.14b). Thioredoxin (Th) proteins are involved in oxidation-reduction reactions. They work in concert with thioredoxin reductases, where the aim is to reduce the thioredoxin protein, thereby allowing reduced thioredoxin to reduce other substrates. Vitamins C and E, for instance, can be regenerated by reduced thioredoxin to their reduced form to take part in further reduction-oxidation reactions. Figure 13.14b shows an example of ascorbate converted to dehydroascorbate by Th protein and TrxR enzymes.

The enzyme **iodothyronine deiodinase** contains selenium. This enzyme converts thyroxine (T_4) to tri-iodothyronine (T_3), a deiodination reaction. T_3 is an active thyroid hormone. There are other, non-selenium-containing, deiodinases that may catalyze this reaction. Type 1 deiodinase contains selenium; in selenium deficiency, the synthesis of this deiodinase is markedly diminished, resulting in the production

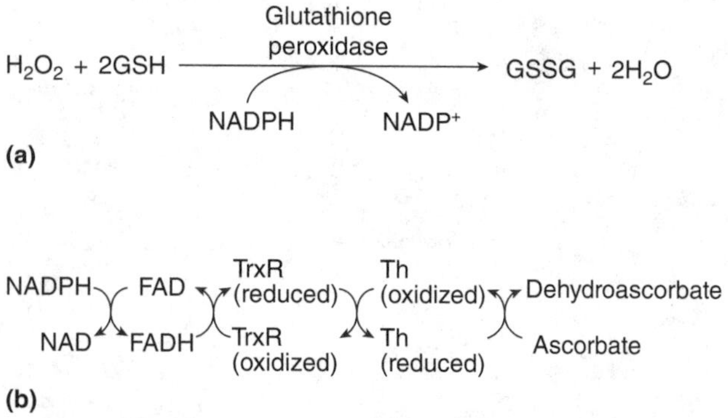

$$H_2O_2 + 2GSH \xrightarrow[\text{NADPH} \quad \text{NADP}^+]{\text{Glutathione peroxidase}} GSSG + 2H_2O$$

(a)

NADPH ⤸ FAD ⤸ TrxR (reduced) ⤸ Th (oxidized) ⤸ Dehydroascorbate

NAD ⤹ FADH ⤹ TrxR (oxidized) ⤹ Th (reduced) ⤹ Ascorbate

(b)

FIGURE 13.14 Reaction Catalyzed by the Selenium-containing Enzymes. (a) Reaction catalyzed by the selenium-containing enzyme glutathione peroxidase. (b) Reaction catalyzed by selenium-containing thioredoxin reductase enzymes and the protein, thioredoxin. G, glutathione; GSH, reduced glutathione; GSSG, oxidized glutathione; NADP⁺, oxidized form of nicotinamide adenine dinucleotide phosphate; NADPH, reduced form of NADP; TrxR, thioredoxin enzymes; Th, Thioredoxin protein; FAD, Flavin Adenine Dinucleotide; FADH, reduced form of FAD.

of less T_3 and an accumulation of T_4. The other deiodinases do not respond as an adaptation to selenium deficiency.

Selenoprotein W is a selenium-containing protein found in muscle. Its weight is slightly less than 10 kilodaltons, and each molecule contains one atom of selenium. This protein was found to be critical in the prevention of white muscle disease in cattle and sheep. White muscle disease is a condition in which the muscle is weakened due to a dietary selenium deficiency in these animals. The expression of the gene for selenoprotein W decreases dramatically in selenium deficiency compared with adequate diet levels. The role of this protein in muscle health remains unknown.

Selenium Incorporation into Proteins

Selenium-containing proteins are different from other metalloproteins in that in many cases, metals are added after translation. Another mechanism that occurs when producing selenium-containing proteins is a process known as **cotranslation**, in which an amino acid that already contains selenium is incorporated into a polypeptide chain (**FIGURE 13.15**). For this process to occur, a unique set of components that function at the molecular level are required:

- Selenophosphate synthetase
- Selenocysteine insertion sequence binding protein 2 (SBP2)
- Eukaryotic selenocysteinyl-tRNA-specific elongation factor (eEFsec)
- Selenocysteine synthase
- Selenocysteine-specific tRNA
- Two unique mRNA elements

The two unique mRNA elements are (1) the codon UGA, which is normally a stop codon, and (2) the selenocysteine insertion sequence. Selenium is incorporated into selenoproteins as selenocysteine. UGA codes for selenocysteine. For this reason, selenocysteine is sometimes called the 21st amino acid.

Another required component is selenocysteine transfer RNA. This transfer RNA is larger than tRNAs for other amino acids and has the amino acid serine bound to it. For cotranslation to occur, selenium is required in the form of selenophosphate, which requires the enzyme selenophosphate synthetase in the following reaction:

$$HSe^- + ATP \rightarrow SeP_3H + AMP + Pi$$

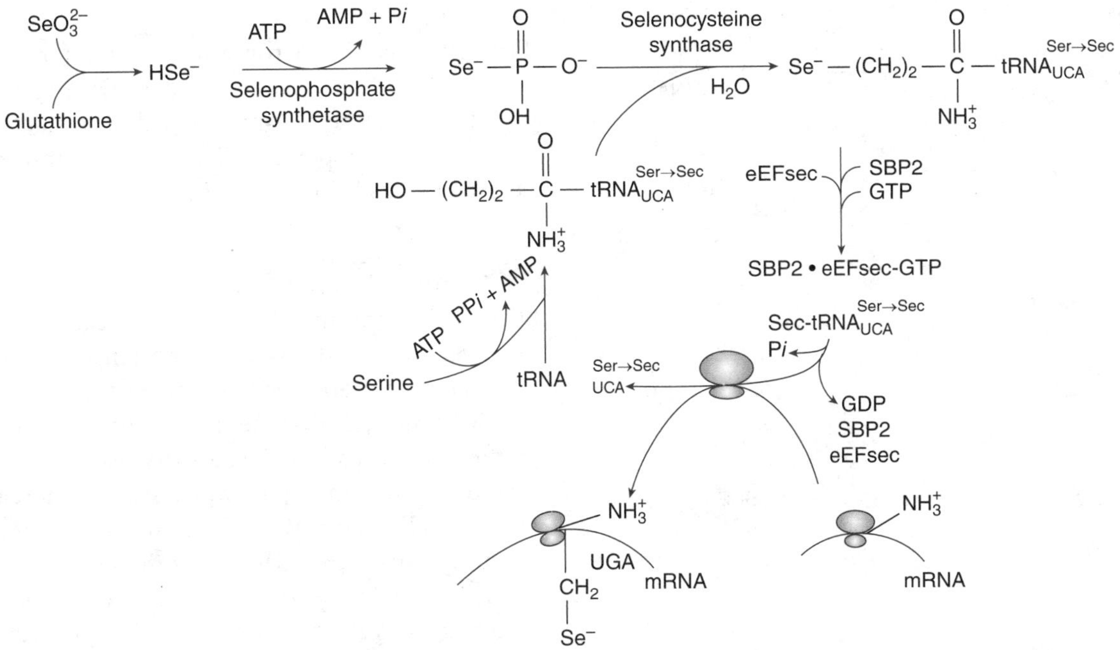

FIGURE 13.15 Cotranslation Cycle for the Incorporation of Selenocysteine into a Polypeptide Chain. Selenium is present in proteins through a process known as cotranslation, meaning it is added to a polypeptide during synthesis. Other metals are added to proteins after synthesis. Selenium is incorporated into selenoproteins as selenocysteine. The codon UGA is normally a stop codon, but not in this case. The presence of selenocysteine insertion sequence binding protein 2 (SBP2) and eukaryotic selenocysteinyl-tRNA elongation factor (eEFsec) will form a SBP2-eEFsec-GTP complex. This complex binds to a tRNA specific for selenium, which recognizes the UGA not as a stop codon but as a codon for selenocysteine, thereby incorporating selenium into the polypeptide.

The selenophosphate next reacts with the tRNA that has serine bound to it in the presence of the enzyme selenocysteine synthase. This converts the serine on the tRNA to selenocysteine. Incorporation of the selenocysteine into the polypeptide chain requires not only the UGA codon but also a structure called the selenocysteine insertion sequence (SECIS) at the 3' end of the mRNA. The cell machinery recognizes the UGA not as a stop codon but as the codon for selenocysteine when the SECIS is present. Next, the eukaryotic selenocysteinyl tRNA–specific elongation factor binds to the ribosome. As this occurs, the selenocysteine insertion sequence-binding protein 2 binds to the SECIS for selenocysteine insertion into the peptide chain (**FIGURE 13.16**).

Relationships Among Selenium and Other Nutrients

Copper deficiency can possibly decrease glutathione peroxidase activity. Although it is still unclear why this occurs, it is probable that the gene for glutathione peroxidase is not expressed to the same extent during copper deficiency.

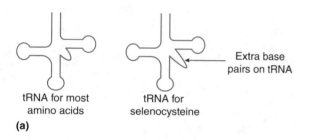

(a)

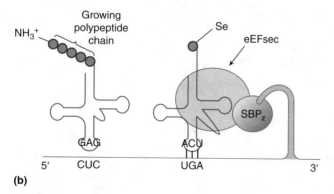

(b)

FIGURE13.16 Cotranslation. (a) Transfer RNA (tRNA) for typical amino acids and for selenocysteine. Notice that the arm for the selenocysteine tRNA is larger because it has more nucleotide base pairs than other tRNAs. (b) Details of how the stem-loop structure, eEFsec, and SBP2 interact with the tRNA for selenocysteine in the addition of that amino acid to a growing polypeptide chain.

Vitamin E has been shown in animals to spare selenium and reduce the amount necessary in the diet. Other factors with such a role have also been identified; these include decreased food intake, high protein intake, high levels of vitamin A and vitamin C, and synthetic antioxidants. In contrast, substances and situations that are known to antagonize dietary selenium, thereby increasing its need, include heavy metals, sulfate, mercaptans, and chlorinated hydrocarbons. Deficiencies of vitamin E, riboflavin, vitamin B_6, and methionine can also increase the need for selenium.

Some substances are known to reduce the potential for selenium toxicity. These substances may act as methyl donors, which synthesize selenium metabolites that are simply excreted. The methyl donors include methionine, betaine, choline, creatinine, and amidinoglycine. Also, the heavy metals mercury, cadmium, lead, silver, and arsenic and the trace elements copper, zinc, and iron substitute for selenium and reduce its toxic potential. Furthermore, antioxidants, such as vitamin E, DPPD, and BHT help the antioxidant function of glutathione peroxidase and thereby reduce the toxic effects of selenium.

Recommended Levels of Intake for Selenium

The RDA is 55 micrograms per day for adults. The UL is 400 micrograms per day. During pregnancy, the RDA is 60 micrograms per day; for lactation, it is 70 micrograms per day. The RDA for those younger than 13 years is lower.

Selenium Deficiency

Cases of selenium deficiency in humans mostly occur in premature infants or in patients receiving protracted total parenteral nutrition for extended periods of time. The disease that results from a selenium deficiency is called Keshan disease. The symptoms include cardiomyopathy, cataracts, increased red blood cell fragility, skeletal muscle degeneration, and impaired growth are some of the symptoms of this deficiency. Residents of areas of China that have selenium-poor soil have a high incidence of Keshan disease. Children are most affected by this condition. Selenium deficiency alone may not be the major factor as coxsackievirus B4 interacts with a selenium deficiency.

Selenium deficiency affects skeletal cartilage, which may lead to Kashin-Beck disease, especially in children. This disease is common in China in areas with low selenium levels. Joints are deformed and may lead to dwarfism. There is evidence that this disease may not be due to selenium deficiency per se, but is, in fact, a mycotoxin. Research indicates that mycotoxins can produce Kashin-Beck disease. In the presence of elevated selenium, the impact of the mycotoxin appears to be attenuated.

Selenium Toxicity

There are three forms of selenium toxicity: acute selenosis, subacute selenosis, and chronic selenosis. Acute selenosis occurs when excess amounts of selenium are ingested over a short period of time. Symptoms of acute selenosis include an unsteady gait, cyanosis of the mucous membranes, and difficulty breathing, which can lead to death. Autopsy reports of acute selenosis describe liver congestion, endocarditis, myocarditis, and smooth muscle degeneration in the gastrointestinal tract, gallbladder, and bladder. Long-bone erosion was also reported in these cases.

When large doses of selenium are ingested over a long time period, subacute selenosis is observed. Symptoms of subacute selenosis include neurologic dysfunction, such as vision impairment, ataxia, and disorientation; respiratory distress is often seen as well. Subacute selenosis is commonly seen in livestock that graze on selenium-accumulating plants. These seleniferous plants are concentrated in western states, such as Montana, Colorado, Wyoming, New Mexico, and Arizona.

Chronic selenosis occurs when moderate doses of selenium are ingested over a considerable length of time. This condition is characterized by skin lesions and dermatitis, such as alopecia and hoof necrosis (in livestock), emaciation, chronic fatigue, anorexia, gastroenteritis, liver dysfunction, and spleen enlargement.

The most toxic forms of selenium are sodium selenite, sodium selenate, selenomethionine, and selenodiglutathione. However, there are wide variations in selenium toxicity with respect to the valence state of the molecule. Recently, a multitude of selenium compounds have been synthesized as chemopreventive, anticarcinogenic substances. These are being tested for their toxic effects.

There is an area of China that has unusually high concentrations of selenium in the soil. Because this selenium becomes incorporated into the food supply, the residents were evaluated for clinical and biochemical indications of selenium intoxication. The average daily selenium intake was estimated to be 1.4 milligrams for adult men and 1.2 milligrams for adult women. Increased clotting time and reduced serum glutathione were observed in this group compared with those whose selenium intakes were 0.07 milligram (men) and 0.06 milligram (women). Clinical signs that were observed consisted of garlic odor in the breath and urine, brittle or lost nails, lowered hemoglobin levels, and nervous system problems, such as peripheral anesthesia, acroparesthesia, and pain in the extremities.

In livestock, symptoms of selenium toxicity are seen in the nervous system as ataxia, tremors, hypersensitivity, and convulsions. In humans, nervousness, chills, numbness, impaired nerve conduction, and peripheral anesthesia are seen. Mottled teeth have been seen in humans with selenium toxicity. In animals intoxicated with selenium, the liver has been demonstrated to show steatosis and necrosis. However, this has not been reported in humans.

Kidney problems such as congestion, necrotizing nephrosis, and calcinosis have only been reported in animals. The heart appears to be affected by selenium toxicity, as manifested by myocarditis in rats and bradycardia in humans. Only livestock have shown respiratory disturbances, such as congestion, edema, respiratory distress, and hydrothorax. The skin is affected by selenium toxicity. This is seen as thick, streaked, brittle nails; dry, brittle hair; hair loss; and red, swollen hands and feet. In animals, cracked hooves are noticed, as well as dermatosis and alopecia. Anemia, increased prothrombin time, and decreased hemoglobin are hematologic manifestations seen in both humans and animals. Decreased immune function has been demonstrated in rats with selenium toxicity. In both animals and humans with selenium toxicity, loose stools, diarrhea, excessive salivation, and dyspepsia have been observed. Deformities of fetal chicks and ducks are seen in selenium toxicity.

● BEFORE YOU GO ON . . .

1. List the forms of selenium that may be found in the diet.
2. What is the role of glutathione peroxidase, Selenoproteins P and W?
3. How can selenium status affect iodine metabolism?
4. Explain Keshan disease.
5. What is Kashin-Beck disease?

Selenium and Cancer Prevention

Research has revealed an inverse association between selenium and several cancers, including prostate, bladder, lung, colorectal, esophageal, and gastric cancers. The most consistent protective effect of selenium is against prostate cancer. In a double-blind study, 974 men with a history of early cancer received either 200 micrograms per day of selenium or a placebo. They were followed for a mean of 4.5 years. The selenium-treated group had 13 prostate cancer cases, compared with 35 cases in the control group, which represented a 63% reduction in prostate cancer. Another study measured plasma selenium levels in 586 men diagnosed with prostate cancer during a 13-year period and compared them with 577 control subjects. Men with increased selenium levels at the beginning of the study had significantly lower prostate cancer risk. Among those with cancer, those with a high level of selenium had a lower rate of progression in their prostate cancer.

Two studies have suggested an inverse association between selenium and bladder cancer. One study revealed an inverse relationship between blood selenium levels and bladder cancer in more than 25,000 people. A second study revealed an inverse association between toenail selenium levels and bladder cancer in a group of 120,852 men and women aged 55 to 69. A meta-analysis from 16 studies reported an inverse association of breast cancer with serum selenium levels. Genetic variations in GPX1 that lowers activity has been reported to increase risk of both stomach and colon cancer, suggesting that genetic mutations of selenoproteins need to be considered.

Data regarding an association between lung cancer and selenium are weak. Survey studies suggest that if a population lives in a low-selenium area, extra selenium in the diet may protect against lung cancer.

Toenail selenium levels were inversely related to the risk of colon cancer. One study of 758 people with colon cancer suggested that they had lower blood selenium levels compared with a group of 767 control subjects that had similar numbers of females and males and a similar racial mix. A 26% reduction in risk for colon cancer was reported for those with higher selenium levels in their blood. Those older than 57 years had an even higher reduction in risk (57%).

A study in China on esophageal and stomach cancer was conducted using selenium, β-carotene, and vitamin E. Those who received the supplements had significantly lower mortality rates from esophageal and stomach cancers than those who did not receive any supplements.

In summary, strong data from human studies appear to support the hypothesis that selenium can decrease cancer risk. However, it may be premature to suggest that individuals should routinely supplement with selenium. It may be that no single nutrient reduces the risk of cancer but rather that a combination of factors, including several nutrients, may act in concert with each other to prevent cancer. The studies do suggest, however, that having an adequate dietary intake of selenium (i.e., at the AI level) would be prudent in reducing a person's risk of cancer.

▶ Fluoride

In nature, the element fluorine exists primarily as a negatively charged ion. Thus, similar to iodide (iodine) and chloride (chlorine), fluorine is commonly referred to as *fluoride*. Fluoride was first recognized as a toxic element in animals in the 1920s when phosphate salts from rocks were used as a source of calcium and phosphorus for farm animals. Some of the rocks contained 1 to 2% fluoride. Animals consuming this feed showed depressed growth and increased mortality from fluoride toxicity. In contrast, in the late 1930s, it was observed that there was a decreased incidence of dental caries in humans in areas where water supplies had large levels of fluoride. Recognition of the link between fluoride and dentition soon followed (**SPECIAL FEATURE 13.4**).

Dietary Sources of Fluoride

Most foods are poor sources of fluoride and probably should not be used exclusively to meet human needs. However, the process of adding fluoride to drinking water (**fluoridation**) has greatly improved human fluoride consumption. Fluoridation, a practice that began in the 1940s in the United States, typically uses sodium fluoride and sodium fluorosilicate at about 1 to 2 parts per million. About 1 milligram of fluoride per day is consumed by Americans through fluoridated drinking water. Thus, fluoridated water and foods prepared with fluoridated water are among the best dietary sources. Infant formulas and foods are made with fluoridated water, thereby improving an infant's intake. Fluoride-containing toothpastes, which typically use sodium fluoride, also account for some fluoride ingestion.

Absorption of Fluoride

In general, fluoride is very well absorbed from most dietary sources. Soluble fluoride sources, such as the aqueous-dissolved sources in fluoridated water, are almost completely absorbed. Fluorides bound to proteins demonstrate moderate absorption. Unlike other minerals, fluoride is absorbed to a great extent in the stomach. Thus, ingested fluoride is represented within the blood within minutes of consumption and achieves maximal levels within a half hour or so. Fluoride is also absorbed along the length of the small intestine. Regardless of the site of absorption, fluoride is probably absorbed by passive diffusion. Like sodium, potassium, and chloride absorption, fluoride absorption does not appear to be hindered relative to physiologic status, nor is it hindered competitively by its fellow halogen anion, chloride.

Metabolism and Function of Fluoride

Blood fluoride levels are rather low, in the part per billion concentration range. Fluoride is stored in calcified tissues (bones and teeth); the levels are proportional to the dietary intake. Excretion is primarily by way of the urine, with small amounts appearing in the feces. Fluoride balance is usually positive in humans, with a slow increase seen with aging. However, fluoride is not efficiently transferred across the placenta. Therefore, a newborn infant has relatively lower levels of fluoride. If the level of fluoride in bones and teeth exceeds 3,000 micrograms per gram tissue, fluoride begins to accumulate in the soft tissues. Fluoride accumulation occurs at the time teeth are being developed.

Fluoride is important for bone and dental health. A lack of dietary fluoride alone is not the sole cause of tooth decay. Sugar and a sticky carbohydrate will adhere to teeth. This provides a medium in which bacteria may grow to form plaque. *Streptococci mutans* is the primary bacteria that will adhere. The bacteria will produce an acid that wears at the protective enamel. The bacteria can enter the tooth and lead to tooth decay. Fluoride can protect the enamel from being worn away. This is the reason that fluoride is incorporated into hydroxyapatite crystal at places that contain hydroxyl (OH^-) chemical groups. This can occur either at the point of initial crystallization or by displacement in mature hydroxyapatite crystals according to the following equation:

$$Ca_{10}(PO_4)_6(OH)_2 + xF^- \rightarrow Ca_{10}(PO_4)_6(OH)_{2-x}F_x^-$$

Such a substitution causes the crystal to become harder and more stable. Therefore, the general effect of fluoride is a hardening of dental aspects, such as enamel. This is the primary mechanism by which fluoride helps to prevent tooth decay.

SPECIAL FEATURE 13.4

Fluoride and Tooth Decay

The association between tooth decay and fluoride was first noticed in the early 1900s. In 1942, a definite link between fluoride and decreased levels of tooth decay was established. Government studies were initiated in 1945 to determine whether fluoride in the water supply could decrease tooth decay. The goal was to add enough fluoride to water to achieve an average concentration of one part per million. The study was conducted in Newburgh and Kingston, New York. These two cities are similar in demographics but are separated by the Hudson River. Fluoride was added to the Newburgh water supply; Kingston served as the nonfluoridated control. The incidence of tooth decay among children was followed for 10 years. Newburgh had a dramatic decrease in tooth decay. The younger the child, the greater the drop in tooth decay, missing teeth, and fillings; there was a 48 to 65% reduction, depending on the age of the child.

Although adding fluoride to public water appeared to be a good thing to do in order to decrease tooth decay, initially, there was much opposition. Very conservative political groups opposed the measures. Many thought that there could be hazards to the program, that it was ineffective, and that medicine was being forced on the public. The issue of individual rights vs the good of the group was central to this debate.

A fluoride level of one part per million in drinking water is safe; toxic effects can be noted at fluoride levels of two parts per million and higher. The amount of fluoride that is added to public water supplies is very safe, and no hardening of soft tissues has been reported at these levels. However, the public has often voted against fluoridation of water; fluoridation has therefore, often been enacted by a legislature and not by a direct public vote. In 2008, 72.4% of the population had access to fluoridated water, according to the Centers for Disease Control and Prevention. The goal of the U.S. government was to give 75% of the population access to fluoridated water by 2010. However, the country has fallen slightly short of that goal, with 73.9% of the current population having access to fluoridated water. Healthy People 2020 sets a goal of 79.6% of the U.S. population being served with fluoridated water by 2020.

Water is not the only source of fluoride; it is also added to toothpaste and mouthwash. Many dentists offer a fluoride treatment to help harden tooth enamel. To learn more about the fluoridation of water, visit the Centers for Disease Control and Prevention website at https://www.cdc.gov/fluoridation/index.html

Recommended Levels for Fluoride Intake and Fluoride Toxicity Concerns

The DRI for fluoride is expressed as an AI: 4 milligrams per day for men and 3 milligrams per day for women. There is no change during pregnancy or lactation. The UL for those older than 8 years is 10 milligrams per day.

Excess fluoride intake may occur, although its incidence is rather rare. Such toxicities may lead to deformed bones and discolored or mottled teeth, a condition called **fluorosis**. Fluoride may also inhibit fatty acid oxidation and the formation of acetyl CoA. Inhibition of glycogen breakdown has also been suggested. Signs of accelerated aging often appear, as well as loss of appetite, loss of body weight, gastrointestinal enteritis, muscular weakness, convulsions, pulmonary congestion, and respiratory and cardiac failure.

● BEFORE YOU GO ON . . .

1. What is a good source of dietary fluoride?
2. How does fluoride help to decrease dental decay?
3. What can excess fluoride intake lead to with respect to teeth, and lipid and glycogen metabolism?

▶ Chromium

Chromium was first discovered to be essential in 1959. It can exist in several oxidation states, ranging from −2 to +6, with the trivalent +3 being the most relevant to humans. Chromium was once thought to primarily serve as a structural component of a complex compound called glucose tolerance factor (GTF). This compound supposedly aided in the function of insulin and was thought to help in insulin binding to membranes. It is unknown whether a glucose tolerance factor actually exists. However, it is widely believed that chromium promotes insulin function in some manner. A deficiency of chromium may result in elevated blood glucose and cholesterol levels.

Dietary Chromium

Scientists have only recently begun to investigate the chromium content of foods. Egg yolks, whole grains, and meats, especially organ meats, are good sources (**TABLE 13.9**). Cheeses, mushrooms, nuts, beer, and wine also make significant contributions. Dairy products are relatively poor chromium sources. Vegetation grown in chromium-rich soils may also make a significant contribution to the human diet. Many multivitamin/multimineral supplements include

TABLE 13.9 Chromium Content of Select Foods

Food	Chromium (μg)
Meat	
Turkey ham (3 oz)	10.4
Ham (3 oz)	3.6
Beef cubes (3 oz)	2.0
Turkey (3 oz)	1.7
Chicken (3 oz)	0.5
Grains	
Waffle (1)	6.7
English muffin (1)	3.6
Bagel, egg (1)	2.5
Rice, white (1 cup)	1.2
Bread, whole wheat (1 slice)	1.0
Fruits and vegetables	
Broccoli (2 cups)	11.0
Juice, grape (1 cup)	7.5
Potatoes, mashed (1 cup)	2.7
Juice, orange (1 cup)	2.2
Lettuce (1 cup)	1.8
Apple, unpeeled (1)	1.4

chromium. Most of the chromium in foods is found as the trivalent form. Brewer's yeast is a good source of chromium.

Absorption of Chromium

The absorption of chromium probably occurs via a carrier-mediated system at lower intakes that is complemented by passive diffusion at higher intakes. The jejunum is the primary site of absorption; however, absorption occurs along the length of the small intestine. If chromium is in an inorganic state, absorption appears to be very low (<5%). However, chromium provided in organic form demonstrates a much higher rate of absorption (15 to 25%). Chromium associated with the molecule picolinate also demonstrates better absorption than inorganic chromium alone. The presence of vitamin C has been thought to enhance chromium absorption based on both rodent and human studies.

Metabolism and Function of Chromium

Tissue levels of chromium are relatively high in infancy and decline with age. The adult body may contain 4 to 6 milligrams of chromium; more concentrated organ tissues include the kidneys, liver, spleen, pancreas, bone, and muscle, including cardiac muscle. The concentrations of chromium in the blood are not well regulated. It appears that excretion of chromium in the urine provides the primary means of disposal. Inorganic chromium is transported in the blood, primarily aboard transferrin because chromium competes with iron for binding sites. Chromium can also be transported via albumin and plasma globulins and, perhaps, lipoproteins.

Chromium is believed to bind to a lower-molecular-weight binding substance that has been given the name **chromodulin** (**FIGURE 13.17**), a protein with a molecular weight of 1.5 kilodaltons. In the cell, chromodulin can bind four chromium atoms

and can facilitate the entry of glucose into fatty acid synthesis. In target cells, chromodulin is in the apo form (without chromium bound to it). Chromium (Cr^{3+}) is brought to the cell via a chromium-transferrin complex and binds to the cell's transferring receptor. The entire complex is then internalized. Once the complex is inside the cell, the chromium is released and binds to apochromodulin to form chromodulin. The activated chromodulin binds to the insulin receptor and a protein kinase is activated, which, in turn, causes increased phosphorylation that mediates the effects of insulin. Thus, the general physiologic significance of chromium is to enhance the actions of insulin. Insulin enhances glycolysis, glycogen synthesis, fatty acid synthesis, and protein synthesis. Another mechanism that is postulated is that chromium may reduce insulin degradation, thus allowing insulin to have a longer time to exert its effect.

There has been recent interest in chromium as a supplement, with reports that increased lean body mass and reduced body fat resulted from chromium supplementation in animals and humans. Early investigations suggested that chromium supplementation increased lean body mass with a decrease in percent body fat in males and females undergoing resistance training. However, later human studies have not supported the claim of a change in body composition.

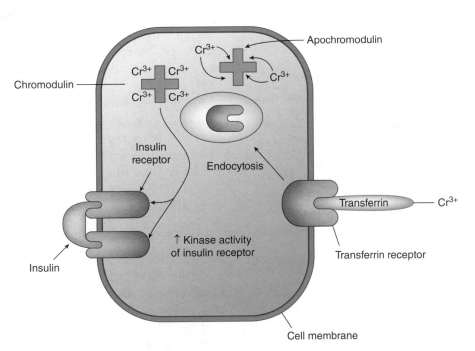

FIGURE 13.17 Proposed Role of Chromium in Modulating Insulin Action Through Interaction with the Cytoplasmic Protein Chromodulin. Chromium is present in cells complexed to a protein termed chromodulin. Chromium binds to a transferrin receptor on a cell membrane and the complex is internalized. Chromium is released from the complex and binds to apochromodulin to form chromodulin. Chromodulin binds to the insulin receptor. This will increase the kinase activity of insulin where it will promote glycolysis and the synthesis of glycogen, fatty acids, and proteins.

Recommended Levels of Intake for Chromium and Chromium Imbalance

The AI for chromium is 35 micrograms per day for men aged 14 to 50 years, decreasing to 30 micrograms per day for those older than 50 years. The AI is 23 micrograms per day for women 19 to 50 years old, and 20 micrograms per day for those older than 50 years. The AI for pregnancy is 29 to 30 micrograms per day, depending on age; it increases to 44 to 45 micrograms per day for lactation. No UL has been established for chromium because toxicity has not been reported.

Patients on long-term enteral feeding where chromium is lacking may develop chromium deficiency symptoms. Chromium deficiency can result in glucose intolerance, which is an inability to properly reduce blood glucose levels after a meal and throughout the day. One consequence of glucose intolerance is hyperinsulinemia. It has been suggested that mild chromium deficiency may be a risk factor for syndrome X, which places an individual at significantly higher risk of heart disease.

● BEFORE YOU GO ON . . .

1. What appears to be the major function of chromium for human health?
2. How does the protein chromodulin function at the cell level?
3. What can a chromium deficiency lead to?

▶ Manganese

Manganese was first identified as an essential nutrient in the early 1930s. Despite its wide distribution in nature, manganese occurs in very low quantities in human tissue. However, its significance to human function cannot be overlooked. It is both an activator and a constituent of several enzymes. In humans, manganese exists in either the +2 or +3 oxidation states.

Dietary Sources of Manganese

Whole grain cereals, fruits and vegetables, legumes, nuts, tea, and leafy vegetables are good food sources of manganese. Animal foods are generally poor contributors of manganese. Additional substances in plants, such as fiber, phytate, and oxalate, along with excessive calcium, phosphorus, and iron, can decrease manganese absorption.

Absorption of Manganese

Relatively little is known about the mechanisms of manganese absorption. It is likely that a saturable, active transport system is involved. It could involve a ZIP transporter or even DMT1. It is clear, however, that manganese is absorbed along the entire length of the small intestine. About 2 to 15% of ingested manganese can be absorbed; however, the presence of dietary factors, such as fibers, phytate, oxalates, calcium, and phosphorus, can decrease the absorption percentage.

Metabolism and Function of Manganese

The total amount of manganese in an adult human is about 12 to 20 milligrams. It is widely and uniformly distributed in tissue. Within cells, it is concentrated in the mitochondria, with relatively larger content in the nucleus as well. Bone, liver, kidney, pancreas, the lactating mammary gland, and the pituitary gland contain higher than average levels, whereas the skeletal muscles are lower by comparison. In bone, manganese is found as part of hydroxyapatite. The levels of manganese in bone and in the liver are 3.5 and 2 milligrams per kilogram, respectively.

Manganese is transported in the blood bound to transferrin or other proteins, notably α2-macroglobulin, at a level approximating 1 to 2 micrograms per 100 milliliters of blood. Its primary route of excretion from the human body is via fecal elimination of unabsorbed manganese, along with that incorporated into digestive secretions. As with intestinal absorption, transport of manganese into cells of organs is thought to involve ZIP proteins and DMT1.

Manganese functions largely as either an activator of specific enzymes or as a key component of metalloenzymes. Manganese is fundamentally important in cartilage tissue formation and remodeling, in particular, for chondroitin sulfate. UDP-glucuronic acid and N-acetyl galactosamine are condensed in the presence of the manganese-dependent enzyme galactosyltransferase, resulting in glycosaminoglycans, which are long polysaccharide chains. The addition of sulfate allows for the formation of chondroitin sulfate in cartilage. Manganese is also used in collagen production as it is a cofactor for prolinase where it produces the amino acid proline. Collagen is high in proline and this can lead to better wound healing, particularly the skin.

Manganese is also involved with aspects of carbohydrate metabolism because it is a cofactor for pyruvate carboxylase as well as an activator for the gluconeogenic enzyme phosphoenolpyruvate carboxylase (PEPCK). Manganese plays a role in the formation of prothrombin. Arginase, which is involved in urea synthesis, contains four atoms of manganese, and the dipeptidase prolidase is activated by manganese. Mitochondrial superoxide dismutase (SOD) is a manganese-dependent enzyme. This form of SOD is found almost exclusively in the mitochondria, thus protecting the organelle from oxidative damage. Finally, manganese may function as a modulator of second messenger systems. For instance, manganese increases cAMP levels in stimulated cells as well as being an activator of guanylate cyclase.

Recommended Levels of Intake and Manganese Imbalance

Manganese has an AI of 1.8 or 2.3 milligrams per day for adult women and men, respectively. In animals, manganese is important for both reproductive performance and bone development. In chickens, for instance, slip tendon is a condition caused by manganese deficiency in which the ridges on the leg bones of chickens are diminished such that a tendon may slide over the ridge. Manganese deficiency in people is rare; however, nausea, vomiting, dermatitis, decreased growth of hair and nails, and changes in hair color can result from deficiency. Manganese toxicity is also rare, although miners inhaling manganese-rich dust can experience Parkinson-like symptoms.

● BEFORE YOU GO ON . . .

1. Why is manganese important in cartilage?
2. For which enzymes is manganese a cofactor?
3. Which proteins bind manganese in the blood?

▶ Ultratrace Minerals

Cobalt

Cobalt occurs regularly in plant and animal tissues and is widely distributed. In humans, cobalt is part of vitamin B_{12}. Therefore, cobalt's presence and function in tissue is really a reflection of vitamin B_{12}. Because humans are unable to synthesize vitamin B_{12}, cobalt itself is not viewed as an essential nutrient, but merely as a component of an essential nutrient.

Cobalt is poorly absorbed as an inorganic element. If cobalt is injected, relative amounts are found in the urine. Small amounts are also found in the saliva. Traces may also be found in bile and pancreatic juices and some in the feces. A deficiency of cobalt can be experienced in ruminant animals. These animals need to ingest cobalt for the synthesis of vitamin B_{12} by their gut microflora. In such animals, emaciation, weakness, and anemia are common signs of cobalt deficiency.

Cobalt can be toxic in the range of 10 to 20 milligrams per kilogram of body weight. Polycythemia, bone marrow hyperplasia, reticulocytosis, and increased blood volume are signs of toxicity. Excessive cobalt depresses oxidative phosphorylation and leads to tissue hypoxia, changes in the nervous system, thyroid hyperplasia, and myxedema. Congestive heart failure from cobalt toxicity has been reported in humans.

Boron

There is a growing body of evidence to argue in favor of the essentiality of boron. Boron has been recognized as essential for plants since the 1920s; however, its essentiality for humans was not really investigated until the 1980s. It currently appears that boron does indeed influence the composition and mechanical properties of bone.

Dietary Sources and Absorption of Boron

Fruits, leafy vegetables, nuts, and legumes are rich sources of boron, whereas meats are among the poorer sources. Beer and wine make a respectable contribution to human boron intake. Boron appears in foods primarily as sodium borate and boric acid, two forms that seem to be readily absorbed (> 90%).

Metabolism and Function of Boron

Although relatively little is known regarding boron transport in the blood, physiologic levels appear to be regulated primarily by urinary excretion. Boron is found in many tissues; however, bone contains the most. In plants, boron is an essential factor for cell maturation and differentiation. This role has not been found in humans to date. Furthermore, flavonoid synthesis in plants depends on boron, whereas flavonoid synthesis does not seem to occur in humans. Boron appears to either directly or indirectly affect the metabolism of calcium in bone and influences the composition and strength of bone. This is an area that has been receiving more and more attention as scientists try to address bone diseases. Interestingly, boron needs are increased during a vitamin D deficiency. Also, boron has been recognized to ameliorate many of the manifestations of magnesium deficiency in bone tissue.

Recommended Levels of Boron Intake and Boron Imbalance

The requirement for boron is probably about 1 milligram daily, although no DRI has been established. The UL for both sexes is 20 milligrams per day. Boron deficiency results in an increased urinary loss of calcium and magnesium, presumably derived from storage primarily in bone. Conversely, taking large amounts of boron may induce nausea, vomiting, lethargy, and an increased loss of riboflavin.

Molybdenum

The essentiality of molybdenum was first identified in 1958; however, molybdenum has been difficult to investigate because it is an ultratrace mineral. In human tissue, molybdenum is typically found in concentrations of less than one part per million (< 1 microgram per gram of wet tissue). Furthermore, researchers have had difficulty inducing molybdenum deficiency in experimental animals both because of its relatively small requirement and because of an inability to purify experimental diets to reduce all traces of molybdenum.

Dietary Sources and Absorption of Molybdenum

Most of the foods humans eat contain a respectable amount of molybdenum, which ultimately reflects the soil content in which the plants were grown. Organ and other meats, legumes, cereals, and grains are among the better sources of molybdenum. Very little is known at this time regarding the absorptive processes for molybdenum. Although the stomach appears to be able to contribute to the absorption of molybdenum, most absorption probably occurs in the proximal small intestine. At lower intakes, molybdenum is probably absorbed by active carrier-mediated transport, which is complemented by passive diffusion at higher intake levels. Molybdenum absorption has been estimated to range from 25 to 80%. Diets high in molybdenum decrease copper absorption and increase copper loss in the urine.

Metabolism and Function of Molybdenum

As mentioned earlier, the molybdenum content of human tissue is typically less than one part per million.

Tissues, such as the liver, adrenal glands, kidneys, and bone, are the most concentrated. Other tissues, such as muscle, lungs, brain, spleen, and small intestine, contain slightly higher concentrations as well.

Molybdenum, as a constituent of molybdoenzymes, participates in certain oxidation-reduction reactions. Molybdenum is a component of a cofactor for the molybdopterin structure that is found at the catalytic site of some enzymes. Xanthine oxidase and xanthine dehydrogenase are found in a variety of tissue, and the dehydrogenase form can be converted into the oxidase form in tissue. These enzymes are fundamental in hydroxylating various purines and pyrimidines, pteridines, and other heterocyclic nitrogen-containing compounds. In this sense, molybdenum is necessary for the transformation of hypoxanthine to xanthine as well as xanthine to uric acid.

The molybdoenzyme sulfite oxidase catalyzes the conversion of sulfite to sulfate. Sulfite oxidase is a mitochondrial enzyme located in several types of tissue and is responsible for the terminal step in the metabolism of sulfur-containing amino acids (cysteine and methionine). Finally, the molybdoenzyme aldehyde oxidase may be important in the metabolism of certain drugs.

Recommended Levels of Molybdenum Intake and Imbalances

The RDA for adults is 45 micrograms of molybdenum daily. Because of molybdenum's widespread availability in the diet, deficiency is somewhat rare. However, people receiving intravenous feedings for several months are at risk. In contrast, molybdenum is fairly nontoxic. However, because molybdenum is involved in the breakdown of bases to the waste product uric acid, which is excreted via the urine, higher intakes of this mineral could place certain prone individuals at greater risk of kidney stones. Excessive uric acid production may also increase the risk of developing gout.

Interestingly, excess molybdenum may result in decreased copper absorption by the small intestine. It is not unusual to combat Wilson disease with compounds containing molybdenum. Copper is crucial for the development and spread of new blood vessels, a process called angiogenesis. In tumors, angiogenesis is enhanced. However, a copper-deficiency will reduce angiogenesis. Molybdenum-like drugs are sometimes used to block copper absorption to impair angiogenesis in cancer.

Vanadium

Vanadium exists in several oxidation states, ranging from +2 to +5. In humans, as well as other organisms, vanadium appears mostly in the pentavalent form, vanadate (VO_3^- or $H_2VO_4^-$), or in the tetravalent state, vanadyl (VO^{2+}). Recently, it has become a popular supplement for weight-training individuals hoping to increase their muscle mass.

Dietary Sources and Absorption of Vanadium

Although still only containing nanograms to micrograms of vanadium, breakfast cereals, canned fruit juices, fish sticks, shellfish, vegetables (especially mushrooms, parsley, and spinach), sweets, wine, and beer are better sources. Although pertinent information is somewhat lacking, vanadium absorption appears to be relatively small: 5 to 40%.

Metabolism and Function of Vanadium

Vanadium is present in trace concentrations in most organs and tissues throughout the human body and has long been questioned in regard to essentiality. It is important to realize that the presence of a substance does not necessarily indicate essentiality. Nevertheless, researchers have discerned that the absence of vanadium from animal diets reduces their growth rate, infancy survival, and hematocrit, despite the inability of researchers to identify specific functions for vanadium.

Vanadium administered in higher quantities exerts numerous effects on human metabolism. However, these activities cannot be considered vanadium dependent because they are observed only when vanadium is administered in excessive amounts. In this manner, vanadium acts as a pharmaceutical agent, not necessarily a nutrient. One such effect that is receiving research attention is vanadium's ability to mimic the activity of insulin. Vanadium appears to be able to affect glucose metabolism in a manner similar to insulin. Promising research with diabetic animals has suggested that vanadium therapy may control high blood glucose levels (hyperglycemia).

Recommended Levels of Vanadium Intake and Vanadium Imbalances

A dietary requirement for vanadium has yet to be established; however, 10 to 25 micrograms of vanadium per day may be appropriate. As mentioned previously, vanadium deficiency may result in reductions in growth rate, infancy survival, and hematocrit. Further, vanadium deficiency may alter the activity of the thyroid gland and its ability to properly use iodide. Signs of vanadium toxicity, such as a green tongue, diarrhea, abdominal cramping, and alterations in mental functions, have been reported in individuals ingesting more than 10 milligrams of vanadium daily over extended periods of time. A UL of 1.8 milligrams per day for adult men and women has been established.

Nickel

In general, plants are more concentrated sources of nickel than are animal foods. Nuts are the most concentrated sources, and grains, cured meats, and vegetables offer respectable amounts. Fish, milk, and eggs are recognized as poorer nickel sources. The absorption of nickel from the gut is probably affected by varying the amounts of copper, iron, and zinc present, and perhaps vice versa. Adult requirements for nickel are most likely about 35 micrograms daily. A UL of 1,000 micrograms per day for both sexes has been established.

The possible essentiality of nickel had not been seriously considered until the last 30 years or so. Defining exact roles for nickel in humans remains somewhat elusive. However, nickel does seem to be involved in the breakdown of the amino acids leucine, valine, and isoleucine (branched-chain amino acids) and odd-chain-length fatty acids. Nickel research is relatively new, and more information about the roles of nickel will probably emerge within the next decade.

Arsenic

As a natural constituent of the earth's crust, arsenic can be found in most soils and is taken up by plants. However, the arsenic content of foods can also be affected by the arsenic content in pesticides and airborne pollutants. Among the most concentrated sources of arsenic are sea animals (fish, shellfish). Dietary requirements for arsenic have not been established, although 12 to 15 micrograms daily is probably sufficient.

Although arsenic has long been regarded as an undesirable substance, it may be an essential component of the human body after all. Although its involvement has not been clearly characterized, arsenic is most likely important in the metabolism of two amino acids, methionine and arginine. Arsenic deficiencies have resulted in a reduced growth rate in animals. Arsenic deficiency may also reduce conception rate and increase the likelihood of death in newborns.

Perhaps, no other constituent of the human body conjures up a stronger notion of toxicity than arsenic. It certainly is the only nutrient that can be fatal in milligram amounts. Arsenic, in the form of arsenic trioxide, can be fatal at doses greater than 0.76 to 1.95 milligrams.

Silicon

Not much is really known about the silicon content of various foods. Plant sources, including high-fiber cereal grains and root vegetables, seem to be better sources than animal sources. Silicon, in the form of quartz, is the most abundant mineral on the planet. However, silicon makes only a minuscule contribution to human body weight. Silicon seems to be involved in the health of connective tissue. In bone, silicon seems to improve the rate of both bone mineralization and growth. The manufacture of collagen, a predominant protein found in connective tissue, relies on an adequate supply of the nonessential amino acid proline and a slightly modified form of proline called hydroxyproline. Silicon is probably required for the optimal synthesis of both proline and hydroxyproline. Silicon is also important for the manufacturing of other proteins and substances vital to proper connective tissue. Silicon deficiency can result in poor growth and development of bone, including decreased mineralization. Not much is known at this time regarding silicon toxicity.

● BEFORE YOU GO ON . . .

1. What appears to be the major function of cobalt? Boron?
2. What enzymatic reactions involve molybdenum as a cofactor?
3. What protein hormone is vanadium thought to function as when given in high enough amounts?
4. What function is nickel thought to play a role in?
5. With what amino acids may arsenic be involved? Silicon?

⚕ CLINICAL INSIGHT

Bariatric Surgery and Micronutrient Deficiency: Impact on Pregnancy Outcomes

In Chapter 2, the various types of bariatric surgery used for weight loss were discussed. Gastric banding, gastroplasty, gastric sleeve, and Roux-En-Y are procedures to reduce either food intake, enhanced satiety, or malabsorption. These procedures may have significant side effects and include potential decreased status of micronutrients such as potassium, copper, iron, zinc, vitamin A, vitamin B_{12}, and folate. Such decreases in status could result from decreased food intake, malabsorption, or a combination of both. With the frequency of such surgical interventions for obesity, including women of child bearing age, one area of concern may be that any subsequent pregnancies could impact micronutrient status of both the mother and infant, either at birth or later. Nutritional requirements are increased both during pregnancy and lactation for the mother. A decrease in nutritional status is not only reflected in maternal health outcomes but also those of the neonate. The question is whether there is evidence to support decreased micronutrient status, deficiencies, or nutrition-related outcomes in mothers and their newborns where the mother has had some type of gastric surgery for weight loss.

While there are few comprehensive studies on this topic, there have been cohort studies and case reports on this subject. Jans and associates published a meta-analysis on this subject in 2015. Using strict guidelines (Preferred Reporting Items for Systematic Reviews and Meta-Analysis, or PRISMA) for selection of published articles, 25 papers were identified in which the 17 were case studies and the remaining 8 were cohort studies, either retrospective, prospective, or a combination of both were studied. Variables that were assessed in these mothers included micronutrient status by assessing a number of micronutrient blood concentrations before the pregnancy, supplements used before and during pregnancy, time between surgery and pregnancy, and any adverse neonatal outcomes.

The nutrients that appeared to be below normal included several of the vitamins, such as vitamin K, vitamin A, vitamin B_{12}, and folate. Vitamin D did not appear to be affected. With respect to minerals, surprisingly, only iron appeared to be low. Copper, zinc, magnesium, iodine, calcium, and magnesium did not appear to be low despite evidence to support malabsorption of these nutrients in some of the bypass procedures used. Not all of these findings can be generalized. For instance, in one case study, a severe case of zinc deficiency in a 38-year-old female who had undergone bypass surgery was reported. The report suggested that those who go through a restricted bariatric surgery, such as gastric banding or gastroplasty, are at less risk for developing a zinc deficiency and other possible deficiencies as opposed to a malabsorptive surgery, such as a Roux-En-Y. While there was no pregnancy involved here, the lack of findings from other studies may be complicated by a lower use of malabsorptive-type bariatric surgeries used for weight loss. It would appear that focusing on micronutrient deficiencies, especially those dealing with the microelements should perhaps focus on Roux-En-Y surgical interventions of females who become pregnant.

At this point, there is only weak evidence to suggest that bariatric surgery has a nutritional impact on pregnant mothers and neonates. However, the clinician should be aware of any possible micronutrient deficiency, especially iron and perhaps zinc, in pregnant women and their offspring who have undergone bariatric surgery.

▶ Here's What You Have Learned

1. Heme iron is much more effectively absorbed by the small intestinal cells than nonheme iron. Valence state plays an important role in uptake of nonheme iron, with the ferrous (+2) state much better absorbed than elemental iron or the ferric (+3) form.

2. Ionic iron is absorbed by divalent metal transporter 1 (DMT1) at the brush border and then is delivered to either ferritin or mobiloferrin in the enterocyte. Iron that will be absorbed into the bloodstream is delivered to the basolateral side of the enterocyte and given to IREG1 (ferroportin) for export. A copper-containing enzyme called hephaestin oxidizes the ferrous to the ferric form of iron so that it can be picked up by serum transferrin, because the ferrous form cannot bind to transferrin.

3. Another regulator in iron absorption is hepcidin, a hormone that is produced by liver cells when stores of liver iron are high. Hepcidin targets the small intestine and blocks the uptake of iron by binding to ferroportin and causes the complex to be internalized by the enterocyte or macrophage.

4. Translation of ferritin and the transferrin receptor is based on iron stores and mediated through iron regulatory proteins. When sufficient iron stores are present, iron binds to the iron regulatory proteins and makes them ineffective. In the absence of iron binding, such as in deficiency states, the iron regulatory proteins allow for the blockage of ferritin synthesis but enhance transferrin receptor synthesis to facilitate greater iron absorption by cells.

5. Iron toxicity has been reported in both humans and animals. The more common human form is an HLA-linked hemochromatosis that appears to be one of the most common inborn errors in metabolism among whites of European descent. In this genetic condition, iron absorption is greatly enhanced because the regulatory protein HFE is defective. This results in increased oxidation in tissues, especially in the liver.

6. Zinc is a cofactor for more than 200 enzymes. It is absorbed by small-intestinal enterocytes via ZIP4 and is ferried to the basolateral portion of the cell and exported via zinc transporter 1. High levels of dietary zinc stimulate the synthesis of a low-molecular-weight protein called metallothionein that effectively traps zinc and prevents its absorption.

7. Iodine acts primarily through thyroxin, a hormone that increases basal metabolic rate as one of its many functions. When iodide is bound to all four positions on the tyrosine residue of the thyroglobin protein, the compound is called thyroxin (T_4). Iodination at the 3, 5, and 3′ ring positions results in a molecule called triiodothyronine (T_3). Collectively, T_3 and T_4 are referred to as thyroid hormone, with T_4 predominating in the blood.

8. Copper absorption may be passive or carrier mediated. One of the copper transporters is Ctr1. DMT1 may also play a role in copper absorption. When copper is in the cell, it must be bound to a protein; otherwise, it will act as a pro-oxidant. These proteins are termed chaperone proteins. The chaperone protein responsible for ferrying copper to copper–zinc superoxide dismutase is CCS; for cytochrome c oxidase, it is Cox17; and for ATP7A, it is Atox1. Cox11, Sco1, and Sco2 are mitochondria chaperone proteins for copper.

9. Two genetic conditions lead to copper-associated diseases. Menkes disease is caused by a defect in the ATP7A protein ATPase responsible for copper absorption in the small intestine. This results in a copper deficiency. Wilson disease affects the ATP7B protein in the Golgi network of the liver, such that copper cannot be exported from liver cells. This results in hepatotoxicity due to increased copper levels, but to a decrease in copper levels in peripheral tissues.

10. Copper plays a role in a wide variety of biochemical pathways, in which it is a cofactor for enzymes such as lysyl oxidase, cytochrome c oxidase, dopamine and tyrosine hydroxylases, and copper–zinc superoxide dismutase.

11. Selenium is often referred to as an antioxidant nutrient because it is a cofactor for the enzyme glutathione peroxidase, which converts hydrogen peroxides produced from a catalase reaction to water. Another antioxidant pathway involves selenium containing enzymes thioredoxin reductases, which reduces oxidized metabolites to take part in further reduction-oxidation reactions. Iodothyronine deiodinase also contains selenium, which converts thyroxine (T_4) to triiodothyronine (T_3) in iodine metabolism.

12. Selenium may be incorporated into proteins through an elaborate process known as cotranslation. Here, the codon UGA, normally a stop codon for protein synthesis, codes for the amino

acid selenocysteine. This amino acid is formed when the amino acid serine is bound to a larger-than-normal tRNA. Special cell proteins and mRNA elements take part in incorporating selenocysteine in a growing polypeptide chain.

13. The major function of fluoride is hardening the teeth. It does this by interacting with hydroxyapatite crystals to form a more rigid structure.

14. Chromium is thought to be required for proper insulin functioning and may require a protein called chromodulin to bind to it in the cell in order for insulin to function correctly.

15. Manganese is found in bone as part of hydroxyapatite. It functions largely as an activator of specific enzymes. It is needed in cartilage tissue formation and remodeling, in particular, of chondroitin sulfate. Manganese is also involved with aspects of carbohydrate metabolism because it is a cofactor for pyruvate carboxylase as well as an activator for the gluconeogenic enzyme phosphoenolpyruvate carboxylase (PEPCK). Manganese plays a role in the formation of prothrombin. Arginase, which is involved in urea synthesis, contains four atoms of manganese, and the dipeptidase prolidase is activated by manganese. Mitochondrial superoxide dismutase is a manganese-dependent enzyme. Manganese may function as a modulator of second messenger systems. For instance, manganese increases cAMP levels in stimulated cells as well as being an activator of guanylate cyclase.

16. The ultratrace minerals whose functions are still being researched include cobalt, boron, molybdenum, vanadium, nickel, arsenic, and silicon. All of these minerals have been demonstrated to play some role in metabolism, but their precise essentiality has not yet been established.

▶ Suggested Reading

Andrews GK. Cellular zinc sensors: MTF-1 regulation of gene expression. *Biometals.* 2001;14(3–4):223–237.

Aschner JL, Aschner M. Nutritional aspects of manganese homeostasis. *Mol Aspects Med.* 2005;26(4–5):353–362.

Babaknejad N, Sayehmiri F, Sayehmiri K, et al. The relationship between selenium levels and breast cancer: a systematic review and meta-analysis. *Biol Trace El Res.* 2014;159(1–3):1–7.

Beard JL, Dawson H, Piñero DJ. Iron metabolism: a comprehensive review. *Nutr Rev.* 1996;54(10):295–317.

Bellinger FP, Raman AV, Reeves MA, Berry MJ. Regulation and function of selenoproteins in human disease. *Biochem J.* 2009;422(1):11–22.

Berry MJ, Tujebajeva RM, Copeland PR, et al. Selenocysteine incorporation directed from the 3′UTR: characterization of eukaryotic EFsec and mechanistic implications. *Biofactors.* 2001;14(1–4):17–24.

Black M, Medeiros DM, Brunnett E, Welke R. Zinc supplements and serum lipids in young adult white males. *Am J Clin Nutr.* 1988;47(6):970–975.

Bost M, Houdart S, Oberli M, Kalonji E, Huneau JF, Margaritis I. Dietary copper and human heath: current evidence and unresolved issues. *J Trace Elem Med Biol.* 2016;35:107–115.

Campbell WW, Joseph LJ, Davey SL, Cyr-Campbell D, Anderson RA, Evans WJ. Effects of resistance training and chromium picolinate on body composition and skeletal muscle in older men. *J Appl Physiol (1985).* 1999;86(1):29–39.

Centers for Disease Control and Prevention. 2008 water fluoridation statistics. Available at: http://www.cdc.gov/fluoridation/statistics/2008stats.htm. Accessed November 17, 2010.

Clark LC, Dalkin B, Krongrad A, et al. Decreased incidence of prostate cancer with selenium supplementation: results of a double-blind cancer prevention trial. *Br J Urol.* 1998;81(5):730–734.

Cousins RJ. Gastrointestinal factors influencing zinc absorption and homeostasis. *Int J Vitam Nutr Res.* 2010;80(4–5):243–248.

Cousins RJ, Blanchard RK, Moore JB, et al. Regulation of zinc metabolism and genomic outcomes. *J Nutr.* 2003;133(5 suppl 1):1521S–1526S.

de Romaña DL, Olivares M, Uauy R, Araya M. Risks and benefits of copper in light of new insights of copper homeostasis. *J Trace Elem Med Biol.* 2011;25(1):3–13.

Duffield-Lillico AJ, Dalkin BL, Reid ME, et al.; Nutritional Prevention of Cancer Study Group. Selenium supplementation, baseline plasma selenium status and incidence of prostate cancer: an analysis of the complete treatment period of the Nutritional Prevention of Cancer Trial. *BJU Int.* 2003;91(7):608–612.

Duffield-Lillico AJ, Reid ME, Turnbull BW, et al. Baseline characteristics and the effect of selenium supplementation on cancer incidence in a randomized clinical trial: a summary report of the Nutritional Prevention of Cancer Trial. *Cancer Epidemiol Biomarkers Prev.* 2002;11(7):630–639.

Duffield-Lillico AJ, Slate EH, Reid ME, et al., Nutritional Prevention of Cancer Study Group. Selenium supplementation and secondary prevention of nonmelanoma skin cancer in a randomized trial. *J Natl Cancer Inst.* 2003;95(19):1477–1481.

Eichholzer M, Tönz O, Zimmermann R. Folic acid: a public health challenge. *Lancet.* 2006;367(9519):1352–1361.

Eide DJ. Zinc transporters and the cellular trafficking of zinc. *Biochim Biophys Acta.* 2006;1763(7):711–722.

Eisenstein RS. Iron regulatory proteins and the molecular control of mammalian iron metabolism. *Annu Rev Nutr.* 2000;20:627–662.

Finley JW, Davis CD. Manganese deficiency and toxicity: are high or low dietary amounts of manganese cause for concern? *Biofactors.* 1999;10(1):15–24.

Food and Nutrition Board, Institute of Medicine. *Dietary Reference. Intakes for Calcium, Phosphorus, Magnesium, Vitamin D, and Fluoride.* Washington, DC: National Academies Press; 1997.

Food and Nutrition Board, Institute of Medicine. *Dietary Reference Intakes for Vitamin A, Vitamin K, Arsenic, Boron, Chromium, Copper, Iodine, Iron, Manganese, Molybdenum, Nickel, Silicon, Vanadium, and Zinc.* Washington, DC: National Academies Press; 2000.

Gerhardsson L, Brune D, Nordberg IG, Wester PO. Protective effect of selenium on lung cancer in smelter workers. *Br J Ind Med.* 1985;42(9):617–626.

Ghadirian P, Maisonneuve P, Perret C, et al. A case-control study of toenail selenium and cancer of the breast, colon, and prostate. *Cancer Detect Prev.* 2000;24(4):305–313.

Harris ED. Cellular transporters for zinc. *Nutr Rev.* 2002;60(4):121–124.

Hashimoto A, Kambe T. Mg, Zn and Cu transport proteins: a brief overview from physiological and molecular perspectives. *J Nutr Sci Vitaminol (Tokyo).* 2015;61(suppl):S116–S118.

Helzlsouer KJ, Comstock GW, Morris JS. Selenium, lycopene, alpha-tocopherol, beta-carotene, retinol, and subsequent bladder cancer. *Cancer Res.* 1989;49(21):6144–6148.

Jans G, Matthys C, Bogaerts A, et al. Maternal micronutrient deficiencies and related adverse neonatal outcomes after bariatric surgery: a systematic review. *Adv Nutr.* 2015;6(4):420–429.

Kambe T. An overview of a wide range of functions of ZnT and Zip zinc transporters in the secretory pathway. *Biosci Biotechnol Biochem.* 2011;75(6):1036–1043.

Kennedy E, Meyers L. Dietary reference intakes: development and uses of micronutrient status of women—a global perspective. *Am J Clin Nutr.* 2005;81(5):1194S–1197S.

Li H, Stampfer MJ, Giovannucci EL, et al. A prospective study of plasma selenium levels and prostate cancer risk. *J Natl Cancer Inst.* 2004;96(9):696–703.

Lönnerdal B. Intestinal regulation of copper homeostasis: a developmental perspective. *Am J Clin Nutr.* 2008;88(3):846S–850S.

Lukaski HC. Chromium as a supplement. *Ann Rev Nutr.* 1999;19:279–302.

Mark SD, Qiao YL, Dawsey SM, et al. Prospective study of serum selenium levels and incident esophageal and gastric cancers. *J Natl Cancer Inst.* 2000;92(21):1753–1763.

Mastrogiannaki M, Matak P, Keith B, Simon MC, Vaulont S, Peyssonnaux C. HIF-2α, but not HIF-1α, promotes iron absorption in mice. *J Clin Invest.* 2009;119(5):1159–1166.

Medeiros DM. Copper, iron, and selenium dietary deficiencies negatively impact skeletal integrity: a review. *Exp Biol Med (Maywood).* 2016;241(12):1316–1322.

Medeiros DM, Wildman R. Newer findings on a unified perspective of copper restriction and cardiomyopathy. *Proc Soc Exp Biol Med.* 1997;215(4):299–313.

Melse-Boonstra A, Jaiswal N. Iodine deficiency in pregnancy, infancy and childhood and its consequences for brain development. *Best Pract Res Clin Endocrinol Metab.* 2010;24(1):29–38.

Meplan C, Hesketh J. The influence of selenium and selenoprotein gene variants on colorectal cancer risk. *Mutagenesis.* 2012; 27:177-186.

Mooney KW, Cromwell GL. Efficacy of chromium picolinate and chromium chloride as potential carcass modifiers in swine. *J Animal Sci.* 1997;75(10):2661–2671.

Nielsen FH. Is boron nutritionally relevant? *Nutr Rev.* 2008;66(4):183–191.

Oshiro S, Morioka MS, Kiluchi M. Dysregulation of iron metabolism in Alzheimer's disease, Parkinsons's disease, and amyotrophic lateral sclerosis. *Adv Pharmacol Sci.* 2011;doi:10.1155/2011/378278.

Pantopoulos K. Iron metabolism and the IRE/IRP regulatory system: an update. *Ann NY Acad Sci.* 2004;1012:1–13.

Papamargaritis D, Aasheim ET, Sampson B, le Roux CW. Copper, selenium and zinc levels after bariatric surgery in patients recommended to take multivitamin-mineral supplementation. *J Trace Elem Med Biol.* 2015;31:167–172.

Peters U, Chatterjee N, Church TR, et al. High serum selenium and reduced risk of advanced colorectal adenoma in a colorectal cancer early detection program. *Cancer Epidemiol Biomarkers Prev.* 2006;15(2):315–320.

Prohaska JR, Gybina AA. Intracellular copper transport in mammals. *J Nutr.* 2004;134(5):1003–1006.

Schomburg L, Köhrle J. On the importance of selenium and iodine metabolism for thyroid hormone biosynthesis and human health. *Mol Nutr Food Res.* 2008;52(11):1235–1246.

Schwarz G, Mendel RR, Ribbe MW. Molybdenum cofactors, enzymes and pathways. *Nature.* 2009;460(257):839–847.

Shah YM, Matsubara T, Ito S, Gonzalez FJ. Intestinal hypoxia-inducible transcription factors are essential for iron absorption following iron deficiency. *Cell Metab.* 2009;9(2):152–164.

Vick G, Mahmoudizad R, Fiala K. Intravenous zinc therapy for acquired zinc deficiency secondary to gastric bypass surgery: a case report. *Dermatol Ther.* 2015;28(4):222–225.

Wang Q, Zhang X, Chen S, et al. Prevention of motor neuron degeneration by novel iron chelators in SOD1^{G93A} transgenic mice of amyotrophic lateral sclerosis. *Neurodegener Dis.* 2011;8(5):310–321.

Wang X, Zhou B. Dietary zinc absorption: a play of Zips and ZnTs in the gut. *IUBMB Life.* 2010;62(3):176–182.

Wei WQ, Abnet CC, Qiao YL, et al. Prospective study of serum selenium concentrations and esophageal and gastric cardia cancer, heart disease, stroke, and total death. *Am J Clin Nutr.* 2004;79(1):80–85.

Zeegers MP, Goldbohm RA, Bode P, van den Brandt PA. Prediagnostic toenail selenium and risk of bladder cancer. *Cancer Epidemiol Biomarkers Prev.* 2002;11(11):1292–1297.

Zhuo H, Smith AH, Steinmaus C. Selenium and lung cancer: a quantitative analysis of heterogeneity in the current epidemiological literature. *Cancer Epidemiol Biomarkers Prev.* 2004;13(5):771–778.

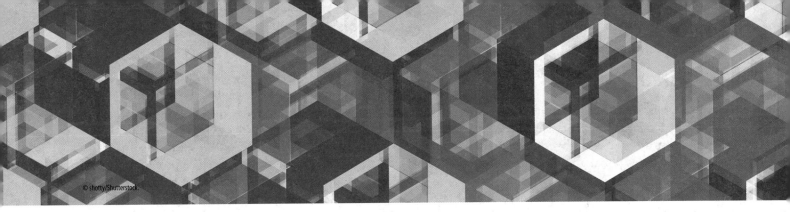

CHAPTER 14

Nutraceuticals and Functional Foods

▶ Introduction

The area of nutraceuticals and functional foods is an exciting one for nutrition professionals. What's more, depending on the report and included food/product type by 2020, the global functional food market is expected to achieve or exceed a value of $100 billion. The term **functional food** has been defined in different ways and is often leveraged in marketing materials for foods. However, in general, a functional food is a food that delivers health or other functional benefit beyond providing energy and nutrients that help people meet their basic requirements for growth and development and prevent deficiency-related disorders. In the United States, the European Union, and other countries, specific guidelines are in place for claims regarding functional foods. A number of functional foods have been defined based on their functional

components, which are called **nutraceuticals**, and many of these are well established and understood. However, numerous other foods and food components are of interest and under investigation. In this chapter, we will explore functional foods and the claims associated with different foods as well as provide an overview for understanding the different subcategories of nutraceuticals and functional foods.

▶ Defining Nutraceuticals and Functional Foods

At this time, the terms *functional food* and *nutraceutical* do not have widely accepted definitions. Different organizations and nations have developed their own definitions, some of which are listed in **TABLE 14.1**. Regardless of the specific definition used,

TABLE 14.1 Definitions of Functional Foods

Organization	Definition
Academy of Nutrition and Dietetics (AND)	The AND classifies all foods as functional at some physiologic level because they provide nutrients or other substances that furnish energy, sustain growth, or maintain/repair vital processes. However, functional foods move beyond necessity to provide additional health benefits that may reduce disease risk and/or promote optimal health. Functional foods include conventional foods, modified foods (i.e., fortified, enriched, or enhanced), medical foods, and foods for special dietary use.
International Food Information Council (IFIC)	The IFIC considers functional foods to include any food or food component that may have health benefits beyond basic nutrition.
Institute of Food Technologists (IFT)	The IFT expert report defined functional foods as foods and food components that provide essential nutrients, often beyond quantities necessary for normal maintenance, growth, and development, and/or other biologically active components that impart health benefits or desirable physiologic effects.
Health Canada	Health Canada defines a functional food as similar in appearance to, or may be, a conventional food that is consumed as part of a usual diet, and is demonstrated to have physiologic benefits and/or reduce the risk of chronic disease beyond basic nutritional functions, i.e., they contain bioactive compound(s).
European Commission[a]	The European Commission Concerted Action on Functional Food Science in Europe regards a food as functional if it is satisfactorily demonstrated to beneficially affect one or more target function in the body, beyond adequate nutritional effects, in a way that is relevant to either an improved state of health and well-being and/or reduction of risk of disease. In this context, functional foods are not pills or capsules, but must remain foods and they must demonstrate their effects in amounts that can normally be expected to be consumed in the diet.
Japan	Known as Foods for Specified Health Use, these are foods composed of functional ingredients that affect the structure and/or function of the body and are used to maintain or regulate specific health conditions, such as gastrointestinal health, blood pressure, and blood cholesterol levels.

[a]Represents member states of the European Union (EU).

most organizations state that nutraceuticals and/ or their food forms should promote health aspects beyond minimal needs for reproduction, growth, development, and progression through a generally healthy lifespan.

The emphases of the field of nutrition have changed over time. From the late 1800s through approximately the 1960s, the emphasis was on identifying essential nutrients, such as water-soluble and fat-soluble vitamins and certain minerals, and on establishing basic nutrient requirements to prevent deficiency. Since then, nutrition research has increasingly focused on the relationship between nutrition and obesity and the role of nutrition in the development of chronic degenerative disorders and diseases, such as heart disease, osteoporosis, and cancer. These investigations have identified the potential of nutrients and nutrition synergies in promoting health and preventing the development of chronic diseases and disorders. This focus on the role of functional foods was highlighted in a 2013 position paper of the Academy of Nutrition and Dietetics:

> It is the position of the Academy of Nutrition and Dietetics to recognize that although all foods provide some level of physiological function, the term, "functional foods" is defined as whole foods along with fortified, enriched, or enhanced foods that have a potentially beneficial effect on health when consumed as part of a varied diet on a regular basis at effective levels based on significant standards of evidence. The Academy supports the U.S. Food and Drug Administration (FDA) approved health claims on food labels when based on rigorous scientific substantiation.

▶ Organizational Systems for Nutraceuticals and Functional Foods

The concept of food as medicine is not new. The use of foods to prevent and/or treat certain diseases can be found in ancient drawings and writings. Perhaps, the most famous statement came from Hippocrates, who said "Let food be thy medicine." However, laboratory and clinical investigations to identify the active substances (nutraceuticals) and to establish efficacy conditions and circumstances began in earnest only a few decades ago. So, what were the first nutraceuticals that nutritionists were able to identify? Among

the first nutraceuticals examined were plant fibers, β-carotene, and the ω-3 polyunsaturated fatty acids (PUFA). Today, the number of purported nutraceuticals is in the hundreds and includes isoflavones, tocotrienols, allyl sulfur compounds, conjugated linoleic acid (CLA), and carotenoids, such as lutein, zeaxanthin, and lycopene. No longer are nutraceuticals only of interest to scientists and healthcare practitioners; today, the concept of functional foods and their nutraceuticals is mainstream. Continued interest in nutraceuticals, particularly regarding the need for nonmedical solutions to prevent and/or treat chronic diseases, means that many organizations have become interested in developing a greater understanding and application of nutraceuticals and the foods that deliver them. Nutraceuticals can be organized by their (1) food sources; (2) mechanism of action; (3) potential health benefits; and (4) chemical, elemental, or molecular structure.

Food Sources

Nutraceuticals can be consumed as components of numerous natural or manufactured foods and supplements. In this sense, nutraceuticals can be part of a food in its naturally harvested stated (e.g., fruits and vegetables), provided after minimal handling/preparation (e.g., meats), or processed to create a short-term viable consumer good (e.g., milk). Although debates continue regarding concepts, such as organic, free range, and GMO (genetically modified organism), these do not change the general classification of functional foods.

Supplements offer the potential for a more concentrated delivery of nutraceuticals, including those extracted from the original source. Supplements are typically in pill (e.g., capsules, tablets, and soft gels), powder, or sometimes a ready-to-drink (RTD) form and have a Supplement Facts panel. The latter point is important because FDA guidelines allow for a Supplement Facts panel to list nutrients in the supplement in addition to those found on the Nutrition Facts panel, which is limited to calories, carbohydrates (total carbohydrate, sugars, and added sugar), protein, fat (e.g., total, SFA, MUFA, PUFA, and *trans* fats), vitamin D, calcium, potassium, sodium and iron (**FIGURE 14.1**).

Another important consideration for many people is the origin of a food or ingredient in functional food recipes or formulas. Here, some distinction can be made for foods from animals vs plants, as well as those of microbial origin or even synthetics of naturally occurring compounds. The polyphenol resveratrol is an excellent example of a nutraceutical that can be

Previous Nutrition Facts

Nutrition Facts

Serving Size 2/3 cup (55g)

Serving Per Container About 8

Amount Per Serving

Calories 230   Calories from fat 72

% Daily Value*

Total Fat 8g	12%
Saturated Fat 1g	5%
Trans Fat 0g	
Cholesterol 0mg	0%
Sodium 160mg	7%
Total Carbohydrate 37g	12%
Dietary Fiber 4g	16%
Sugars 1g	
Protein 3g	
Vitamin A	10%
Vitamin C	8%
Calcium	20%
Iron	45%

*Percent Daily Values are based on a 2000 calorie diet. Your daily value may be higher or lower depending on your calorie needs.

	Calories:	2,000	2,500
Total Fat	Less than	65g	80g
Sat Fat	Less than	20g	25g
Cholesterol	Less than	300mg	300mg
Sodium	Less than	2,400mg	2,400mg
Total Carbohydrate		300g	375g
Dietary Fiber		25g	30g

New Nutrition Facts (2018)

Nutrition Facts

8 servings per container

Serving size   2/3 cup (55g)

Amount Per Serving

Calories   **230**

% Daily Value*

Total Fat 8g	10%
Saturated Fat 1g	5%
Trans Fat 0g	
Cholesterol 0mg	0%
Sodium 160mg	7%
Total Carbohydrate 37g	13%
Dietary Fiber 4g	14%
Total Sugars 12g	
Includes 10g Added Sugars	20%
Protein 3g	
Vitamin D 2mcg	10%
Calcium 260mg	20%
Iron 8mg	45%
Potassium 235mg	6%

*The % Daily Value (DV) tells you how much a nutrient in a serving of food contributes to a daily diet. 2,000 calories a day is used for general nutrition advice.

FIGURE 14.1 Comparison of Previous and New Nutrition Facts Panels.

Reproduced from Food and Drug Administration. Nutrition Labeling. 2017. Available at: www.fda.gov/Food/GuidanceRegulation/GuidanceDocumentsRegulatoryInformation/LabelingNutrition/ucm064904.htm; Food and Drug Administration. Dietary Supplement Labeling Guide. 2017. Available at: www.fda.gov/Food/GuidanceRegulation/GuidanceDocumentsRegulatoryInformation/DietarySupplements/ucm070597.htm. Accessed July 15, 2013.

synthesized or derived from a natural origin, such as Japanese knotweed, grape skins, or red wines, or produced via genetically modified yeast. **TABLE 14.2** provides an overview of various nutraceuticals and whether they are of plant, animal, or microbial origin.

Several nutraceuticals are found in higher concentrations in specific foods or food families. For instance, **capsaicinoids** are found primarily in peppers, whereas allyl sulfur (organosulfur) compounds are particularly concentrated in onion and garlic.

TABLE 14. 2 Examples of Nutraceuticals Grouped by Food Source[a]

Plant

Allicin	Gallic acid	Lignin	Potassium
Ascorbic acid	Genestein	δ-Limonene	Quercetin
Capsaicin	Geraniol	Lutein	Resveratrol
β-Carotene	β-Glucan	Luteolin	Pterostilbene
Cellulose	Glutathione	Lycopene	Selenium
Choline	Indole-3-carbonol	Nordihydrocapsaicin	α-Tocopherol
Daidzein	β-Ionone	Pectin	γ-Tocotrienol
Hemicellulose	Lecithin	Perillyl alcohol	Zeaxanthin

Animal

Calcium	Docosapentaenoic acid (DPA)	Sphingolipids	Creatine
Conjugated linoleic acid (CLA)	Eicosapentaenoic acid (EPA)	Ubiquinone (coenzyme Q10)	
Docosahexenoic acid (DHA)	Selenium	Zinc	

Microbe

Bacteria

Bifidobacterium bifidum	B. infantis	L. acidophilus (NCFB 1748)
B. longum	Lactobacillus acidophilus (LC1)	Streptococcus salvarius (subs. thermophilus)

Yeast

Saccharomyces boulardii

[a]The substances listed in this table include those that are either accepted or purported nutraceutical substances.
Data from Wildman REC. Classifying nutraceuticals. In: Wildman REC and Bruno RS (3rd ed.), *The Handbook of Nutraceuticals and Functional Foods*. Boca Raton, FL:, Taylor & Francis Group; 2018.

TABLE 14.3 provides a listing of some nutraceuticals that are considered unique to certain foods or food families. Interestingly, the list of food sources for some nutraceuticals can be long and include numerous, seemingly unrelated foods. For instance, citrus fruits contain the isoflavone **quercetin**, as do onions. These foods are quite different; citrus fruits grow on trees, whereas the edible bulb of the onion

plant (an herb) develops at ground level. Other plant foods with higher quercetin content are red grapes, broccoli (which is a cruciferous vegetable), and the Italian yellow squash. Again, these foods appear to bear very little resemblance to citrus fruits, or onions for that matter. Indeed, there are no guarantees that closely related or seemingly similar foods contain the same nutraceuticals. For example, both onions

TABLE 14.3 Examples of Foods That Have Higher Content of Specific Nutraceuticals[a]

Nutraceutical Substance/Family	Foods of Remarkably High Content
Adenosine	Garlic, onion
Anthocyanates	Grapes, red wine
Allyl sulfur compounds	Onions, garlic
3-*n*-Butyl phthalide	Celery
β-Carotene	Citrus fruit, carrots, squash, pumpkin
Capsaicinoids	Pepper fruit
Carnosol	Rosemary
Catechins	Teas, berries
Cellulose	Most plants (component of cell walls)
CLA	Beef and dairy
Curcumin	Turmeric
Ellagic acid	Grapes, strawberries, raspberries, walnuts
EPA and DHA	Fish oils, algae, krill
β-Glucan	Oat bran, barley
Indoles	Cabbage, broccoli, cauliflower, kale, Brussels sprouts
Isoflavones	Soybeans and other legumes, apios
Isothiocyanates	Cruciferous vegetables
Lycopene	Tomatoes and tomato products
Quercetin	Onion, red grapes, citrus fruit, broccoli, Italian yellow squash
Resveratrol	Grapes (skin), red wine
Creatine	Animal meat

[a]The substances listed in this table include those that are either accepted or purported nutraceutical substances.

Data from Wildman REC. Classifying nutraceuticals. In: Wildman REC and Bruno RS (3rd ed.), *The Handbook of Nutraceuticals and Functional Foods*. Boca Raton, FL: Taylor & Francis Group; 2018.

and garlic are perennial herbs arising from a rooted bulb and botanically are members of the Lily family. However, although onions are loaded with quercetin, with some varieties containing up to 10% of their dry weight of this flavonoid, garlic does not contain any quercetin.

Mechanism of Action

Another means of classifying nutraceuticals is by their mechanism of action. Nutraceuticals can be grouped together, regardless of food source, based on their proven or purported physiologic actions on humans.

Classifications could include antioxidants, antibacterials, hypotensives, hypocholesterolemics, platelet aggregate antagonists, anti-inflammatories, anticarcinogenics, osteoprotectives, and so on. **TABLE 14.4** offers an example of nutraceuticals categorized by mechanism of action. Such a model would be helpful to an individual who

TABLE 14.4 Examples of Nutraceuticals Grouped by Mechanisms of Action[a]

Anticancer		
Ajoene	Ellagic acid	Limonene
Capsaicin	Enterolactone	Lutein
Carnosol	Equol	Pterostilbene
CLA	Genestein	Sphingolipids
Curcumin	Glycyrrhizin	α-Tocopherol
Daidzein	*Lactobacillus bulgaricus*	α-Tocotrienol
Diallyl sulfide	*Lactobacillus acidophilus*	γ-Tocotrienol
Positive Influence on Blood Lipid Profile		
β-Glucan	Resveratrol	δ-Tocotrienol
MUFA	Saponins	δ-Tocotrienol
ω-3 PUFAs	β-Sitosterol	
Quercetin	Tannins	
Antioxidant		
Ascorbic acid	Gingerol	Lycopene
β-Carotene	Glutathione	Oleuropein
Catechins	Hydroxytyrosol	Polyphenolics
Chlorogenic acid	Indole-3-carbonol	Tannins
CLA	Lutein	Tocopherols
Ellagic acid	Luteolin	Tocotrienols
Anti-inflammatory		
Capsaicin	DHA	Linolenic acid
Curcumin	EPA	Quercetin
Osteogenic or Bone Protective		
Calcium	Daidzein	Soy protein
CLA	Genestein	Creatine

[a]The substances listed in this table include those that are either accepted or purported nutraceutical substances.

Data from Wildman REC. Classifying nutraceuticals. In: Wildman REC and Bruno RS (3rd ed.), *The Handbook of Nutraceuticals and Functional Foods*. Boca Raton, FL: Taylor & Francis Group; 2018.

is genetically predisposed to a particular medical condition or to scientists trying to develop powerful functional foods for just such a person. The information in this model would be helpful in planning a diet to help manage a chronic condition or to prevent one from developing. However, note that many issues related to toxicity, synergism, and competition associated with nutraceuticals and their foods are not yet known.

Several nutraceuticals have more than one mechanism of action. One of the seemingly most versatile nutraceutical categories is the ω-3 PUFA. The nutraceutical properties of ω-3 PUFA are direct as well as indirect. For example, ω-3 PUFA are used as precursors for eicosanoid substances that promote local vasodilation and bronchodilation and deter platelet aggregation and clot formation. These roles can be prophylactic for asthma and heart disease, respectively. ω-3 PUFA may also reduce the activities of protein kinase C and tyrosine kinase, both of which are involved in a cell growth signaling mechanism. Here, the direct effects of these fatty acids may reduce cardiac hypertrophy and cancer cell proliferation. ω-3 PUFA also appears to inhibit the synthesis of fatty acid synthase (FAS), which is a principal enzyme complex involved in de novo fatty acid synthesis. Furthermore, one fatty acid, eicosapentaenoic acid (EPA), may have a positive influence on the mTOR (mammalian target of rapamyocin) signaling pathway in muscle, which supports muscle protein synthesis operations. Based on these roles in fat and muscle protein metabolism, chronic consumption of fish or fish oils, which are particularly high in EPA, could theoretically support a healthier body composition and, in turn, have an impact on obesity.

Health Claims

The true test of the beneficial role of a nutraceutical on human health is for the results of numerous scientific studies to support the use of the nutraceutical in achievable, practical amounts without concern for toxicity. Based on these and other parameters, government agencies have developed health claims as guidelines for food companies to communicate effectively and accurately about specific nutrients. A **health claim** is any claim made on a food label, including a dietary supplement, that expressly or by implication, characterizes the relationship of any substance to a disease or health-related condition. Implied health claims include those statements, symbols, vignettes, or other forms of communication that suggest that a relationship exists between the presence or level of a substance in the food and a disease or health-related condition.

Furthermore, health claims are limited to claims about disease risk reduction; they cannot make claims about the diagnosis, cure, mitigation, or treatment of disease. Health claims are required to be reviewed and evaluated by FDA prior to use. An example of an authorized health claim is: "Three grams of soluble fiber from oatmeal daily in a diet low in saturated fat and cholesterol may reduce the risk of heart disease. This cereal has 2 grams per serving." A full listing of the health claims allowed by the FDA for use on nutrition product packaging can be found on the FDA's website: https://www.fda.gov/food/ingredientspackaginglabeling/labelingnutrition/ucm2006876.htm.

Health claims are not the same as **structure/function claims**. Structure/function claims may describe the role of a nutrient or dietary ingredient intended to affect the normal structure or function of the human body, for example, "calcium builds strong bones." Structure/function claims must be truthful and not misleading. Unlike health claims, however, structure/function claims are not pre-reviewed or authorized by the FDA. Both structure/function and health claims can be used on the labels of conventional foods and dietary supplements.

A good example of the impact of functional foods and nutraceuticals can have on health is the story of olive oil, as detailed in **SPECIAL FEATURE 14.1**.

SPECIAL FEATURE 14.1

Olive Oil as a Functional Food

Olive oil is now being promoted as a functional food. However, several types of olive oils are on the market, and they may vary in their health benefits. Consumers who are looking to olive oil as a functional food should choose those that are labeled as being "extra virgin oil," or EVO. EVO is the oil first pressed under light pressure during processing and is not subjected to further refinement. Although all olive oil is high in PUFA and MUFA, which have been shown to reduce the risk of coronary heart disease, EVO has added benefits beyond its fatty acid composition. Other types of olive oil are good sources of MUFA and PUFA, just like EVO, but apparently, they are less effective at reducing the risk of coronary heart disease and certain cancer types.

Consumption of EVO is high in the Mediterranean diet, which is a likely reason why this diet can prevent the development of certain diseases. When other oils are used in place of EVO, the Mediterranean diet does not have the same effectiveness. Why is this? Apparently, EVO has a number of compounds that act as antioxidants. The Mediterranean diet is high in antioxidants, particularly phenolic compounds. EVO is particularly high in phenolic compounds (**TABLE 1**), such as hydroxytyrosol, tyrosol, oleuropein, and vanillic and caffeic acids. Oleuropein impacts the bitterness of olives, and other phenols may also impart some bitterness. EVO also has lignans, which may have beneficial health effects, such as (+)-1-acetoxypinoresinol, (+)-pinoresinol, and (+)-1-hydroxypinoriesinol. Some EVO has as much as 100 milligrams of lignin per kilogram.

EVO is thought to be protective against the development of coronary heart disease. In addition to its high levels of MUFA and PUFA, the antioxidants in EVO can reduce the presence of oxidized LDL, which is a highly atherogenic form of LDL. Specifically, oleuropein and hydroxytoluene are highly effective in reducing the oxidation of LDL.

The phenolic compounds in EVO have also been found to reduce the body's inflammatory response. Cytokines, which are important mediators of inflammation, are inhibited by the presence of phenolic compounds. For example, oleuropein and caffeic acid can decrease the concentration of the cytokine interleukin-1β. Studies on human subjects have demonstrated that the Mediterranean diet can decrease serum levels of tumor necrosis factor-α and vascular cell adhesion molecule (VCAM)-1.

With regard to cancer, the two cancer types where EVO may be most protective appear to be breast cancer and prostate cancer. Case-control studies have suggested that EVO has a protective effect against the development of breast cancer. EVO is high in the monounsaturated fatty acid oleic acid, which is thought to protect against the development of breast cancer. However, EVO is more effective in protecting against breast cancer than other oils high in oleic acid, suggesting that the antioxidant compounds that EVO may provide have a protective effect. A European study examined the fatty acid profiles of postmenopausal women with breast cancer and controls in various countries. Consumption of oleic acid had a strong inverse relationship with breast cancer in Spanish cultures, but not among subjects from Berlin, Northern Ireland, the Netherlands, and Switzerland or non-Spanish residents. One reason for the lack of a relationship between oleic acid and breast cancer among non-Spanish cultures could be that EVO contains other compounds, such as phenolics and flavonoids, both of which are good antioxidants. The Spanish subjects obtained their oleic acid from EVO, whereas the residents of other countries obtained theirs from other sources.

TABLE 1	Possible Nutraceuticals in Extra Virgin Olive Oil
Phenolics	
Caffeic acid	
Hydroxytyrosol	
Oleuropein	
Tyrosol	
Vanillic acid	
Lignans	
(+)-1-acetoxypinoresinol	
(+)-pinoresinol	
(+)-1-hydroxypinoriesinol	

A link has been suggested between EVO intake and reduced incidence of prostate cancer. Men from Southern Europe, such as Greece, Italy, Portugal, and Spain, have a lower incidence of prostate cancer. This is thought to be due to the high EVO content in the Mediterranean diet. One case-controlled study compared 858 men younger than age 70 with prostate cancer with 905 age-matched men in Australia. The researchers found that those on diets with high levels of EVO, tomatoes, and allium-containing vegetables had a reduced rate of prostate cancer, but the relationship with EVO was weak.

EVO might have other health benefits. Some evidence suggests that the Mediterranean diet may prevent metabolic syndrome. A consensus report on the health benefits of EVO suggested that EVO may prevent cognitive decline and increased incidence of Alzheimer disease as people age.

● BEFORE YOU GO ON . . .

1. What is the practical difference between a nutraceutical and a functional food?
2. What is a Supplement Facts panel?
3. In what ways can nutraceuticals be classified?
4. Discuss a nutraceutical that has multiple mechanisms of action.

▶ Organization of Nutraceuticals by Molecular Structure

As scientific investigation continues, several hundred substances will probably eventually be deemed nutraceuticals. Many of these nutraceuticals have characteristic molecular structures such that they can be classified into several chemical families (**TABLE 14.5**). The following presents some of the more important nutraceutical categories.

TABLE 14.5 Classification of Nutraceuticals Based on Chemical Composition

Isoprenoids (terpenoids)	Fatty Acids and Lipids
Carotenoids	Conjugated linoleic acid (CLA)
Saponins	Lecithin
Simple terpenes	Monounsaturated fatty acids (MUFA)
Tocopherols	ω-3 Polyunsaturated acids (PUFA)
Tocotrienols	Sphingolipids
Phenolic Compounds	**Protein, Amino Acid & Derivatives**
Anthrocyanins	Leucine
Coumarins	Creatine
Flavonols	**Minerals**
Isoflavones	Calcium
Lignin	Copper
Stilbenes	Potassium
Tannins	Selenium
Carbohydrates and Carbohydrate Derivatives	Zinc
Ascorbic acid	**Microbial**
Nonstarch polysaccharides	Prebiotics
Oligosaccharides	Probiotics

Isoprenoid Derivatives (Terpenoids)

The terms **isoprenoid** and **terpenoid** refer to the same class of molecules. These substances are without question the largest groups of secondary metabolites. Secondary metabolites are substances produced by plants that serve roles generally outside of the plants' basic needs. Isoprenoid derivatives include carotenoids, tocopherols, tocotrienols, and saponins. This group derives its name from its principal molecular building block—isoprene (**FIGURE 14.2**).

Most plants contain so-called essential oils, which contain a mixture of volatile **monoterpenes** and **sesquiterpenes**. **Limonene** is found in the essential oils of citrus peels; **menthol** is the chief monoterpene in peppermint essential oil (**FIGURE 14.3**). Two potentially nutraceutical **diterpenes** in coffee beans are **kahweol** and **cafestol**. Both of these diterpenes contain a furan ring, which might be an important starting point for some of the potential anti-neoplastic activity of these compounds. Meanwhile, several **triterpenes** (**FIGURE 14.4**) have been reported to have nutraceutical properties. These compounds include plant sterols (eg. Sitosterol); however, some of these structures may have been modified to contain fewer than 30 carbons. One of the most recognizable groups of triterpenes is the **limonoids**. These triterpenes are found in citrus fruit and impart most of their bitter flavor. **Limonin** and **nomilin** are two triterpnoids that may have nutraceutical applications based on preliminary studies that these compounds might have antineoplastic properties. **Saponins** are triterpene derivatives whose nutraceutical potential is attracting interest. Based on preliminary investigations, saponins have been noted to potentially lower cholesterol levels, decrease cancer risk, and enhance the immune system.

The carotenoid family includes the carotenes and xanthophylls and **tetraterpenoids**. Tetraterpenoids contain 40 carbons composed of four monoterpene units. The name *carotenoid* is derived from carrots (*Daucus carota*). The carotenoids are perhaps the most recognizable pigment within the isoprenoid class. The carotenoids generally produce colors of yellow, orange, and red. Carotenoids are very important in photosynthesis and photoprotection in plants.

Carotenes and xanthophylls differ only slightly. Carotenes are purely hydrocarbon molecules (i.e., lycopene, α-carotene, β-carotene, γ-carotene), whereas the xanthophylls (i.e., lutein, capsanthin, cryptoxanthin, zeaxanthin, astaxanthin) contain oxygen in the form of hydroxyl, methoxyl, carboxyl, keto, and epoxy groups. With the exception of **crocetin** and **bixin**, the naturally occurring carotenoids are tetraterpenoids,

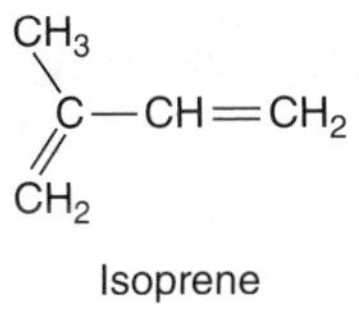

FIGURE 14.2 Isoprene. This is the basic building block of all isoprenoid and terpenoid derivatives.

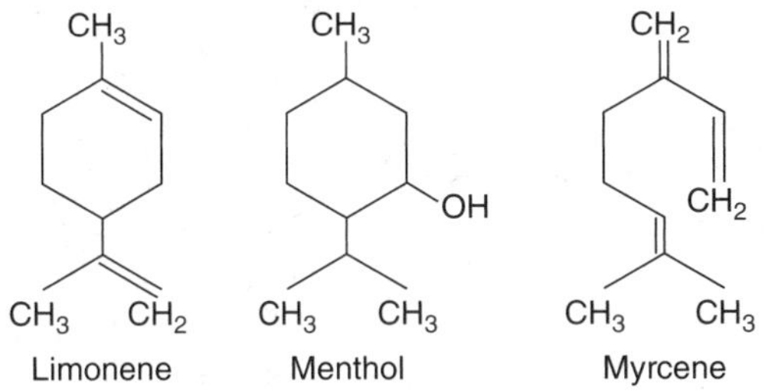

FIGURE 14.3 Select Monoterpenes. These are selected structures of monoterpenes. Liminone is an oil found in citrus fruit peels. Menthol is an oil in peppermint. Myrcene is present in plants and herbs, including mangoes, hops, bay leaves, thyme, and basil.

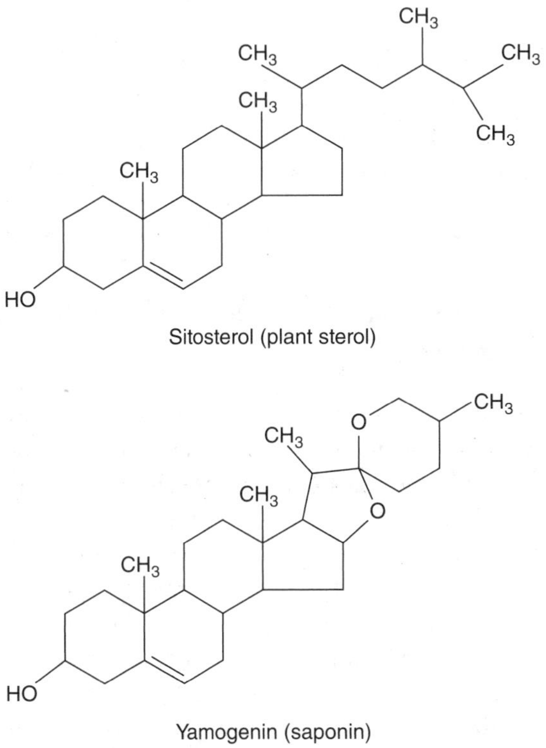

FIGURE 14.4 Select Triterpenes. Triterpenes include plant sterols (top structure) and saponins (bottom structure). Saponins, such as yamogenin, in some studies, suggest that these compounds may lower blood cholesterol, decrease cancer risk, and enhance the immune system. Dietary sources include legumes, such as chickpeas, kidney beans, soybeans, lentils, and peanuts. Sitosterols have a structure similar to cholesterol but can be used to treat elevated blood cholesterol levels. They are found in wheat germ, soybeans, and corn oil. Fruits, vegetables, nuts, and seeds are also sources.

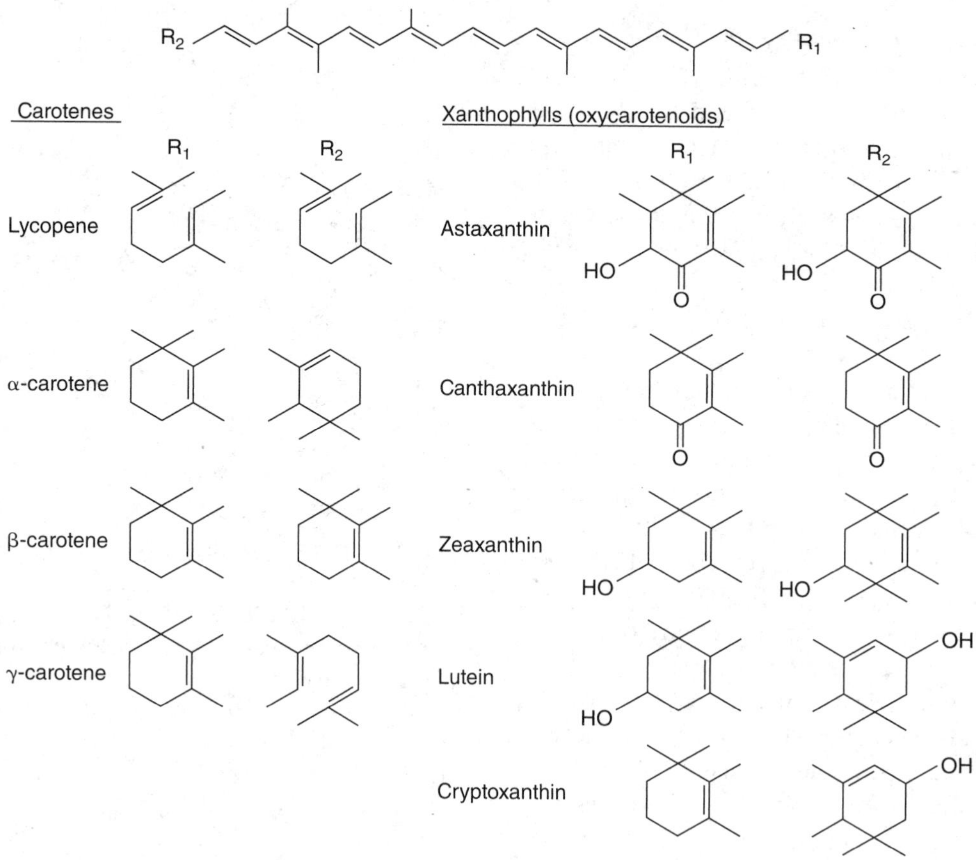

FIGURE 14.5 Select Carotenoids (tetraterpenoids). Select carotenoids, include carotenes and xanthophylls. Carotenes are hydrocarbon molecules whereas xanthophylls contain oxygen in various forms, such as hydroxyl, methoxyl, and carboxyl groups on the ring structures. A wide variety of vegetables contain carotenoids.

having a basic structure of 40 carbons with unique modifications (**FIGURE 14.5**).

Different foods have different kinds and relative amounts of carotenoids. Also, the carotenoid content can vary seasonally and during the ripening process. For example, peaches contain violaxanthin, cryptox-anthin, β-carotene, persicaxanthin, neoxanthin, and as many as 25 other carotenoids; apricots contain mostly α-carotene, β-carotene, and lycopene; and carrots contain about 50 to 55 parts per million of carotene in total, mostly α-carotene, β-carotene, and z-carotene, as well as lycopene. Many vegetable oils also contain carotenoids, with palm oil containing the most. For example, crude palm oil contains up to 0.2% carotenoids.

Phenolic Compounds

Like the terpenoids, phenolic compounds are also considered secondary metabolites. The base for this very diverse family of molecules is a phenol struc-ture, which is a hydroxyl group on an aromatic ring. From this structure, larger and more interest-ing molecules are formed, such as anthocyanins, coumarins, phenylpropamides, flavonoids, tannins, and lignin. Phenolic compounds perform a variety of functions for plants, including defending against herbivores and pathogens, absorbing light, attract-ing pollinators, reducing the growth of competitive plants, and promoting a symbiotic relationship with nitrogen-fixing bacteria.

A number of biosynthetic pathways form phe-nolic compounds. The predominant pathways are the **shikimic acid pathway** and the **malonic acid pathway**. The shikimic acid pathway is named as such because an intermediate of the pathway is shi-kimic acid. The shikimic acid pathway is more sig-nificant in higher plants, although the malonic acid pathway is also present. The malonic pathway is the predominant source of secondary metabolites in lower plants, fungi, and bacteria and this chemical pathway begins with acetyl CoA.

In the shikimic pathway, simple carbohydrate intermediates of glycolysis and the pentose phosphate path-way (PPP) are used to form the aromatic amino acids phenylalanine and tyrosine (**FIGURE 14.6**). A third aromatic amino acid, tryptophan, is also a deriv-ative of this pathway. Because animals do not have the shikimic acid pathway, these aromatic amino acids are essential amino acids in the diet. The basic flavonone

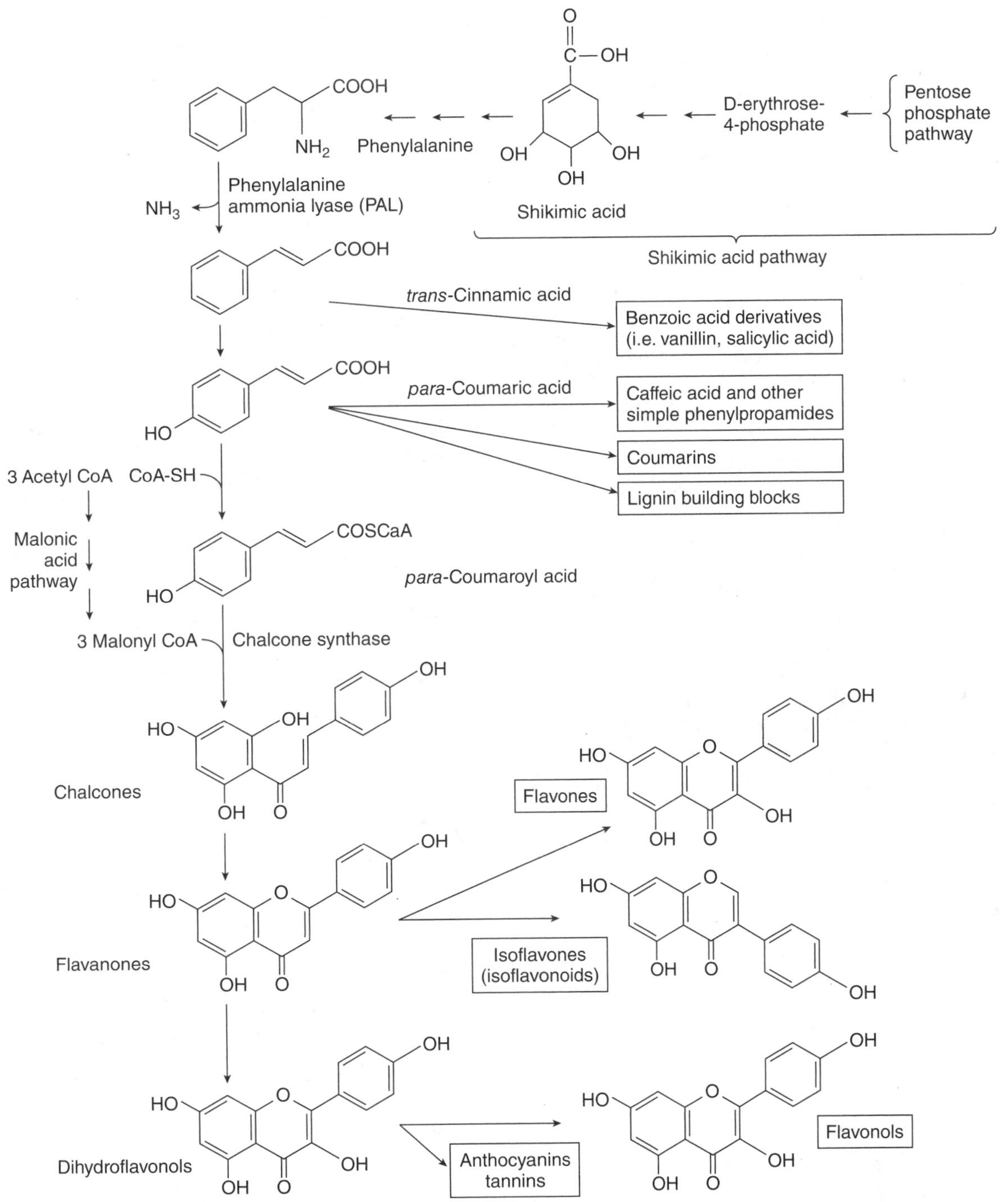

FIGURE 14.6 Production of Phenolic Compounds from Phenylalanine and Acetyl CoA. The basic structure of phenolic compounds is the presence of a hydroxyl group on an aromatic ring. The two biochemical pathways that produce this are the Shikimic acid pathway (found in plants only) and the Malonic acid pathway. The Shikimic acid pathway produces phenylalanine, but this pathway is not present in animals and thus phenylalanine must be provided by the diet. Malonic acid is produced from Acetyl CoA as a precursor. Both pathways lead to the production of a flavonone structure, which acts as a precursor to flavones, isoflavones, and flavonols.

structure produced by the pathway is the precursor for the flavones, isoflavones, and flavonols. Flavonones can also be used to make anthocyanins and tannins via dihydroflavonols (**FIGURES 14.7** and **14.8**).

The flavonoids are one the largest classes of phenolic compounds in plants. Perhaps the most ubiquitous flavonoid is quercetin. Hesperidin is also a common

flavonoid, especially in citrus fruits. Flavonoids have 15 carbons and are endowed with two aromatic rings linked by a three-carbon bridge (**FIGURE 14.9**). The rings are labeled A and B. Although the simpler phenolic compounds and lignin building blocks result from the shikimic acid pathway and are phenylalanine derivatives, formation of the flavonoids requires some

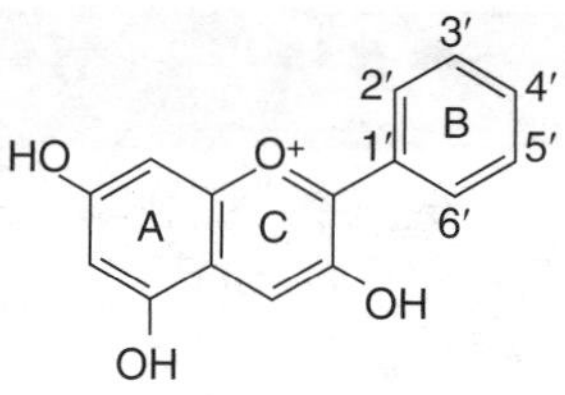

Anthocyanidin

Anthocyanidin derivatives and pigment color

Anthocyanidin	Substitutes	Color
Perlargonidin	4'–OH	Orange–Red
Cyanidin	3'–OH, 4'–OH	Purple–Red
Delphinidin	3'–OH, 4'–OH, 5'–OH	Blue–Purple
Peonidin	3'–OCH$_3$, 4'–OH	Rose–Red
Petunidin	3'–OCH$_3$, 4'–OH, 5'–OCH$_3$	Purple

(a)

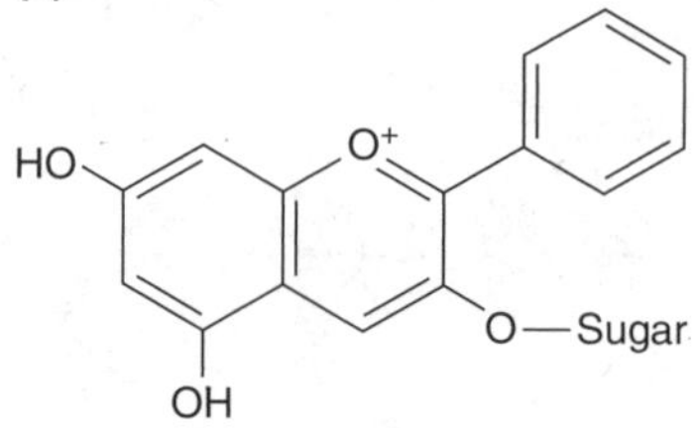

(b)

FIGURE 14.7 Anthocyanidins and Anthocyanin. These are pant flavonones as synthesized in Figure 14.6. (a) Generalized structure of an anthocyanidin. The table details chemical substitutions on specific carbons of the B ring to produce a particular anthocyanidin. (b) Chemical structure of anthocyanin. Anthocyanin is an anthocyanidin derivative with sugar moieties on the "C" ring.

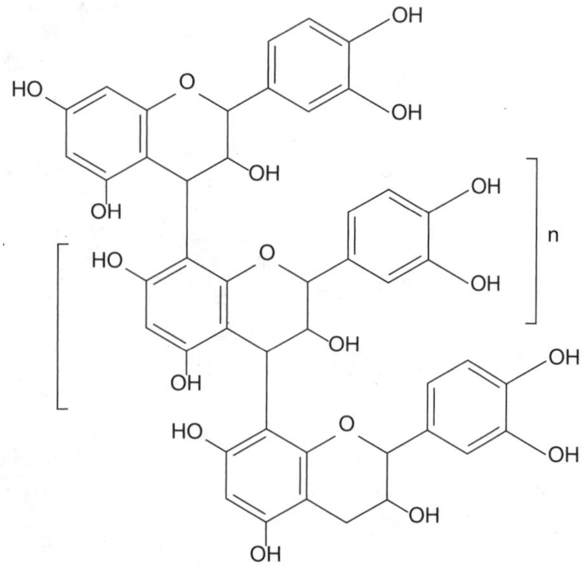

FIGURE 14.8 Basic Tannin Structure Formed from Phenolic Units. Tannins are produced from flavonones (see Figure 14.6).

FIGURE 14.9 Flavonoids. (a) Basic flavonoid carbon structure. (b) Carbons 5 through 8 are derived from the malonic acid pathway and carbons 2 through 4 and 1' through 6' are derived from the shikimic acid pathway via the amino acid phenylalanine. Carbons 2 through 4 comprise the three-carbon bridge.

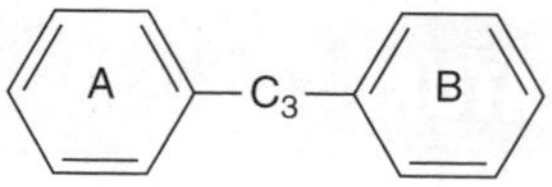

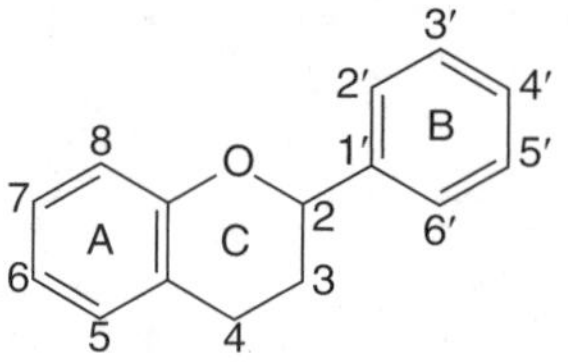

Ring B and the three-carbon bridge are derived from the shikimic acid pathway. The flavonoids are subclassified based primarily on the degree of oxidation of the three-carbon bridge.

Flavonoids typically have hydroxyl groups at carbon positions 4, 5, and 7, as well as other locations. The majority of naturally occurring flavonoids are actually glycosides, meaning that a sugar moiety is attached. The attachment of hydroxyl groups and sugars will increase the hydrophilic properties of the flavonoid molecule, whereas attachment of methyl esters or modified isopentyl units will increase the lipophilic character. The primary structural feature that separates isoflavones from the other flavonoids is a shift in the position of the B ring.

Some plants produce the flavonoids known as **anthocyanins** and **anthocyanidins**, which function largely as pigments. Basically, anthocyanins are anthocyanidins but with sugar moieties attached at position 3 of the three-carbon bridge between rings A and B (ring C). These compounds are responsible for the red, pink, blue, and violet coloring of many fruits and vegetables, including blueberries, apples, red cabbage, cherries, grapes, oranges, peaches, plums, radishes, raspberries, and strawberries. Only about 16 anthrocyanidins have been identified in plants, and they include pelargonidin, cyanidin, delphinidin, peonidin, malvidin, and petunidin.

Another group of phenolic compounds is stilbenes, which have health benefits. **SPECIAL FEATURE 14.2** details the structure, health benefits, and mechanisms by which they promote health. Two compounds that have been promoted and studied extensively are **resveratrol** and **pterostilbene**. These compounds are found in grapes, berries, and red wine and afford positive health benefits.

assistance from both the shikimic acid pathway and the malonic acid pathway. Ring A is derived from acetic acid (acetyl CoA) and the malonic acid pathway.

SPECIAL FEATURE 14.2

The Stilbenes: Resveratrol and Pterostilbene

Stilbenes are a class of nonflavanoid polyphenolic compounds that are often found in some foods. Different types of plants produce these compounds. There are a number of stilbenes but two of them that have nutritional and health significance are resveratrol and pterostilbene. These chemicals are similar to one another with pterostilbene having two methyl groups whereas resveratrol does not have any (**FIGURE 1**).

Pterostilbene is present in grapes and blueberries. Resveratrol is also found in grapes and blueberries, and other berries. Resveratrol is widely known as a component of wine, particularly red, and has received much attention from both the scientific and lay communities. Pterostilbene has not received as much attention, but research suggests it may exert more positive health benefits compared with resveratrol. Both of these stilbenes are produced in plants in response to stress and injury and have antifungal properties.

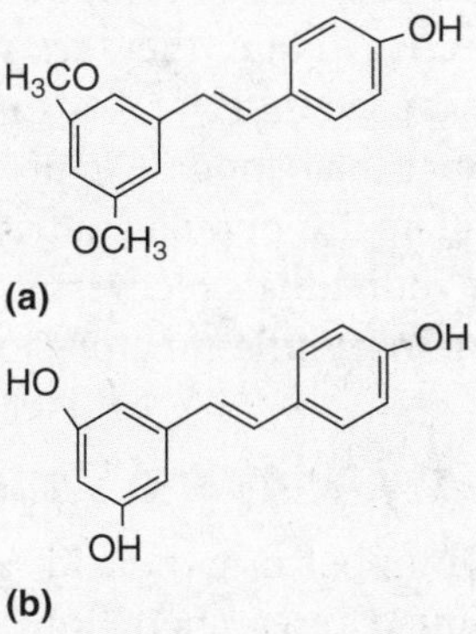

These stilbenes are known as having both antioxidant and anti-inflammatory properties; and protect against cardiovascular disease, cancers, and improve cognitive function. Some studies suggest that pterostilbene has stronger properties on some of these functions compared with resveratrol. As mentioned, blueberries are a good source or anthocyanins, which also has health effects, but the presence of pterostilbene in blueberries may exert a more powerful health effect. For instance, both stilbenes offer chemopreventive activities but pterostilbene is much more powerful as it takes less quantity compared with resveratrol.

Stilbenes, particularly pterostilbene, are effective in combating various cancer types. In animal models, less pterostilbene was required compared with resveratrol to combat cancers. The inhibitory effect is thought to be due to an increase in enzymes (Phase II enzymes), which enhances the excretion of carcinogens.

FIGURE 1 Chemical structure of (a) pterostilbene and (b) resveratrol.

Stilbenes increase antioxidant enzymes, such as glutathione S-transferase and glutathione in colon cancer cells. Oxidative stress, which can lead to cancer, is attenuated by both stilbenes. An enhanced erythroid 2-related factor 2 (Nrf2) expression is evident with pterostilbene and resveratrol. Nrf2, a transcription factor, will lead to the expression of antioxidant enzymes. Additionally, these stilbenes are anti-inflammatory. Inducible nitric oxide synthase (iNOS) is proinflammatory in colon cancer cells, but pterostilbene can block the expression of iNOS.

Increased apoptosis and decreased cell proliferation is another mechanism that can decrease cancer. Studies with pterostilbene indicate both increased apoptosis and decreased cell proliferation in breast, bladder, lung, colon, prostate, and stomach cancers.

Stilbenes can improve cognitive function and decrease both Parkinson's and Alzheimer's diseases. Pterostilbene crosses the blood brain barrier more easily than resveratrol. The neuroprotection proposed by these compounds is upregulation of Mn-SOD. Moreover, it appears that the increase in Mn-SOD depends on the upregulation of the transcription factor PPARα. Many of the studies demonstrating improved brain function were with blueberry feeding studies.

Cardiovascular disease is decreased with stilbene intake. Myocardial infarcts and hypertension are decreased with animals fed blueberries; and function is improved. Atherosclerosis may be decreased as LDL-cholesterol levels decline. This is likely due to the upregulation of PPARα, which leads to increased synthesis of enzymes involved in fatty acid β-oxidation. Leptin and PPARγ, which promote fat biosynthesis, are both decreased. However, not all studies have demonstrated an impact upon LDL-cholesterol levels, particularly in humans.

Stilbenes can prevent diabetes as decreased glucose and glycosylated hemoglobin (HbA1c) and increased insulin levels result from pterostilbene feeding. Furthermore, pterostilbene may enhance peripheral utilization of glucose and liver hexokinase activity. The latter results in greater uptake of glucose.

There are clear lines of evidence that stilbenes, especially pterostilbenes, and blueberries have a positive health benefit on a variety of diseases that are of public health concern. In some instances, pterostilbenes and resveratrol can be found as a supplement. The safety of the levels of these compounds that can be consumed in such forms have not been fully addressed. At the least, it would appear that the grapes, blueberries, and other berries are functional foods that should be consumed.

Carbohydrates and Carbohydrate Derivatives

Carbohydrates are also sources of nutraceuticals. The glucose derivative ascorbic acid (vitamin C) is perhaps one of the most recognizable nutraceutical substances and is a very popular supplement. Ascorbic acid functions as a nutraceutical compound—primarily as an antioxidant.

Fibers are also carbohydrate-based nutraceuticals. Fibers are digestion-resistant polysaccharides that are grouped together with the phenolic polymer compound lignin to form one of the most recognizable nutraceutical families. By and large, fiber plays a structural role in plants. For example, cellulose and hemicellulose are major structural polysaccharides found within plant cell walls. Beyond providing structural characteristics to plant tissue, another interesting role of certain fibers in plants is in tissue repair after trauma, somewhat analogous to scar tissue in animals.

Another family of polysaccharides that is worthy of discussion is the glycosaminoglycans (GAGs). Although these compounds are found in animal connective tissue, they are important to this discussion because they are also potential components of functional foods. At present, GAG and chondroitin sulfate are popular nutrition supplements being used by individuals recovering from joint injuries or suffering from inflammatory joint disorders.

Fatty Acids and Structural Lipids

A number of fatty acids and/or their derivatives have piqued researchers' interest for their possible nutraceutical potential. These include the ω-3 PUFA found in higher concentrations in plants, fish, and other marine animals and the **conjugated linoleic acid (CLA)** produced by bacteria in the rumen of grazing animals, such as cattle. The formation of CLA probably serves to help control the vitality of the releasing bacterial population in the rumen. The ω-3 PUFA in plants and fish probably play an important role in their membranes. Some plants also use ω-3 PUFA in a second-messenger system to form jasmonic acid when plant tissue is under attack (i.e., by insect feeding).

Plants primarily produce fatty acids in order to form triglycerides to serve as energy stores (oils). Fatty acids are also components of plant cell membrane glycerophospholipids and glyceroglycolipids, which serve similar roles as phospholipids in humans. In fact, several of the plant glycerophospholipids are structurally similar to phospholipids. Some of the major fatty acids produced include palmitic acid (16:0), oleic acid (18:1 ω-9), linoleic acid (18:2 ω-6), and linolenic acid (18:3 ω-3). Grazing animals ingest linoleic acid from plants, which is then metabolized to CLA by rumen bacteria. Herbivorous fish also ingest these fatty acids when they consume algae and other seaweeds and phytoplankton. Carnivorous fish and marine animals then acquire these PUFA and their derivatives from the tissue of other fish and marine life. Fish will further metabolize the PUFA to produce longer and more unsaturated fatty acids, such as DHA (docosahexaenoic acid, 22:6 ω-3) and EPA (eicosapentaenoic acid, 20:5 ω-3). The elongation and further unsaturation yields cell membrane fatty acids that are better suited for the colder temperatures and higher hydrostatic pressures associated with deep-water environments. CLA is found mostly in the fat and milk of ruminant animals, which indicates that beef, dairy foods, and lamb are major dietary sources.

CLA has been noted to potentially impact body composition and might have antineoplastic properties.

Protein, Amino Acids, and Amino Acid Derivatives

This class of nutraceuticals may include intact or hydrolyzed proteins (i.e., whey protein), polypeptides, amino acids, and nitrogenous and sulfur amino acid derivatives. Food proteins exhibit different digestion kinetics, peptide products, and amino acid composition, which might lead to nutraceutical and functional food benefits. For instance, whey protein is rapidly digested and a potent stimulator of body (and muscle) protein synthesis and is insulinogenic. Some of these properties are based on the leucine–rich, amino-acid content and peptide products that increase incretin levels, which have an impact on the pancreatic tissue.

At this time, a few amino acids are being investigated for their nutraceutical potential outside of sports nutrition, including leucine (and Branched Chain Amino Acids [BCAA]), arginine, taurine, and aspartic acid. Arginine, whose precursor, citrulline, is often purported to be cardioprotective because it is a precursor molecule for nitric oxide (NO), promotes vasodilation. Some speculate that it may also reduce atherogenesis. Taurine may have blood pressure–lowering properties as well as an antioxidant role. Meanwhile, the amino acid derivative creatine, which naturally occurs in meats and is produced endogenously, has been recognized for its potential nutraceutical benefit to the musculoskeletal system and neurological tissue, especially during aging. However, research on the nutraceutical benefits of these amino acids is inconclusive, and the effects of supplementation of these amino acids on other aspects of human physiology are unclear.

Several important plant molecules are formed via amino acids, including isothiocyanates, indole-3-carbinol, allyl sulfur compounds, and capsaicinoids. One important nutraceutical amino acid–derived molecule is folic acid, which is believed to be cardioprotective in its role of minimizing homocysteine levels. Other members of this group would include the tripeptide glutathione and choline.

Minerals

Several minerals have been recognized for their nutraceutical potential and thus have become candidates for inclusion in functional foods. Among the most obvious mineral with nutraceutical properties is calcium. Calcium has a strong role in promoting bone health, but it may also have a role in preventing colon cancer, hypertension, and cardiovascular disease. Potassium has also been purported to reduce hypertension and thus improve cardiovascular health. A couple of trace minerals have also been purported to have nutraceutical potential. These include copper, selenium, manganese, and zinc. Their nutraceutical potential is usually discussed in relation to their possible role as antioxidants. Copper, zinc, and manganese are components of superoxide dismutase (SOD) enzymes, whereas selenium is a component of glutathione peroxidase. Certainly more investigation is required in the area of trace elements in light of their metabolic relationships to other nutrients and the potential for toxicity.

Microbes (Probiotics)

Whereas the other groupings of nutraceuticals involve molecules or elements, probiotics involve intact micro-organisms. Most probiotic organisms are bacteria. In order to be classified as a probiotic a microbe must be resistant to acid conditions of stomach, bile, and digestive enzymes normally found in the human gastrointestinal tract; be able to colonize human intestine; be safe for human consumption; and have scientifically proven efficacy. Among the bacterial species recognized as having functional food potential are *Lactobacillus acidophilus*, *L. plantarum*, *L. casei*, *Bifidobacterium bifidum*, *B. infantis*, and *Streptococcus salivarius* subspecies *thermophilus*. Some yeast have also been noted as being probiotics, including *Saccharomyces boulardii*. Probiotics may help alleviate symptoms of gastrointestinal disorders, such as irritable bowel syndrome (IBS), diarrhea, Crohn disease, ulcerative colitis, and lactose intolerance through the reduction of pathogenic bacteria in the gut.

● BEFORE YOU GO ON . . .

1. What are the roles of the shikimic acid pathway and the malonic acid pathway in the production of phenol-based nutraceuticals?

2. List some examples of nutraceuticals that are isoprenoid derivatives.

3. Provide an example of a nutraceutical from each of the following categories: (a) carbohydrate (b) fatty acid (c) mineral (d) probiotic.

🩺 CLINICAL INSIGHT

What is the Role of Nutritionists and Dietitians in Advising Use of Functional Foods and Nutraceuticals?

The use of functional foods and nutraceuticals have made it into dietetic and nutrition curricula. There have been ample and convincing publications on the positive health effects of these compounds and foods in promoting a healthy diet. It is important that practitioners remain aware of the literature and advances in this field.

There are some words of caution that should be considered. It would appear that most of the positive data on these foods and compounds demonstrate that they can prevent the onset or delay many chronic diseases. From a public health perspective, this is important to promote within reason. However, in many instances, treating a disease that is chronic or advanced may not be as efficacious. Stated another way, a distinction should be made in distinguishing public heath aspects from clinical aspects in the field. It would be inappropriate for the practitioner to encourage the use of these products and foods in the place of prescription medications or other evidence-based treatments. Food labeling does not allow nutrition and disease claims; however, it does allow for structure and function claims. This is appropriate.

Foods, such as berries, fruits, whole grains, cold water fish, and vegetables, are functional foods and are already encouraged as part of a healthy diet. Other foods produced by food manufacturers are important. A good example is calcium-fortified orange juice, perhaps the most popular functional beverage, which is beneficial to most women and even males for promoting either peak bone mass or decreasing the loss of bone. Historically, nutrition focused on studying "required nutrients" in which deficiency signs were present when they were lacking in the diet. This is still the case today. However, the paradigm shift for functional foods and nutraceuticals is to optimize nutritional health and is less concerned about nutrition deficiencies.

Unfortunately, not all claims about functional foods are always accurate and often, a review of websites where some foods are advocated as having specific benefits need to be reviewed with caution. A good example is the issue of gluten-free diets where foods have wheat and rye removed. Gluten-sensitive enteropathy is a disease whereby patients have an immune response by their gastrointestinal track and leads to inflammation and malabsorption of nutrients. The role of such products has been advocated to benefit health for those not diagnosed with gluten sensitivity. There have been ad hoc reports that consumers of gluten-free products use them to "feel better" or lose weight. A problem with this, especially advocating it as a weight loss food, is that the evidence for such a claim is lacking. Gluten-free foods are higher in fat and sugar. Many of the products are higher in calories and often lead to weight gain and not weight loss. With new functional foods and nutraceuticals being developed and/or advocated, evidence-based studies need to confirm their benefit. It is, therefore, critical that dietitians and nutritionists study each item on its own merit before offering an opinion to a client or consumer. In most cases, functional foods and nutraceuticals have a place in a well-balanced diet.

▸ Here's What You Have Learned

1. Experts have developed a variety of definitions of what a functional food is. The most common definition of a functional food is that it is a food that provides a health benefit beyond basic nutrition. Nutraceuticals are the chemical components of functional foods that provide the particular health benefit.

2. Nutraceuticals can be of plant, animal, or microbial origin. Oftentimes, a particular nutraceutical can be found in a variety of different foods. Some foods that have the same nutraceuticals may have little relation with one another.

3. Nutraceuticals may be classified based on (a) their chemical, elemental, or molecular aspects; (b) the food sources in which they appear; (c) their mechanism of action; and (d) their proposed health benefits.

4. Nutraceuticals classified on the basis of mechanism of action are sometimes grouped as follows: anticancer, positive blood profile indicators, antioxidants, anti-inflammatories, and osteogenic protective properties.

5. Isoprenoid derivatives include nutraceuticals, such as carotenoids, tocopherols, saponins, and limonoids. Some of these derivatives are present in plant oils. Even coffee beans may offer cancer protection by the presence of the diterpenes, kahweol and cafestol.

6. Phenolic-derived nutraceuticals include a variety of aromatic compounds, such as anthocyanins, coumarins, flavonoids, tannins, and lignins. These compounds have two aromatic rings linked by a carbon bridge. In the case of flavonoids, two metabolic pathways are involved in the production of each ring: ring A is produced by the malonic acid pathway and ring B is produced by the shikimic acid pathway.

7. A variety of nutraceuticals are derived from essential nutrients that, although needed for growth and maintenance, also offer health benefits. Ascorbic acid, fiber, and glycosaminoglycans are carbohydrate-derived nutraceuticals; ω-3 PUFA and CLA are examples of fatty acid–based nutraceuticals; some amino acids, such as arginine, ornithine, taurine, and aspartic acid, may serve as amino acid–based nutraceuticals; and calcium, as well as other minerals, are mineral-based nutraceuticals.

8. Probiotics are a class of microbial nutraceuticals that have received a great deal of attention in recent years. Probiotic species include *Lactobacillus acidophilus*, *Bifidobacterium bifidum*, and *Streptococcus salivarius* subspecies *thermophilus*. Some yeast also have probiotic properties. Probiotics may be effective in the treatment of several gastrointestinal disorders, such as irritable bowel syndrome (IBS) and Crohn disease.

9. Protein, peptides, and amino acids can have specific application based on rate of digestion, potency to promote protein synthesis in muscle, and other tissue. Certain amino acids, including nonproteogenic ones, can have unique roles, including circulation support and cell buffering.

▸ Suggested Reading

Crowe KM, Francis C. Academy of Nutrition and Dietetics. Position of the Academy of Nutrition and Dietetics: functional foods. *J Acad Nutr Diet*. 2013.113(8):1096–1103.

Daliri EB, Oh DH, Lee BH. Bioactive Peptides. *Foods*. 2017;6(5):pii: E32.

Distrutti E, Cipriani S, Mencarelli A, Renga B, Fiorucci S. Probiotics VSL#3 protect against development of visceral pain in murine model of irritable bowel syndrome. *PLoS One*. 2013;15;8(5):e63893.

Health Canada. 2013. Available at: http://www.agr.gc.ca/eng /industry-markets-and-trade/statistics-and-market-information /by-product-sector/functional-foods-and-natural-health -products/functional-foods-and-nutraceuticals-canadian -industry/?id=1170856376710.

Hodge AM, English DR, McCredie MR, et al. Foods, nutrients and prostate cancer. *Cancer Causes Control*. 2004;15(1):11–20.

Huang WY, Davidge ST, Wu J. Bioactive natural constituents from food sources-potential use in hypertension prevention and treatment. *Crit Rev Food Sci Nutr*. 2013;53(6):615–630.

Hui C, Qi X, Qianyong Z, Xiaoli P, Jundong Z, Mantian M. Flavonoids, flavonoid subclasses and breast cancer risk: a meta-analysis of epidemiologic studies. *PLoS One*. 2013;8(1):e54318.

International Food Information Council. 2013. Available at: http:// foodinsight.org.

Institute of Food Technology 2013 Website. Available at: http:// www.ift.org/knowledge-center/focus-areas/food-health-and -nutrition/functional-foods.aspx

International Life Science Institute. 2013. Available at: http://www.ilsi. org. http://www.ilsi.org/Europe/Pages/TF_FunctionalFoods.aspx

Lai CS, Li S, Miyauchi Y, Suzawa M, Ho CT, Pan MH. Potent anti-cancer effects of citrus peel flavonoids in human prostate xenograft tumors. *Food Funct*. 2013;4(6):944–949.

Kosuru R, Rai U, Prakash S, Singh A, Singh S. Promising therapeutic potential of pterostilbene and its mechanistic insight based on preclinical evidence. *Eur J Pharmacol*. 2016;789:229–243.

Leonardi T, Vanamala J, Taddeo SS, et al. Apigenin and naringenin suppress colon carcinogenesis through the aberrant crypt stage in azoxymethane-treated rats. *Exp Biol Med (Maywood).* 2010;235(6):710–717.

Medeiros DM, Hampton M. Olive oil and health benefits. In: Wildman RED (ed.), *Handbook of Nutraceuticals and Functional Foods.* 2nd ed. Boca Raton, FL: CRC Press, Taylor and Francis Group: 2009;297–308.

Miles EA, Zoubouli P, Calder PC. Differential anti-inflammatory effects of phenolic compounds from extra virgin olive oil identified in human whole blood cultures. *Nutrition.* 2005;21(3):389–394.

Miller EG, McWhorter K, Rivera-Hildalgo F, Wright JM, Hirsbrunner P, Sunahara GI. Kahweol and cafestol: inhibitors of hamster buccal pouch carcinogenesis. *Nutr Cancer.* 1991;15(1):41–46.

Owen RW, Mier W, Giacosa A, Hull WE, Spiegelhalder B, Bartsch H. Identification of lignans as major compounds in the phenolic fraction of olive oil. *Clin Chem.* 2000;46(7): 976–988.

Patel S, Santani D, Shah M, Patel V. Anti-hyperglycemic and anti-hyperlipidemic effects of *Bryonia laciniosa* seed extract and its saponin fraction in streptozotocin-induced diabetes in rats. *J Young Pharm.* 2012;4(3):171–176.

Perez-Jimenez F, Alvarez de Cienfuegos G, Badimon L, et al. International conference on the healthy effect of virgin olive oil. *Eur J Clin Invest.* 2005;35(7):421–424.

Pierre AS, Minville-Walz M, Fèvre C, et al. Trans-10, cis-12 conjugated linoleic acid induced cell death in human colon cancer cells through reactive oxygen species-mediated ER stress. *Biochim Biophys Acta.* 2013;1831(4):759–768.

Simonsen NR, Fernandez-Crehuet Navajas J, Martin-Moreno JM, et al. Tissue stores of individual monounsaturated fatty acids and breast cancer: the EURAMIC study. European Community Multicenter Study on Antioxidants, Myocardial Infarction, and Breast Cancer. *Am J Clin Nutr.* 1998;68(1):134–141.

Taiz L, Zeiger E. *Plant Physiology.* 2nd ed. Sunderland, MA: Sinauer Associates;1998.

Visioli F, Galli C. The effect of minor constituents of olive oil on cardiovascular disease: new findings. *Nutr Rev.* 1998;56(5 pt 1): 142–147.

Visioli F, Bellomo G, Montedoro GF, Galli C. Low density lipoprotein oxidation is inhibited in vitro by olive oil constituents. *Atherosclerosis.* 1995;117(1):25–32.

Wattenberg LW, Lam LKT. Protective effects of coffee constituents on carcinogenesis in experimental animals. *Banbury Rep.* 1984;17:137–145.

Whelan K, Quigley EM. Probiotics in the management of irritable bowel syndrome and inflammatory bowel disease. *Curr Opin Gastroenterol.* 2013;29(2):184–189.

Wildman REC, Kelley M. *Nutraceuticals and foods.* In: Wildman REC (ed.), *Handbook of Nutraceuticals and Functional Food.* 2nd ed. Boca Raton, FL: CRC Press, Taylor and Francis Group: 2009;1–21.

Yue R, Yamada A, Watanabe K, et al. Production of eicosapentaenoic acid by a recombinant marine cyanobacterium, *Synechococcus* sp. *Lipids.* 2000;35(10):1061–1064.

Glossary

A

α-ketoadipic aciduria A genetic defect in a gene that encodes for the enzyme α-ketoadipic dehydrogenase that converts α-ketoadipic acid to glutaryl-CoA. α-ketoadipic acid accumulates and in infants this disease can lead to difficulty with motor skills and may have seizures.

abetalipoproteinemia A recessive genetic disorder that results in the malabsorption of fat and fat-soluble vitamins from food. It is due to a failure to produce apolipoprotein B, which is needed for the formation of chylomicrons and very low-density lipoproteins.

acetoacetate A type of ketone body.

acetone A type of ketone body.

acetyl CoA carboxylase A key enzyme that begins fatty acid synthesis by catalyzing the carboxylation of acetyl CoA to produce malonyl CoA.

acrodermatitis enteropathica A recessive genetic disorder in which zinc uptake by the small intestine is markedly diminished due to a defect in the transporter ZIP4 protein, leading to signs of zinc deficiency.

actin Thin contractile protein of muscle tissue.

action potential Rapid and specific change in the electric properties of a plasma membrane in response to a stimulus.

active transport Energy-requiring movement of a substance across a membrane, via a transport protein, against a gradient (e.g., concentration, electric).

adipocyte Another name for a fat cell that composes adipose tissue.

aerobic Requiring oxygen for energy metabolism.

alanine–glucose cycle A series of reactions between muscle and the liver, whereby amino acids in the muscle are converted to alanine, which is transported via the blood to the liver, where the alanine is converted first to pyruvate and then to glucose, which can then circulate back to muscle.

albumin A blood protein that is water soluble and carries a variety of salt and nutrients; it helps to maintain osmotic pressure of the blood.

alcoholic liver disease A general term that is used to describe alcohol-related liver diseases, such as fatty liver, hepatitis, fibrosis, and cirrhosis.

aldosterone A steroid hormone produced by the adrenal glands that helps regulate blood pressure and increases the reabsorption of sodium and secretion of potassium from the kidney tubules.

alkaptonuria An inborn error of metabolism in which a tyrosine breakdown product, homogentisate, is unable to be converted to the next product, maleyl-acetoacetate, due to a defect in the enzyme homogentisate dioxygenase. Accumulation of homogentisate leads to problems with joints and connective tissue.

amine oxidase Copper-containing enzyme that catabolizes certain amino acids, such as histidine and tyramine.

amino acid A compound that contains a central carbon that has an amine group, a carboxyl group, and a hydrogen atom and has a side chain (R) bonded to it. It is the building block of proteins.

amino acid score See *chemical score.*

amylase Enzyme found in saliva and pancreatic juice that digests amylose and straight chains in amylopectin.

amyloid-β peptides Plaques and neurofibrillary tangles in brain tissue found in Alzheimer's disease.

amyloid precursor protein Precursor to amyloid-β peptides found in brain tissue of Alzheimer's disease.

amylopectin Starch consisting of straight chains of glucose with branching.

amylose Starch consisting of straight chains of glucose.

anaerobic Energy systems that do not have an oxygen requirement.

android A pattern of adipose tissue accumulation, mainly in the trunk and upper body; often referred to as "apple-shaped" or central obesity. Android fat accumulation is more common in males and increases the risk of obesity-related diseases.

anemia A decrease in the number of red blood cells, a decrease in the amount of hemoglobin, or any other condition leading to a decrease in the oxygen-carrying capacity of blood.

angiotensin I A liver protein produced from angiotensinogen through the actions of the kidney enzyme renin.

angiotensin II A product of angiotensin I that is produced in the lung by angiotensin-converting enzyme. Production of angiotensin II results in the release of aldosterone from the adrenal cortex and antidiuretic hormone from the pituitary gland.

angiotensin-converting enzyme (ACE) An enzyme in the lung that converts angiotensin I to angiotensin II.

angiotensinogen An inactive or precursor liver protein that, when activated, may lead to a series of compounds that are involved in water and sodium regulation as well as blood pressure.

antidiuretic hormone (ADH) A peptide hormone produced by the hypothalamus that facilitates the reabsorption of water by the kidney tubules. Also known as vasopressin.

anthocyanidin A class of purple to blue plant flavonoid pigments without sugar moieties attached that have potential health benefits such as cancer prevention as well as anti-aging and anti-inflammatory effects.

anthocyanin A purple to blue plant flavenoid pigment present in many foods, such as blueberries, that have potential health benefits, such as cancer prevention as well as antiaging and anti-inflammatory effects. They are essentially anthocyanidins with sugar moieties attached.

aorta The major blood vessel exiting the heart at the left ventricle to carry blood to the body.

avidin A protein found in egg whites that binds tightly to biotin.

B

Barrett's syndrome A precancerous esophagus condition.

basal metabolic rate (BMR) The measurement of basal metabolism during a specific period of time (such as an hour or a day).

basal metabolism The energy expended during nonactive time (rest) at a comfortable environmental temperature and at least 12 hours after the consumption of a meal.

beriberi A disease affecting the nervous system that is caused by a thiamin deficiency.

β-glucan A polysaccharide composed of D-glucose units linked by β-glycosidic bonds.

β-hydroxybutyrate A type of ketone body.

bioelectrical impedance analysis (BIA) Procedure for assessing body composition in which an electric current is passed through the body. The resistance to current flow reflects the relative amount of fat present.

biological value (BV) The amount of nitrogen from protein digested, absorbed, and used by the body but not excreted.

Bitot spot The build-up of keratinized tissue on the conjunctiva of the eye due to a vitamin A deficiency.

bixin A carotenoid-like compound with antioxidant and anticarcinogenic effects.

blood pressure The pressure of blood against the vessel walls.

body composition The relative contributions to a person's mass made by different substances or tissues. Body composition can be broken down in various ways, such as fat mass and fat-free mass, or as water, bone mineral mass, other fat-free mass, and fat mass.

body mass index (BMI) An index of a person's weight in relation to height; determined by dividing the weight (in kilograms) by the square of the height (in meters).

body weight The total mass of a person, expressed in pounds (lb) or kilograms (kg).

brown adipose tissue (BAT) Specialized adipose tissue that can generate additional heat to maintain body temperature. Typically found in infants but not in significant amounts in adults.

Brown-Vialetto-Van Laere syndrome A disorder of the nervous and muscle systems due to genetic defects in the genes encoding riboflavin transporters RFVT2 and 3.

C

cafestol A molecule found in coffee that is thought to have strong anticancer properties but that may also elevate blood cholesterol levels.

calbindin A vitamin D–dependent calcium-binding protein present in the mucosal cells of the small intestine and in kidney cells.

capsaicinoid An amino acid–based nutraceutical found primarily in peppers that can be used in topical ointments and nasal sprays to relieve pain.

carbamoyl phosphate A negatively charged compound that is a key compound in the urea cycle necessary to convert ammonia to urea for disposal.

carbohydrate response element-binding protein (ChREBP) A transcription protein activated by a high-carbohydrate diet that upregulates genes that promote enzymes used in lipid synthesis.

carbonic anhydrase Enzyme that reversibly catalyzes the formation of carbonic acid (H_2CO_3) from CO_2 and H_2O.

cardiac output Product of stroke volume multiplied by heart rate in a minute (e.g., 5 L/min).

celiac sprue Autoimmune disorder of the small intestine that leads to diarrhea, abdominal distension, and malabsorption of nutrients. Sometimes used interchangeably with gluten-sensitive enteropathy.

cell The smallest functioning living unit.

cell membrane structure The outer portion of a cell, composed of lipid and protein.

cell receptor A protein on the surface of a cell membrane to which other proteins can bind to initiate a specific cell reaction.

cell signaling Biochemical processes in a cell responsible for communication and coordination of events.

cellulose Fiber component and main structural polysaccharide in plant cell walls that is composed of repeating glucose units with a β1–4 linkage.

central fatigue Fatigue that results from problems with the central nervous system resulting from the effects of hypoglycemia on the brain and nerves during prolonged exercise.

chaperone protein A protein that can fold or unfold other molecules. These proteins bind reactive trace elements and ferry them to different parts of the cell for delivery.

chemical score The amount of a limiting amino acid in a particular protein or diet in relation to the requirement or need by that organism. Also known as amino acid score.

chitin A carbohydrate that is a polymer of N-acetyl-glucosamine and composes the shells or exoskeletons of insects and crustacean. It is considered a type of human dietary fiber.

chloride shift The movement of chloride ions from the plasma into red blood cells when carbon dioxide is transferred from tissues to the plasma, which allows blood pH to be maintained.

cholangitis Inflammation of bile ducts.

cholelithiasis Production of gall stones.

cholestasis Little or no bile secreted.

cholecystitis Inflammation of the gallbladder.

chondroitin sulfate Glycosaminoglycan found in joint connective tissue, such as cartilage.

chromodulin An intracellular chromium-binding polypeptide that interacts with insulin at the cell membrane level by binding to the insulin receptor.

Cirrhosis Hardening and scarring of the liver.

cis On the same side of a double bond. In terms of fatty acids, each hydrogen atom is on the same side of a double bond.

clotting factor Substance in the blood that promotes clot formation.

colon The large intestine.

complete protein A protein that contains all essential amino acids capable of promoting growth and maintenance. Also known as a high biologic value protein.

computerized axial tomography (CAT or CT) scan Sophisticated form of low-intensity x-ray received by a detector across the tissue that produces a "slice" image of the body. Slices can be pieced together using a computer to provide a three-dimensional image.

conjugated linoleic acid (CLA) An ω-3 fatty acid with a single bond separating a pair of double bonds. It is found in meat and dairy products and is known for its strong anti-carcinogenic activity. CLA has been used to treat inflammatory bowel disease and is thought to facilitate weight loss by reducing fat and increasing lean tissue.

connective tissue A fibrous tissue that is involved in connecting other structures with one another and is composed of predominantly collagen protein.

core body temperature Temperature at the core of the body in and around vital organs.

Cori cycle The phases in the metabolism of carbohydrate: (1) glycogenolysis in the liver; (2) passage of glucose into the circulation; (3) deposition of glucose in muscles as glycogen; and (4) glycogenolysis during muscular activity and conversion to lactate, which is converted to glycogen in the liver. Also called the lactic acid cycle.

cotranslation The addition of a mineral-containing amino acid through the process of translation in polypeptide synthesis via a triplet codon. In most cases, this refers to the addition of selenocysteine to a polypeptide.

co-transport A transport mechanism in cells in which two compounds or substances are simultaneously transported across a membrane by the same carrier protein. Co-transport may or may not require ATP.

cretinism A congenital condition due to low maternal iodine intake during pregnancy that leads to stunted mental and physical growth.

CRISPR A strand of DNA with short repeats of DNA called "spacers" that is used as a gene editing tool.

crocetin A carotenoid found in saffron. It may reduce physical fatigue and improve sleep quality. It is better known for its potential to combat cancer.

Crohn's disease Chronic inflammation of the bowel, particularly the ileum of the small intestine.

CTR1 Copper transport protein 1; a membrane bound copper-binding protein that imports copper into cells.

cupric The inorganic form of copper with a +2 charge.

cuprous The inorganic form of copper with a +1 charge.

cyclooxygenase An enzyme that is important in the production of a group of powerful biochemical compounds called prostanoids, which include such compounds as prostaglandins, prostacyclin, and thromboxane.

cytochrome c oxidase A copper-containing multi-subunit polypeptide enzyme complex in the electron transport chain that is involved in the production of ATP and water.

D

DASH (Dietary Approaches to Stop Hypertension) eating plan A diet developed in conjunction with the National Heart, Lung and Blood Institute to control high blood pressure. The diet is low in sodium and encourages the consumption of nuts, whole grains, fish, poultry, fruits, and vegetables while lowering the consumption of red meats, sweets, and sugar. It is also abundant in potassium, magnesium, and calcium.

de novo lipogenesis The synthesis of complex lipids from simple compounds.

deamination The removal of amino groups from compounds, particularly amino acids, with the production of urea.

dehydration A loss of body fluids in excess.

denaturing The process by which a protein loses its complex tertiary and quaternary structure by heat, acids, salts, or solvents.

densitometry Method of assessing body composition based on body density assessment, including underwater weighing and plethysmography.

desaturation The biochemical process of removing a bond to create a double bond or unsaturated bond in a fatty acid.

diabetes insipidus A condition characterized by extreme water loss leading to extreme thirst. Normally caused by the lack of antidiuretic hormone.

diastolic blood pressure The lowest blood pressure exerted by the blood against the walls of the blood vessels when the heart is in relaxation.

dietary fiber A class of carbohydrates that is resistant to digestion.

dietary folate equivalent A unit of measure used to indicate the conversion of folic acid to folate. Folic acid is more potent than the folate that occurs naturally in foods, so the amount of folic acid consumed is multiplied by a factor of 1.7 to give the dietary folate equivalent.

dimerization An event in which two molecular complexes interact and proceed to perform a purposeful function.

diterpene A class of terpenoids found in plants that have antibacterial, antiviral, antifungal properties.

digestible indispensable amino acid score (DIAAS) A numerical term to compare relative protein quality with the level of essential amino acids present in a food.

direct calorimetry A method to assess whole-body energy expenditure; heat energy released by the body warms a layer of fluid surrounding a specialized room (metabolic chamber), and the change in fluid temperature is the energy expended.

disaccharide Carbohydrate molecule composed of two monosaccharides linked by a chemical bond.

distal convoluted tubule (DCT) The part of the renal nephron between the loop of Henle and the collecting duct system.

divalent metal transporter 1 (DMT1) A protein on the small-intestinal absorptive surface that is responsible for the absorption of iron and copper in their inorganic forms.

diverticulitis A condition where diverticula, or outpocketings, of the colon become inflamed and infected.

diverticulosis A condition in which there are outpocketings (diverticula) of the colon.

DNA Deoxyribonucleic acid; the genetic blueprint from which proteins are synthesized. A double-stranded helix of nucleotides.

dopamine hydroxylase A copper-containing enzyme that converts dopamine to norepinephrine.

doubly labeled water (DLW) Tool used to assess energy expenditure based on estimations of CO_2 production; uses water molecules with isotopes of hydrogen ^2H and ^{18}O.

dual-energy x-ray absorptiometry (DXA) Assesses body composition using low levels of x-rays; includes assessment of bone tissue.

duodenum First of three segments in the small intestine. Major site of absorption of nutrients.

E

edema Swelling of interstitial spaces with fluid that results in excess of accumulation of water in the tissues.

eicosanoid A powerful biochemical produced by long-chain fatty acids that has profound effects on physiology.

electrolyte A compound that ionizes when dissolved in water.

electron transport chain A series of enzymatic complexes associated with the inner membrane of the mitochondria and serving as the site of oxidative phosphorylation.

elongation The addition of carbons, usually two for each reaction, in the synthesis of fatty acids.

endoplasmic reticulum Membranous portion of a cell where protein synthesis and lipid synthesis occur.

endosome Cell structures that transport a variety of compounds to either lysosomes for degradation or to the cell membrane surface for recycling.

energy (calorie) balance The balance between energy consumed (and absorbed) and energy expended by the body.

enteric nervous system (ENS) One of the main divisions of the autonomic nervous system; its primary role is to support and regulate the function of the gastrointestinal system.

enterocyte A cell lining the wall of the small intestine that is involved in the absorption of nutrients.

enzyme A protein that facilitates a biochemical reaction by lowering the energy required.

epithelial A type of tissue or cell that may line surfaces or cavities of various structures and organs in the body.

epithelial cell A type of cell that composes tissues that line the surfaces of structures or cavities in organisms.

erythrocyte Another name for a red blood cell, or the oxygen-carrying cell of the blood.

erythropoiesis The cellular events involved in the production of red blood cells.

essential amino acid An amino acid needed for health and maintenance and that must be ingested because the tissues of the body cannot synthesize it.

essential fat Body fat associated with bone marrow, the central nervous system, internal organs, and, in women, the mammary glands and pelvic region; considered indispensable.

essential fatty acid A fatty acid needed by the body that must be supplied by the diet because the tissues are unable to synthesize it.

essential hypertension High blood pressure in the absence of any known cause.

euglycemia Achievement of an optimal fasting blood glucose level by hormonal regulation.

eukaryotic initiation factor (eIF) A combination of proteins needed to initiate translation and protein synthesis on the ribosomes.

excitable cell A cell capable of generating action potentials of electric current.

exon The portion of RNA transcribed from the DNA that is translated into a protein.

extrinsic pathway In blood clotting, the process by which prothrombin is activated through a series of reactions. Factor VII (a vitamin K–dependent protein) is activated by a tissue factor called thromboplastin. Activated factor VII then activates factor X, which activates prothrombin.

F

facilitated diffusion Movement of a substance across a membrane, via a transport protein, down a gradient (e.g., concentration, electric).

factorial method A method to determine the amount of nitrogen needed to take in to keep the body in nitrogen balance. This method determines obligatory nitrogen losses (the nitrogen loss in urine, feces, sweat, nails, and dermal sources) when a protein-free diet is given to test subjects.

farsenoid X receptor (FXR) A nuclear receptor that binds to a promoter of genes involved with bile metabolism.

fat-free mass (FFM) The mass of the body that is not fat, including muscle, bone, skin, and organs.

fatigue Reduction in athletic performance that stems from physiologic events in muscle (peripheral fatigue) or the central nervous system (central fatigue).

fatty acid A hydrocarbon chain with a carboxyl group as the terminal carbon. The chain may have double bonds or be completely saturated.

fatty liver Fat infiltration and inflammation of the liver.

fatty acid oxidation The breakdown of fatty acids two carbons at a time in the presence of oxygen.

fatty acid synthase A complex of multiple enzymes involved in the synthesis of fatty acids.

fatty acid synthesis The production of fatty acids two carbons at a time from acetyl CoA.

ferric The inorganic form of iron with a +3 charge.

ferritin A large and complex molecule consisting of 24 polypeptides that functions to store 4,500 atoms of iron for each molecule.

ferroportin A membrane protein that transports iron from inside a cell to the outside.

ferrous The inorganic form of iron with a +2 charge.

ferroxidase A copper-containing enzyme (e.g., ceruloplasmin) that has a profound effect on iron metabolism by promoting the conversion of the ferrous form of iron to the ferric form.

fiber Indigestible fibrous structural molecule found in plant tissue; includes indigestible straight and branched-chain polysaccharides as well as lignin.

fibrin A fibrous protein that serves as the foundational network of a blood clot.

fibrinogen A protein produced by the liver that forms a fibrin clot following the action of prothrombin.

fibroblast growth factor 23 (FGF23) A protein that works in tandem with the Klotho protein that decreases serum phosphate levels when elevated.

fluoridation The addition of the mineral fluoride to water to help prevent dental caries.

fluorosis The appearance of white specks or streaks on tooth enamel due to excess fluoride intake.

folium A Latin term meaning "leaf"; folic acid derives its name from this word because leafy vegetables are high in this water-soluble vitamin.

Forkhead box protein 01 (FOX01) A transcription factor that controls both mitochondria fatty acid metabolism and protection from oxidative stress.

fructan A class of fructose-based polymers of varying length that includes inulin, oligofructose, and fructooligosaccharides (FOS).

fructose Monosaccharide found in fruits and honey and as half of the disaccharide sucrose.

functional fiber A fiber that consists of isolated, nondigestible carbohydrates that have beneficial physiologic effects in humans.

functional food A food that provides health benefits beyond basic nutrition.

G

galactose Monosaccharide found, to a limited degree, in foods and as half of the disaccharide lactose.

gastric Refers to the stomach.

Gastric banding A type of bariatric surgery. A silicon band is placed around the top portion of the stomach to leave a small volume pouch, which allows for a greater sense of "fullness"

Gastric bypass A type of bariatric surgery in which the upper portion of the stomach is stapled to prevent food from entering the distal portion of the stomach, and an opening is created from the stomach to the small intestine in which a portion of the duodenum is bypassed to decrease absorption. Roux-En-Y bypass is another name.

Gastroplasty A type of bariatric surgery where the upper portion of the stomach is stapled to a reduced fixed size.

Gastric sleeve A type of bariatric surgery in which a portion of the stomach is stapled so that food passes from the esophagus, through the stomach sleeve, and enters the small intestine.

gene A portion of DNA that encodes for a specific protein.

glucogenic Normally refers to the production of glucose with the breakdown of certain amino acids.

glucosamine A basic building block of glycosaminoglycans; consists of glucose with an attached amine group.

glucose The most abundant monosaccharide in food carbohydrate and the primary carbohydrate that circulates in the blood.

glucose tolerance The ability to appropriately reestablish euglycemia following meal-induced hyperglycemia.

glucose transporter (GLUT) A family of proteins that transport glucose across cell membranes.

glucose transporter 5 (GLUT5) A family of transport proteins that shuttle fructose across cell membranes.

glucose-6-phosphate Created in the first reaction of glycolysis; can be used to make glycogen, to enter the pentose phosphate pathway, or to continue glycolysis.

glutaric aciduria type 1 An inborn error of tryptophan metabolism resulting from a defect in the enzyme glutaryl CoA dehydrogensase, which is involved in the breakdown of tryptophan. An intermediate breakdown product, glutaryl CoA, is converted to glutaric acid, which accumulates in fluids. This accumulation of glutaric acid may lead to seizures, acidosis, and an enlarged head.

glutathione A tripeptide of glutamic acid, cysteine, and glycine involved in antioxidant activities.

glutathione peroxidase A selenium-containing antioxidant enzyme that functions to convert hydrogen peroxide (produced by the enzyme catalase) to water.

gluten-sensitive enteropathy Sometimes referred to as celiac disease. Inflammation of the small intestine due to an autoimmune inflammatory disease precipitated by the ingestion of the wheat protein, gluten.

glycemia The level of glucose in the blood.

glycemic index The glycemic response of a food relative to a standard carbohydrate-containing food.

glycemic load The glycemic index of a food normalized for a standard serving size for a food.

glycemic response The degree and duration of elevation of blood glucose level that is produced by eating a specific food.

glycogen Carbohydrate storage molecule consisting of branching chains of glucose.

glycolysis The breakdown of glucose to pyruvate in a cell in the absence of oxygen.

glycosaminoglycan (GAG) A structurally unique polysaccharide that includes amino sugar (glucosamine or galactosamine); found in joints and connective tissue.

goiter Hypertrophy of the thyroid gland, caused by a deficiency of iodine.

goitrogen A substance, normally present in food, that interferes with iodine utilization by the thyroid gland.

Golgi apparatus Cellular organelle that packages macromolecules, such as lipids and proteins destined to become part of plasma membrane or released from the cell.

gum Water-soluble polysaccharides derived from plants, seaweed, or bacterial fermentation that are used as thickeners, gels, emulsifiers, and stabilizers in food.

gynoid A pattern of adipose tissue accumulation, mainly in the lower body, including the legs, hips, and buttocks; it is often referred to as "pear-shaped" obesity. More common in females.

H

health claim Allowable claim regarding the relationship between a nutrient or food and an aspect of health or function. Health claims are provided by the FDA in the United States and European Commission in the EU.

healthy weight For a particular gender, height, and build, the body weight associated with a lower risk of disease.

hematocrit The percentage of blood that is composed of red blood cells.

heme carrier protein (hcp1) A protein in the small intestine mucosal cells that transports a heme molecule from the gut lumen into an enterocyte.

heme iron A form of iron. Heme is a large heterocyclic organic molecule that contains an iron atom at the center of a prosthetic ring structure, known as a porphyrin ring.

heme oxygenase A mucosal enzyme that is able to break down the heme molecule and liberate iron.

hemicellulose A fiber component composed of pentose and hexose sugars covalently bonded in a $\beta 1-4$ linkage with branching side chains.

hemoglobin The iron-containing pigment within red blood cells that binds oxygen for efficient transport.

hepatic lipase A liver enzyme that cleaves the fatty acids of a triglyceride; it is involved in the production of low-density lipoproteins.

hepatic portal vein Principal vein that drains blood from the digestive tract and the pancreas and circulates blood through the liver before going to the heart. Also known as the portal vein.

hepatitis Inflammation of the liver.

hepatocyte Highly specialized liver cell that is involved in the metabolism of energy nutrients, including the storage of glycogen, gluconeogenesis, and urea production.

hepcidin A liver peptide hormone that functions to block iron export from mucosal cells by blocking the action of ferroportin.

hephaestin A copper-containing protein that transports iron from the mucosal cells of the small intestine to the blood circulation. It has ferroxidase activity, whereby it oxidizes iron to the ferric form.

heterogeneous nuclear RNA (hnRNA) The original RNA synthesized in the nucleus as a copy of the DNA before any modification.

HFE A gene involved with iron metabolism. The HFE protein regulates iron absorption.

high biological value protein See *complete protein.*

high-energy bond Cellular chemical bond (normally phosphate) by which energy is stored and subsequently released to drive a biochemical reaction.

high-energy phosphate A molecule that can quickly release phosphate for ATP production (e.g., guanosine triphosphate, creatine phosphate).

high-fructose corn syrup (HFCS) Enzymatically processed corn starch whereby some of the glucose is converted to fructose to achieve a desired sweetness. HFCS is used as a commercial sweetener and is popular in sport foods.

holo-RBP A complex of all-*trans* retinol bound to retinol-binding protein (RBP) that is responsible for transporting vitamin A in a cell and in the blood.

hormone A chemical produced by one part of the body that has a biochemical effect on a different part of the body.

hyaluronic acid A glycosaminoglycan found in joints.

hydroxyapatite The calcium-containing crystalline unit of bone.

hyperglycemia Elevated blood glucose level.

hyperglycinemia Increased blood levels of the amino acid glycine.

hyperinsulinemia Elevation of the level of insulin in circulation in response to an increase in blood glucose.

hyperkalemia An electrolyte imbalance characterized by high levels of blood potassium.

hypermethioninemia A condition resulting in an increase in the amino acid methionine, accumulating in the blood often due to a defect in the enzyme methionine adenosyl transferase, which converts methionine to S-adenosyl methionine.

hypernatremia An electrolyte imbalance characterized by high levels of blood sodium.

hypertension High blood pressure.

hypertrophy Increase in cell size.

hypochromic microcytic anemia A type of anemia characterized by red blood cells that have less hemoglobin per cell and smaller cell size.

hypoglycemia Blood glucose concentration that is below fasting level.

hypokalemia An electrolyte imbalance characterized by low levels of blood potassium.

hyponatremia An electrolyte imbalance characterized by low levels of blood sodium.

hypoxia inducible factors (HIF) Transcription factors or proteins produced when tissue oxygen is low and that targets the promoters of genes involved in improving oxygen availability in the cell. An example is when oxygen levels are low in cells; these factors can upregulate those genes that promote iron absorption.

I

in vivo A Latin word meaning "within a living organism."

indicator amino acid oxidation (IAAO) method A newer method used to determine dietary protein requirements. Uses a radioactive labelled essential amino acid (eg phenylalanine) whereby increased dietary protein results in a decrease in oxidation of the essential amino aicd. The point at which no further change in oxidation occurs with increased dietary protein is the dietary protein requirement.

indirect calorimetry A method to estimate whole-body energy expenditure that is based on measuring the amount of oxygen used and carbon dioxide produced during energy metabolism.

inflammatory bowel disease A general term in reference to Crohn's disease or ulcerative colitis.

insensible water loss The daily loss of water through the lungs, skin, and feces.

insoluble fiber Fiber that is insoluble in water, such as cellulose, hemicellulose, lignin, and modified cellulose.

intervention trial An experimental study in which a factor under study is modified and a number of variables measured to determine the response.

intraluminal phase The digestion of lipids within the lumen of the gastrointestinal tract (mainly the small intestine).

intrinsic pathway In blood clotting, the process by which prothrombin is activated via the interaction of factor XII with collagen fibers of a damaged blood vessel. Sometimes referred to as the contact activation pathway or tissue factor pathway.

intron The portion of RNA transcribed from the DNA that is not eventually translated into a protein. Sometimes called junk RNA.

iodothyronine deiodinase A selenium-containing enzyme that is involved in the conversion of thyroxin into the metabolically active triiodothyronine by removal of an iodine atom.

IREG1 A membrane protein that transports iron from inside a cell to the outside. Also known as ferroportin.

iron deficiency anemia An anemia that occurs when hemoglobin levels fall below 7 grams per 100 milliliters of blood.

iron-responsive element-binding protein (IREP) A protein involved in iron metabolism that interacts with messenger RNA to either inhibit translation of iron storage proteins (e.g., ferritin) or enhance the stability of iron transporters such as transferrin receptors. IREPs are active proteins in iron deficiency.

isoprenoid A class of chemical structures that function as pigments, vitamins, and precursors to sex hormones. Sometimes referred to as terpinoids.

isoprostane A prostaglandin-like compound with anti-inflammatory action derived from long-chain fatty acids (such as arachidonic acid) that have been oxidized.

isozyme An enzyme that has more than one form.

J

jejunum The second segment of the small intestine.

juxtaglomerular apparatus A group of kidney arteriole cells of the glomerulus that produce the enzyme renin.

K

kahweol A molecule found in coffee beans that may have several health benefits, including preventing bone breakdown. May also have anticancer and anti-inflammatory properties.

ketogenic Refers to the production of ketone bodies with the breakdown of certain amino acids.

ketone body A by-product of fatty acid breakdown that is water soluble and can be used for energy by the brain and heart.

ketosis A physiologic state in which ketone body production exceeds metabolism, resulting in an accumulation of ketone bodies in the blood and tissue.

kilocalorie (kcal) Measurement of energy; the amount of energy required to raise the temperature of 1 kilogram of water by 1 °C; equal to 4.184 kilojoules (kJ).

Klotho A protein that works in tandem with FGF23 in lowering serum phosphate levels when elevated.

Kruppel-like factor 4 (KLF4) A transcription factor that binds to a gene promoter to up-regulate the mRNA transcription for transporter ZIP4 when zinc deficiency is present.

kwashiorkor Historically known as protein undernutrition, but more recently recognized as a disease caused by lack of both protein and energy; the symptoms in a child include edema, fatty liver, dermatitis, irritability, depigmented hair, and anorexia. It is a specific type of protein–calorie malnutrition.

L

lactase Digestive enzyme produced by the small intestine that splits the disaccharide lactose.

lactose Disaccharide found in milk and dairy; it is digested by the enzyme lactase.

lactose intolerance Symptoms such as bloating, cramping, and diarrhea experienced by people who produce an insufficient amount of lactase.

lean body mass (LBM) Sum of the body's fat-free mass and essential fat.

leukocyte White blood cell; part of the immune system that fights infections.

lignin A noncarbohydrate component of insoluble dietary fiber composed of aromatic polymers.

limonoid A triterpene found in citrus fruits that imparts a bitter flavor. It is thought to have anticancer, antifungal, antibacterial, and antimalarial properties.

limiting A term used to describe a lack of certain dietary amino acids to make a protein due to insufficient levels in foods or diet.

limiting amino acid The essential amino acid present in the smallest amount in a protein food.

limonene A monoterpene found in citrus peels that is thought to relieve gastroesophageal reflux disease and heartburn. May detoxify certain cancer-causing compounds by increasing the activity of liver enzymes.

limonin A limonoid found in citrus fruits. It is a powerful anticancer agent for cancers of the colon, stomach, breast, lung, and mouth. It also has anti-HIV properties.

lipoprotein A complex in which proteins, triglycerides, phospholipids, and cholesterol are packaged to allow them to be water soluble so they can be transported in the blood.

lipoxygenase An enzyme that is involved in the metabolism of longer-chain fatty acids into powerful biochemicals.

liver X receptor (LXR) A nuclear receptor that binds to gene promoters that up-regulate transporters for cholesterol transfer to HDL-cholesterol, transporters that regulate cholesterol absorption, and transporters that facilitate cholesterol and phospholipid export from the liver.

loop of Henle A structure in the kidney nephron, within the medulla, that connects the proximate convoluted tubule to the distal convoluted tubule.

lysosome Structure of a cell that contains digestive enzymes.

lysyl oxidase A copper-containing enzyme that promotes the cross-linking of collagen and elastin fibrils by promoting the production of aldehydes and lysine residues that form bonds in these tissues.

M

magnetic resonance imaging (MRI) Method for determining tissue density by using a large electromagnet that creates a magnetic field. After radio waves are introduced, the magnetic field realigns hydrogen atoms that give off their excess energy at different rates depending on the type of tissue. Emitted energy is then analyzed by a computer, which constructs an image.

major mineral A mineral whose estimated average daily dietary need is 100 milligrams or more and that represents more than 0.01% of total human mass.

malonic acid pathway A biochemical pathway whereby three molecules of acetyl CoA are biochemically converted into three molecules of malonyl CoA, which are eventually used in the synthesis of flavones, isoflavones, and flavanols from metabolites of the aromatic amino acids phenylalanine, tyrosine, and tryptophan.

maltase Digestive enzyme produced by the small intestine that splits the disaccharide maltose.

maltodextrin A polysaccharide that consists of small links of glucose with a branch point. Can be produced by partially digesting starch.

maltose Disaccharide found in limited amounts in the diet; produced when starch is broken down. Maltose is digested in the small intestine by the enzyme maltase.

maple syrup urine disease An inborn error of metabolism where the branched-chain amino acids are unable to be catabolized due to a defect in the enzyme branched-chain α-keto acid dehydrogenase complex. The inability to degrade the amino acids results in the accumulation of ketoacids in tissues and plasma, which leads to a number of brain-related disorders.

marasmus A type of protein–calorie malnutrition characterized by severe calorie deficiency leading to extreme emaciation with muscle wasting and dry, loose skin.

megaloblastic macrocytic anemia A type of anemia in which the red blood cells are immature and larger than normal. It is usually caused by a deficiency of folate or vitamin B_{12}.

menthol A monoterpene found in peppermint oil that can create a cooling sensation when it comes into contact with skin or mucus membranes.

metabolic cart Instrument that measures the volume of gas exchanged between an individual and the environment; measures O_2 used and CO_2 produced.

metabolic rate The energy expended in a certain period of time (such as kilocalories per hour).

metabolic syndrome A set of blood and anthropometric conditions that increase the risk of diseases, in particular, cardiovascular disease and Type 2 diabetes.

metabolism The energy-releasing processes of cells, tissues, or the human body; may be measured in kilocalories expended.

metal transcription factor-1 (MTF-1) A transcription factor that binds to gene promoters that regulate zinc-containing proteins, such as ZnT-1 and metallothionein.

metallothionein A polypeptide produced by the small intestine as well as other tissues, such as the liver and kidney, that functions to bind trace minerals.

methylmalonic acidemia An inborn error of metabolism in which an enzyme needed for threonine breakdown,

methylmalonyl-CoA mutase, is defective, leading to an accumulation of methylmalonic acid.

micro RNA (miRNA) A type of RNA composed of a few nucleotide base pairs that are encoded by genomic DNA. miRNA blocks translation by binding to the complementary sequences of mRNA. Also enhances mRNA degradation.

microvilli Projections of enterocyte plasma membrane on the villi of the small intestine. Microvilli enhance the enterocyte surface to bring nutrients into the cell for metabolism and absorption.

minor mineral A mineral present in the human body as less than 0.01% of total mass. Minor minerals may act as cofactors in human tissues or may be part of various compounds, or both. Also known as a trace element or mineral.

Mitochondrial biogenesis Birth and multiplication of mitochondria organelles.

mitochondrion Unit of a cell that is responsible for the aerobic generation of energy in the form of ATP.

mobiloferrin A cytoplasmic protein in cells that is capable of binding and transporting iron.

monosaccharide The simplest carbohydrate molecule.

monoterpene A plant-based essential oil found in fruits, vegetables, and herbs. Can prevent initiation and progression of cancer and can also be used as a cancer treatment.

monounsaturated A fatty acid in which there is one double bond in the hydrocarbon chain.

motor cortex Region of the brain that initiates voluntary skeletal muscle contraction.

motor unit The combination of a motor neuron and all of the muscle fibers it innervates.

mRNA (messenger RNA) A single-stranded copy of DNA synthesized in the nucleus of a cell; enters the cytoplasm to direct the correct assembly of amino acids composing a protein.

mTOR An enzyme involved in a metabolic signaling pathway found in muscle that supports protein synthesis and regulation of cell growth, cell proliferation, cell motility, and cell survival, among other functions. The term is an acronym for mammalian target of rapamycin.

mucosal phase The digestion of lipid breakdown products within the mucosal cells of the small intestine. The synthesis of medium-chain triglycerides and the re-esterification of cholesterol occurs in this phase.

muscle Contractile tissue of animals.

muscle cells The unit of muscle responsible for contraction of movement of the human body.

muscle fiber An alternative term for a muscle cell based on the thin, elongated appearance of muscle cells; the unit responsible for contraction.

myofibril Bundle of myofilaments forming an internal subdivision of skeletal and cardiac muscle.

myosin Thick contractile protein of muscle tissue.

N

nephron The microscopic functional unit of a kidney.

nervous tissue Type of tissue composed of nerve cells (neurons) that transmits electric impulses throughout the body.

net protein utilization (NPU) A measure of how efficiently protein is used by an organism; the NPU is the biological value (BV) multiplied by the digestibility of the protein.

neuromuscular junction The anatomic structure (synapse) intersecting a muscle fiber and nerve fiber.

neuron A nerve cell.

neurotransmitter Chemical produced by the body to transmit an electric signal to another cell type of structure in the body, usually across a synapse.

Niemann-Pick C1-Like 1 (NPC1L1) Refers to a protein on the brush border of the small intestine enterocyte that is thought to be responsible for cholesterol absorption. It is also thought to be present in hepatocytes.

nitrogen balance The amount of nitrogen exiting a body compared with the amount entering.

nitrogen balance method A method to determine the minimum amount of dietary protein needed to keep a subject in nitrogen equilibrium.

nomilin A limonoid found in citrus fruits. Has been found to have anti-HIV properties and possible antiobesity and antihyperglycemic properties.

nonalcoholic fatty acid liver disease or nonalcoholic steatohepatitis A nonalcohol related liver disease characterized by fatty liver. Diabetics, obesity, and genetic propensity individuals are candidates for this disease.

nonheme iron All dietary iron that is not in the heme form.

NPC1L1-flotillan-cholesterol membrane microdomain NPC1L1 binds cholesterol on the gut lumen side and subsequently transfers it to the area of the small intestine enterocyte membrane that becomes cholesterol enriched, which is referred to as a microdomain.

nutraceutical The functional or chemical component of a food that provides a health benefit beyond basic nutrition.

O

obesity State of excessive body fat; body fat of 25% or more of total mass for men and 33% or more for women.

Obestatin A hormone produced by stomach cells that produced an anorectic response.

oligosaccharide Short, indigestible chain of monosaccharides, found mostly in legumes.

opsin Light-sensitive protein of the photoreceptor cells in the retina of the eye. Opsins convert light in the form of photons into an electrochemical signal.

organelle A structure within a cell with a specialized function.

organic matrix The carbon-containing material between cells or within the mitochondria.

orphan receptor A cellular nuclear receptor in which a ligand-activating compound was originally not known. The receptors bind to promoters of genes to initialize gene transcription.

osteoblast Bone cell responsible for bone synthesis.

osteoclast Bone cell responsible for bone breakdown.

osteomalacia Loss of mineralization, resulting in decreased bone density.

P

pancreatitis Inflammation of the pancreas.

pectin A polysaccharide composed of repeating methylated or nonmethylated galacturonic acid subunits covalently bonded with a $\beta 1$–4 linkage.

pellagra Disease caused by a niacin deficiency in which diarrhea, dermatitis, dementia, and, eventually, death, can result.

pentose phosphate pathway A biochemical pathway that generates both NADPH and pentose sugars. Sometimes called the hexose monophosphate shunt.

pernicious anemia A megaloblastic macrocytic anemia caused by the lack of intrinsic factor that leads to a vitamin B_{12} deficiency.

peroxisome Structure of cells that facilitates the metabolism of fatty acids and various toxins.

phenylketonuria (PKU) An inborn error of metabolism in which phenylalanine is unable to be metabolized to tyrosine due to a defect in the enzyme phenylalanine hydroxylase. If untreated, PKU can lead to mental retardation, epileptic seizures, and skin lesions.

phospholipid A lipid in which two fatty acids are bound to carbons 1 and 2 of a glycerol molecule and a phosphate moiety is bound to the third carbon.

photophobia Excess sensitivity or aversion to light.

phytase An enzyme that can break down the monosaccharide phytic acid and can bind up trace minerals.

phytochemical A plant-derived substance (nutraceutical) that may help support the prevention or treatment of disease processes, such as atherosclerosis and inflammation.

plasma The noncellular component of blood composed primarily of water with dissolved substances, such as proteins, glucose, electrolytes, and clotting factors.

plasmin A blood enzyme that is responsible for degrading the blood-clotting protein fibrin.

plasminogen A precursor to the blood protein plasmin.

platelet Small blood cell that is involved in blood maintenance and in blood clotting.

plethysmography Method of estimating body composition based on densitometry. Body volume is based on air displacement.

point of unsaturation Place on the fatty acid hydrocarbon chain where a double bond occurs between adjacent carbon atoms.

polydextrose A polysaccharide polymer of glucose and sorbitol used as a bulking agent in foods to bolster fiber claims and to impart sweetness in order to reduce the amount of sugar in foods.

polysaccharide Complex carbohydrate containing hundreds of monosaccharides; polysaccharides include starch, fiber, and glycosaminoglycans.

polyunsaturated A fatty acid in which there are two or more double bonds in the hydrocarbon side chain.

post-transcriptional modification The process by which heterogeneous nuclear RNA is changed into mature messenger RNA.

preformed vitamin A The type of vitamin A found in animal sources of food; it is absorbed in the form of retinol.

previtamin A The type of vitamin A found in plants; it needs to be converted to active vitamin A and can be converted to retinol by the body.

primary structure The sequence of amino acids composing a polypeptide linked together via peptide bonds.

probiotic Live digestive tract bacteria that are beneficial to health.

propionic acidemia An inborn error of metabolism in which an enzyme needed for threonine catabolism, propionyl CoA carboxylase, is defective, leading to an accumulation of propionic acid.

protein digestibility corrected amino acid score (PDCAAS) A measure of protein quality that takes into account both the quality as determined by its individual amino acid score and the percent digestibility of the protein.

protein efficiency ratio (PER) A method of evaluating protein quality by the weight gain of a growing animal in relation to its protein intake when energy is ample and a protein source is fed at an adequate level.

protein structure One of the four basic structures that the polypeptide chains of proteins assume to achieve their intended function: primary, secondary, tertiary, and quaternary.

protein–energy malnutrition (PEM) A general term used to describe a condition caused by a lack of both protein and calories. Types include kwashiorkor and marasmus.

Proton-coupled folate transporter (PCFT) A large intestine transport protein for folate absorption.

proximal convoluted tubule (PCT) A kidney tubule that connects the Bowman capsule to the loop of Henle of the nephron unit.

psyllium A name applied to several members of the plant genus *Plantago*, whose seeds are used commercially for the production of mucilage.

Pterostilbene A nutraceutical that can be synthesized or derived from a natural origin such as grape skins and berries, particularly blueberries. It has a wide range of possible health benefits, including antiaging, cardioprotective, antidiabetic, neuroprotective, and cancer prevention effects.

pulmonary artery The major blood vessel that exits the right ventricle to carry blood from the heart to the lungs.

pyloric sphincter A smooth muscular ring that separates the stomach from the duodenum.

Q

quercetin An isoflavone class of nutraceuticals common in citrus fruit, red wine, onions, green tea, apples, and berries. It has been promoted for treating a variety of diseases, such as heart disease; preventing certain cancers; reducing inflammation; and lowering blood cholesterol levels.

R

rebound scurvy A condition in which an infant develops scurvy because during pregnancy the mother consumed large amounts of vitamin C, causing the enzymes that break down vitamin C to accumulate both in the mother and fetus. Upon birth, the newborn continues to break down vitamin C, leading to scurvy.

Reduced folate carrier (RFC) An intestinal transport protein for several water-soluble vitamins, including thiamin and folate.

reference protein A high-quality protein, such as milk or egg, that is used to compare the quality of other proteins.

renal system The organs that are involved in the production of urine.

renin An enzyme produced in the kidney glomerulus in response to low blood volume, decreased blood pressure, or low sodium levels to stimulate a series of biochemical reactions to correct these changes.

resistant dextrins The indigestible components of starch breakdown products resulting from heat/acid and enzymatic (amylase) treatment.

resistant starches Naturally occurring starches that are not completely hydrolyzed by amylases in the upper digestive tract.

respiratory exchange ratio (RER) The ratio of carbon dioxide expired to oxygen consumed at the level of the lungs.

respiratory quotient (RQ) Ratio of carbon dioxide produced and oxygen consumed at the cell or tissue level.

resting energy expenditure (REE) Is similar to basal metabolic rate and is the calories expended while at rest; but the subject does not have to be fasting as one does for basal metabolic rate.

resting metabolic rate (RMR) Level of energy expenditure during nonactive rest at a comfortable environmental temperature and 4 hours after the consumption of a meal; tends to be about 10% greater than basal metabolic rate.

resting potential The resting electric charge of an excitable cell.

resveratrol A nutraceutical that can be synthesized or derived from a natural origin, such as Japanese knotweed, grape skins, and red wines or from genetically modified yeast. It has a wide range of possible health benefits, including antiaging, cardioprotective, antidiabetic, neuroprotective, and cancer prevention effects.

retinol activity equivalent (RAE) A standardized unit to indicate the relative potency of various forms of vitamin A. One retinol activity equivalent is equal to 1 microgram of retinol, 12 micrograms of β-carotene, or 24 micrograms of other carotenoids.

reverse cholesterol transport The removal of cholesterol from peripheral body tissues and transport to the liver for breakdown. The process normally uses high-density lipoproteins.

rhodopsin The pigment of the retina that forms photoreceptor cells. Sometimes called visual purple.

ribose A five-carbon monosaccharide that serves as a component of RNA, DNA, and ATP.

ribosomal RNA (rRNA) The RNA found in the ribosomes, a cell structure in which protein synthesis occurs in the cell cytoplasm.

rickets A bone condition, most often seen in children, resulting from vitamin D deficiency that is associated with a failure of growing bone to mineralize. As the epiphyseal cartilage of bone continues to grow, it is not properly replaced with matrix and hydroxyapatite. This results in a bowing of longer weight-bearing bones such as the femur, tibia, and fibula of the legs, deformations of the knee region, and curvature of the spine.

RNA (ribonucleic acid) Nucleic acid that is similar to DNA but is single stranded. The three main types of RNA are ribosomal, transfer, and messenger RNA.

RNA interference (RNAi) A class of RNA molecules that silence gene expression.

Roux-En-Y A type of bariatric surgery where the upper portion of the stomach is stapled to prevent food from entering the distal portion of the stomach, and an opening is created from the stomach to the small intestine where a portion of the duodenum is bypassed to decrease absorption. Gastric bypass is another name.

RFVT1, RFVT2, RFVT3 different intestinal riboflavin transport proteins.

S

S-adenosyl methionine (SAM) A compound that acts as a donor of methyl groups for a number of biochemical reactions.

saponin A class of chemical compounds referred to as glucosides that are present in many plants. Health benefits are thought to include cholesterol reduction, reduced cancer risk, immune system enhancement, prevention of bone loss, and antioxidant activity.

sarcolemma The plasma membrane of a muscle fiber.

sarcomere The contractile unit of a muscle, composed of myosin and actin, among other proteins.

sarcoplasmic reticulum Tubules and vesicles in a cell that regulate calcium levels.

saturated A fatty acid that does not contain any double bonds in the hydrocarbon chain.

scurvy A disease characterized by bleeding gums and pinpoint skin bleeding due to a vitamin C deficiency that causes defective collagen to form.

secretory phase The phase of lipid digestion in which lipid products are expelled into the lymph or portal vein.

selenoprotein P A selenium containing protein that transports and stores selenium and is thought to function as an antioxidant. It appears to be involved in selenium homeostasis in both brain and testes.

Selenoprotein W A selenium containing protein that is critical in preventing certain muscle disease in cattle and sheep.

sesquiterpene A class of plant-based essential oils similar to monoterpenes; have antiseptic and anti-inflammatory properties.

shikimic acid pathway A biochemical pathway where simple carbohydrate intermediates of glycolysis and the pentose phosphate pathway (PPP) are converted to the aromatic amino acids phenylalanine, tyrosine, and tryptophan. Further chemical modifications lead to the synthesis of phenolic compounds such as flavones, isoflavones, and flavanols.

SIRT Groups of proteins sometimes referred to as silent information regulator 2 or Sir2. It has roles in various critical metabolic pathways by activating enzymes. It is under the control of increased levels of NAD^+ that result in increased expression of SIRT.

SIRT1-AMPK-PGC1α complex A complex whereby activity of a group of enzymes and regulatory transcription factors improves insulin sensitivity, enhanced fatty acid oxidation, and decreased lipogenesis. Dietary leucine intake may activate this complex and lead to decreased obesity.

sirtuins Referred to as "silent information regulator 2", works with niacin in affecting those enzymes involved with insulin secretion, gluconeogenesis, mitochondrial biogenesis, endothelial function, lipid metabolism, cell cycling, and apoptosis.

skeletal muscle One of three types of muscle; skeletal muscle is controlled voluntarily by the central nervous system.

skeleton A rigid framework that provides structure and protection to an organism.

small hairpin RNA (shRNA) A type of RNA that functions in a manner similar to miRNA. It is used in experiments where it is introduced into cells using a vector, such as a plasmid or virus. It can either block translation or lead to mRNA degradation.

small heterodimer partner (SHP) A gene product that inhibits the transcription of the mRNA for 7 α-hydroxylase, a rate-limiting enzyme in the conversion of cholesterol to bile acid.

small interfering RNA (siRNA) Synthetic molecules that are similar to miRNA and are used in biological experiments to silence genes.

SMVT An intestinal transport protein for biotin and pantothenic acid absorption.

Sodium-ascorbate co-transporter 1 (SVCT1) and 2 (SVCT2) A transporter for vitamin C absorption in the small intestine.

soluble fiber Fibers that are soluble in water, such as pectins, gums, and mucilages.

splicing The removal of nonsense RNA sequences (introns) from the RNA immediately after transcription to join portions of RNA (exons) that code for particular amino acids.

SREBP cleavage-activating system (SCAP) A protein located in the endoplasmic reticulum that responds to cell cholesterol levels. When cell cholesterol levels decline, SCAP will escort SREBP to the cell nucleus in order to enhance expression of enzymes involved with cholesterol biosynthesis.

starch A digestible polysaccharide consisting of straight chains of glucose that can have branching.

steap3 An enzyme that removes transferrin-bound iron that has been engulfed by a liver endosome and converts it from the ferric form of iron to the ferrous form.

steatorrhea Presence of fatty stools due to fat malabsorption.

stellate cell The major liver cell type involved in the development of liver fibrosis. Stellate cells are also early lipid storing cells of the liver.

sterol A class of organic compound classified as a lipid. The biochemical structures are composed of four rings; an example is cholesterol.

sterol regulatory element-binding protein (SREBP) A transcription factor that has several isoforms, all of which are involved in lipid or cholesterol biosynthesis.

Stilbenes A class of nonflavanoid polyphenolic compounds that are often found in foods.

stroke volume The volume of blood pumped with each heartbeat.

structure/function claim Describes the role of a nutrient or dietary ingredient intended to affect normal structure or function in humans.

subcutaneous Beneath the skin.

sucrase Digestive enzyme produced by the small intestine that splits the disaccharide sucrose.

sucrose Disaccharide derived from the sugar cane plant that is used as a sweetener in recipes; it is digested in the small intestine by the enzyme sucrase.

superoxide dismutase An antioxidant enzyme that promotes the dismutation of superoxide into hydrogen peroxide and oxygen. It may contain a mineral, such as copper or manganese.

sweat Fluid secreted by special glands in the skin that is composed mostly of water and dissolved salts.

sweat water The water component of sweat.

synapse The space between adjacent neurons (nerve cells) in which the impulse is transmitted from one neuron to another neuron.

synthesis of amino acids The process of the production of amino acids by the body from other compounds.

systolic blood pressure The maximum blood pressure exerted by the blood against the walls of the blood vessels composing the cardiovascular system when the heart contracts.

T

tau Abnormal protein in the neurofibrillary tangles present in Alzheimer's disease.

tendon Connective tissue that connects muscle to bone.

terpenoid A class of chemical structures that function as pigments, vitamins, and precursors to sex hormones. Sometimes called isoprenoids.

tetraterpenoid A class of compounds that have 8 isoprene molecules (or 4 monoterpene molecules) and 40 carbons. Carotenoids are a type of tetraterpenoid.

thermic effect of activity (TEA) A component of total energy expenditure; includes not only skeletal muscle activity during obvious movements such as walking, running, bicycling, climbing stairs, or vacuuming the floor, but also skeletal muscle activity associated with the maintenance of position and posture.

thermic effect of food (TEF) A component of total energy expenditure; the increase in energy expenditure associated with the digestion, absorption, processing, and storage of food and its components.

thermogenin An uncoupling protein found in brown adipose tissue that is involved in increasing metabolism via nonshivering thermogenesis. Also known as uncoupling protein 1 (UCP1).

thio-ester A chemical compound formed from an esterification of a thiol (sulfur) group and a carboxyl group.

thioredoxin reductase Selenium containing enzymes that reduce the protein thioredoxin to reduce other compounds as part of an oxidation-reduction cycle.

thirst A craving for fluids, leading to the intake of water.

thromboplastin Sometimes referred to as factor III. It is found in white blood cells, tissues, and platelets. In the presence of calcium, it can facilitate the conversion of prothrombin to thrombin.

THTR1, THTR2 Small intestinal transport proteins for thiamin.

thyroglobin The storage form of iodine, in which iodine is incorporated into the globulin protein.

thyroxin (T_4) A thyroid prohormone that contains four atoms of iodine per molecule of zinc; affects basal metabolism.

tocopherols A class of vitamin E molecules with saturated phytyl side chains.

tocotrienols A class of vitamin E molecules with unsaturated phytyl side chains.

total energy expenditure (TEE) Sum of all energy-releasing processes of the human body.

total fiber The sum of dietary fiber plus functional fiber.

TPP-riboswitch An mRNA molecule whereby thiamine pyrophosphate binds to the molecule and expresses thiazole synthase to produce thiazole, a compound known for its anti-inflammatory and neuroprotective properties.

trans On opposing sides of a double bond. In terms of fatty acids, each hydrogen atom is on opposite sides of a double bond.

transaminase Enzyme that transfers amine groups from amino acids to α-keto acids, such as pyruvate and α-ketoglutarate.

transamination A biochemical reaction that transfers an amino group from one amino acid to an α-keto acid to produce a new amino acid, while producing a new α-keto acid with the remaining carbon skeleton of the original amino acid.

transcription The process by which messenger RNA directs the cell to assemble amino acids in a particular order as specified by the DNA code.

transcription factor A protein that binds to the promoter of DNA or a gene that controls the transcription of the gene or the synthesis of mRNA from the DNA.

transcuprin A plasma protein that transports copper.

transfer RNA (tRNA) The RNA found in the cytoplasm that is responsible for bringing specific amino acids to the ribosomes in the process of protein synthesis.

transferrin A glycoprotein in the plasma that transports iron from the tissues and bloodstream to the bone marrow, where it is reused in the formation of hemoglobin.

translation The synthesis of protein by the reading of the messenger RNA code for the correct amino acids.

transport Process by which substances and molecules are transferred from one area of the body to another, or from outside a cell to inside a cell.

transporter ZIP4 A protein in the mucosal cells of the small intestine that transports zinc from the gut lumen into an enterocyte.

triglyceride A lipid composed of one glycerol molecule bonded with three fatty acid molecules.

triiodothyronine (T_3) A thyroid hormone produced from thyroxin by the removal of an iodine atom; it is metabolically active, affecting many reactions, including increasing the basal metabolic rate.

triterpene Precursors to plant sterols that contain six isoprene rings.

tropical sprue Inflammation of the small intestine that occurs in people living in tropical regions.

tropocollagen A helical structure of three polypeptides that is the basic unit of all collagens.

tropomyosin A muscle protein that binds to actin during muscle contraction.

troponin A complex of three regulatory proteins that assists in regulating muscle contraction.

TRPM6 A membrane channel protein on enterocytes of the ileum for magnesium absorption via a saturable mechanism. Sometimes referred to as "transient receptor potential melastatin divalent cation-permeable channel protein."

TRPM7 A magnesium channel protein that is expressed ubiquitously on most cells for magnesium absorption. It is similar to TRPM6.

TRPV6 A membrane channel for calcium absorption by small intestine enterocytes. Sometimes referred to as "transient receptor potential cation, subfamily V, member 6."

turnover The replacement of existing biochemicals or cells with new ones.

tyrosine A non-essential amino acid involved with protein synthesis and an intermediate in the production of acetyl CoA and neurotransmitters.

tyrosine hydroxylase A copper-containing enzyme that converts the amino acid tyrosine into dihydroxyphenylalanine (DOPA), which is subsequently converted to dopamine.

tyrosinemia type II An inborn error of metabolism in which tyrosine accumulates due to a defect in the enzyme tyrosine aminotransferase, which converts tyrosine to p-hydroxyphenol-pyruvate. Can lead to mental retardation and skin and eye lesions, if left untreated.

U

ulcerative colitis Inflammation and ulcers of the colon.

ultrafiltrate A solution produced by passage through a semipermeable membrane.

uncoupling protein 2 Family of mitochondrial proteins that may increase thermogenesis by uncoupling electron transfer from oxidative phosphorylation.

underwater weighing (UWW) Technique for assessing body composition (fat mass and lean body mass) by applying a person's weight underwater as an estimator of volume.

unsaturated A fatty acid that contains one or more double bonds.

urea cycle A series of biochemical reactions by which ammonia is converted to urea for excretion. The process occurs mainly in the liver, with some activity in the kidney.

urinary water The water that composes urine.

V

vasopressin See *antidiuretic hormone (ADH).*

villi Tiny fingerlike projections lined with enterocytes in the intestinal mucosa of the small intestine. Villi constitute one of the three levels of folding that greatly expands the surface area of the small intestine.

vitamin An organic compound required for an organism to live, that either cannot be synthesized or is not synthesized enough by the organism and thus needs to be obtained from the organism's diet.

vitamin K carboxylase The enzyme responsible for the carboxylation of glutamic acid residues to form γ-carboxyglutamic acid in key proteins.

vitamin K cycle A series of coupled reactions by which vitamin K converts glutamate to γ-carboxyglutamate.

VO$_2$ Volume of oxygen consumed.

VO$_2$max Maximum volume of oxygen consumed in a given time period. Also termed peak VO$_2$.

W

Wernicke-like syndrome A brain disorder due to thiamin deficiency.

X

xerophthalmia A disease of the eye caused by vitamin A deficiency. It is characterized by a dry and thickened conjunctiva and ulceration of the cornea that leads to blindness.

Z

zinc finger protein A DNA-binding, fingerlike polypeptide projection caused by zinc binding to specific histidine and cysteine residues. Allows for proteins to bind to DNA promoters.

zinc transporter 1 (ZnT-1) A protein on the basolateral portion of a mucosal cell that binds zinc for export to the blood.

Index

Note: Page numbers followed by *f* or *t* indicate material in figures or tables, respectively.

A

abetalipoproteinemia, 296
absorption, 69
  boron, 411–412
  calcium, 347–349, 347*t*
  chloride, 362–364
  chromium, 408–409
  copper, 395–396, 396*t*, 397*f*–398*f*
  fluoride, 406–407
  folic acid, 328–329
  iodine, 392
  iron, 374–378, 374*f*, 375*t*
  magnesium, 357–358
  manganese, 410
  molybdenum, 412
  monosaccharides, 70
  niacin, 321
  nickel, 413
  pantothenic acid, 339
  phosphorus, 354–355
  potassium, 363
  riboflavin, 318
  selenium, 401
  sodium, 363
  thiamin, 313–314
  vanadium, 413
  vitamin B_6, 324
  vitamin B_{12}, 332–333
  vitamin C, 308–309
  zinc, 386–389
Academy of Nutrition and Dietetics (AND), 420*t*
Acceptable Macronutrient Distribution Range (AMDR), 69
ACE. *See* angiotensin-converting enzyme
acetoacetate, 135, 165
acetone, 135
acetyl CoA, 120, 182*f*, 219, 338
  carboxylase, 114, 338
acetylcholine, 41, 49, 248
acid detergent method, 104, 104*t*
acid–base balance, 162
aconitase, 88
ACP. *See* acyl carrier protein
acrodermatitis enteropathica, 388
ACTH. *See* adrenocorticotropin hormone

actin, 25, 162, 248
action potential, 24, 364
active transport, 19
acyl carrier protein (ACP), 340
acyl CoA, 263
adaptive thermogenesis (AT), 213–216
adenosine diphosphate (ADP), 86
adenosine monophosphate (AMP), 87, 339
adenosine triphosphate (ATP), 7, 14*f*, 86–87, 208, 255, 256*t*, 339
  contribution during early exercise, 256*f*
  electron transport chain and, 13–17
Adequate Intake (AI), 69, 284
  for water, 201
ADH. *See* antidiuretic hormone
adipocytes, 3
  glucose uptake and utilization, 222*f*
  hyperplasia *vs.* hypertrophy, 239–240, 239*f*
  regulation in energy balance, 238–239
adipose tissue, glucagon in, 79
adolescence, body fat, 226
ADP. *See* adenosine diphosphate
adrenocorticotropin hormone (ACTH), 253*t*, 255
aerobic training, 262
AI. *See* Adequate Intake
ALA. *See* α-aminolevulinic acid
alanine, 173
alanine cycle, 259, 259*f*
alanine–glucose cycle, 169, 171*f*
albumin, 161
aldosterone, 196, 253*t*
aliphatic amino acids, 148
alkaptonuria, 178
allyl sulfur compounds, 421
α-adrenergic agonists, 77
α-aminolevulinic acid (ALA), 378
α-amylase, 48, 69
α-carotene, 275
α-dextrinase, 69
α-keratin, 162
α-ketoadipic aciduria, 180
α-tocopherol, 292–294
Alzheimer disease, 386
  vitamin B_{12}, folate, and homocysteine in, 336

AMDR. *See* Acceptable Macronutrient Distribution Range
amino acid score, 159
amino acid–derived substances, 163, 163*t*
amino acids, 3
  carriers, 156
  catabolism of, 166*f*
  chains, 12
  classification of, 148–150, 149*f*
  composition, 196, 198*f*
  and derivatives, 434
  in enterocytes, active absorption, 156, 156*f*
  in human body, 148, 148*t*
  links of, 150
  metabolism
    alanine–glucose cycle, 169, 171*f*
    degradation, 165–168
    disposal of amino acid nitrogen, 173
    exercise and, 263–266
    glutamine, 168–169, 168*f*–170*f*
    inborn errors, 178–182
    and neurotransmitters, 169–173, 171*f*–173*f*
    proteins and, 10–12
    synthesis, 165
    transamination and deamination, 164–165, 164*f*
    urea cycle, 173, 174*f*
  nitrogen, disposal of, 173
  requirements, 176–177
  role in metabolism, 160–163
  structure of, 148*f*
  transport systems, 157, 157*t*
amino transferases, 164
aminolevulinic acid (ALA), 325
aminopeptidases, 157
ammonia, 173
AMP. *See* adenosine monophosphate
amylopectin, 64, 65, 68
amylose, 64–65
AND. *See* Academy of Nutrition and Dietetics
android obesity, 237
anemia
  megaloblastic macrocytic, 331
  pernicious, 332, 335

angiotensin I, 196
angiotensin II, 196
angiotensin-converting enzyme
        (ACE), 196
angiotensinogen, 196
animal flesh (skeletal muscle), 67
animal glycogen, 65
animal meat proteins, 152
"animal starch," 65
anomers, 62
anthocyanidins, 432, 432f
anthocyanins, 432
antidiuretic hormone (ADH), 196, 253t
    structure, 197, 198f
    urine volume and plasma osmolality
        by control of, 199f
antioxidant function of vitamin A, 283
AOAC. See Association of Official
        Analytical Chemists
AOAC 2011, 104t, 105
aorta, 28
appetite, mediators of
    hormonal influences, 45–46
    neuroendocrine influences, 46–47
arginine, 165, 434
arsenic, 414
ascorbic acid. See vitamin C
aspartate, 165
Association of Official Analytical
        Chemists (AOAC), 104t, 105
AT. See adaptive thermogenesis
athletic performance, caffeine and, 254
ATP. See adenosine triphosphate
atrioventricular (AV) node, 28
avidin, 337

B

Baker's yeast, 101
Barrett syndrome, 44
basal metabolic rate (BMR), 212
    equations for, 213
basal metabolism, 212–213
basic amino acids, 156
BAT. See brown adipose tissue
BCAAs. See branched-chain amino acids
BCKAD. See branched-chain α-ketoacid
        dehydrogenase
beef, 152
Bendectin, 327
beriberi, 316
    types of, 316
β-carotene, 275, 276, 421
    absorption of, 276
β-glucans, 101
β-hydroxybutyrate, 135
β-lactoglobulin, 152
BGP. See bone Gla protein
BIA. See bioelectrical impedance analysis
bile, 52–53

biocytin, 337
bioelectrical impedance analysis (BIA),
        231–232, 231f
biological value (BV), 158
biotin, 274, 337–338, 337f
    deficiency and toxicity, 338
    metabolism and function of, 337–338
    RDA for, 338
    sources of, 337
bitot spots, 284
bixin, 429
Blackfan-Diamond syndrome, 384
blindness, xerophthalmia and, 284
blond plantago seed, 102
blood, 26–29
    clotting, 161
    glucose regulation, 72
blood plasma, 193
blood pressure, 29
BMI. See body mass index
BMR. See basal metabolic rate
BOD POD, 229, 229f
body composition, 182–184
    assessment, 228–232, 228t
    BIA, 231–232, 231f
    body densitometry, 228–229
    DXA, 230, 230f
    plethysmography, 229
    skinfold, 230–231, 231f
    TOBEC, 231–232, 231f
body densitometry, 228–229
body mass index (BMI), 225–226, 225t
    calcium intake, 354
body water, 227
    components of, 227t
    definition, 227
    elements and molecules, 226
    fat mass and fat-free mass,
        226–227
    loss on physiologic performance, 267t
    minerals (ash), 227
body weight, 199, 200
    active people, 226
    BMI, 225–226
    definition, 224
    and health, 224–226
bone, 22–23
bone Gla protein (BGP), 300
bone marrow cells, heme synthesis,
        379f–381f
boron, 411–412
brain damage, 185
branched-chain α-ketoacid
        dehydrogenase (BCKAD), 315
    complex, 179
branched-chain amino acids (BCAAs),
        263
    body composition and obesity,
        182–184
    metabolism of, 180f
    transaminase reaction, 266

brown adipose tissue (BAT), 232
BV. See biological value

C

C peptide, 77
cafestol, 429
caffeine and athletic performance, 254
calbindin, 287–288, 349
calcitonin, 349, 350f
calcium
    absorption, 347–349, 347t
    blood level and regulation, 349
    deficiency, 353–354
    dietary sources, 346–347, 347t
    intake, recommended levels of, 353
    in muscle fiber contraction, 249, 249f
    parathyroid hormone role in
        homeostatic control of, 289f
    physiologic roles of, 349–353
    toxicity, 354
calcium citrate malate (CCM), 346
calcium oxalate, crystals, 311
calcium-binding protein (CBP),
        287–288, 349
calmodulin, binding with calcium, 353
caloric sweeteners, 68
calorimetry
    direct, 206, 206f
    indirect, 209–210, 209f
cAMP. See cyclic AMP
cancer, vitamin A role in, 282–283
capsaicinoids, 422
carbamoyl phosphate, 173
carbohydrate response element binding
        protein (ChREBP), 91, 91f
carbohydrates, 5, 428t
    absorption, 69
    circulation and cellular uptake
        blood glucose regulation, 72
        GLUT, 74–75, 75t
        glycemic index, 72, 72t
        glycemic load, 72–73
        monosaccharide activation, 75–76
    consumption, 67–68
        before, during and after exercise,
            260–261
    definition of, 60
    derivatives, 428t, 433–434
    digestion, 67, 70f
        starch and disaccharides, 69–70
    hormones in metabolism
        insulin, 76–79, 76t
        insulin-to-glucagon molar
            ratios, 80
    metabolic pathways for. See metabolic
        pathways
    metabolism, 256–258
    monosaccharides, 72
    oxidation during exercise, 260

recommendations, 69
supercompensation, 260
types and characteristics
dietary fiber, 68
disaccharides, 62–63
monosaccharides, 60–63
polysaccharides. *See* polysaccharides
carbon skeleton, 165
carbonic anhydrase, 28
system, 211, 211*f*
carbonyl carbon, 62
carboxylase enzymes, biotin and, 338
carboxypeptidase, 155
cardiac enlargement, beriberi characteristics, 316
cardiac output, 28
cardiac sphincter, 37
cardiomyopathy, 9
cardiovascular system, 246
carnitine, vitamin C and, 309
carotenes, 275, 429
carotenoids, 275, 421, 429–430, 430*f*
structure, 276*f*
vitamin A and. *See* vitamin A, and carotenoids
carrier-mediated transport, 19
carriers, amino acids, 156
casein proteins, 152
CAT. *See* computerized axial tomography
catecholamines, 80, 252–254
neurotransmitter synthesis, 171*f*
cation exchange capacity, 108
CBG. *See* corticosteroid-binding globulin
CBP. *See* calcium-binding protein
CCK. *See* cholecystokinin
CCK-A receptors, 233
CCK-B receptors, 233
CCM. *See* calcium citrate malate
cell, 3
binding proteins, vitamin A storage and, 280
differentiation, 281–285
membrane
proteins, 4
structure, 4*f*, 17
receptors, 17
structure, 3–9, 3*f*
cell signaling, 4, 18
cellular metabolism, 217–218
cellular protein functions, 17–21
cellular retinoid-binding protein (CRBP), 277
cellulose, 97–98, 98*t*
cellulose synthase, 98
cephalic phase, digestion, 47
cereal grains, 68
cGMP. *See* cyclic guanosine monophosphate
chaperone proteins, 396
chaperones, 9, 17

chemical mediators, energy homeostasis, 233–234
CCK, 233
insulin and ghrelin, 233
leptin, 233–234
NPY and galanin, 234
chemical score, 159
chemoelectrical potential force, 16
chemotherapy, vitamin C and, 312
chitin, 101
chitosan, 101
chloride
absorption, 362–364
dietary sources, 361
intake, recommended levels of, 365
physiologic functions of, 364–365
tissue, urinary, and sweat content, 364
chloride shift, 365
chlorophyll, magnesium in, 357
cholecalciferol, production of, 286
cholecystokinin (CCK), 43, 45–46, 233
cholesterol, 4
binding, 107
synthesis, 120, 121, 121*f*
cholinergic fibers, 41
chondroitin sulfate, 6, 101
ChREBP. *See* carbohydrate response element binding protein
chromium
absorption of, 408–409
dietary sources of, 408
intake, recommended levels of, 410
metabolism and function of, 409, 409*f*
chromodulin, 409
chylomicrons, 277
chyme, 50
chymotrypsinogen, 155
circulation, 26–29
citrate, 219
citrate synthase, 88
citric acid cycle, 87–88
CLA. *See* conjugated linoleic acid
clotting factors, 161
cobalt, 411
CODEX Alimentarius Commission, 105
coenzyme, 315
function, 306
riboflavin and, 317*f*
thiamine as, 315, 315*f*
coenzyme A, 338, 338*f*
pantothenic acid and, 338, 338*f*
coenzyme Q (CoQ), 17
collagen, 150, 162
vitamin C and, 309
colon, 39
complete proteins, 158
computerized axial tomography (CAT), 228
conjugated linoleic acid (CLA), 421, 434
connective tissue, 21
protein, 162

constipation, 107–108
contractile proteins, 162, 266
Cook, James, 306
copper
absorption of, 395–396, 396*t*, 397*f*–398*f*
deficiency, 399
dietary sources of, 395
genetic anomalies, 399–400
intake, recommended levels of, 399
metabolism and function of, 397–399
CoQ. *See* coenzyme Q
core body temperature, 215
cori cycle, 258–259
coronary heart disease, 141
risk, homocysteine and, 164
corrin ring, 332
corticosteroid-binding globulin (CBG), 81
corticotropin-releasing factor (CRF), 46
and leptin, 233–234
cortisol, 76*t*, 79–81, 253*t*, 255
fasting state, 222
co-transport mechanism, 19
CRBP. *See* cellular retinoid-binding protein
creatine kinase, 359–360
creatine phosphate, 255–256
system, 249*f*
cretinism, 395
CRF. *See* corticotropin-releasing factor
cristae, 16
crocetin, 429
crude fiber method, 103, 104*t*
Cunningham equation, 213
cupric, 395
cyanide (CN) group, 332
cyanocobalamin, 332, 332*f*
cyclic AMP (cAMP), 18, 20, 80, 254
cyclic guanosine monophosphate (cGMP), 281
cyclooxygenase, 135, 136
cystathionine, 167
cysteine, 165, 166
cystinuria, 157
cytochrome c oxidase, 9, 17, 396
cytochrome P450 system, 6
cytoplasm, 5
cytosine, 10
cytosine triphosphate (CTP) synthase, 168
cytosol, 5

D

daily water loss, 199
DBH. *See* dopamine β-hydroxylase
DBP. *See* vitamin D-binding protein
DCT. *See* distal convoluted tubule
de novo lipogenesis, 114

deamination reactions, amino acids, 164–165, 164*f*
deficiency
 biotin, 338
 copper, 399
 folic acid, 331
 iodine, 394–395
 iron, 383
 niacin, 322
 pantothenic acid, 340–341
 riboflavin, 319
 selenium, 404–405
 thiamin, 316
 vitamin B_6, 327
 vitamin B_{12}, 335–336
 vitamin C, 311
 zinc, 391
dehydration, 204, 205*t*
 and performance, 267, 267*t*
dehydroascorbic acid, 307
 chemical structures of, 308*f*
dementia, 322
denaturing, 154
densitometry, 228
deoxyribonucleic acid (DNA), 3, 9–12
dephosphorylation of proteins, 18
desaturation, 114–115
diabetes insipidus, 197
diabetes mellitus, 241
diarrhea, 204
diastolic blood pressure, 366
dicarboxylic acids, 156
diet, hypertension and, 366, 366*t*
Dietary Approaches to Stop Hypertension (DASH) eating plan, 366, 367*t*
dietary fat, 276
dietary fiber, 60, 66, 69
 cholesterol binding and reduction of lipids, 107, 107*f*
 classification system, 96
 daily intake and recommendations, 108–109
 description, 96
 fecal bulking, constipation and diverticulosis, 107–108, 108*f*, 108*t*
 gastrointestinal fermentation and health, 106
 metal binding, 108
 satiety and reduced glycemic effect, 107
 types and characteristics
  β-glucans, 101
  cellulose, 97–98, 98*t*
  chitin and chitosan, 101
  fructans, 101
  glycosaminoglycans, 101
  gums, 100
  health benefits and structural carbohydrates, 103, 105*t*

hemicellulose, 98–100
 lignin, 100, 100*f*
 oligosaccharides, 102
 pectins, 100
 polydextrose, 102
 psyllium, 102
 resistant dextrins, 102
 resistant starches, 102–103, 105
dietary folate equivalent, 331
Dietary Guidelines for Americans, 224
dietary lipids
 digestion
  intraluminal phase, 129–130, 129*f*
  mucosal phase, 130–132
  secretory phase, 132
 food sources
  cholesterol, percentage and weight, 125, 126*t*, 127*t*
  food triglycerides, 125, 125*t*
  linoleic and linolenic acid, 128, 128*t*
 oils, 125, 126, 127, 128
 P/S ratio, 125
 requirements, 128
dietary protein
 excess, 185
 quality of, 158–159
Dietary Reference Intakes (DRIs), 68, 284
 for vitamin K, 300
dietary sources
 biotin, 337
 boron, 411
 calcium, 346–347, 347*t*
 chloride, 361
 chromium, 408
 copper, 395
 fluoride, 406
 folic acid, 328, 329*t*
 iodine, 391–392
 iron, 374–378
 magnesium, 357, 358*t*
 manganese, 410
 molybdenum, 412
 pantothenic acid, 339
 phosphorus, 354, 355*t*
 potassium, 361, 363*t*
 riboflavin, 317–318, 318*t*
 selenium, 401
 sodium, 361, 362*t*
 thiamin, 313, 314*t*
 vanadium, 413
 vitamin B_6, 323–324, 324*t*
 vitamin B_{12}, 332–333, 334*f*
 vitamin C, 308, 308*t*
 zinc, 386
diet-induced thermogenesis (DIT). *See* thermic effect of food (TEF)
digestibility, of proteins, 158
digestion
 niacin, 321
 pantothenic acid, 339
 phases, 47

digestive enzymes, 53
 small intestine, 53
digestive tract
 fiber processing in, 107*f*
 movements, 41–42
 wall, structure of, 37*f*
dihydroxyacetone phosphate, 82
dimerization, 281
dinucleotides, 61
dipeptidases, 157
direct calorimetry, 206, 206*f*
disaccharides, 62–63, 63*f*, 67, 69
 carbohydrate digestion, 69
distal convoluted tubule (DCT), 196
disulfide bond, 76, 77*f*
diterpenes, 429
divalent metal transporter 1 (DMT1), 377
diverticulitis, 108
diverticulosis, 108, 108*f*
DLW. *See* doubly labeled water
DMT1. *See* divalent metal transporter 1
DNA. *See* deoxyribonucleic acid
Donath, Willem, 313
dopamine, 80
dopamine β-hydroxylase (DBH), 80
doubly labeled water (DLW), 210–211
drinking water, 200
DRIs. *See* Dietary Reference Intakes
"dry" beriberi, 316
dual-energy x-ray absorptiometry (DXA), 230, 230*f*
duodenum, 39
DXA. *See* dual-energy x-ray absorptiometry
dyslipidemia, 241

E

EAA. *See* essential amino acid
EAR. *See* estimated average requirement
early refeeding, 219–220, 221*f*, 222*f*
edema, 162
 etiology of, 202
 formation mechanisms for, 202, 202*t*
 heart failure, 203, 203*f*
 in pathologic states, 202–204
EFA. *See* essential fatty acid
egg proteins, 153
eicosanoids, 135–136
eicosapentaenoic acid (EPA), 426
eIF. *See* eukaryotic initiation factor
Eijkman, Christiaan, 312
elastin, 162
electrolytes, 24, 364
 balance of, 196
 composition in extracellular and intracellular fluid, 365*t*
 regulation of, 197
 saliva, 48–49
electron microscopy, 262

electron respiratory chain, 8
electron transport chain, 8, 16*f*
    and oxidative phosphorylation, 13–17
elements of human body, 2–3, 3*t*
elongation, 114–115
Elvehjem, Conrad, 320
enantiomers, 62
endocrine organs, 19
endocrine system, 252
endomysium, 25
endoplasmic reticulum, 6, 6*f*
    rough *vs.* smooth, 6
endorphins, 253*t*
endosomes, 7
endurance training, 251
    energy sources during, 262*f*
    hormonal responses, 253*t*
energy balance
    adipocyte regulation in, 238–239
    scale, 236*f*
energy expenditure. *See* metabolism
energy gap, 235
energy homeostasis, chemical mediators,
    233–234
energy intake
    chemical mediators of energy
        homeostasis, 234
    futile cycle systems, 232–233
energy of activation, 18
energy-requiring process, 329
energy-thrifty genes, 240
ENS. *See* enteric nervous system
enteric nervous system (ENS), 40–41
enterocytes, 39, 53, 69, 72
enterohepatic circulation, 52
entero-oxyntin, 47
enzymatic method, 104*t*, 105
enzymes, 8, 18, 48
    classes of, 160–161, 161*t*
EPA. *See* eicosapentaenoic acid
epimysium, 25
epinephrine (adrenalin), 80–81, 252, 253*t*
epithelial cells, 21, 21*f*
ergocalciferol, production of, 286
erythrocytes, 28
erythropoiesis, 23
esophageal sphincter, 49
esophagus, 49
essential amino acid (EAA), 150, 158,
    176*t*
essential fat, 226
essential fatty acid (EFA), 117–118
essential hypertension, 366
estimated average requirement (EAR)
    vitamin E, 295
estrogen, 253*t*
euglycemia, 72
eukaryotic initiation factor (eIF), 177
European Commission, 420*t*
EVO. *See* extra virgin oil
excitable cells, 24, 364

exercise
    blood glucose levels during, 258–259
    carbohydrate
        consumption, 260–261
        metabolism and, 256–258
        oxidation during, 260
    different fuel sources during, 259*f*
    muscle amino acid metabolism during,
        266
    muscle and basics of, 246–255
    protein and amino acid metabolism,
        263–266
    stores and, 261–263
        glycogen stores and, 260
        utilization and, 263
    triglyceride and fatty acid metabolism,
        261
    vitamins, minerals, and, 268, 269*t*
    water and, 267–268
exons, 11
extra virgin oil (EVO)
    phenolic compounds in, 427
    possible nutraceuticals in, 427*t*
extrinsic pathway, 300

F

facilitated diffusion, 18–19
factorial method, 175
FAD. *See* flavin adenine dinucleotide
FAO. *See* Food and Agriculture
    Organization
farnesoid X receptor (FXR), 124
FAS. *See* fatty acid synthase; fatty acid
    synthesis
fascicles, 25
fasting, 222–223
fat
    stores and exercise, 261–263
    utilization, exercise and, 263
fat mass, 226
    distribution in obesity, 237
fat metabolism, molecular control
        mechanisms of
    non-nuclear receptors, 124
    nuclear receptors
        FXR, 124
        LXRs, 123, 124
        PPARs, 121–124
fat-free mass (FFM). *See* lean body mass
fat-soluble vitamins, 306
    vitamin A, 274–285
    vitamin D, 285–291
    vitamin E, 292–297
    vitamin K, 297–302
    water and, 274
fatty acid synthase (FAS), 114, 340, 426
fatty acid synthesis (FAS), 114–115
fatty acids, 3, 428*t*
    acetic acid, 113

cis *vs.* trans, 116–117, 117*f*
EFA, 117–118
elongate and desaturate, 114
linoleic and linolenic acids, 112, 112*f*
metabolism, exercise and, 261, 262*t*
oxidation, 15
    in muscle, 263
pentose phosphate pathway, 114,
    116, 116*f*
and structural lipids, 434
synthesis, 114–115
FBPs. *See* folate-binding proteins
fecal bulking, 107–108, 108*f*, 108*t*
fecal nitrogen, 158
fed state, 219, 220*f*
    longer, 221
ferric, 309
ferritin/mobiloferrin, 377
ferroportin, 377
ferrous, 309
fetal hemoglobin, 161
fibers, 60, 65, 68, 433
    analysis in foods, 103, 104*t*
    consumption, 68
    definition, 96
    health benefits, 103–106, 105*t*
fibers types, 25
fibrin, 161
fibrinogen, 161
fibrous proteins, 150
FIGLU. *See* N-formiminoglutamic acid
fish proteins, 152
five-carbon pentoses, 61
5-methyl THF, 331
flavin adenine dinucleotide (FAD), 16,
    317, 317*f*, 318
flavin mononucleotide (FMN), 17, 317,
    317*f*, 318
flavonoids, 432, 432*f*
fluid balance, protein, 162
fluoridation, 406
fluoride
    absorption of, 406–407
    dietary sources of, 406
    intake, recommended levels, 408
    metabolism and function, 407
    tooth decay, 407
    toxicity, 408
FMN. *See* flavin mononucleotide
folate. *See* folic acid
folate-binding proteins (FBPs), 329
folic acid, 328–331
    absorption of, 328–329
    activation of, 330*f*
    deficiency, 331
    dietary sources of, 328, 329*t*
    in mental disorders and Alzheimer
        disease, 336
    metabolism and functions
        of, 329–331
    methyl–folate trap, 331

folic acid (*continued*)
  one-carbon moieties attached to
    THF, 330*f*
  RDA for, 331
  structure of, 328*f*
  toxicity, 331
Food and Agriculture Organization
  (FAO), 184, 184*t*
Food and Nutrition Board, 201
food proteins, 152, 152*t*
food sources
  examples of nutraceuticals grouped
    by, 423*t*
  higher content of specific
    nutraceuticals, 424*t*
foot drop syndrome, 316
FOS. *See* fructo-oligosaccharides
four-carbon tetroses, 61
free amino acids, 156
French psyllium seed, 102
fructans, 101
fructo-oligosaccharides (FOS), 101
fructose, 61, 67, 72
functional fibers, 96–97
functional foods, 420
  defining, 420–421, 420*t*
  olive oil as, 426–427
  organizational systems for, 421
    food sources, 421–424
    health claims, 426–427
    mechanism of action, 424–426
Funk, Casimir, 274, 313
futile cycle systems, 232–233
FXR. *See* farnesoid X receptor

G

G proteins, 18
GABA. *See* γ-aminobutyric acid
GAGs. *See* glycosaminoglycans
galactose, 61, 62, 67, 72
galanin, 47, 234
gallbladder, 52–53
γ-aminobutyric acid (GABA), 325
γ-carotene, 275
gastric emptying, 50–51
gastric glands, 38
gastric inhibitory peptide (GIP), 43–44
gastric juice, 50
gastric phase, digestion, 47
gastric-releasing peptide (GRP), 41
gastrin, 42–43
gastroesophageal reflux disease
  (GERD), 44
gastrointestinal fermentation and
  health, 106
gastrointestinal system, 37
  heme and nonheme iron, absorption
    of, 377
gastrointestinal tract

anatomy
  digestive tract wall structure, 37
  large intestine, 39
  mouth, 37
  small intestine, 38–39
  stomach, 37–38
endocrine and paracrine functions
  cholecystokinin, 43
  gastrin, 42–43
  GIP, 43–44
  histamine, 45
  motilin, 44–45
  peptide YY, 45
  secretin, 43
  somatostatin, 43
movements, 41–42
vasculature, 42
GDP. *See* guanosine diphosphate
gene expression, retinoic acid
  receptors and vitamin
  A interaction on, 282*f*
genes, 9–12
  silencing, 12
GERD. *See* gastroesophageal reflux
  disease
ghrelin, 46, 233
GIP. *See* gastric inhibitory peptide
global protein undernutrition, causes of,
  185–186
globular proteins, 150
glomerular capillary pressure, 195
glucagon, 76*t*, 79–80, 253*t*, 255
  breakdown, 222, 223*f*
glucan, 64
glucogenic amino acids, 163
glucokinase, 78, 83
gluconeogenesis, 88–89, 90*f*
glucose, 53, 61, 67, 72, 78
  transport into cells, 74–75
  uptake and utilization in
    adipocytes, 222*f*
  use, brain, 218
glucose tolerance factor (GTF), 321, 408
glucose transport proteins (GLUT),
  74–75, 75*t*
Glucose Transporter 5 (GLUT5), 70
glucose-6-phosphate, 18, 76,
  82, 87, 258
GLUT. *See* glucose transport proteins
GLUT1 protein, 75
GLUT2 protein, 75
GLUT3 protein, 75
GLUT4 protein, 75, 75*f*, 78
GLUT5 protein, 75
GLUT7 protein, 75
glutamate, 165, 167, 325
  dehydrogenase, 165
glutamine, 153, 165
  metabolism, 168–169, 168*f*–170*f*
glutaric aciduria type 1, 180
glutathione, 87

glutathione peroxidase, 404
gluten proteins, 153
glycemic effect, satiety and
  reduced, 107
glycemic index, 72, 72*t*
glycemic load, 72–73
glycemic response, 72, 72*f*
glyceraldehyde-3-phosphate, 82
glycine, 148, 156, 162, 163, 165, 166
  metabolism, 181–182
glycocalyx, 5
glycogen, 5
  in animal tissue, 65
  degradation, 86–87
  exercise, 260
  loading, 260, 262*t*
    protocol, 262*t*
  turnover, 84–85
glycogenolysis, 86, 87*f*
glycolipids, 4
glycolysis, 14, 83–84, 83*f*, 430
  early refeeding, 219–220
glycoproteins, 5, 13, 283
glycosaminoglycans (GAGs), 60, 63,
  65–66, 101, 434
glycosidic bonds. *See* disaccharides
goiter belt, 394
Goldberger, Joseph, 319
Golgi apparatus, 6–7, 6*f*, 77
grains, cereal, 67
ground substance, 23
growth hormone, 253*t*, 255
GRP. *See* gastric-releasing peptide
GTF. *See* glucose tolerance factor
GTP. *See* guanosine triphosphate
guanosine diphosphate (GDP), 281
guanosine triphosphate (GTP), 13, 281
gums, 96, 97, 98*t*
gynoid obesity, 237
György, Paul, 323

H

H2 blockers, 44
hair follicles, 194*f*
Harris and Benedict equation, 213
Hartnup disease, 157
Haworth, Norman, 306
HCl. *See* hydrochloric acid
hcp1. *See* heme carrier protein 1
HDL. *See* high-density lipoproteins
health, 226
  body weight and, 224–226
  gastrointestinal fermentation
    and, 106
Health Canada, 420*t*
health claims, 426–427
healthy weight, 224
heart, 26–29
  chambers, 28

heart disease, elevated blood homocysteine and, 336
heart failure, edema, 203, 203f
hematocrit, 28
heme carrier protein 1 (hcp1), 377
heme iron, 374
heme oxygenase, 377
heme production, 325, 327f
hemiacetal group, 62
hemicellulose, 98–99
hemoglobin, 28, 161
hemolytic anemia, 311
heparin, 101
hepatic lipase, 141
hepatic portal vein, 42
hepatic tocopherol transfer protein (HTTP), 293
hepatocytes, 5, 78, 79
hepcidin, 378
hephaestin, 377
hesperidin, 431
heterogeneous nuclear RNA (hnRNA), 11
hexokinase, 83
hexose monophosphate (HMP) shunt, 169
hexoses, 63
    six-carbon, 60
HFE, 377
HIF. See hypoxia inducible factors
high biological value proteins, 158
high-density lipoproteins (HDL), 124, 137
high-energy bonds, 14
high-energy phosphate, 61
high-protein diets, weight loss, 160
high-quality protein, 158
histamine, 45
HMG. See 3-hydroxy-3-methylglutaryl
HMP shunt. See hexose monophosphate shunt
hnRNA. See heterogeneous nuclear RNA
holo-RBP, 278–279
homocysteine, 335
    and coronary heart disease risk, 164
    in mental disorders and Alzheimer disease, 336
homopolysaccharides, 64, 65, 100
hormonal adaptation to acute and chronic exercise, 252–255
hormone aldosterone, 195
hormones, 7, 19–21, 233, 234
hormones in metabolism
    insulin receptors, 79
    insulin-to-glucagon molar ratios, 80
hormone-sensitive lipase (HSL), 134, 261
hox genes, 282
HSL. See hormone-sensitive lipase
HTTP. See hepatic tocopherol transfer protein
human body, 1–30
    electron transport chain, 13–17

elements of, 2–3, 2t
molecules of, 2–3, 2t
nucleus and genetic aspects, 9–12
organ systems, 22–30
oxidative phosphorylation, 13–17
protein. See protein
tissue, 21–22
human breast milk, 201
human calorimetry. See direct calorimetry
hunger-stimulating hormone, 46
hyaluronic acid, 6, 101
hydration, while exercising, 200
hydrochloric acid (HCl), 50, 154
hydrogen gas, 106
hydrolases, 161t
hydrostatic pressure, 202, 203
hydroxyapatite, 23, 350, 350f
hydroxylase, 309
hydroxylation, reaction, 309
hydroxylysine, 163, 165
3-hydroxy-3-methylglutaryl (HMG), 120
hydroxyproline, 156, 162, 163, 165
hyperglycemia, 72
hyperinsulinemia, 74
hyperkalemia, 365
hypermethioninemia, 179
hypernatremia, 365
hypertension, 141, 241
    and diet, 366
        DASH eating plan, 367t
hyperthyroidism, 294
hypertrophy, 232
hypervitaminosis, signs of, 284
hypochlorous acid, 383
hypochromic microcytic anemia, 383
hypoglycemia, 72
hypohydration, of plasma/hypovolemia, 267
hypokalemia, 368
hyponatremia, 368
hypothalamus, 197, 199f
    food intake and weight regulation, 232
hypoxia inducible factors (HIF), 378

I

IBW. See ideal body weight
ideal body weight (IBW), 224, 225t
IDL. See intermediate-density lipoprotein
IF. See intrinsic factor
IGF-1. See insulin-like growth factor-1
IGFs. See insulin-like growth factors
IgG. See immunoglobin G
IMCBP. See intracellular membrane calcium-binding protein
imino acids, 156
immunoglobin G (IgG), 388
IMP. See inosine monophosphate

incomplete protein, 158
Indian plantago seed, 102
indigestible dextrins, 102
indirect calorimetry, 209–210, 209f
inosine monophosphate (IMP), 169
inositol phospholipids, 4
inositol-P_3, 18, 19f
insensible water losses, 200
insoluble fiber, 97, 98t, 103
Institute of Food Technologists (IFT), 420t
insulin, 45, 72, 76, 233, 253t, 255
    insulin-mediated glucose uptake, 77–78
    metabolic roles of, 78
    production, 76–77, 78f
    receptors, 79
    role in fed state, 219
    secretion, 77
insulin-like growth factor-1 (IGF-1), 253t
insulin-like growth factors (IGFs), 239
insulin-mediated glucose uptake, 77–78
insulin-to-glucagon molar ratios, 80
integrated energy metabolism, metabolic states and, 216–223
intermediate-density lipoprotein (IDL), 137
International Food Information Council (IFIC), 420t
intestinal phase, digestion, 47
intracellular edema, 199
intracellular membrane calcium-binding protein (IMCBP), 287, 349
intrinsic factor (IF), 50, 332
intrinsic pathway, 300
introns, 11
inulin, 101
iodine
    absorption of, 392
    deficiency, 394–395
    dietary sources of, 391–392
    intake, recommended levels, 393–394
    metabolism and function of, 392–393
iodothyronine deiodinase, 402
ionization, of sodium chloride into water, 193f
IREG1, 377
IREP. See iron-responsive element-binding protein
iron
    absorption, 309, 374–378
    deficiency, 383
    dietary sources of, 374–378
    intake, recommended levels of, 383
    iron toxicity (overload), 383–385
    metabolism and function of, 378–383
iron deficiency anemia, 383
iron-responsive element-binding protein (IREP), 382
isocitrate dehydrogenase, 88
isoflavones, 421

isoleucine metabolism, 178–179, 180f
isomaltase, 69
isomerases, 161t
isoprene, 429, 429f
isoprenoid derivatives, 429–430
isoprostanes, 135
ispaghula husk, 102

J

Jansen, Barend, 313
Japan, 420
jejunum, 39
juxtaglomerular apparatus, 196

K

kahweol, 429
Kashin-Beck disease, 426–427
Kearns-Sayre syndrome, 9
Keshan disease, 404
ketogenic amino acids, 163
ketone body, 133–135
    formation of, 134, 135f
ketosis, 68
KGP. *See* kidney Gla protein
kidney Gla protein (KGP), 300
kidney nephron unit, 195, 195f
kilocalories, 14
kinky-hair disease. *See* Menkes disease
KLF4. *See* Kruppel-like factor 4
Krebs cycle, 8, 14, 15f, 87–88, 89f, 165,
    166f, 258, 263, 314f, 315
Kruppel-like factor 4 (KLF4), 390
kwashiorkor, 185

L

lactase, 69
    deficiency, 71
lactate, 85, 258, 259f
lactate dehydrogenase (LDH), 84
Lactobacillus acidophilus, 71
lactose, 63
lactose intolerance, 71, 106
large intestine, 53–55
LBM. *See* lean body mass
LDH. *See* lactate dehydrogenase
LDL. *See* low-density lipoproteins
LDL-cholesterol, 241
lean body mass (LBM), 213, 226, 229, 231
    African Americans, 227
    BIA, 231–232
    and RMR, 213
lecithin. *See* phosphatidylcholine
legumes (beans), 63, 67, 102
Leigh syndrome, 9

leptin, 46, 233–234
LES. *See* lower esophageal sphincter
leucine, 168
    body composition and obesity,
        182–184
    metabolism, 178–179, 180f
leukocytes, 28
ligases, 161t
lignans, 427t
lignin, 100, 100f
limonene, 429
limonin, 429
limonoids, 429
Lind, James, 306
lipids, 428t
    cholesterol binding and reduction of,
        107, 107f
    dietary lipids. *See* dietary lipids
    fat metabolism, molecular control
        mechanisms of
        non-nuclear receptors, 124
        nuclear receptor, 121–124
    fatty acids, 434
        acetic acid, 113
        cis *vs.* trans, 116–117, 117f
        EFA, 117–118
        elongate and desaturate, 114
        linoleic and linolenic acids,
            112, 112f
        pentose phosphate pathway, 114,
            116, 116f
        synthesis, 114–115
    metabolism
        eicosanoids, 135–136, 136f
        fatty acid oxidation, 132–133, 133f
        ketone body production, 133–135
        lipoproteins, 136–141
    phospholipids, 119–120, 119f
    sterols, 120–121
    triglycerides, 118–119, 118f
lipid-soluble substances, 53
lipogenesis, 79, 91
lipoprotein lipase (LPL), 261
lipoproteins, 39, 136–141, 196
    health implications and interpretation,
        141
    metabolism of
        chylomicrons, 138, 139f
        HDL, 140, 141f
        VLDL and LDL, 138, 140f
    types of, 136–138
lipoxygenase, 135
liver, 81
    arginosuccinate synthetase, 177
    cell, pyridoxal metabolism in, 324f
    early refeeding, 219–220
    effects of cortisol in, 81
    heme synthesis, 379f–381f
    parenchymal cells, vitamin A
        metabolism in, 280f
liver X receptors (LXRs), 123, 124

loop of Henle, 196
low-density lipoproteins (LDL), 137
lower esophageal sphincter (LES), 37
low-quality protein, 158
LPL. *See* lipoprotein lipase
lung cancer and retinoids, 282–283
LXRs. *See* liver X receptors
lyases, 161t
lymphatic system, 203
lysine, metabolism, 181–182
lysosomes, 7
    functions of, 5t

M

magnesium
    absorption, 357–358
    ATP stabilization, 359, 359f
    deficiency and toxicity, 360–361
    dietary sources, 357, 358t
    intake, recommended levels for, 360
    involvement in hexokinase activity,
        359f
    physiologic roles, 359–360
    tissue content and excretion, 358–359
magnetic resonance imaging (MRI), 228
major minerals
    calcium. *See* calcium
    chloride, 361–368
    of human body, 346t
    magnesium, 357–361
    phosphorus, 354–357
    potassium, 361–368
    sodium, 361–368
    sulfur, 368–369
malate dehydrogenase, 88
malnourished adults, 186
malnourished children, 186
malonic acid pathway, 430
maltase, 69
maltose, 63
mammalian target of rapamyocin
    (mTOR), 426
manganese
    absorption of, 410
    dietary sources of, 410
    imbalance, 411
    intake, recommended levels, 411
    metabolism and function of, 390,
        410–411
mannose, 61, 62
MAO. *See* monoamine oxidase
maple syrup urine disease (MSUD),
    178–179, 180f, 315
marasmus, 185
mast cells, 101
matrix Gla protein (MGP), 300
meat proteins, 152
mechanism of action, 424–426, 425t
medications, GERD, 44

megaloblastic macrocytic anemia, 331
Meissner plexus, 41
melatonin, 172, 172f
membranes
    fluid mosaic, 4f
    of tissue, 294
menaquinones, 297
Menkes disease, 399
mental disorders, vitamin B$_{12}$ role
    in, 336
MERRF. See myoclonus epilepsy with
    ragged red fibers
messenger RNA (mRNA), 11
MET. See metabolic equivalent
metabolic cart, 209
metabolic crossroads, 219
metabolic equivalent (MET), 246, 246t
metabolic pathways for
    carbohydrates, 83
    glycogen turnover, 84–85
    glycolysis, 83–84, 83f
    Krebs cycle, 87–88, 89f
    lipogenesis, 79, 91
    pentose phosphate pathway, 83–84
metabolic rate, 208
metabolic states
    and integrated energy metabolism,
        216–223
        cellular and tissue metabolism,
            217–218
        early refeeding, 219–220, 221f, 222f
        fasting, 221–223, 223f
        fed state, 219, 220f
        intermediate to longer fed state,
            221
        metabolic crossroads, 219
        obligate glucose utilization, 218
        starvation, 223
    transitional, 218–219
metabolism, 9
    adaptive thermogenesis, 213–216
    amino acids
        alanine–glucose cycle, 169, 171f
        degradation, 165–168
        disposal of amino acid
            nitrogen, 173
        glutamine, 168–169, 168f–170f
        inborn errors of, 178–182
        and neurotransmitters, 169–173,
            171f–173f
        synthesis, 165
        transamination and deamination,
            164–165, 164f
        urea cycle, 173, 174f
    basal, 212–213
    biotin, 337–338
    branched-chain amino acids, 180f
    cellular, 217–218
    crossroads, 219
    folic acid, 329–331
    glutamine, 168–169, 168f–170f

lysine, glycine and threonine, 181–182,
    183f
methionine, 179–180, 181f
niacin, 321–322
pantothenic acid, 339–340, 340f
pyridoxal in liver cell, 327f
riboflavin, 318–319
    in skeletal muscle, 212
thermic effect
    of activity, 213–214
    of food, 214
thiamin, 314–315
tissue, 212–213
tryptophan, 180, 182f
tyrosine, 178, 179f
valine, leucine and isoleucine,
    178–179, 180f
vitamin B$_6$, 324–327
vitamin B$_{12}$, 333–335
metal binding capacity, 108
metal transcription factor-1 (MTF-1),
    390
metallothionein, 388
methionine metabolism, 179–180, 181f
methotrexate, 330–331
methylcobalamin, 332, 333
methyl-folate trap, 331
methylmalonic acid, 339
methylmalonic acidemia, 180
methylmalonyl CoA, 335
MGP. See matrix Gla protein
Michaelis-Menton constant, 177
micro RNA (miRNA), 12
microbes. See probiotics
microbial, of nutraceuticals based
    classification, 428t
microcytic anemia, 284
microvilli, 39
Mifflin–St. Jeor equation, 213
milk proteins, 152–153
minerals, 227, 268, 428t, 434–435
    major. See major minerals
    minor/trace. See minor minerals
    vitamins and, related to
        exercise, 269t
minor minerals
    chromium, 408–410
    copper, 395–400
    fluoride, 406–408
    iodine, 391–395
    iron. See iron
    manganese, 410–411
    selenium, 401–406
    ultratrace minerals, 411–414
    zinc, 386–391
miRNA. See micro RNA
mitochondria, 7–9, 7f
    cardiac myocyte, 16f
    functions of, 5t
mitochondria transcription factor A
    (mtTFA), 8

mitochondrial biogenesis, 8
mitochondrial diseases, 9
mixing movements, gastrointestinal tract,
    42
molar ratios, insulin-to-glucagon, 80
molecules
    of human body, 2–3, 2t
    water
        dipolar nature of, 192
        held together by hydrogen
            bonds, 192f
molybdenum, 412
monoamine oxidase (MAO), 171
monosaccharides, 60–62, 67–68, 72, 98
    absorption of, 70
    activation, 75–76
    d and l isomers, 62, 62f
    derivatives, 62
    epimers, 62
    structures, 62
monounsaturated fatty acid (MUFA), 113
monoterpenes, 429, 429f
mortality rate and incidence of
    xerophthalmia, 284
motilin, 44–45
motor cortex, 249
motor neuron, 247
motor unit, 247
    recruitment, 249–251, 251f
mouth, anatomy, 37
MPB. See muscle protein breakdown
MPS. See muscle protein synthesis
MRI. See magnetic resonance imaging
mRNA. See messenger RNA
MSUD. See maple syrup urine disease
MTF-1. See metal transcription factor-1
mTOR, mammalian target of
    rapamyocin
mtTFA. See mitochondria transcription
    factor A
mucilages, 97, 98t
mucopolysaccharides, 65, 101
mucous type of protein secretion, 48
MUFA. See monounsaturated fatty acid
muscle protein breakdown (MPB), 265
muscle protein synthesis (MPS),
    264–265
muscles
    action potentials, 248
    adaptation
        endurance exercise, 251
        strength training, 251–252
    amino acid metabolism, during
        exercise, 266
    carbohydrate utilization, 258
    cells, 5
        contraction, 71
    contraction, 250f
        calcium role in, 351–353, 352f
        smooth muscle, 40
    fatty acid oxidation in, 263

fibers types, 249, 252
   characteristics of, 250*t*
   and endurance adaptation, 252
function of, 162
glycogen, 258
human body, 247*f*
hypertrophy, 251
   exercise-related events support, 251*f*
   motor unit recruitment,
      249–251, 251*f*
   neuromuscular junctions, 247–248
   sarcomeres and contraction, 248–249
   structure of, 162, 248*f*
   tissue, 21–22
myenteric plexus, 41
myoclonus epilepsy with ragged red
   fibers (MERRF), 9
myofibrils, 25, 248
myoglobin, 382
myosin, 25, 162, 248

N

NAD. *See* nicotinamide adenine
   dinucleotide
NADP. *See* nicotinamide adenine
   dinucleotide phosphate
National Health and Nutrition
   Examination Survey (NHANES),
   201, 235
natural gums, 100
NEAT. *See* nonexercise activity
   thermogenesis
nephrons, 29, 30*f*
nervous tissue, 21, 23–25
net protein utilization (NPU), 158
neurodegenerative disorders, iron and,
   385–386
neuromuscular junctions, 247–248
   with acetylcholine as neurotransmitter,
      248*f*
neurons, 23
   of ENS, 40–41
neuropeptide Y (NPY), 46–47, 234
neurotransmitters, 24, 41
   amino acids and, 169–173, 171*f*–173*f*
   formation of, 325, 326*f*
neutral amino acids, 156
neutral detergent method, 104, 104*t*
N-formiminoglutamic acid (FIGLU), 330
NHANES. *See* National Health and
   Nutrition Examination Survey
niacin, 274, 319–323
   active forms of, 320*f*
   deficiency, 322
   digestion and absorption of, 321
   metabolism and functions of, 321–322
   pharmacologic use of, 322–323
   RDA for, 322
   sources of, 320–321, 320*t*, 321*f*

structures of, 320*f*
   toxicity, 322–323
nickel, 413
nicotinamide, 320, 320*f*, 321
nicotinamide adenine dinucleotide
   (NAD), 320, 321, 321*f*
nicotinamide adenine dinucleotide
   phosphate (NADP), 320–322,
   320*f*
nicotinic acid. *See* niacin
Niemann-Pick C1-Like 1 (NPC1L1), 132
nitrogen balance, 174
nitrogen balance method, 175
nitrogen, removal of, 165
nomilin, 429
noncellulose polysaccharides, 108
noncontractile proteins, 266
nonessential amino acids, 165
nonexercise activity thermogenesis
   (NEAT), 213–214
nonheme iron, 374
nonmarine gums, 100
nonpitting edema, 204
nonshivering thermogenesis (NST),
   216
nonstarch polysaccharides (NSPs), 66, 96
norepinephrine, 80, 193, 252, 253*t*
NPC1L1. *See* Niemann-Pick C1-Like 1
NPC1L1-flotillan-cholesterol membrane
   microdomain, 132
NPU. *See* net protein utilization
NPY. *See* neuropeptide Y
NRF-1. *See* nuclear respiratory factor-1
   (NRF-1)
NSPs. *See* nonstarch polysaccharides
   (NSPs)
NST. *See* nonshivering thermogenesis
nuclear envelope, 5, 9
nuclear respiratory factor-1 (NRF-1), 8
nucleosides, 10
nucleotide, 10
nucleus and genetic aspects, 9–12
nutraceuticals, 429
   classification of, 428*f*
   and functional foods. *See* functional
      foods
   by molecular structure, isoprenoid
      derivatives (terpenoids), 429–430
nutrition
   vs. supplement facts panels, 423*t*
   vitamin A and carotenoids
      relationships, 284

O

OAA. *See* oxaloacetate
obese diabetic mouse, 46
obesity, 182–184, 235
   and age, 240
   in children, 240
   definition, 237

   distribution of fat mass, 237–238
   financial impact of, 237
   genetic influences on, 240
   history, 237
   men *vs.* women, 240
   prevalence, 237
   and related diseases, 240–241
obligate glucose utilization, 218
oligosaccharides, 63, 102, 105*t*
   straight-chain, 85
olive oil, as functional foods, 426–427
opsin, 280
oral cavity, 48–49
oral hygiene, saliva, 48
organ systems, 22–30
   blood pressure, 29
   bone, 22–23
   heart, blood and circulation, 26–29
   nervous tissue, 21, 23–25
   renal system, 29–30, 29*f*, 30*f*
   skeletal muscle, 3, 25–26
   skeleton, 22–23
organelles, 3–9
   and cell membranes, 17
   functions, 5, 5*t*
      endoplasmic reticulum, 6, 6*f*
      endosomes, 7
      Golgi apparatus, 6–7, 6*f*
      lysosomes, 7
      mitochondria, 7–9, 7*f*
      peroxisomes, 7
organic matrix, 23
organizational systems for nutraceuticals
   and functional foods, 428
   food sources, 421–424
   health claims, 426–427
   mechanism of action, 424–426
ornithine, 163
orphan receptors, 121
osmoreceptors, 197
osmotic pressure, 202
osteoblasts, 23
osteoclasts, 23
osteomalacia, 291, 353
osteoporosis, 353
overweight, body mass index,
   225–226, 225*t*
oxalate, 347, 348*f*
oxaloacetate (OAA), 89
oxidative deamination, 164, 164*f*
oxidative phosphorylation, electron
   transport chain and, 13–17
oxidoreductase, 161*t*
oxygen consumption, 246
oxyntic glands, 38
oxythiamin, 313

P

PABA. *See* para-aminobenzoic acid
PAL. *See* physical activity level

pancreatic digestive juice, 51–52
pantothenic acid, 338–341, 338*f*
  deficiency and toxicity of, 340–341
  digestion and absorption of, 339
  food sources of, 339
  metabolism and function of,
    339–340, 340*f*
  RDA for, 340
para-aminobenzoic acid (PABA), 328
parasympathetic innervation, 41
parathyroid hormone (PTH), 287, 349, 350*f*
Parkinson disease, 386
passive diffusion, 18
Pauling, Linus, 311, 312
PCM. *See* protein-calorie malnutrition
PCT. *See* proximal convoluted tubule
PDCAAS. *See* protein digestibility
    corrected amino acid score
pectins, 97, 98*t*, 100
pellagra, 319, 320
PEM. *See* protein-energy malnutrition
pentose phosphate pathway (PPP),
    83–84, 116, 116*f*, 315, 430
pentoses, five-carbon, 61
PEPCK. *See* phosphoenolpyruvate
    carboxykinase
pepsin, 50, 154
pepsinogens, 50
PEPT1, 157
peptide bonds, 148, 148*f*
peptide YY (PYY), 45, 47
PER. *See* protein efficiency ratio
peripheral proteins, 4
pernicious anemia, 332, 335
peroxisomal proliferating activating
    receptor-γ co-activator
    (PGC-1), 8
peroxisome proliferator activator receptors
    (PPARs), 121–124, 239
peroxisome proliferator-activated
    receptor alpha (PPARα), 21
peroxisomes, 7, 21, 165
Peyer patches, 39
PGC-1. *See* peroxisomal proliferating
    activating receptor-γ
    co-activator
phenolic compounds, 428*t*, 430–433, 431*f*
phenolics, 427*t*
phenylalanine, 167, 167*f*, 178
  metabolism, 178
phenylalanine hydroxylase, 309
phenylethanolamine-N-
    methyltransferase (PNMT), 80
phenylketonuria (PKU), 168, 178
phosphate (PO$_4$), 119
phosphatidylcholine, 277
phosphoenolpyruvate carboxykinase
    (PEPCK), 89, 123
phosphofructokinase, 83–84
phosphofructokinase 1 (PFK1), 83–84
phosphofructokinase 2 (PFK2), 83–84
phospholipids, 4, 119–120, 119*f*

phosphorus, 354–357
  deficiency and toxicity, 357
  dietary sources, 354, 355*t*
  digestion and absorption of, 354–355
  intake, recommended levels of, 357
  physiologic roles of, 356–357
  serum levels, 355–356
phosphorylase a, 86
phosphorylation, of proteins, 18
photophobia, 319
photosynthesis, 60
physical activity level (PAL), 214, 214*t*,
    246, 246*t*
phytase enzyme, 354
phytate, 347–348, 348*f*
phytochemicals, 68, 109
pitting edema, 204
PKU. *See* phenylketonuria
plant starch, 63–64
Plantago ovata, 102
plasma, 26
plasma membrane, 4–5
plasma osmolality, 201
  regulation of, 199*f*
plasma proteins, 162, 196, 203
plasma transport of vitamin A and
    carotenoids, 278–279
plasma volume, 267
  physiologic effects of reduced, 268*f*
plasmin, 161
plasminogen, 161
platelets, 28
plethysmography, 229
pleural effusion, 204
PLP. *See* pyridoxal phosphate
PNMT. *See* phenylethanolamine-
    N-methyltransferase
points of unsaturation, 113
polydextrose, 102
polymorphism in vitamin D receptor
    gene, 290
polysaccharides, 63–66, 101
  animal glycogen, 65
  dietary fiber, 66
  glycosaminoglycans, 65–66
  oligosaccharides, 63
  plant starch, 63–64
polyunsaturated fatty acids (PUFA), 113,
    421
posterior pituitary gland, 196, 197
post-transcriptional modification, 11
potassium
  absorption, 363
  deficiency, 365, 368
  dietary sources, 361, 363*t*
  intake, recommended levels of, 365
  physiologic functions of, 364–365
  tissue, urinary and sweat
    content, 364
  toxicity, 368
PPARα. *See* peroxisome proliferator-
    activated receptor alpha

PPARγ, 239
PPARs. *See* peroxisome proliferator
    activator receptors
PPP. *See* pentose phosphate pathway
preadipocyte factor-1 (Pref-1), 239
preadipocyte factor-1 preadipocyte
    factor-1 respiratory exchange
    ratio (RER)
  galanin, 234
precursors, biochemical compounds,
    163, 163*t*
preeclampsia, 353–354
Pref-1. *See* preadipocyte factor-1
preformed vitamin A, 274
previtamin A, 275
prilosec, 44
primary structure, of protein, 150, 151*f*
probiotics, 54, 435
procarboxypeptidase, 155
proinsulin, 76, 77
proline, 156, 165, 309
propionic acid, 339
propionic acidemia, 179
propionyl carboxylase, 338
propulsive movements, gastrointestinal
    tract, 41
Prosky method, 105
protein α–helix, 150
protein digestibility corrected amino acid
    score (PDCAAS), 159
protein efficiency ratio (PER), 158–159
protein turnover
  during endurance exercise, 265–266
  during resistance exercise,
    264–265, 265*f*
protein-calorie malnutrition (PCM), 185
protein-energy malnutrition (PEM), 185
protein-malnourished females, 185
proteins
  amino acids. *See* amino acids
  blood components, 161
  carbon and methyl donors, 163
  cellular functions, 17–21
  concentration, 202
  deficiency, 184–185
  digestion and absorption, 153–157
    154*f*, 155*t*
  endocrine functions, 162
  energy supply, 163
  estimated daily loss of, 175*t*
  excess, 184–185
  exercise and, 263–266
  fluid balance, 162
  history of, 148
  hormones. *See* hormones
  immunity, transport carriers and
    membrane receptors, 162–163
  intakes by food source, 177, 184–185
  malnutrition, 284
  noncontractile *vs.* contractile, 266
  plasma membrane, 4–5

proteins (*continued*)
  precursors, 163, 163t
  quality of, 158–159, 184–185
  quantity of, 153
  recommendations, 266–267
  requirements, 174–176
  role in metabolism, 160–163
  saliva, 48
  selenium incorporation into,
      403–404
  structures of, 150–151, 151f
  synthesis, 11–13, 177, 177f
  transmembrane, 4
  transport, 17–19, 53
  undernutrition, 185–186
proton-motive force, 17
proximal convoluted tubule (PCT), 196
psyllium, 102
PTH. *See* parathyroid hormone
PUFA. *See* polyunsaturated fatty acids
pulmonary arteries, 28
purine bases, 10
purine nucleotide bases, synthesis of, 169f
pyloric sphincter, 38
pyridoxal metabolism, in liver cell, 327f
pyridoxal phosphate (PLP), 323–325
  in heme biosynthesis, 327f
  Schiff base mechanism for,
      324–325, 325f
pyridoxamine, 323, 324
pyridoxine, 323, 324
pyrimidine bases, 10
pyrimidine nucleotide bases, synthesis
      of, 169f
pyrithiamine, 313
pyruvate, 83, 89, 315
  as crossroad intermediate, 219
pyruvate carboxylase, 89
pyruvate dehydrogenase, 84
pyruvate kinase, 84
PYY. *See* peptide YY

Q

quercetin, 423

R

R group, 148
R proteins, 333
racemases, 62
radiation, vitamin C and, 312
RAE. *See* retinol activity equivalents
raffinose, 63, 102, 105t
RBCs. *See* red blood cells
RDA. *See* Recommended Dietary
      Allowance
reabsorption, water, 196
rebound scurvy, 311

receptors
  cells, 17
  transmembrane proteins, 17f
Recommended Dietary Allowance
      (RDA)
  biotin, 338
  folic acid, 331
  niacin, 322
  pantothenic acid, 340
  riboflavin, 319
  thiamin, 316
  vitamin A, 284
  vitamin B$_6$, 327
  vitamin B$_{12}$, 335
  vitamin C, 311
  vitamin D, 290
  vitamin E, 295
red blood cells (RBCs), 218
reference proteins, 158
  safe levels of, 184, 184t
renal parenchyma, 30
renal system, 246
renal tubule system, 196
renin, 196
  secretion, 201
renin-angiotensin mechanism, 201
renin-angiotensin-aldosterone system, 197f
reproduction, vitamin A role in, 283
RER. *See* respiratory exchange ratio
resistant dextrins, 102
resistant maltodextrins, 102
resistant starches, 102–103, 105
respiratory exchange ratio (RER),
      46, 210, 210t
respiratory quotient (RQ), 209
  NPY, 233
resting metabolic rate (RMR), 212
  equations for, 213
resting metabolism. *See* basal metabolism
resting potential, 24
resveratrol, 421
retinoic acid receptors (RXRs), 122
  interaction on gene expression, 282f
retinoid X receptors (RXR), 393
retinoids, 282
retinol, 275
  conversion of retinal to, 280
retinol activity equivalents (RAE), 284
retinyl esters, 275
  fatty acids removal of, 275
retinyl palmitate, 275, 277
retrogradation, 103
reverse cholesterol transport, 140
rhodopsin, 280–281
riboflavin, 316–319
  absorption and transport of, 318
  deficiency and toxicity, 319
  dietary sources of, 317–318, 318t
  metabolism and roles of, 318–319
  RDA for, 319
  structure of, 317f

ribonucleic acid (RNA), 3, 9–12
  types of, 12
ribose, 11, 61
ribose-5-phosphate, 169
ribosomal RNA (rRNA), 11
rickets, 290
ripened fruits, 67
RMR. *See* resting metabolic rate
RNA interference (RNAi), 12
RNAi. *See* RNA interference
rough endoplasmic reticulum, 6, 6f
roughage. *See* dietary fiber
rugae, 39
rule of thumb, 213

S

43S preinitiation complex formation,
      177, 177f
S-adenosyl homocysteine (SAH), 163
S-adenosyl methionine (SAM), 163, 179
SAH. *See* S-adenosyl homocysteine
saliva, 48
SAM. *See* S-adenosyl methionine
saponins, 429
sarcolemma, 248
sarcomeres, 26, 26f
  and contraction, 248–249
  definition, 248
sarcoplasmic reticulum, 26, 248
saturated fatty acids (SFA), 113
SCAP. *See* SREBP cleavage-activating
      protein
Schiff base mechanism, for PLP,
      324–325, 325f
SCO2, 9
scorbutic rosary, 311
scurvy, 306, 311
  rebound, 311
seaweed gums, 100
sebaceous glands, 194f
secondary structure, of protein, 150
secretin, 43
secretory glands, 194f
secretory granules, 7
secretory vesicles, 7, 77
selective serotonin reuptake inhibitors
      (SSRIs), 173f
selenium
  absorption of, 401
  and cancer prevention, 406
  deficiency, 404–405
  dietary sources, 401
  incorporation into proteins, 403–404
  intake, recommended levels of, 404
  metabolism and function of, 401–403
  relationships with other
      nutrients, 404
  toxicity, 405
serine, 165

serotonin, 172, 172f, 173f
serous type of protein secretion, 48
sesquiterpenes, 429
SFA. *See* saturated fatty acids
SGLT1. *See* sodium/glucose cotransporter 1
shikimic acid pathway, 430
short-chain fatty acids, 106
SHP. *See* small heterodimer partner
shRNA. *See* small hairpin RNA
sickle cell disease, 384
side group, 148
silicon, 414
siRNA. *See* small interfering RNA
skeletal, 25–26
skeletal muscle, 3, 25–26
    cells, 266
    fibers, 25
skeletomuscular system, 246
skeleton, 22–23
skinfold assessment, 230–231, 231f
    sites, 230t
slow-moving protease, 50
small hairpin RNA (shRNA), 12
small heterodimer partner (SHP), 124
small interfering RNA (siRNA), 12
small intestine, 51
    absorption, 53
    anatomy, 38–39
    digestive enzymes of, 53
    hydration of fiber, 107
smooth endoplasmic reticulum, 6
smooth muscle, 40
    contraction, calcium role in, 351–353, 352f
SOD. *See* superoxide dismutase
sodium
    absorption, 362
        routes of, 364f
    deficiency, 204, 365
    dietary sources, 361, 362t
    hypertension, 365
    intake, recommended levels of, 365
    physiologic functions of, 364
    reabsorption, 195
    tissue, urinary, and sweat content, 364
    toxicity, 365
sodium/glucose cotransporter 1 (SGLT1), 70
sodium-gradient hypothesis, 70
sodium-to-potassium ratio, 365
soluble fiber, 97, 98t, 108
somatostatin, 43
Southgate fractionization system, 104–105
soy protein isolate (SPI), 153
soy proteins, 153
Spanish psyllium seed, 102
specific dynamic action (SDA). *See* thermic effect of food (TEF)
SPI. *See* soy protein isolate

splicing, 11
SREBP. *See* sterol regulatory element binding protein
SREBP cleavage-activating protein (SCAP), 124
SSRIs. *See* selective serotonin reuptake inhibitors
stachyose, 63, 102, 105t
starch, 47
    carbohydrate digestion, 69
    plant, 63–64
starvation, 223
Steap3, 377
stellate cells, 280
steroid hormones, 19, 21
sterol regulatory element binding protein (SREBP), 124
sterols, 120–121
stomach
    anatomy, 37–38
    digestion, 49
    in protein digestion, 154
stroke volume, 28
structure/function claims, 426
subcutaneous adipose tissue, 230
submucosa plexus, 41
succinic acid, 339
succinyl CoA, 335f
sucrase, 69
sucrose, 64
sugars, 65, 68
    sweetness and alternative sweeteners, 64t
sulfur, 368
sulfur-containing amino acids, 149, 163
summit metabolism, 216
superoxide dismutase (SOD), 294, 411
    components of, 435
swallowing, act of, 49
sweat, 193
    glands, 193–195, 194f
    water, 193–195
sympathetic innervation, 41
synapse, 24
synthesis, 86, 86f
synthesis of amino acids, 165
systolic blood pressure, 366
Szent-Györgyi, Albert, 306

T

taurine, 163, 170, 434
TEA. *See* thermic effect of activity
TEE. *See* total energy expenditure
TEF. *See* thermic effect of food
tendons, 6
terpenoids derivatives, 429–430
tertiary structures, of proteins, 150, 151f
testosterone, 253t
tetrahydrofolate (THF), 329, 330f

tetrapeptidases, 157
tetraterpenoids, 429
tetroses, four-carbon tetroses, 61
thermic effect of activity (TEA), 213–214
thermic effect of food (TEF), 214
thermogenin, 232
THF. *See* tetrahydrofolate
thiamin, 312–316
    vs. thiamin pyrophosphate, role of, 314f
    deficiency, 316
    dietary sources of, 313, 314t
    digestion, absorption, and transport of, 313
    metabolism and functions of, 314–315, 315f
    phosphates, 313, 313f
    RDA for, 316
    role of, 315f
    structure of, 313f
    toxicity, 316
thiamin pyrophosphate (TPP), 314, 314f, 315
thio-ester, 339
thirst, 201
three-carbon trioses, 61
threonine, metabolism, 181–182, 183f
thromboplastin, 300
thyroglobin, 392
thyroid hormones, 392
    effects of, 393, 394t
thyroid receptor (TR), 393
thyroid-stimulating hormone (TSH), 216, 253t, 393
thyrotropin-releasing hormone (TRH), 216, 393
thyroxine (T_4), 253t, 392, 393, 394t
tissue, 21–22
    metabolism, 217–218
TOBEC. *See* total body electrical conductivity
tocopherols, 292, 292f
    excretory pathway for, 295f
tocotrienols, 292, 292f, 421
total body electrical conductivity (TOBEC), 231–232, 231f
total dietary fiber, 105
total energy expenditure (TEE), 208–216, 246
    direct calorimetry, 206, 206f
    doubly labeled water, 211–212
    energy metabolism
        adaptive thermogenesis, 214–216
        basal, 212–213
        food, thermic effect, 214
        thermic effect of activity, 213–214
    indirect calorimetry, 209–210, 209f
    and measurement, 208
total fiber, 96
toxicity
    biotin, 338

toxicity (*continued*)
  calcium, 354
  fluoride, 408
  folic acid, 331
  iron, 385–386
  magnesium, 360–361
  niacin, 322–323
  pantothenic acid, 340–341
  phosphorus, 357
  potassium, 365, 368
  riboflavin, 319
  selenium, 405
  sodium, 365
  thiamin, 316
  vitamin B_6, 327
  vitamin C, 311
  zinc, 391
TPP. *See* thiamin pyrophosphate
TR. *See* thyroid receptor
trace elements, 374
trace metals, 374
transaminase, 161
transamination, 324, 325
  amino acids, 164–165, 164f
transcobalamin I, 333
transcobalamin II, 333
transcription, 11
  factors, 389–390
transcuprin, 398–399
transfer RNA (tRNA), 11
transferases, 161t
transferrin, 377
transitional metabolic states, 218–219
translation, 12
transmembrane proteins, 4
transport proteins, 17–19, 53, 161
transport systems, amino acids, 157, 157t
transporter ZIP4, 387
TRH. *See* thyrotropin-releasing hormone
tricarboxylic acid (TCA) cycle. *See* Krebs
    cycle
triglyceride, 3
  exercise and, 261
  intramuscular stores of, 263
  structure of, 118, 118f
triiodothyronine (T_3), 253t, 393
trioses, three-carbon, 61
tripeptides, 157
triterpenes, 429, 429f
tropocollagen, 162, 309
tropomyosin, 25, 162, 249
  in muscle fiber contraction, 249, 249f
troponin, 25, 249
  in muscle fiber contraction, 249, 249f
TRPM6, 358
trypsin, 155
  inhibitor, 51, 155
trypsinogen, 155
tryptophan, 163, 170, 171f, 172, 172f
  metabolism, 180, 182f
TSH. *See* thyroid-stimulating hormone

turnover, 23
tyrosine, 165, 167, 178
  hydroxylase, 398
  metabolism, 178, 179f
  vitamin C and, 309
tyrosinemia type II, 178

U

ubiquitin, 340
UDP-glucose. *See* uridine diphosphate
    glucose
ultrafiltrate, 30, 195
ultratrace minerals
  arsenic, 413
  boron, 411–412
  cobalt, 411
  molybdenum, 412
  nickel, 413
  silicon, 414
  vanadium, 412–413
UMP. *See* uridine monophosphate
uncooked starch, 103
uncoupling protein, 232
undernutrition, proteins, 185–186
underwater weighing (UWW), 228, 229f
undigested starch, 103
uracil, 11
urea cycle, 163, 173, 174f
uridine diphosphate (UDP), 168
uridine diphosphate glucose (UDP-
    glucose), 86, 86f, 168
uridine monophosphate (UMP), 168
uridine triphosphate (UTP), 168
urinary system. *See* renal system
urinary water, 195–199
urine volume, regulation of, 199f
U.S. Department of Agriculture (USDA), 68
UTP. *See* uridine triphosphate
UWW. *See* underwater weighing

V

valine, metabolism, 178–179, 180f
Van Soest method, 104, 104t
vanadium, 412–413
vasopressin, 196
  structure, 197, 198f
VDR. *See* vitamin D receptor
verbascose, 63, 102, 105t
very low density lipoproteins (VLDL),
    137, 294
villi, 39, 42
vision, 280–281
  vitamin A as *cis*-Retinal in, 282f
vital amine, 313
vitamin A
  and carotenoids
    dietary sources of, 275

  digestion and absorption of,
      275–277
  in enterocyte, digestion, absorption,
      and processing, 278f
  excretion of, 284
  functions of, 280–283
  nutrient relationships for, 284
  plasma transport of, 278–279
  as *cis*-Retinal in vision, 282f
  deficiency, 284
  definition, 274
  food sources of, 277t
  intake, recommended levels of, 284
  interaction on gene expression, 282f
  isomers of, 275f
  metabolism in liver parenchymal cells,
      280f
  storage and cell binding proteins, 280
  structures of, 275f
  toxicity, 284–285
vitamin B_1. *See* thiamin
vitamin B_2. *See* riboflavin
vitamin B_3. *See* niacin
vitamin B_6, 323–327, 324f
  absorption of, 324
  deficiency, 327
  food sources of, 323–324, 323t
  metabolism and function of, 324–327
  RDA for, 327
  toxicity, 327
vitamin B_{12}, 50, 332–336, 332f
  absorption of, 332–333
  deficiency, 335–336
  digestion of, 332–333
  food sources, 332–333, 333f
  in mental disorders and Alzheimer
      disease, 336
  metabolism and function of, 333, 335
  RDA for, 335
vitamin C, 306–312, 307f, 433
  absorption of, 308–309
  deficiency of, 311
  in disease prevention, 312
  food sources of, 308, 308t
  functions of, 309, 310f
  RDA for, 311
  structures of, 308f
  toxicity, 311
  treatment, 311
vitamin D, 349, 353–354
  calcium absorption, 347–349, 348f
  deficiency, 291
    children and adolescents suffering
        from, 291
  dietary, 285–286
    absorption and transport,
        285–286
  exertion actions on genes, 289f
  food sources of, 286, 287t
  hydroxylation reactions of biological
      significance, 288f

intake, recommended levels, 290
   for children and adolescents, 291
magnesium absorption, 357–358
metabolism of, 286–287, 288f, 289f
phosphorus absorption, 354–355
vitamin D receptor (VDR), 287
   and functions, 287–290
vitamin D–binding protein (DBP), 287
vitamin E, 292
   absorption and transport, 293
   deficiency, 296
   food sources of, 292–293, 293t
   function of, 294
   intake, recommended levels,
      294–295
   isomers, 292f
   storage and excretion, 293–294
   toxicity, 297
vitamin H, 337
vitamin K, 274, 284
   absorption and transport of,
      285–286
   deficiency and toxicity, 301–302
   functions of, 298–300, 298f, 299f
   intake, recommended levels,
      300–301
   sources of, 297–298
   structures of, 298f
vitamin K carboxylase, 298, 298f
vitamin K cycle, 300, 301f
vitamins, 268, 274t. See also specific
      vitamins
   definition, 274
   fat-soluble. See fat-soluble vitamins
   and mineral related to exercise, 269t
   water-soluble. See water-soluble
      vitamins
VLDL. See very low density lipoproteins
VO₂ max, 255, 258, 259
volatile fatty acids, 106

W

WAT. See white adipose tissue
water
   AI for, 102
   balance, 199–201
      from intake and output, 199, 199t
   chemical and physical properties of,
      192
   content of various foods, 200, 201t
   deficiency (dehydration) and
      intoxication, 204, 205t
   and electrolytes, 196
   and exercise, 267–268
   and fat solubility, 274
   in human body, distribution of,
      193, 193t
      sweat water, 193–195
      urinary water, 195–199
   ionization of sodium chloride
      into, 193f
   metabolic generation of, 200
   molecules, 192, 192f
   properties, 192
   reabsorption, 196
   recommendations for athletic
      performance, 267–268
water-packed tuna, 152
water-soluble vitamins, 306–342
   biotin, 337–338, 337f
   folic acid, 328–331
   niacin, 319–323
   pantothenic acid, 338–341, 338f
   riboflavin, 316–319
   thiamin, 312–316
   vitamin B₆, 323–327, 323f
   vitamin B₁₂, 332–336, 332f
   vitamin C, 306–312, 307f
weight loss, high-protein diets, 160

"wet" beriberi, 316
wheat proteins, 153
whey proteins, 152–153
white adipose tissue (WAT), 232
WHO. See World Health
      Organization
Williams, Robert, 313
Wills factor, 328
Wills, Lucy, 328
Wilson disease, 399–400
World Health Organization (WHO), 69
   safe levels of protein intake,
      184, 184t

X

xanthophylls, 275, 429
xerophthalmia, 284
xylose, 61

Y

yeast, 101

Z

zinc
   absorption of, 386–389, 388f
   deficiency, 391
   dietary sources of, 386
   intake, recommended levels of,
      390–391
   metabolism and function of, 389–390
   toxicity, 391
zinc finger proteins, 390
zinc transporter 1 (ZnT-1), 388